PLANNING FOR HEALTH

Development and Application
of Social Change Theory

HENRIK L. BLUM, M.D.

Professor of Health Planning
School of Public Health and
Department of City and Regional Planning
University of California, Berkeley

HUMAN SCIENCES PRESS ● NEW YORK
A division of Behavioral Publications, Inc.

Library of Congress Catalog Number   74-722

ISBN: 0-87705-149-6

Printed in the United States of America
56789   98765432

Library of Congress Cataloging in Publication Data

Blum, Henrik L
  Planning for health; development and application of social change theory.

  1. Medical policy—United States. 2. Planning. 3. Social change. I. Title. [DNLM: 1.
Health and welfare planning. 2. Social change. WA525 B658p 1974]
R854.U5B56   362.1   74-722

To Marian

Contents

PART III: PLANNING TO DETERMINE WHAT IMPROVEMENTS ARE WANTED

LIST OF FIGURES

Preface

This book was undertaken as an attempt to portray the application of planning theory to health concerns. To most people, planning for health suggests a straightforward attempt to put the most appropriate available technology to work in the hope of preventing or ameliorating various states of ill health. Our approach is from a broader view. The process of applying health care to overcome or avoid illness, disability, and death is only one input to health. Heredity, environmental factors, and behavior patterns have far greater influence on man's well-being or health than medical care.

The task of creating and then applying planning theory to this broad definition of health was approached much as a planner would attack any other analysis. To begin, it was necessary to define the purposes planning was meant to serve. For me, this purpose was identified with the creation of intended or deliberate change, and consequently, the further constraints of democratic selection and achievement of change in our society were seen as an integral part of the problem. Next, an analysis of the dynamics of social changes was undertaken. This led to the recognition of four major determinants. Planning was then examined to see how it could best affect the four determinants by means of which desired social changes would be brought about. An eclectic developmental mode of planning was derived as a result of scrutinizing many approaches to planning. The various phases of this planning process and the concepts, structures, methodologies, and functions needed to activate them were developed accordingly. These were then applied to goals and problems from the larger system of health and from the smaller system of health care. In either case the interests of the encompassing society in what transpired in both systems were held in focus.

Unless otherwise stated, the general tenor of our concerns is addressed to the scene and the needs of the United States, where, it must be pointed out, broad scope planning is more a matter of discussion than practice. In these circumstances the role of the health planner is undeniably lonely, yet potentially it is enough of a trailblazing one to be rewarding. In other countries, where general socioeconomic planning is well accepted, health planning may be readily integrated. Health planning is beginning or going on with varying degrees of sophistication and complexity in almost all parts of the globe and under every form of government. The logic, nature and choice of the approaches offered by the planning process presented here have carefully taken into account the need of adapting to the values and the political, social and economic situations in which the planning is to take place. It is for this reason that I believe that much of the material will have wide relevancy—even in the presence of more advanced stages of planning and among different political and value systems.

Acknowledgments

Many diverse sources of information and conceptualization helped in the formulation of my ideas. Where I was able to identify the source of specific elements it has been acknowledged in the text. The book grew out of many earlier attempts by myself and my immediate faculty colleagues to capture the nature, significance, and applicability of planning processes to health. Mary Arnold, Richard Bailey, Robert Biller, Allan Blackman, Leonard Duhl, Elizabeth Jolly, George Keranen, Peter Maris, Alberta Parker, Edward Rogers, Cyril Roseman, Frank Stead and Melvin Webber contributed repeatedly and continuously to my thinking, as have staff members Harold Hibbard, Elaine Walbroek, Helen Mortenson, and Eleanor Sully.

Innumerable students also contributed to my thinking about various aspects of the work. Lucy Jones, Pekka Pitkanen, and Agnes Rovnanek in particular, opened rather significant key conceptual or applications areas. My office colleagues, particularly Mrs. Evelyn Brovelli, Jan Gerkin, Leslie Hausman, Amy Siemens, and Paula Wiggins, contributed to the production. Above all, I extend my appreciation to Maggie Hall who undertook to edit and supervise the production of the manuscript. She pointed out errors of content as well as style and construction, and suggested and carried out some of the most meaningful rearrangements. She used cajolement, evidence, and completed improvements to move me along.

Three people in particular provided me not only with ideas, references, and criticisms but undertook to review the entire effort as a gesture of friendship as well as of professionally shared interest. I feel an unlimited debt to Sarah Archer of the University of California at San Francisco, Erich Jantsch of Vienna, Austria, and Ritva Kaje of Helsinki, Finland. Their efforts contributed to major and extensive conceptual concerns and revisions, some of which I dared not take back to them.

I am indebted to Messrs. Nicholas Parlette and William Manning of the Western Regional Office, American Public Health Association, for the opportunity to assemble and distribute earlier versions of many ideas and tools in many kinds of situations with planners, interested citizens, health professionals, and politicians.

Some of the materials here have been "surfaced" over the past few years for attempted applications and criticisms. Chapter 3 grew out of a working paper entitled "Working Definitions of Health for Planners: Merging Philosophies in Public Health," commissioned by the Office of Comprehensive Health Planning for the state of California. Chapter 9 grew from a similar paper entitled "Purposes, Roles and Functions of a Comprehensive Health Planning Body." Chapter 6 grew out of a paper entitled "Priority Setting for Problems, Solutions, and Projects by Means of Selected Criteria," which appeared in the *International Journal of Health Services.* Modification of Figures 1.1, 1.2, 2.3, 2.4, and 7.2 and related discussions also first appeared in the *International Journal of Health Services* in my Review of *Approaches to National Health Planning* by H. E. Hilleboe, A. Barkuus, and W. C. Thomas, Jr. We wish to thank the editors of the *International Journal of Health Services* and the Baywood Publishing Co., Inc. for permission to use these materials.

I have, from time to time, dipped into the pool of our earlier materials published as *Health Planning 1969* by the Western Regional Office, American Public Health Association, whose kind permission enabled us to use various figures and materials.

And finally, this work could not and would not have been undertaken without support from the Department of Health, Education and Welfare, Public Health Service, Health Services and Mental Health Administration, Comprehensive Health Planning Service through project grant 95501.

Part I

INTRODUCTION

1. Health and the Systems Approach

The assumption underlying the creation of health care services is that better health will result—that some improvement in health not otherwise attainable will result—from effectively applied health care services. From this, the seriously confused conclusion has been drawn that good health is primarily dependent upon good health services. As a corollary, more extensive and, by implication, better health care services have come to be seen as leading to the achievement of better health. Yet it can be argued that these notions are more nearly aligned with social misdirection and disaster than with improved health.

INPUTS TO HEALTH

The range of factors consequential for health (see Figure 1.1), suggests that interventions in areas such as education or employment may have to precede, accompany, or replace traditional health care services. These other approaches, or inputs, may work more effectively, cost less, be more desirable generally, and in addition serve other widely desired goals. Moreover, the health of people, including those yet to be born, may be improved most significantly if nonhealth interventions are set in motion today to avoid many of the problems of ill health that otherwise will face the health care sector in the future—a future almost certain to be overburdened by the rising expectations, demands, and needs of populations with greater numbers of aging persons than we now have, and probably living a more trying existence.

THE SYSTEMS APPROACH

At the beginning of a career in health planning, I encountered the terminology for the activities commonly undertaken by planners—assessment, forecasting, problem definition, system analyses, goal setting, alternative interventions, cost-benefit comparisons, implementation, and evaluation. I was seeking a model of planning, for my guidance. What appealed most was learning how to arrange these activities into systems that could be utilized to improve understanding and the transmission of ideas, and could be used to formulate an

2

effective strategy for doing what was wanted. And this brought back memories of my medical training.

A considerable part of the physician's training has traditionally been devoted to taking case histories. The data about the patient's bodily subsystems are supported by information about his family tree (genetics), about his life at work and with his family, and about his habits, education, and culture. Starting with the patient's immediate complaint, the physician puts together a model of a full-body system comprised of interacting subsystems built around a genetic constitution. This system is seen to be totally reactant to an environment of general cultural and social constraints and of specific work and family constraints, and is visualized as further acted upon by aspirations, education, and habits. A future state of potential well-being is then projected, along with any threatening problems.

Competent practicing physicians have had long and extensive experience in planning future health goals. In the process they immerse themselves in the definition of problems, case by case. Unlike the plan-

FIGURE 1.1
INPUTS TO HEALTH

POPULATION
size distribution,
growth rate, gene pool

NATURAL RESOURCES

HEREDITY

CULTURAL SYSTEMS

ENVIRONMENT
fetal
physical (natural and man-made)
socio-cultural
education, employment, means

PSYCHO-SOCIO-SOMATIC HEALTH (well being)

HEALTH CARE SERVICES
prevention, cure, rehabilitation

ECOLOGICAL BALANCE

BEHAVIOR

MENTAL HEALTH
emotional satisfaction, intellectual efficiency, adaptability

The width of the four huge input-to-health arrows indicates my assumptions about the relative importance of the inputs to health. The four inputs are shown as relating to and affecting one another by means of an encompassing matrix which could be called the "environment" of the health system.

ner, who never has enough comparable cases to determine whether his practices are based on sound theory, the physician has evidence before him as to how his theories of diagnosis, prognosis, therapy, and evaluation are borne out in his practice. In addition, he gets confirmation in his knowledge of particular bodily subsystems and their interrelationships with other subsystems.

In defining a health problem, the physician must assess its origins and its potentials for damage. His prognosis for the whole patient must cover the probabilities of outcome without therapy, with therapy A, with therapy B, and so on. The costs and benefits of each alternative intervention are weighed, using the well-documented actual probabilities of specified outcomes, whether or not they are formally expressed.

Each medical problem is seen as occurring in a whole body system composed of many subsystems interacting in a rather individually characteristic way, no matter what the generic similarities. Each patient's body system differs from that of others because of age, sex, attitudes, genetics, prior damage, and so on. Each system lives under different external constraints. As a result, not only are the diagnosis and prognosis highly individual, but the probabilities and the costs and benefits must be calculated anew for each intervention for each patient, even if he presents a problem superficially identical with that of many previous patients. Generally speaking, no two patients get identical therapy for the identical condition unless they have much in common. Even the general outlook of the physician has predictable relationship to the therapy or guidance system that he provides for the patient.

Thinking back to my most distinguished medical mentor, A. L. Bloomfield, and his famous Stanford grand rounds, it becomes clear that he was not necessarily the best examiner or history taker, and that he could and did make do with the measuring efforts of a student or an intern. His forte and his brilliance lay in putting the evidence together and in clarifying the problem and relating it to the entire system (patient). He used the odds (probabilities) skillfully, forecast which other evidences should be present if his "fix" on the problem was correct, sought the required collateral evidence cheaply by circumspect, pinpoint testing, and thus verified his diagnosis (analysis). He even developed the probabilities of being in error using the collaborative evidence he chose, and of whether other possible but less likely diagnoses deserved the expense or hazards of being explored.

Bloomfield moved on to alternative courses of action, weighing each in the light of the whole system and of environmental logic. With the feedback from the forecasts he made of the projected alternative futures, he decided either on inaction or on his course of therapy. True to good practice, he even concerned himself with implementation and particularly with follow-up evaluation. By measuring the achieved results against the intended ones, he kept track of his patient's well-being and also was able to draw conclusions about the soundness of his entire planning effort. He learned from each failure and each success, and both added to his store of probabilities.

Bloomfield was doing what all competent physicians mean to do, but he saw more clearly than others the scope and functioning of the system, and how to intervene. He saw the significance of forecasting, of cost-utility (even of discounting), of using probabilities to increase his accuracy, and of evaluation as a means of improving his understanding of the system he worked with and the targeting processes he employed to create desired changes.

A systems approach as applied to one area of endeavor is portrayed in Figure 1.2, in which the medical care approach is compared step by step with the outline of the developmental approach to planning. I propose to develop this approach to the achievements of health goals and the amelioration of health problems. Figure 1.3 gives some sense of the dynamic movement of the forces at work in the planning cycle. The nodes represent the steps in the planning process numbered 1 through 7 in Figure 1.2. The cycle is pictured as reiterative. The arrows connecting each node to those preceding portray graphically that the planning process as outlined in the text—which can be thought of as a formal succession of steps—may in fact return the process to any prior step at any time. The planning process may also start at any step in the reiterative cycle.

ROLE OF THE COMMUNITY HEALTH PLANNING BODY

The community for which health planning is to be undertaken may be a tiny neighborhood, a valley or river basin, a state, or even the nation itself. Although I do not doubt that planning principles derived and applied for the community level can then be applied to lesser levels of concern, I am not sure that the reverse follows as easily. I am therefore concentrating on how the community through its health planning agency plans for itself rather than on how some delivery system inside the community plans to get its particular output delivered.

The community health planning body converts the general goals and the health aims of the community into the specific objectives and criteria for health and health services which the community's operating or delivery systems will be asked to meet. These objectives or criteria for outputs are attained by means of another phase of planning, which takes up and organizes the detailed concerns of men, machines, facilities, finances, and consumers to meet the community's specified objectives. Angus Brownfield, in his introduction to the San Francisco Bay Area Comprehensive Health Planning Agency Plan of 1972

FIGURE 1.2
THE DEVELOPMENTAL HEALTH PLANNING PROCESS: A SIMULTANEOUS COMPARISON WITH PATIENT CARE

Goals and Purposes, Including Those of Health

Values

The Health Planning Process*

1. General Policies and Aspirations for Health

   ├─1a. via measurement, forecasting, feedback and assessment

2. Determine desired aspirations and problems, resources, values and political climates; select goal** directions and problems to be studied

   ├─2a. via ecologic and epidemiologic analysis

3. Participatively determine nature of goals and origins of and inputs to problems, possible points of intervention, postulate rational health objectives. List possible interventions

   ├─3a. via socio-economic and political analysis of possible interventions; consider gains and losses from each and give priority rating

4. Design better alternative plans and suggest priorities for goals, objectives, interventions and plans and lay out strategy for presentation and obtaining decision

   ├─4a. via exposure to community and policy makers

The Patient Care Process

Accepted credo—one must use the doctor to restore his health

history and examination given

Manifestations described and most important needs specified

deductions and further confirmatory tests

Etiology and nature of illness and prognosis determined. List possible treatments.

health and socio-economic outcomes considered under each proposed treatment

Select better courses of therapy, outline and lay out strategy for presentation and obtaining decision

patient, doctor (and family) debate courses of action

Each step may introduce cause for reconsideration of preceding steps

6

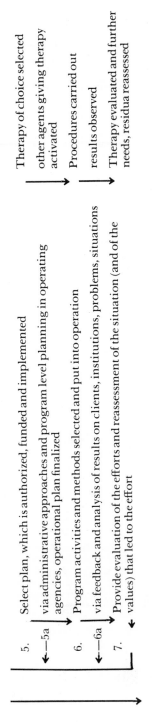

Therapy of choice selected
other agents giving therapy activated

Procedures carried out
results observed

Therapy evaluated and further needs, residua reassessed

5.   Select plan, which is authorized, funded and implemented

—5a   via administrative approaches and program level planning in operating agencies, operational plan finalized

6.   Program activities and methods selected and put into operation

—6a   via feedback and analysis of results on clients, institutions, problems, situations

7.   Provide evaluation of the efforts and reassessment of the situation (and of the values) that led to the effort

Levels of expectation by which to evaluate accomplishment

* Arrows pointing downward indicate a theoretic flow of planning steps, each step by means of specified activity leads to the next step. The arrows pointing to the left indicate that during the considerations carried out at each step, concerns may be generated which call for reconsideration of preceding steps. This upward flow of concern may stop at any relevant step (arrows pointing to the right) for reiteration of planning at that step. *Although the motivating energy is always traceable back to values, the formal planning process can start at any step or steps to get the entire planning cycle into motion.* The discrepancies between the often unstated goals, and the equally unstated levels of expectation, both of which arise from one's hierarchy of values, usually get called problems or unfilled "wants."

** Goals are used in the sense of aspirations and general directions, objectives as more specific elements going to make up progress towards a goal.

pointed out that "community level health planning becomes one of the primary specifiers of the outcomes of health achieving or maintaining activities, but not the designer of systems to organize these activities." Of course, it is the institutional-level planning that will result in the actual outputs which produce the desired effects in the community. However, to plan in behalf of the whole community is much more difficult than to plan at the smaller systems levels after the community has determined its objectives. I therefore concentrate on community level planning.

THE DEVELOPMENTAL APPROACH

If planning theory is to be applied to the improvement of health, we must know the set of purposes that planning is to serve. These can be summarized as (1) defining the desired improvements, (2) achieving them, and (3) measuring this attainment. Because these purposes re-

FIGURE 1.3
DYNAMICS OF THE HEALTH PLANNING PROCESS

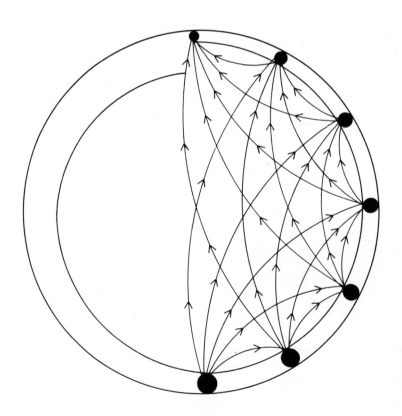

flect a central concern for obtaining major social changes, the nature of social change is conceptualized and the constraints of obtaining it democratically and deliberately must be defined and appended. This is accomplished by adopting an eclectic mode of planning which, although borrowing from many other modes, in particular derives from two: a normative (or idealistic) future-building mode, and an articulated (or systems-oriented) problem-solving mode which is guided by the long-range goals or aims established by the normative one. This eclectic mode I call "developmental."

The developmental mode permits us to focus simultaneously on planning for problem solving (short-term amelioration of problems) and planning for attainment of long-range goals (desired futures). Fortunately, the planning techniques needed for problem solving and for attaining long-range goals are startlingly complementary when tackled by the systems approach, even though the specific techniques and strategies differ and need to be interrelated into a combined strategy, that of developmental planning. (This mode has been previously implied under such names as "middle bridge planning," by Meyerson, and "mixed scanning," by Etzioni.)

In the United States there is a dearth of public long-range goal commitments, and even of willingness to work toward defining them. Planning for public concerns is itself often suspect. Therefore, those who wish to use the developmental mode of planning will find it imperative to promote long-range, direction-setting planning. At the same time, we find that we are generally forced to introduce the subject of planning for health in terms of solving obvious and currently pressing health problems.

When we work in a more goal-oriented society, we concentrate on analyzing how to obtain an established set of goals. In such a society, we watch for current problems as a set of constraints on long-range planning; that is, problems should be favorably affected if severe, not significantly worsened if felt to be tolerable, and ameliorated in the course of long-term goal attainment.

Thus, the society's orientation toward future desires or present hurts determines whether the planners give major concentration to attaining immediate or long-range goals.

This introduction to the systems approach of planning for health may help to explain biases or blind spots. But it is really intended to fulfill other purposes: first, to point out that we do have a conceptual model; second, to indicate that the art and science of planning has reached a very elegant stage for some smaller systems, and to offer hope to those of us who wish to work with more complex and larger systems; and third, to make it clear that medically trained persons should not regard themselves as basically unprepared to work as planners or with planners.

JUSTIFICATION FOR INTERVENING BY PLANNING

The possibility of significantly altering future outcomes by using our desires as guides often raises questions. The most common is: "What right do we have to intervene?" I claim that in our culture we are all interveners. Yet many oppose planning for health on the grounds that planners infringe on the rights of those to be made healthy, of those who pay the major share of the costs, and those who make a living selling health services. There are few who doubt, however, that we must spend our resources and use clubs and guns to maintain law and order when those on the short end of everything are driven to riot. What is so noble about interventions based on fear, hatred, and force? There are those who feel that other interventions, such as education, employment, and early health care should be brought to bear through planning, so that there will be no need to resort to measures of desperation. I, too, opt for the interventions that make it possible to avoid the too-little and the too-late measures that supposedly spare us the necessity of planning for anything but disasters.

A second question is: "How can we be certain we are planning wisely, considering all reasonable options, and not prejudicing the future of various individuals and groups?" We can never be certain, because no group of planners could even conceive of all the options that might be offered to a community. Nor, without extensive participation, could those involved understand the ramifications of the various options. For these reasons, I strongly advocate that planning be undertaken at the neighborhood level as soon as it is begun at city-county, metropolitan, state, and national levels. The greatest possible number of persons and viewpoints must be involved, so that deleterious options do not go unchallenged, nor conceivably desirable alternatives go uninvestigated. Speed is not the prime consideration in these deliberations; emphasis should be on scope, effectiveness, and equity. Also, I am aware that, unless reasonably comprehensive planning sets the stage for a more thorough effort, decisions will continue to be made on the basis of scanty information.

While trying to answer this second question, I came to feel that facing up to the inevitable diversities of value positions may be of the greatest utility, not only for guidance but also for survival. Participation in planning should teach all of us more about our own values, as we struggle to reconcile them with the values of others. We need to learn that we may well hold some "foreign" values ourselves on other issues or at other times. A return to widespread participation in the resolution of issues and the reconciliation of differences may, in fact, be more crucial to our well-being than any health measures. The development of the ability to work together and understand one another may help to wean us away from the interclass, interethnic, and international paranoias that threaten not just to postpone or undo measures for well-being but to bring our world to a sudden stop.

A third question is: "Can health be planned for if planning for public concerns is limited primarily to what goes on in the health sector?" Such restricted health planning—euphemistically known as "comprehensive health planning" in the United States—is not particularly promising. Without significant interrelated planning, sector by sector, I doubt that health can be planned for, even though isolated health sector planning activities might be carried out and might modestly improve health care delivery.

However, a justification for undertaking such planning is that it is a beginning. If we use the systematic approach to problem-solving and insist on guidance from normative goals, planning for health may allow us to make a more meaningful approach to goal achievement and problem-solving. Health is an area of high political, social, and individual interest. It may offer an ideal ground on which to thrash out new and old values and work out the experimental processes of comprehensive planning. Many areas of health concern are shared by persons of all shades of political belief and degrees of economic well-being. The extension of thinking about cause and effect and the development of timely and acceptable interventions formulated around health issues may make possible the utilization of newly designed processes and the reestablishment of meaningful sharing of political concerns and actions.

Part II

ENVIRONMENT FOR
PLANNING

2. Planning:
A Preferred Instrument of Deliberate
and Democratically Achieved Social Change

Planning, it can be assumed, is devoted to directing and attaining social changes of a specific and desired nature. Although present theories about the causes of change are much in dispute and firm evidence is scarce, people who plan believe that ordered change is possible and that at least some control can be exerted over the variables which produce change. Blackman[1] has contrasted beliefs about the causality of social change with the ways the holders of divergent beliefs would view deliberate attempts to provoke social change. One of his contrasting pairs of beliefs opposes "change is easy and good" to "change is difficult and dangerous." An individual's responses to such concepts can define him as an optimist or pessimist in regard to planning, and can reveal whether he would acknowledge planning to be a useful tool.

Another pair of beliefs contrasts the "truly long" and the "comparatively short" view of the significance of change. Here, rather interestingly, those who have very long-term and resigned views about, for instance, ecological controls, may find themselves allied with those who want only very short-term gains and little formal societal or global planning. They might even be joined by those who take the natural-history or Spenglerian view of a life-to-death progression of societies and do not believe that planning can do much good, if any at all, in changing the course of events.[2] Those who take a normative and very long view and want a willed future that is not only bearable but is kept desirable over all time, of course opt for an elaborate scheme of continued feedback from the past and from desired images of the future.[3]

Assuming that there is desire among the public for deliberate change, and that the desire signifies belief in the possibilities for its realization, we can turn to the question of how to apply planning. Blackman's contrasting pairs of beliefs about causality bring out the issues which we must surmount in choosing a set of planning directions. "Changing individuals" versus "changing institutions" is a pair with obviously divergent implications for the interventions to be chosen. "Order" versus "conflict" is a pair that sharpens the issue of how to deal with departures or deviances from usual behavior patterns.

14

Are interventions to be designed to return the deviant to an ordered system (if necessary even by repression and at the risk of promoting conflict)? Or should interventions engage the deviant in conflict, in the belief that society needs such conflict ordeals if it is to consider reordering its priorities and reorganizing its institutions (for example, changing education and its instrumentalities, the schools)? [4]

Another contrast pair, "coercion" versus "consensus," focuses attention on the means that are believed best for getting people to agree on a set of directions. "Elitist change" versus "mass change" focuses on beliefs about the extent to which citizens must be involved in considering direction and change. Differing opinions about roles of consumers' advocates, lobbyists, experts, and indigenous leaders represent differing beliefs about the desirability of popular involvement in selecting and securing change. By scrutinizing past successes and failures in attempts at social change, perhaps we can learn about the nature of change and find guidance for our future attempts to plan for and achieve deliberate and democratic social change. [5]

ORIGINS OF SOCIAL CHANGE

Smelser,[6] who writes that the "most exciting theories of social change are lacking scientific adequacy," has suggested the basis for a method of planning deliberate and democratic social change which, with some modification, I propose to develop. Borrowing freely from Smelser, one can put in skeletal form a theory for planning which will take fairly explicit notice of the many aspects of planning practice which must be faced in any comprehensible approach to achieving publicly intended social change.

Relevance of Concepts of Traditional and Modern Societies

Traditional societies are supposedly distinguished by a value system that does not conceive of departures from the status quo. The values of such a society operate to provide an overwhelming negative feedback (return to prior status quo) in response to any external force or nonconforming acts. No systemic changes occur from generation to generation; even the replacement of a ruler by death or usurpation, unless by conquest from the outside, finds in his place another who is equally and similarly traditional. The position of individuals is inherited rather than attained. Behavior is inertial and prescriptive rather than acquisitive. It is custom-bound, self-oriented, and authoritarian. Creativity is absent. Tradition sets precedent and solves problems, whether by authority or by consensus.[7]

Modern societies are supposed to be change oriented and operate on a positive feedback basis. Significant cultural changes may occur not only from generation to generation, but nowadays seemingly almost from one annual cohort to the next. Behavior is energic, acquisitive, impersonal, and organization oriented. Innovation and creativity are constantly shaping reality into new relationships whenever the new is seen to serve the purposes of the innovator better than the old.[8]

Another theory proposes that resource poor societies come to appear to be anti-change or traditional through beliefs in limited good, and casts doubt on real differences between so-called traditional and modern societies.[9]

Transitional societies are the ones wherein value systems of the traditional are pitted against the modern, the modern usually being superimposed by external forces which sooner or later win internal support.[10] In the transitional society a schism is set up by the value systems of those native to the culture who come to want change and those who continue to oppose it, and the schism is in itself probably a major force for further change.

I suspect that we, as planners, need not be concerned with traditional societies, if there are any, for they will not seek our services; we, therefore, can concentrate on the transitional and modern societies. However, Hagen's work on how change slowly enters the traditional society through situations which destroy the status of significant numbers of adult males offers a very satisfying explanation of the origins of change in a non-change society.[11] McClelland provides another psychologic theory of change based on how child-rearing practices affect the need for achievement, but this would seem to depend on prior, and largely unexplained by him, impetus for change in those practices.[12]

In a society such as ours in the United States, are there any significant groups that hold traditional or ambivalent transitional views? We are repeatedly told that our society is in great part post-industrial.[13] Are we possibly, in part, also post-modern? If so, what does this mean in terms of the possibilities for social change?

Innumerable kinds of groups, many communities, and even some states are holding on to an anti-change ethic. And other groups are acquiring this attitude; they often emerge by detaching themselves from very sophisticated change-oriented environments. These two forces—the historically firmly anti-change "intellectual hillbillies" and the new anti-change adherents—are returning our society, even if ever so slightly, toward a transitional or ambivalent level. These two forces are maintained primarily by the feedback from activities within our own country, secondarily from feedback about our adventures among our international neighbors, and, to some extent, as a result of our travel among the planets.

This diversion into the attitudes toward change among modern social groups was not prompted by any suspicion that the underlying primal energy stream is particularly different among men or societies anywhere. However, the nature of the issues which trigger change is different enough in the modern group and in its two encompassed anti-change elements—one more nearly traditional, one perhaps post-modern—that we must keep in mind that even in our own society the energy or impetus for changes may be quite differently aroused. Moreover, once aroused, the direction taken may be quite variable. For the traditional anti-change segment the only acceptable change means turning the clock back; for the post-modern segment it may mean halting the current streams of change; for the modern segment and its planners, change signifies harnessing primal energies to desired new ends.

Society as an Open System:
The Four Major Determinants of Change

Social functioning can be conceived as the working of an open system that interacts with its environment and with its own subsystems.[14] Changes in one factor result in changes in others, or in the relationships between them. This concept of social functioning avoids the notion of a homeostatic or stable equilibrium social system in the modern society. In the stable system of the hypothesized traditional society, any factor alteration or impingement from the outside would lead to a negative (or return to the prior position) kind of feedback—much like many physiologic functions. By contrast, as a result of alterations of internal factors and deviancies or from exposure to new or altered external factors, change-oriented cultures have ample positive feedback and are very tolerant, if not desirous, of a drift to new sets or states or, rather, evanescent equilibria. Some of these states last long enough to be described and to provide behavioral and institutional guidance, but usually continue to alter so rapidly as to be a source of surprise and shock to many.

Such a system is open, of course; the factors at work are rarely well defined and their relationships are not very clear. Moreover, the internal workings of the open system are not free from influences that are external to the system as we delineate it. Buckley's book on sociology and modern systems theory, already referred to, was invaluable in arranging a theoretical base from which planning could satisfactorily be seen as a means of democratically producing deliberate and publicly agreed upon social change.

Search for the most deep-seated origins of change has led to theories about the processes which are at the root of change,[15] such as:

Stress and reaction to stress.
Multiple and conflicting role demands.

Long-term social development, accumulation of knowledge, inventions, etc.

Long-term social disintegration, a predetermined cultural rise and fall.

Changes in economics, e.g. circumstances of production, consumption, distribution (there is an impressive array of economic type theories, none of which individually looks remarkably potent).

Impingements on a specific society by "outside" knowledge, inventions, behaviors, etc.

Innate attributes of a society which carry the seed of change, e.g. race, religion, etc.

Cataclysmic changes such as result from natural disaster, climatic changes, diseases, and ecologic shifts, whether man-made or not.

Population growth and resulting imbalances with the environment or with society's institutions.

Extensions of logic and reasoning.

Natural and social selection.

Coleman concludes that there are two major groups of social change theories: those which assume it starts with change in individuals, and those which assume it starts with changes in social conditions. He further points out that radicals and conservatives are found in both camps.[16] In change-oriented societies there is a continuous and conscious search for advantage through change. The United States is generally accepted as the extreme case where change is valued for its own sake by a large proportion of the population. The array of variables that are associated with change in modern societies is testimony either to the power of the change orientation, or to the innumerable forces capable of making change occur in a change-susceptible society, or in one that has the affluence to afford choice and risk.

In addition to the alleged change-causing processes already listed, such occurrences or forces as improved education, effects of mass media, religious aberrations, revived nationalism, new technological discoveries, environmental changes, improved health status, affluence or economic growth, political movements, charismatic leaders, and war are all said to be causally responsible for significant social changes.

Smelser[17] takes us considerably further by organizing all the situational variables related to change into what he calls the four determinants of change:

the structural setting for change.
the operation of social controls.
mobilization for change.
the impetus to change.

Structural Controls

Smelser views the structural setting for change as carrying aspects of opportunity as well as obstacle, and uses such examples as whether there are agencies or systematized activities which play into or prevent events such as stock market collapses, or agencies and activities which sidetrack grievances or channel them into responsive and competent sources able to respond. I would add specific control mechanisms such as laws, police, courts and sanctions, which are highly structured means of control. In our society we have a system of so-called free enterprise, embracing a credo which encourages the "rational" approach to attaining what one wants. It is matched by a set of political machinery which—by its very extensive system of checks and balances, as well as easy means of getting legislative change—indicates how much change in structure was anticipated.

Societal System Pressures and Self-Regulation

System pressures are made up of the existence and operation of informal pulls and hauls as the society goes about its work and as the parts of the system impinge upon one another.[18] Lax for some issues, stern for others, ignored in some communities, but repressive in others for the same issue, these informal pressures are part of the configuration of forces critical to the desire for change and repression of changes. These are built-in forces which support some changes and resist others. Some of these pressures are almost institutionalized whether privately or publicly expressed, as by mass media, churches, voluntary organizations and leaders.

Nadel's *self regulation*[19] similarly speaks to the desired, but not formally controlled, pressures that are exerted when someone steps out of line, but more particularly to the problems caused by not doing the customary and accepted things. Nadel uses many examples, such as the "disadvantages" that accrue to bachelors in some societies; and although not specifically intended, keep the pressures on every person to get married.

Mobilization

Marshalling the forces for change is in part an explanation of why charismatic leaders and political movements seem, and in fact are, so important to social change. In our society, we can see that the cult of "success and all honor to those who succeed," combined with a relatively freely mobile society, carries all the ingredients for the fairly easy development of highly visible leaders. They may earn their status and even a mantle of authority from success in invention, industry, the market, labor, politics, sports, arts, or academia. Moreover, authority won in one area may be easily transferred (even through inheritance) to other fields.

Impetus

The fourth determinant, impetus, is practically built into our culture by our Judeo-Christian social justice ethic and by our poor performance relative thereto. Our United States credo of equality, justice, fairness, liberty, one citizen-one vote, education, rationality, etc.,[20] and our exaggerated belief, so transparent to foreigners—such as de Tocqueville[21] or Myrdal[22]— that these are all in operation, could be considered a staging platform for change. Such values are attained only with great difficulty, particularly when placed in the context of the market place, where "free" enterprise, such as it is, offers not only a competitive sphere of concerns, but also a perpetual source of discrepancy between achievement and value-based expectations.

The widely divergent standards by which values are enforced or prevented from being enforced, and the inequality of their application, when combined with national braggadocio and wide discussion on these subjects disseminated by every form of mass media, surely constitute a constant and potent source of pride, aggravation, and frustration to most citizens of the U.S.A. The dissonances generated by the discrepancies among values, and between values and practices, provide no small set of continuing forces for change. The origins and roles of dissonance will be discussed extensively later in the chapter.

Impetus obviously has two major components, energy and direction. It is hard to agree with Smelser[23] that direction of change derives principally from the means or source of control. It seems more reasonable to assume that direction is inherent in the source of the energy or impetus. Probably each of the three other determinants also helps shape the ultimate direction impetus takes.

My hypothesis is that impetus is the main ingredient, that it arises from dissonances created by conflicts between values, and from discrepancies that are seen, felt or believed to exist between accomplishments attained under pursuit of value-derived goals and the value derived standards of expectation. Dissonance releases primal energy in pursuit of improving or lessening dissonance.

Deliberate, publicly and democratically agreed-upon change (new goals) will further act to create awareness of new discrepancies between what we currently have and what we believe we want in the future. New dissonance results; and the impetus for change is generally increased in order to lessen that dissonance. Dissonance may cause changes in structure, system pressures, or mobilization. These I regard as typically of secondary importance to the main determinant, impetus. Rarely can the planner deliberately and agreeably change these three secondary determinants only by what he does directly to them. It is by his play on impetus for what is wanted that he can usually change the three determinants of structure, mobilization, and control. Changes in structure and systems pressures, however, are the epitome of deep-seated social change. Of course, changes in structure, mobilization, and control do alter the levels and directions of strains that produce impetus, the key determinant which caused the changes in the first place.

Alterations in the four determinants are very likely to be high priority objects of deliberate social change. However, stress and impetus do not inevitably lead to desires for deliberate or democratic change. They also lead to apathy, paranoia, hatred, and crippling fear. Planning must reorganize and channel impetus, and open vistas attractive enough to overcome paralysis as well as to compete with demands of less pressing values that appear more easily achieved.

Apparently the key effort of planning (which we see as the happiest means of introducing publicly desired change into our democratic society) must be directed to harnessing and guiding the energies which create the impetus for change.

A Model of Social Change

Outline of a Proposed Model of Social Change from Which My Planning Theory and Methodology Are Derived

Primal needs or natural drives release and direct innate or primal energy to effectuate their satisfaction. Drives exist in a constantly shifting hierarchy dependent in great part on how well each is satisfied at the moment.

The overall environment determines how primal needs are actually best met, and as a result valued behavior patterns emerge.

In any given society, human interaction and survival or valued behavior patterns have resulted in a well structured value hierarchy, even though innumerable subsocietal units have somewhat different hierarchies. New environmental demands (external forces) and changes in societal sub-group behavior and relationships (internal forces) create a constantly shifting hierarchy of values.

The innate energies available for meeting primal needs are transferred to the pursuit of values, which may bear little more than symbolic relationships to the primal needs themselves.

Because of the desire to reach certain achievements which will fulfill these values, the values set goals, and thus behavior.

Values also set expectations or standards by which the value holder can decide whether the achievements were in fact adequate to reach the goals and satisfy the value.

Discrepancies are observed when what is perceived or believed to have been achieved toward reaching the desired goal set by a value is compared with the standard of what was acceptable as set up by the same value. Such discrepancies are the source of dissonance and thus of strain for the value holder. The situation applies to individuals as much as to groups. Discrepancies also arise between values or value systems and role demands. Individual behavior is packaged into roles which must respond to many subsets of values and to many societal subsystems. Many of the roles necessary for one person can be seen as congruent only with the greatest difficulty; the effort to achieve congruence sooner or later leaves most individuals in a state of tension, strain, or readiness for change.

Awareness of discrepancies or degrees of failures is the means by which value holders come to feel the dissonance between achievement and expectation and, therefore, the means through which they become desirous of change. Dissonance is intolerable to the value holder, and it releases primal energies in amounts consonant with the intensity or degree of the failure felt and the hierarchical position of the unsatisfied value among all the values held.

Values also make up the steering mechanism which guides impetus for change.

Once the concept of change is accepted by a society, social change is the response stimulated by dissonance with the intent of changing the situation or values to lessen dissonance.

The change-oriented society commonly attempts, at least initially, to improve the performance of its activities or alter the environment so that current expectations and goals are met and values are reasonably satisfied.

To lower dissonance, the change-oriented society may alter its goals, lower its norms for behavior or accomplishment, remodel or abandon unsatisfied values, or even adopt opposite ones.

There is no evidence that the wellsprings of innate energy for achieving primal drives (now directed to achieving value set goals) ever dry up.

In the modern society there is no evidence that quieting dissonance by removing perceived discrepancies between achievement and expectation causes cessation or necessarily even a long-term, major slowdown in the evolution of new dissonances. The pace of growth and invention and their creation of new needs and environmental obstacles—as well as the intellectual production of new vistas and new values—continues to set the stage for dissonances produced by satisfied old values and by the challenges of meeting new ones.

The key determinant of social change is the impetus created by dissonance.

Three secondary determinants of social change are: the structural or formalized social control setting; informal social system pressures or "self-regulation"; and mobilization for change.

The energy exerted by the impetus is heavily directed towards altering or revising the three secondary determinants to allow satisfaction of unsatisfied values, or resolution of the unacceptable role burdens or conflicts. As a result, changes in the three secondary determinants themselves may become the major immediate resultant social changes. These in turn become the instrumentalities from which a whole stream of other social changes may emerge.

No model can do justice to such a complex reality as social functioning. But enough seems known about how an open system operates and enough experience exists on planning as a means of introducing social change, that a model can be derived to serve as a means of guidance to planners. The model used to describe social change is built on our perception of the open-system concept of society, in which its environment and all of its parts affect, control, or influence all other parts. Changes introduced from outside (environment of the system), new awareness of old states, or awareness of new states may all lead to a reaffirmation of old goals (negative feedback) or the seeking of new goals (positive feedback). The term *states* might include the perception of things, of relationships, of means, or of desired situations, whether in existence or conceptualized as good or bad possibilities for the future.

Buckley[24] carries the idea of endless modifications of the system further by quoting Strauss[25] to the effect that organizational order is a result of shared agreements which are never conclusively, totally, or permanently accepted or bought; they are continuously being renegotiated and the order continually reconstituted—that is, social change in small or even large increments is continuous.

Buckley[26] examines the significance of norms and institutionalization and, quoting Coleman,[27] tries to demolish the idea of norms solely as governors of social behavior. He comes up with a richer configuration: that norms are major social forces, and that man is guided by them in the sense that he not only internalizes them but also learns the long-term consequences to himself of his strategies of action, including those which violate the collectivized values, norms, goals and expectations. I, too, would go further and suggest that the ambivalences set up by differences between socially approved norms and social gains, as opposed to personal norms about desired behavior, are a potent source of individual strain or permanent dissonance and tension. This tension can best be reduced by altering one or both forces that create the dissonance, for example, by attempting to alter the widely-held values or modifying personal behavior, or doing some of both. If dissonances are to be kept low, the behavior called for by the norms of society must make individuals feel gratified—it is not enough for society's spokesmen to say that society is satisfied.

No model ever does justice to a system, and the one amplified below does not, but it seems to be useful to planners as a guide to where and how interventions can be directed so as to be effective. Moreover, the model helps account for the legitimacy of the innumerable modes of planning, because there should indeed be many ways in which publicly desired social change can be brought about if this model is useful as a guide to planning.

Man's Inner Needs as the Primal Source of Energy Toward Goals of Any Kind (The Origins of Energy for Impetus to Change)

Some common threads from Hagen,[28] Malinowski,[29] Maslow[30] and Etzioni[31] come together reasonably well into a statement that there are powerful needs or inner forces typical of man which have attributes of their own not determined by the social structure, cultural or socialization patterns. Hagen chooses the psychological forces, emphasizing: (1) manipulative, (2) agressive, (3) possessive, and (4) succorant-nurturant needs. Malinowski derives a group of basic needs such as: (1) metabolism, (2) reproduction, (3) bodily comforts, (4) safety, (5) movement, and (6) growth. Maslow lists: (1) physiologic, (2) safety, (3) belongingness and love, (4) esteem, (5) self-actualization, and (6) aesthetic.

Satisfaction of these forces takes on certain forms in given environments. For example, metabolism is manifested in a given culture by specific food and commissariat habits. These are of interest because they represent satisfying and reasonably successful matching of needs with the environment, and thus come to make up the configuration of what is valued for satisfying the need. It is clear that man is capable of the expenditure of unbelievable amounts of energy to satisfy his primal needs, and that, as his culture develops, his energies are transferred to value configurations of his choosing.

The Value System as the Current-Day Holder and Releaser of Primal Energies Which Are the Basis for Impetus to Change

Satisfaction of inner needs and drives becomes imbedded in the value system. The inner needs or drives portrayed by Malinowski, Hagen, Maslow or Etzioni, have the capacity, when unsatisfied, to release man's energy in the direction of seeking a change. They provide the impulse, or impetus, for an act which will satisfy the currently most urgently felt need or drive. As already discussed, cultures channel the satisfying acts into a dependable and recognizable pattern of behavior. Moreover, value constructs arise around each of these needs and around the entire collection, so that complete artifactual behavior patterns come into existence from the need to accommodate and arrange all these behavioral responses in accordance with overall needs of survival within the environment constraints and nurturance possibilities.

What are the origins of values? What are values? What is a value system? Values provide a stimulus to action (goal setting), on the one hand, and impose criteria or standards of expectation by which results may be judged, on the other. Values come into existence through a continuing process of creation as man acquires a basic set of "rules for living" from surviving his encounters with the environment. They also emerge from his imaginings and esthetic impulses about how things could or should be. Values are then transmitted generationally. A high proportion of the most fondly held values relate to the past and are currently irrelevant, often inimical to survival. No two persons in a culture are likely to acquire precisely the same hierarchy of values, but some values are more commonly held than others in any given time, country, and society.

"The capacity of man to sense value in the quality of his experience is probably the most fundamental and unique characteristic of man. All human needs, desires, and aspirations are permeated with value attributes."[32] Values have been defined in many ways and analyzed in terms of their significance for those engaged in activities such as Public Health.[33] I have been most heavily influenced by the brilliant presentation on "Individual and Group Values" by Williams,[34] which in many ways illuminated the full role of values in the planning schema presented here.

Values are conceptions of what is desirable or worthy, and are utilized as criteria for choice or preference, or as justification, for choice of action. Values are reflected in human behavior, but not all behavior reflects values. Physiologic and reflex acts, even social reflex acts, need not be expressions of values.

Values are not themselves needs, desires, motives, or interests. One may personally desire what he classifies as without value, or value for others what he does not desire for himself. Values channel and define the desires that arise in biological or environmental exigencies, but values are in no way synonymous with the immediate biological demands that create needs for survival, reproduction, and so on. They can even be in gross conflict with such needs, and alter them in remarkable ways (lifelong chastity vows, risking or giving one's life for the protection of one's society, are examples).

Values are based on historical, cultural, biological, and socioeconomic facts of living and survival, and they are transmitted to off-spring accordingly. Values also grow from rationalized conflicts among values, or between values and environmental demands. Because values are rooted in past personal, archetypal, and cultural experiences, some may be inappropriate in the context of the present and even, if critical to survival, highly dangerous. Values arise, grow, extend, elaborate, specify, explicate, limit, shrink, or are otherwise altered by current life experience and contemplation.

Values test, and are tested by, confrontation with the behavior or activity that they create, thereby setting in motion the stimulus for further change, which is again measured in terms of survival relevance. Standards for behavior (norms) usually become the criteria for testing the character of the behavior rather than for testing its utility in survival—many widely held values no longer relevant to survival are never tested in any rational or conscious way. In this manner, traditional values may continue to influence behavior in such a way that they are prejudicial to other values of current importance and may threaten well-being, or even survival itself. James Reston has said this very well:

> In a world of change the leaders in all institutions in a democratic country have to keep asking whether what they are doing is really relevant to present day realities. The history of the world is strewn with habits and credos which were essential in one age and disastrous in another.[35]

And to the *habits* and *credos* I would add *values*. As an example, the carryover from colonial days of certain beliefs about self-reliance and mutual support probably serve us poorly in an era when industrialization has made the survival of individuals highly interdependent and the creation of job opportunities and job training more important than neighbor helping neighbor.

Fortunately for survival, but unfortunately for the ease of the planner, values constantly change.[36] They change with information and experience, by restatements of propositions, and in light of how they are juxtaposed. They change with exposure to issues, as life position or work changes, and as new elements come into roles. Old values come to have new meanings; priorities shift for this reason and also because of the changing costs of holding to old values. The marginal utility of a value may decline rapidly beyond a particular point. As a consequence, an unstable value structure is the rule, and innumerable poorly resonating value hierarchies have to be dealt with in any given modern society. For those who doubt that values do change, evidences and forecasts of significant value changes have been presented by Wilson in the form of a present versus future profile,[37] and by Harman,[38] who points out the fundamental incompatibility between the values of the person-centered society and the industrial state.

Values exist in a constantly changing hierarchy and, therefore, create a hierarchy of goals. In a given culture there is general agreement on the desirability of many goals, such as expanding education or reducing infant mortality. Traditional approaches directed toward achieving such goals have often overlooked the values which gave rise to the goals. If narrowly conceived programs are set up which block or threaten the same or other equally treasured values and goals, they are not likely to get much support, even if put into operation. In our present state of unsophistication, it is still necessary to work from or toward tangible health or other well-being goals. But higher level societal goals, such as justice, equity, fairness, democracy, or self-fulfillment, must always be kept in view as assurances that our programs are guided by these goals, or at least do not violate them.

A hierarchy of values undoubtedly exists, and is probably not dissimilar to the hierarchy of value-derived goals suggested in Figure 2.1. (The figure carries no connotation of control from the top, nor of each goal necessarily corresponding to a particular value.) Examination of each value or its goals reveals how often it carries the seeds of conflict with other values, even within the same person or among persons holding the same values. Security as a value, extended through all the logical steps of goal and program setting to make it a total reality, soon leads to a loss of equally valued personal liberty. Full liberty and justice for an individual may similarly demand anarchistic freedom to pursue self-expression at the expense of the same valued attributes or activities of his neighbors.

Davidoff and Reiner make a very explicit application of values to planning, pointing out that values are usable as criteria or preference items for goals, as well as being the origins of goals.[39] They note that goals can be compared in terms of their intrinsic value and also in terms of their instrumental worth to other goals, particularly higher level ones, because of the hierarchical arrangement of values.

The explicit definition and extension of a value usually opens the door to its reformulation. "Freedom of choice" may well turn out to be two quite different things. For example, in the question of open housing legislation, it may turn out to be liberty to purchase or not to purchase real estate irrespective of race, or it may be liberty to sell or not to sell real estate to anyone regardless of his race. When this confrontation (Proposition 14 in the California general election of 1966) is further examined in the light of another value, equality of opportunity, some remarkable qualifications may have to be introduced into one's value system in regard to the concepts of freedom and liberty. How could liberty be such a treacherous value? Both contestants claimed that they sought liberty but, actually, one party wanted equity, the other freedom from intrusion. The nature of values is not always apparent from what is proclaimed as the value position. True,

FIGURE 2.1
GOAL HIERARCHY

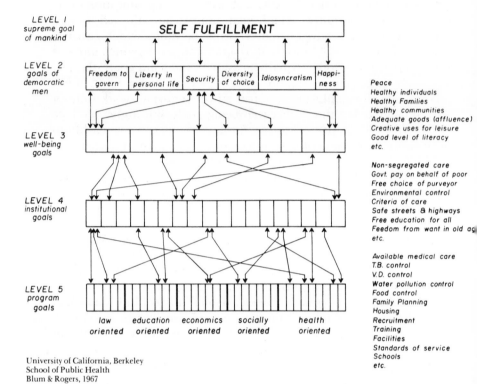

University of California, Berkeley
School of Public Health
Blum & Rogers, 1967

Sample of well-being goals in ascending levels of importance, and in inverse order of tangibility. Arrows represent direct or indirect relationships between goals and different levels which may be positive or negative forces acting upward or downward. Although not shown, goal forces may act on other goals at same level or skip over one or more levels.

in order for values to be discussed they must be consciously held, but their true nature needs careful exploration.

To sum up the definition of values, two different contributions are presented. Kluckhohn defines values as "a conception, explicit or implicit, distinctive of an individual or characteristic of a group, of the desirable, which influences the selection from available modes, means, and ends of action."[40] With the deletion of the word "available," this definition suits the planner's purposes. Skinner phrases the matter quite differently, although we see in his concept utility for our purposes. He says: "People act to improve the world and to progress toward a better way of life for good reasons, and among these consequences are the things people value and call good. . . . Things are good (positively reinforcing) or bad (negatively reinforcing) presumably because of the contingencies of survival under which the species evolved.''[41]

Several other terms are either confused or heavily associated with the concept of values. The following brief paragraphs will help to clarify these terms as I use them.

Goals are descriptions of aspirations which represent fruition of the ideals established by values. They are generally given a more definite set of dimensions when inserted into plans, but their nature may be spiritual or essentially unattainable, as well as practical and attainable. For this reason, in part, they must be broken down into more tangible sub-elements—the objectives. (These definitions of goals and objectives are commonly reversed in the literature.)

Objectives and sub-objectives are the specific endpoints established for the programs which are to bring realization of goals. The time, place, quantity, and quality of change in persons or things constitute objectives or targets. For purposes of programming, organizing, controlling, and evaluating, plans must deal with such items as the division of labor, and must pinpoint the time, spot and mode of impact for program efforts. As a result, objectives are further broken down into sub-objectives, which spell out the points of impact and what is to be accomplished at each point. Sub-objectives do for objectives what objectives do for goals. As they are further refined or limited, sub-objectives may specify accomplishments that represent what is to be delivered, rather than the effects of the delivery on the recipients.

Expectations or value standards are the generally accepted and sanctioned group prescriptions to be applied to outcomes, situations, behaviors, beliefs, or feelings which stem from values held by the group. They are requirements or limits or situation-bounded specifications derived from values, and they reflect the standards of attainment called for by the values. They presume to tell us what stimuli should be attended and what schemes or concepts are acceptable or appropriate. We are less concerned with their provision of prescriptions or sanctions for behavior which is the definition of a *norm*, than with their utility in telling us how well our values are being fulfilled. This is pointed up graphically by Figure 2.2. Nevertheless, in their prescription for behavior, expectations or value standards are clearly a strong anti-change or negative feedback influence, whereas when they tell us of our failure to meet our values, they are a strong force for change.

Interests are determining frames for attitudes resulting from a combination of various values, environmental pressures, and beliefs which have acquired saliency for an individual, group, or organization. They may represent central or peripheral concerns, but in any case are distinguished by saliency to their holder, who has a general tendency to be attracted by anything perceived as involving those concerns. Typically, interests are directed toward concerns of survival, toward what one has learned to do or would like to do, and toward what are felt to be more desirable pleasures, causes, services, or socializing activities. Whether directly or indirectly, correctly or mistakenly, consciously or unconsciously, interests are directed to promoting or facilitating goals high on a priority list.

Beliefs concern the existence of something, whether falsely perceived or not, which stems from either hidden or explicit values or value conflicts. Beliefs may be true or false or untestable. They are not values,

FIGURE 2.2
VALUES AND CHANGE

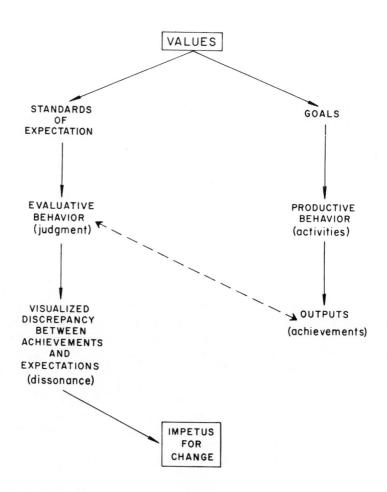

but may in turn give rise to values, and vice versa. Beliefs are not good or bad. They are existential perceptions or presumptions of what is. Beliefs usually carry a normative or value-guided base, as well as perceptual content. Knowledge of facts, as well as of errors, is combined with beliefs to make up the cognitive culture.

Ideology, religion or credo results when many beliefs fall into a pattern or stable cluster and become integrated with values. The ideology may be simple or complex, and may use clichés as symbolic rallying points (racial supremacy, freedom from exploitation for the working man, or liberty). As an ideology achieves saliency, it may become the basis of social, religious or political movements.

Institutions are organized sets of accepted and strongly supported obligatory norms or patterns of how to behave or respond. They are made up from values, knowledge, and beliefs—correct or erroneous. These institutions are the basis upon which rest the mutuality of kinship, social stratification, and the structure of society. One mainstay organized institution of our culture is education; another is religion. These institutions act through approved means or agents, such as schools or churches. Institutions and their agents are instrumentalities for attaining socially valued ends.

Culture is the total pattern of interrelationships of human behavior, organization, and their products, embodied in the activities, beliefs, knowledge, ideologies, institutions, governance, religion, education, and groups. The word is also used to describe a large society, such as the "Western World," in terms of outlooks held in common, or to describe a small isolated group that is characterized by almost total consistency of behavioral and belief attributes from person to person. The term suggests shared appreciative as well as communications systems. Perhaps a culture is most distinctively characterized by particular constellations of its inconsistencies and irrelevancies. The columnist Art Hoppe capitalizes on pointing out the inconsistencies between what we do, what we say, and what we mean in our culture.

A *society* is an enduring and cooperating social group whose members have developed organized institutions or patterns of personal and institutional relationships through interaction with one another. A community, nation or broad grouping of people having common traditions, institutions, and collective activities and interests may be called a society.

With these definitions in mind, let us return to the discussion of values. Values are the initiators of concern. Borrowing from Williams[42] it can be seen (Figure 2.2) that values take us, or more imperatively, drive us, in two directions simultaneously: (1) toward the establishment of goals for action which in turn lead us to productive behavior and activity, and thus achievements; and (2) toward the establishment of societal expectations (criteria or standards) by which to judge the suitability of the action which occurs. These expectations lead to evaluative, appreciative or judgmental behavior. It is the act of judgment or evaluation which brings together for a reckoning the achievements made on behalf of the goals and the expectations held out for them. The evaluation tells us what the values involved have led to, whether the values are being actualized in a consistent way, even whether these values are still desired in the light of their results.

Unsatisfied values or discrepancies are the potential sources of dissonance or strain which, in turn, mobilizes energies toward change. The discrepancy between achievements and expectations is, of course, also the definition of a problem, and if it is visualized or felt, the dissonance it creates provides the impetus for change.

In this view, the stream of energy that is always available to be tapped for social change as part of man's innate makeup is aroused whenever the object of his values (goals) has produced a product or achievement which falls painfully short of the expectations his values had set. The discrepancy between achievement and expectation (or of what one wants to have in reference to some other group) is the source of strain or initiation for change.[43] As a result, it is not the raw needs alone, but also the behavioral configurations (and even the symbols of what have become the accepted and desirable ways of surviving in a culture) that share with the raw needs and probably supersede them in the capacity to heat up or cool off the primal energy to create a change in an unsatisfactory situation.

Goode[44] makes a strong case for the concept that even well-accepted values are not sufficient guides for the individual's behavior, because one person may have to or want to carry out many roles. Social structures are made up of relationships which in turn are made up of role transactions, and one may have to bargain away conflicting role demands. So the role conflicts and inadequacies of response of individuals may end up altering subunits of the social structure, such as churches, schools, and unions. These never ending inter-role dissonances or strains are also forces for change,[45] and social structures are continually and inadvertently altered as a consequence. These may begin as small-scale alterations, but can quietly add up.

Awareness of discrepancies triggers dissonance and action to change. Festinger makes a firm case that the existence of dissonance makes a person uncomfortable and motivates him to try to reduce the dissonance and achieve consonance. (With dissonance present the person may, however, actively avoid situations and information which would likely increase the dissonance,[46] and thus oppose change. This is a key point for planners, and one to which we will return.) Festinger defines *cognition* as any knowledge, belief, or opinion about the environment, about oneself or about one's behavior. He describes *dissonance* as arising from non-fitting relations among cognitions, such as would arise from conflicts among values, beliefs, role conflicts, desires, attitudes, new information, or new events. He cites evidence that cognition is at work, whether exposed to public gaze or not, and that it will create a force commensurate with the intensity of the dissonance to reduce that dissonance.

Factors such as information, internal or external forces, and intellectual or technological achievements are the sources of our awareness of discrepancies between what we want and what we have, between what we want and what we might want. It is that awareness of discrepancies, whether correct or erroneous, that creates the dissonance and releases the energy (impetus) to be used to force change. It is not the stress of slow traffic per se that forces the construction of another freeway, or of a rapid transit system, a move to a dwelling nearer the job, or to a new job. It is the awareness of the dissonance between the painful reality and our values, goals, and expectations about how one should be able to travel that leads to the change. In the traffic example, dissonance as a disturbing force often seems to affect noncommuters more than commuters. Similarly, it is not the stress of hunger per se that leads to riots or revolts, for hunger more often leads to apathy. It is the awareness of the presence of hunger as being contrary to values, goals, or norms that forces bystanders more often than victims to want to correct the dissonance between reality and values.

The more elaborate the valued behavior code, the more the value system may in itself become the center for the energy for social change. Our small and great wars are fought over ideologic beliefs and concepts of general welfare, and not in terms of obtaining identifiable food, lodging, sexual or ego satisfaction as such. In this sense we disagree with Smelser's position when he asserts that impetus arises as the result of the outcome of an encounter with a specific situation, rather than as a result of the dissonance between what the particular situation represents in terms of unfulfilled standards for expectations and goals set by the value system.[47]

Why is it so important to reiterate that it is the value-based dissonance that "gets" to us? Planners have to consider deliberate social change as their goal; unless they are able to deal with the discharge and the direction of the stream of energy that will permit change, they will not know how to plan even if they can describe and design what is wanted. Only by taking into account the well-ensconced values, goals, and standards for expectations can we see who is offended by what, what alternatives the value systems offer various value holders, and what value holders might be inclined to do or to tolerate, or which modified or new values, goals, and norms they could absorb. (A compelling statement issued by Lisle C. Carter makes clear the natures of discrepancies that are at the heart of our multiple crises.[48]

Through perception of what is called for by cherished values, goals, and norms and how much dissonance exists because of them, the planners can determine where and how to proceed. Perhaps in a more Machiavellian mood, the planner also needs to know what new kinds and amounts of dissonance or anxiety might be created to move the various value holders to acceptance of new programs or of new values, goals, and expectations standards. We do remarkably and consistently well in responding in a stereotyped fashion to the word *communism*, and great numbers of us are currently learning to react somewhat predictably to the cry of *pollution*. Because our values, goals, and expectations standards dictate when, how fast, with what intensity, and in what direction we are going to desire changes, choosing the means of arousing stress and of selecting the area of impetus becomes a key area through which planners can help create social change. By directing or channeling impetus, planners can then bring about changes in structured controls and societal pressures, two of the three secondary determinants. These changes in turn become significant long-term social changes in themselves. Mobilization is also heavily influenced by the nature of the impetus as well as by structured controls and societal pressures.

Festinger points out the possibilities for the reduction of dissonance by forced compliance (change of structural controls), if carried through successfully.[49] Using desegregation as an example, dissonance is reduced when those forced to comply or desegregate see the change happening and hasten to alter their belief and value structure toward desegregation so that their thinking will not be dissonant with their enforced actions. Festinger also notes that if the structural control is successfully evaded, opinions will swing against the issue (desegregation) in order to avoid dissonance—which, in this case, would mean support for segregation and strong pro-segregation thinking.

Values are also the *guiding* mechanisms for social change. Intimately interconnected with the preceding concept of triggering energy discharge is the concept of guidance for the discharge. Malinowski starts with the position that psychobiological (he says biological) determinism holds the foundation of culture. Human psychobiological pressures or impulses encounter the environment which must yield what is psychobiologically needed. The pressures are shaped into a series of valued actions which become frozen into the behavior patterns which define a given culture.[50] For example, reproductive impulses end up with cultural responses of kinship, while those of growth become the cultural responses of training. The psychobiological imperatives are first altered by the nature of the environment and, once stereotyped, they are determined by the demands of the society in which they are occurring. From the expectations of the society are formed the cultural imperatives, such as knowledge, which society provides and supervises in the form of education, or authority, which society channels into governmental or other political organizations.

The value hierarchy represents the esteem accorded the various cultural manifestations of the psychobiological imperatives.

The Mechanisms by Which Values Initiate and Direct or Obstruct Change

Anti-change situations come to exist where valued goals passed on by tradition are apparently achieved adequately or meet the expectation standards set up for them. As a minimum, goal and standards achievement typically results in a state of no interest in change in the subject area. It can easily be imagined, however, that an area of concerns providing satisfaction for one group may not be providing much satisfaction for another. For example, in a racially discriminating, less-than-full employment environment, the dominant group may be anti-change and the minority group pro-change on the issue of job opportunity.

Festinger[51] has already been cited as describing how fear of increasing dissonance leads to an avoidance of dissonance-producing information or situation. This assumes that a sense of dissonance already exists. However, awareness coming from unexpected sources is much more likely to be "granted a hearing." Influences that reduce or seem to reduce dissonance are also more likely to be heeded. These may be "justifier" kinds of forces which are likely to be anti-change.

Pro-change situations may occur in various ways:

Awareness of the possibility of establishing more meaningful goals.

Awareness of the inadequacy of current standards of expectations.

Awareness of the failure to meet current standards of expectations in the presence of adequate resources.

Awareness that achievements have come to exceed expectations.

Awareness that achievements fall short of the standards of expectations and that the environment is probably incapable of allowing them ever to be reached.

Awareness of new knowledge or technological breakthroughs that enable entire new approaches to previously unreachable standards or to heretofore only vaguely entertained goals.[52]

Awareness of the availability of unused resources that might allow new goals, new standards, new achievements, or all three.

Awareness of the inutility or destructiveness of current goals (the irrelevance or incompatibility of current values and their goals for survival).

Growing awareness of values and goals observed at work in other cultures that somehow seem to promise new horizons or happiness.

Awareness of new hurts from whatever source, whether they be external, as from the activities of other countries, large or small, or internal, from our own uneven progress and resulting imbalances.

Awareness of the desirability of new life styles, altered family size, new goals and modes of education, altered sex prerogatives or behavior—that is, desirability of new values.

Awareness of changes in the society's status as compared to other societies (for example, that it is slipping behind or passing others on one or many valued parameters).

Awareness of expectations held out for incumbents of various roles.

An Example of Pressures for Change from the Health Care Field. If one takes the present medical care delivery system of the United States as an example, one can see how many gap factors or sources of dissonances have appeared and how these have combined to press for change. The list includes:

Awareness of the equity shortcomings of the health care delivery system, particularly when compared to that of other countries.

Awareness of the Nation's technologic capacity.

Awareness of what is possible in the way of delivery.

Awareness that quality goals traditionally espoused by medical purveyors are not relevant or good enough criteria by which to distribute care fairly, now that everyone is thought to be entitled to that good care.

Awareness that present standards of service for large portions of the population are also inadequate (the poor want more than the customary charity or the county hospitals' provision of slow, unpleasant care, and the middle classes also want improvements in availability and safety).

Awareness that delivery achievements at large county facilities and charity institutions have dropped below even the current pathetic standards, and that many urban and rural areas can hardly get any public or private services.

Awareness that customary manpower resources have "evaporated" from many urban and rural areas, although potential manpower is ample.

Awareness that new levels of health care have recently been delivered to the aged, and that health care resources could be increased so that higher levels of health care could be provided for all segments of society.

Awareness that health care costs are increasing uncontrollably, and that catastrophic level needs are still bankrupting great numbers of people each year.

Awareness that high levels of health care are being delivered in many other countries at lower costs.

Awareness that new resources in the form of new kinds of less expensively trained purveyors are very promising, and the belief that the cost of better care could be less or no greater than the cost of the present often poor care.

Beliefs, mostly erroneous, that our comparatively poor health standing internationally can be improved by better health care.

All of the above suggest many additive if not multiplying forces behind the impetus for change in health care delivery, and promise that major changes will be forthcoming until these dissonances are lessened significantly.

What then is the role of planning? The long-range, generally accepted purposes of planning are to define and introduce publicly intended social change which secures for society what its value systems call for. That is, planning is intended to make changes which *reduce dissonance*. In a change-oriented democratic society with many differing but basically related value systems and value hierarchies, planning appears to be an ideal means of democratically defining and introducing publicly desired, deliberate or intended social changes and of avoiding publicly unexpected, unwanted, or unpleasant changes.

Designing the means and strategy of attaining social change is the major expected activity of planning. Success probably requires an arousal of general awareness of current or impending discrepancies. This will create the dissonance necessary for a powerful societal impetus towards change, thus creating widespread desire for planning. Because there will be no shortage of dissonances, desire for publicly selected social change should result in a sustained demand for planning, once planning has demonstrated adequate utility as well as freedom from unwanted side effects, which often are of more consequence than the benefits produced.

DELIBERATE SOCIAL CHANGE IN MODERN SOCIETIES

In the United States, the basic value arrangements for most groups did not until recently appear to be grossly different, except for Native Americans, Chicanos, and a few small religious communities. Thus, there has been an assumption that if all were brought to a comparable awareness of areas of dissonance, the underlying group of comparable major values would steer us in the same direction. Particularly so if the key values were laid on the table in the form of criteria for selection of ends and means, and weighted in accordance with their position in the hierarchy of values.

Several further issues arise which suggest that the role of planning as visualized here, may be a lot more complicated than the model of social change suggests. It is possible that some sizable groups have so altered their value hierarchies as a result of their special vulnerabilities to certain influences, or because of their continued abuse under the present confused public planning and the dog-eat-dog mode of pursuing intended change privately—that they cannot participate in planning. The first such group that comes to mind are young people who see their world being eroded and their survival seriously threatened by continuation of the historic pursuit of—to them—meaningless affluence. Another group is the domestic Third World, which knows from bitter experiences that gestures toward equity reordering commonly result, intentionally or unintentionally, in a relative, and often an actual, worsening of their lot. At the very least, and perhaps more importantly, a greater expectation gap has been created because the hopes and standards of expectations of Third World people have been intentionally or unintentionally raised beyond any intent of fulfillment by the larger society. (See Chapter 3 for a Third World view of health.)

As a result, these groups—particularly the first—have an inverted value hierarchy and can hardly be brought to a planning or bargaining table. The "People's Park" debacle in Berkeley is an example of how two groups could no longer communicate usefully because their value hierarchies had few bases in common. The situation blew open when the University of California asked for but could not obtain representatives of the street people. None of them felt free to come, because they did not believe in representation.

This situation is probably not so aggravated among the black Third World groups, whom I believe still to be interested mostly in a fair share, rather than in a new scheme. But even if there is adequate value homogeneity among most of our population groups, might there not still be a critical disagreement over the desirability of planning? We know that our sterner conservative leaders (including many industrialists) and their adherents, regardless of their posture in the private sector, are generally opposed to planning for concerns in the public sector. Have they altered very much? Probably not. Are these conservatives about to be joined by counter culture and Third World movements? The latter two groups are aware of planning only as a tool of the private sector, and they are quite convinced that planning has been responsible for bringing us close to disaster on many fronts. Because they also see the private sector as thoroughly controlling the public one, counter culture and the Third World movements have become ambivalent if not outright opposed to planning as well as to technology. They fear that public planning controlled by private interest will once and for all, put every activity in the hands of planners whom they believe are dedicated to little more than using government as the puppet of the controlling industrial and financial interests. Our contacts with both these groups on planning issues lends credence to this supposition. There are, however, observably dissident splinter groups.

One such group would learn to plan or to do professional work so as to assist the populace by infiltrating the established planning system. Another, would learn to plan so as to do advocacy work directly with those having the least share of the society's benefits or opportunities. These two types of activists are offset by a larger group consisting of those who will not assist or participate in the larger society's doings in any fashion, and a few of these actually mean to destroy what they don't like.

Avenues of Intervention: Traditional Applications

New interventions are evident in the form of such magnificently permissive experiments as university admission of "unqualified" minorities and off-campus degrees, new sex behavior standards, new Women's Lib breakthroughs, new gains (and losses) for minorities in general opportunities for jobs, housing, services, amenities, etc., and even the predilection of troops to make decisions about whether to fight or to obey authority. Recent legislative and judicial outpourings have been reviewed for their bearing on planning.[53]

Keeping in mind the four determinants through which applications of effort for change can be directed, it is of interest to see which tools have customarily been used to induce deliberate change. Some of the tools that will be described release energy but have little sense of direction; others are highly directed but may capture little energy; some are democratic, and some are dictatorial. Chin and Benne[54] list a series of strategies for change that, like those listed below, are based on empirical observations rather than on any concepts of determinants of social change. They are widely inclusive and could serve as a good reminder of possible interventions. Other articles in the book containing the Chin and Benne essay offer other views on how to effect change.

Education

Our democratic society has been associated with a dominant belief that education per se is the most significant contribution to informed democratic participation and thus, to the survival of our democracy through change.

Political Action

Political action is another favorite American recipe for getting intended change. In the health field in the United States, political action has certainly not shown itself as a satisfactory substitute for a more result-directed way of achieving desired change. This suggests that political action needs to be partnered with planning rather than be a substitute. Deliberate planning, with citizen, consumer, and victim involvement constitutes a redistribution of power, and power to the people can become a critical force for change.[55]

Uses of Power, Authority, and Leadership

Since these means of introducing desired changes are heavily involved with political action, they share many of the same comments, even though these methods are more directed to mobilization of forces for change than to changes in structure or system pressures. Because the uses of power, authority, and leadership occupy an important place in the concept of planning, they will be taken up as a part of, rather than as a substitute for, planning in the attainment of desired change.

Technologic Achievements

In many quarters, there is remarkable faith in technology as the means of solving all the problems we face.[56] The notion that we are on an endless upward, exponential curve of technologic outpourings[57] which can only bring us good things has been a constantly reinforced belief in the Western World. An uninterrupted exponential growth curve does not match many phenomenologic observations. Even the rate of production of technology is likely to plateau. Support from J. Salk, Boulding and others adds to our conviction.[58] The probable slowing down is, in fact, the only encouraging thing about the unguided technological outpouring. We can be sure that rewards of fame and fortune are not guarantee enough that technology is a wise substitute for deliberate change. Others have seen the need for selective retardation or advance of technological developments to suit social needs, instead of undirected technology which inevitably comes to dictate social change.[59]

Environment as a Change Factor

The environment, in particular the physical environment, is perceived as a source of change in cultures. To quote Allan Blackman:

> There are many theories which assert that changing the design of the city, or the density of cities or the design of housing can produce significant changes in human behavior and social relationships. These physicalist theories of change have appeal at least in part because physical variables are generally easier to manipulate

than social variables. Also, the city planners and health professionals who favor these theories do so in part because their expertise focuses on the physical, not the social, variables. Physical design undoubtedly can have marginal influences on behavior. But its influence has often been exaggerated; and, more dangerous, concern with physical design has sometimes been a substitute for grappling with social and economic problems.[60]

Growth

Until very recently, many, if not most of us in the United States, saw growth of output, if not of population, as a happy means of solving the nation's problems and, by extension, the problems of the whole world. The notion of sharing more generously the increased products of growth with the have-not peoples and causes at home and abroad was a very attractive idea for all but the most fervent free-enterprisers. Now that the consequences of our growth to the livability of our earth have been seriously questioned, and the ethic of no-growth widely popularized, unplanned growth no longer appears to be a desirable substitute for deliberate change.

Citizen Participation and Community Organization

Many among us have leaned heavily on the belief that new and wider based kinds of citizen participation and decision making or even citizen involvement in advisory capacities would serve as a new means to spread knowledge, change attitudes, and come up with the right ways of proceeding with social change. Duhl and Volkman describe networks of participation as a strategy for change, with loyalty given to ideas, issues, or values rather than to leaders.[61]

Conflict

Sharpened and articulated conflict are advocated by some planners to bring about the needed tensions as impetus for change. Generally the vigorous proponents of conflict also have a sense of direction, as towards the right or left. Conceiving of conflict as violent, they anticipate that with enough energy flowing, there will be ample opportunity for something good to emerge under their guidance. History is not at all clear on this score. Because conflict embraces every degree of opposition—from a debate to a life-threatening encounter—it is of interest that our present value system does indeed countenance every form of conflict at some point or another. As a result, planning will no doubt also countenance the use of all degrees or types of conflict when it appears relevant to the desired ends and means.

Coercion

As a mode of producing change, coercion may embrace any extreme from criticism or ostracism to the levying of fines or even to the total loss of property, liberty, and life. At present, structural controls and systems pressures work in great part through these means. But frequently they work in a very indiscriminate way that harms many other than the targeted deviants, often even harming those who are to be protected. Coercion could be a significant part of intended planning. In our country, we prefer to think of coercion as a tool reserved for governmental use alone, but experience tells us that it is utilized in labor, minority, community, business and other group settings, even quite illegally. Coercion remains the major ultimate means available for carrying out governmentally adopted political interventions.

Incentives

The incentive mode of obtaining deliberate change is the obverse of coercion. It therefore carries strong overtones of approval to which most of us are likely to succumb if the price is not more than the intended change is worth. Of course, incentives cannot be used as a reward to the criminally inclined to desist from carrying out a threatened illegal act. Incentives can be part of structural control and a major feature of politically obtained and governmentally institutionalized interventions. Incentives are applicable to individuals, to groups and organizations, and to private and public interests.

Health as an Instrument of Social Change

Health, which is presumably valued for itself or for what it allows people to do, can also be viewed as an instrument for promoting or preventing change. Blackman says that a reasonable argument can be made that some health improvement (or death reduction) campaigns have hindered economic growth in underdeveloped countries.[62] In part, this happened because health was viewed as an end in itself, and the instrumental effects of health toward other ends were not evaluated. Whether health is seen as a means or an end is another question related to our beliefs and knowledge about causality. (There is evidence that ill health causes poverty, but also evidence that poverty causes ill health.)[63]

Various elements of the government's poverty program have begun to use health services as a means of changing people, either to eliminate blocks to learning or blocks to working ability. (Family planning services probably became more acceptable because they were seen as a means for reducing the welfare roles). If America's health resources were used primarily as a means for promoting education, increasing productivity, and eliminating poverty, health resources would probably be allocated in a considerably different way than they are at present.

Images of Man as Change Factors

Earlier in this discussion those approaches to change which focus on people were contrasted with those which focus on institutions. To quote Blackman:

> The stimulus-response image stems from behaviorist psychology and has had considerable impact on political commercial advertising. In grossly simplistic terms, this image says that people can be moved by the repetitive rewarding or punishing of simple associations. In the field of mental health, this image has been successfully used to change the behavior of mental hospital patients.

Further to quote Blackman:

> The rationalist image says that men change when made aware of facts and logic. Etzioni recently proposed a program for changing attitudes toward welfare programs based on the rationalist image. He suggested that conservative opposition to welfare programs was based at least in part on lack of knowledge about the percentage of welfare patients capable of working. (The percentage is very low.) He suggested that private foundations should promulgate this information among those specific groups opposed to welfare.[64]

Blackman further points out that the emotional image of man suggests that men are controlled by powerful drives and feelings and that they can be moved by appeal to these motivating forces. The use of sex in advertising and of scare campaigns in health, both reflect belief in the emotional image of man.

Planning as the Social Change Agent of Choice

Planning as we envision it is our preferred means of achieving deliberate change. Planning may take many alternative approaches. It can devote itself to overcoming current or imminent problems. It may simply sit back and take advantage of a future whenever it finds a forecast of a rosy one. It may take the leadership in preparing society to be ready to cope with a forecast of a dire future. It may direct its efforts to reaching a future in accordance with what is currently desired, with what it is believed will be desired, or go so far as to assist in the reordering of values required to make a new future. To do any, and probably all, of these functions, planning is being asked to be the designer, engineer, and measurer of social change. It should no doubt try to achieve goals with the least expenditure of resources, and will according-

ly try to shift any or all of the four determinants of social change—
impetus, structures, systems pressures, and mobilization—to produce desired improvements as painlessly as possible.

Concepts of "Democratic" and "Deliberate" as Applied to Planning

The complexities of the pluralism of changing value hierarchies in
our value scheme call for a democratic way of introducing satisfying
social change. Of course, democratic procedures may not make the
process particularly easy.

Let us examine the concept of *democratic* as I shall use it: decisions
are subject to reasonably broad-based participation under due process
of law, whether done by current modes of representation, plebiscite, or
methods utilizing an in-between level of participation. The term is
used in contrast to the decision making done by: an elite, an oligar-
chy, an autocracy, or a totalitarian ruler; by internally or externally
based coercive forces; or by deception of whatever origin. The concept
speaks to a breadth of legitimacy in decision making that leaves few of
the citizens with a sense of imposition or frustration because their
views or positions have not received recognition or consideration. It
does not imply consensus, nor does it imply ruthless imposition of the
will of the majority on the minority, for the concept also carries a sense
of justice, fairness, or equity for all individuals which must be part of
the decision.

Deliberate changes are those which, having been defined and
wanted, have been knowingly engineered and are not accidental or
casually promulgated activities.

Planning for the Public Good and Public Planning

We now come to a question raised by Ozbekhan:[65] For whom will
the deliberate planning output be an improvement? First, let us exclude public planning so rigged as to be carried out for the benefits of a
few. Genuine public planning creates benefits for many, with minimal
or no pain to those who do not immediately benefit. By contrast, traditionally acceptable private planning leaves it up to the public sector to
provide measures to counter the consequences of pollution, damages
from delayed medical care, and so on. However, public planning to
date is not always significantly better than private planning. It too
puts out pollutants and poor medical care which hurt individuals and
whole segments of the public in a manner usually attributed only to
private planners. Moreover, the logic of governmentally sponsored
plans for private gains is well accepted in the public sphere.

Private planning needs to take into account only the planner's own gains and any evident legal restrictions. Public planning should take into account all the aspects of the system involved and all persons or groups affected by the proposed changes. Public planning has two types of outcomes to consider: (1) the effects on individuals or small groups, and (2) the effects on society as a whole or on the social system itself. Thus there are two conceptual levels against which each major recommendation coming out of the public planning process must be measured—one is concerned with the individual and the other with the community or society of individuals.

At the first level we ask: How does this recommendation affect man as an individual? How does it affect different men, each with his own idiosyncrasies and interests? Is the recommended option inimical to any significant numbers of people? If so, would implementation result in a superficial short-run harm for individuals in one group which will be more than offset by the ultimate advantages to those individuals and to others? By contrast, is the recommended course life-depriving to some in giving a minor advantage to many (for example, lower cost of coal as a result of unsafe mining practices)? Since it is for man that planning is done, the short- and long-run advantages and disadvantages for various individuals will be the key criteria for the validity of plans at this level. Such planning strives for equitability. (Equitability does not mean returns proportionate to holdings; rather, it means a fair distribution of opportunities for all to be healthy, to get health services, or to participate in decision making and changing the status quo.)

The second conceptual level for confrontation, of equal concern, is concerned with the probable outcome of planning to men in the aggregate—the communities, major subsystems or societies which might be affected. This is important because what is seen as valuable to each man in a society may be destructive to his society, and thus eventually to him. The allocation of resources necessary to achieve high levels of health services may diminish the ability of an economy to create the educational, industrial, or agricultural bases from which to move to new levels of productivity necessary to increase nutrition, education or further health services. Even the most affluent country may decide to harvest its easily available resources in order to give each consumer an immediate satisfaction. But this action may be at the price, after one or two generations, of depriving a whole society of what might then be of greater value in a more crowded world. Examples of such short-sighted goal setting are the fast and careless destruction of fossil fuel deposits, which make up a large share of the actual wherewithal to run the economy, or the destruction of the redwoods which might be a significant source of future esthetic enjoyment.

The possible viewpoints of people not yet alive about a world we cannot yet visualize are hard to conceive, except as each of us imagines himself transported to some future time. Would we then care if the forests were denuded, the temperature raised by a blanket of carbon dioxide, the oceans polluted, or the crops poisoned by chemical residues? The effects on man and society, each as a yardstick against which to measure our public plans over time, should be of help in balancing these perspectives. Some plans will be found wanting on one score, some on the other. Plans that measure up on both scores are the ones to choose.

Public planning, which we shall call planning, is only now coming into consideration as a tool by which we can create futures for ourselves and posterity. It is becoming harder all the time to ignore the mounting evidence that we foul our nest and despoil our world as we go about day-to-day living. Of course, a reverse situation can also be postulated in which, because of an exaggerated spirit of devotion to the future society (or, as recorded in history, to life in the hereafter), living in the present is held to the meanest level of survival.

Repeated reference has been made to the unfailing capacity and drive of men to create systems of values and to strive for attainment of a social order which satisfies them. Man's behavior is purposefully goal-seeking, and he means to achieve power or control over his environment so that his desires can be fulfilled. The larger, modern, change-oriented society is made up of men with many kinds of value sets and correspondingly many sets of goals, and no man lives in an environment free of the effects of other men. Thus, the only hope for goal attainment is perceived to be a cooperative society which leaves as much leeway as possible to strive for goals within a mutually acceptable larger framework. This umbrella of major goals assures achievement to a reasonable level of those goals which are held most in common, and at the same time it allows the greatest leeway for a galaxy of divergent ones.

The slow moving, pluralistically operative, unaided political resolution of differences and advancement of commonalities is now seen as inadequate to carry us forward under the impact of fast moving, disjointed, technological changes which drastically and unevenly alter perceptions of time, distance, place, culture, and desirable goals. Planning is now seen as the device most likely to provide the insight to political decision making that will optimize the achievement of common goals while minimizing the infringement on pursuit of personal goals within the general framework.

At least in the Western nations, planning done by one man for himself is quite a different affair than planning for a society. For himself, a man has to acquire the means, the power, or the degree of control over his environment commensurate with the ends he chooses. Generally, as he approaches each new end, he has enlarged his means and perceives new ends which call for a further enlargement of means. If a society pursues this same path, many large groups of individuals may be forgotten, because the situation is not comparable to an individual who overlooks certain personal ends to achieve his most salient goals. In the non-planning societal situation, individuals and even large groups of individuals, have been overlooked totally so that little in their life is satisfying (in the U.S.A., Appalachia and many ghettos), while the nation pursues a rising GNP and glaring consumption. The larger society cannot act as an individual does and regard these failures as though they were some minor personal objectives being neglected in the thrill of achieving more valued ends.

Can planning help us look after the broader spectrum of interests of all the people who make up our society? This is the intent of Public Law 89-749 for comprehensive health planning in the U.S.A. That law provides that the consumer is to have a 51% direct voice in the planning decisions. Planning for good social ends must encompass the notion of sufficient sagacity, power, control, and resources to alter the future accordingly. It must also encompass planning for means.

It also follows that purposive goal seeking (planning) is a highly desired human end, even though we technically describe it as a means. The process is so much a part of the product we desire (control over our destiny) that it is no surprise that the most aggressively change-oriented societies accept planning as a necessary and wise private activity. But they are often propagandized to wish to restrict use of planning to the private sector, for in the public sector it could well be used in the common good and thereby be a serious threat to the immediate or short-run goals of the most enterprising (planning prone) individuals. Kahn provides an extensive review of the American antipathy to public planning, especially the longer range versions.[66]

MULTIPLE PURPOSES OF PLANNING

There are many different ideas about what the purposes of planning are or ought to be. Few statements of planning purpose are comprehensive. Some are more concerned with the "oughts" of the process itself, but most direct attention to one or several aspects of social change. Some single out the *who, why, what, how, when,* or *where* of goals or goal changes. Others single out one of the same six specifiers in relation to means, and others use the six specifiers in terms of implementation. What is worse, some definitions look at only one level of concern—for example, operational planning.

Blackman has done us a great service in assembling published purposes and definitions of planning so that their varying thrusts can readily be compared.[67] Few statements speak to a single major purpose; some combine half a dozen or more. This confusion of purposes does little to facilitate conversations among planning practitioners, but some lucid insights about this complicated situation are available from Davidoff and Reiner,[68] and Dyckman.[69] What are the purposes of planning to which we should subscribe? Myrdal provides one of the more comprehensive definitions of planning:

> A determined effort through our democratic institutions for collective decisions to make very much more intensive, comprehensive and long-range forecasts of future trends than have been customary, and thereafter to formulate and execute a system of coordinated policies formed to have the effects of bending the foreseen trends toward realizing our ideals, spelled out in advance as definite goals for planning.[70]

Another useful definition is given by Friedman,[71] who also describes and contrasts the nature, consequences, and uses of developmental, adaptive, allocative, and innovative models of planning. In essence, for him, planning is "guidance of change within a social system." As a self-guidance system, planning:

Confronts the expected with intended performance.

Sets up controls to accomplish the intended.

Observes variances from intended path of changes.

Initiates a new cycle to cope with significant variations from the intended.

Petersen,[72] speaking of other purposes of planning, describes other models as deductive, utopian, and inductive. Davidoff[73] describes what he calls "advocacy planning." Ackoff emphasizes the purposes of planning as "anticipatory decision-making required when what we desire involves a system of decisions."[74] This is called for when decisions:

Are too large to handle at once.

Cannot be subdivided into independent subsets.

Produce one or more future states which are desired but not expected to occur unless something is done.

Tinbergen has a similar formulation of circumstances when planning is desirable.[75]

This suggests that the demands for planning are dependent on the complexities of the problem to be handled. I tend to agree and do not hesitate to advocate a laissez faire or marketplace approach for lesser transactions, even though the marketplace itself may have to be designed or rigged by means of planned interventions. One also hears a lot about the degree of satisfaction that should be achieved from planning. If it is *satisficing*, or attainment of a reasonable level of satisfaction of selected criteria much less planning may be involved than with *optimizing*, where the attempt is made to obtain the most of the best balanced mixture of what the goals or selected criteria call for.

Another contrasting pair of planning purposes is the willingness to plan for *coping* with, or adapting to, what is to come, versus planning to *make* the future come out as desired.

Gunnar Myrdal[76] provides another set of considerations about operating the system that involves the issue of optimizing but really centers around the need for speed in attaining change. He makes the demand for "bigger" and "more rapid" changes by means of resolutely altering institutions within which people live and work, instead of by designing interventions directed to induce changes in attitudes, and hoping that in time they will bring appropriate alteration to institutions. Comparisons of alternative interventions should take into account speed of results, and discounting has been created to do just that.

A totally different way of describing planning is offered by Navarro:[77] "The purpose of planning is to rationalize the activities on which planning is imposed, to make subject to calculation what was previously left to chance, and to replace spontaneous adjustment by deliberate control." This places emphasis on the intent to rationalize more than on the nature of outcomes. Galbraith[78] points out that the marketplace and its prices have to give way as decision makers to the practices of planning in the industrial era because of the long lead times required for development, production, costly machinery, and extensive public preparation for the product.

It is of interest to present some of the diversity of purposes which have been prescribed for planning. They might be fitted under several rubrics as is attempted here.

Planning as an aid or replacement to political decision-making:
> A substitute for political decision making.
> A method for reaching decisions.
> Devising and enlarging the selection of choices among goals.
> Devising and enlarging the selection of choices among solutions.
> Improving the wisdom of allocations.
> Defining, achieving, and evaluating improvements (goals) and/or standards for their achievement.
> A means of making clear the extent and operant times of many kinds of costs and benefits in order to enable more efficient, economical and rational choices among both goals and means.
> A means of improving rationality in decisions or making choices.

Planning as a means of anticipating or looking ahead:
> Ability to anticipate and therefore cope with the future.
> Anticipatory decision making when what is desired involves a change in a complex system.

Ability to forecast so as to exploit the future.

Ability to forecast so as to make the future come out as desired.

Planning as a means of improving social justice:

A substitute for "the market" as decision-maker.

A means of improving social welfare in contrast to private gains.

A means of democratizing decisions about goals and means.

Translation of preference into action.

Organizing for action, whether goals or means are available or not.

Design of a pattern for behaving.

Planning as a means of improving the logic, science, or intellectual caliber of efforts applied to our problems:

A means of improving the quality of action.

Solving problems.

The application of logic, science, or intelligence to making decisions.

To replace chance.

Planning as the design efforts and machinery used to turn ideas into blueprints for action:

Translation of policy into operation, creation of a course of action, or a blueprint for action.

Translation of policy into operation.

Designing the means that will carry out any particular intervention.

Planning as the gentle, persuasive route to getting good, democratic, equitable decisions made:

Coordination and cooperation.

A means of preplanning anything, provided the issues of implementation are not approached.

Planning as a means of control:

Planned designs will limit choice of individual, group, or organization actions to activities selected by planners.

Planned designs will limit wasteful competition or explorations which do not show evidence of being directed at desired ends.

Planned designs will guide, in the sense of constrain, decision makers.

Mary Arnold tries to find a few common threads among this welter of planning purposes.

For some of us, planning means the specification of a plan of action; for others, it means determination of the most efficient allocation of resources; for still others it involves the means by which we determine the kind of a future we would like to have. At times, when we use the term planning, we are talking about managerial planning within a circumscribed system such as an agency; at other times we are concerned with planning for an open system such as a state or nation. There is one commonality to all these approaches to planning—the application of scientific reasoning to problem-solving.[79]

Selecting a Set of General Purposes for Planning as a Basis for Designing a Methodology of Planning

Having begun this book with the proposition that the single major purpose of planning is the introduction of desired social changes in desired ways, I have reacted eclectically, sensing good in many formulations of purposes for planning. I find it necessary, however, to subscribe to one particular set of purposes, for it is from these that I will design a planning scheme to carry the purposes of planning that were selected.

Let us set up a hierarchy of ideas about planning that can lead us to a planning model from which the individual steps of the process can be fashioned. This concept of planning is asked to democratically introduce desired social change, and specifies the three major purposes of planning as follows: (1) defining desired improvements; (2) achieving desired improvements; (3) measuring the attainment of the desired improvements.

Defining desired improvements.   Facets of this purpose include:
Definition of general and health aims (goals).
Analysis of goals to understand their origins and the means of attaining them.
Definition of current problems (inadequately achieved goals), including a clarification of why and by whom they are perceived as problems.
Analysis of problems to understand their origins and the means of interrupting or overcoming them.
Improving the relevance of proposed objectives to values (what we claim to desire as opposed to what we claim is desirable).
Offering and improving the definition, design or texture of a "better" future or of specific objectives (setting new goals), clarifying, altering or creating new values and goals.
Part III of this book, Chapters 5, 6, 7, and 8, is devoted to how this aspect of planning is carried out. Planning effort devoted to this aspect

of intended change (making the system work better) is often called normative. Because the open system we live in will increasingly change, so will the galaxy of improvements desired, but in order to plan they must be prioritized and operationalized periodically.

Achieving desired improvements. Facets of this purpose include:
Designing necessary plans to carry out what has been selected as necessary improvements.

Designing implementation and follow through to assure implementation.

Guiding social change. This involves introduction of a suitable breadth of public comprehension and participation.

Expanding of individual and institutional operational capacities (expanding democratization of public policy formation by wider participation, by wider choice among alternative plan options, and by offering a diversity of life style opportunities).

Planning efforts devoted to this aspect of intended change are often seen as a mixture of several distinguishable activities. The first, which may be called *creative planning*, makes tangible the first purpose or definition of desired improvements in that it creates or provides the design for proceeding, that is, a plan. In no way is it implied that this plan is for all time, but it does specify what needs to be done today and tomorrow while adhering to the goals that gave birth to this plan. It represents the statement or packaging in proposal form how desired ends can be achieved by acceptable means (developed in Chapter 8).

The second activity, which may be called *organizational planning*, speaks to how the planning body must comport itself to get the planning done. This is developed in Chapters 9 and 10, which, devoted as they are to the roles, activities, and organization of planning bodies, also carry the beginnings of the strategy for adoption of planning output. Such strategy is required because of the need for planning bodies to be properly situated in the larger society.

The third activity is *strategic planning*, or how to get the products of the planning body politically accepted as an integral part of the general societal machinery (Chapter 11).

The planning activity which secures the improvement might be called *operational* (administrative, program) *planning*. It operationalizes the machinery designed by the planners so that the assignments are correctly made; suitable tools, resources, and manpower are organizationally engaged, so that the encounter with the consumer takes place in a way that is conducive for the service to be appropriately consumed and for the desired results to come to pass. This is also elaborated upon in Chapter 11, in so far as this phase is carried out by the community planning body. (Most of this activity falls into the domain of operating agencies.)

Measuring attainment of the desired improvements. Aspects of this purpose include:

Incorporation of feedback in plan design and implementation.

Evaluation and general reassessment of health status concentrating on results of planned for activities.

Evaluation of the quality of planning undertaken to date, which is critical to further improving the planning capacity and quality.

Evaluation of the quality of cause and effect information available and extension of new knowledge to improve future analysis and design.

This aspect of planning is usually called *evaluation* and sometimes research. It is elaborated upon in Chapter 12.

If there were to be a fourth purpose in our scheme of things it would probably be to arouse adequate impetus—to make planned-for-change desired.

Specific Purposes Assigned to any Given Planning Agency

Not to be confused with the general thrust, or with the three general purposes of planning, are the more specific purposes which any given planning body is called upon to serve. These include abiding by nationally important goals, and carrying out the assignment for which the planning body is legislated or chartered, or which in its freedom it "selects" for itself. In any given society a variety of fairly specific purposes will be expressed as a national sense of direction—for example, medical care for everyone, or full employment. Where there is enabling or enforcing legislation to implement those aims, every public planning body would presumably attempt to promote them.

A fairly detailed set of specific purposes accrues to most planning bodies when they are established, whether by the enabling legislation or by the terms of their own incorporation papers. These purposes may be as specific as planning suitable new facilities, coordinating existing services, or planning comprehensive financing of health care services. The specific purposes which are often used to justify the creation of a given planning body may be nothing more than widely felt (although often erroneous) statements of problems or possible solutions which the community wishes the planning body to investigate. Sometimes they are expressions of desire for heartfelt long term goals.

In the course of time, the planning body continues to add specific purposes which become relevant to the community. New understanding, both of the societally important general goals and of the community, may lead to dropping or modifying many of the planning body's specific purposes.

Assignment of specific purposes does not in any way erode the general purposes which conceptually define what planning bodies are for. In fact, the general purposes help keep the planning body "honest" and focused on the things a planning body can and must do if it is to be more than a program designer.

MODES OR METHODOLOGIES OF PLANNING

There are innumerable ways to affect the four determinants of change—impetus, mobilization, structural controls, and societally promoted self-regulation. Planning to produce social change offers hopes for a reasonable and peaceful means of defining, securing agreement on, and introducing change. It may operate by affecting any or all of the four determinants. Because there are so many styles or modes of planning, each typically focusing on one particular aspect of planning, many with quite misleading names, I introduce names of my own invention to describe specific kinds of planning. Selected are eight rather important options which vary from one another in many ways. They are presented in Figures 2.3 and 2.4. The eclectic "developmental" model which will emerge utilizes one or another part of six of these modes.

Prototypic Modes of Planning

Although described in Figures 2.3 and 2.4 by means of a matrix utilizing fairly specific rubrics, we can briefly contrast the eight modes in terms of their approach to, and their anticipated effects on, democratically achieving deliberate social change.

Laissez Faire

Blackman characterizes the nature of this mode well.

> The laissez-faire model is very difficult to do justice to in a chart because its popular version is so different from its intellectual version. The term is popularly used as an ideological weapon in defense of private profits reaped through an economic system that in no way meets the requirements of the intellectual model. In contrast the intellectual model, in the hands of social scientists, continues to be a very refined tool for making economic and political decisions. For example, it is from this approach that proposals have come for a "negative income tax." The core of this approach, of course, is the perfectly competitive market, which is supposed to provide the consumer with a number of alternatives from which to choose and to encourage greater efficiency and consumer orientation on the part of the suppliers. Even if it is not possible to establish a "perfectly competitive market," making markets more competitive may still help the consumer and stimulate suppliers

in the direction the model suggests. Christopher Jencks has illustrated how this might work in the field of education. [80] He suggests that the behemoth of American education could be moved by government grants to parents which would allow them to send their children to private schools. The grants, he suggests, would encourage the development of a variety of types of schools competing both in philosophies of education and in pedagogic competence.[81]

The values which underlie the laissez faire model (individual freedom to choose among real alternatives, individual liberty, individual initiative, and competition as a motivating mechanism) are still approved by many persons of either liberal or conservative orientations. Not infrequently, the desire to change people or to reform or control them conflicts with freedom of choice. Thus, some of those who favor tight regulation of the lives of welfare recipients are also proponents of the free market ideology.[82] Moreover, perhaps more than 99% of all interactions and exchanges can go on most happily and inexpensively under a relatively uncontrolled approach, provided that some forces are applied to the "free market" system which compel it to act overall in specific desired ways.

As an exclusive mode, laissez-faire offers little choice of futures to other than a handful of hereditary leaders, industrialists, merchant princes, and a diverse collection of celebrities; nevertheless, it still has a major role. Its utility can best be seen by observing those societies where absolutely nothing is supposed to be left to the market place. This leads us to scrutinize the total planning approach, which on occasion has seemed to offer great possibilities. In this situation, the government does the planning and requisitions and distributes the total output (allowing, of course, little consumer choice). But the most highly programmed of all the economies, that of the USSR, has had serious problems shifting from the production of heavy industrial goods with one customer (the government), to the production of consumer goods for many customers. Consumers are not devoid of personal preferences, and the total planners have found that many of their technically planned consumer goods can be disposed of only with the greatest difficulty. Unless total planning succeeds in turning the people into automatons, in the long run, it cannot meet the needs for the production and distribution of consumer goods and services.

One concludes that the market place could well serve the myriad of transactions that hardly seem plannable. Just to feed the people of New York City on a planned basis would put an unbelievable burden on planners (and, apparently, on the city as well, if its planning capacity is to be judged by its current ability to perform other functions, even those as simple as removing the garbage). What is needed is normative direction and suitable interventions impinging on the market

Figure 2.3. COMPARISON OF PLANNING MODES, I (modified from Ritva Kaje)

	Laissez Faire	Disjointed Incrementalism, Problem Amelioration	Allocative	Articulated & Guided Incrementalism, Problem Solving
Planning Outlook	No planning	Minimal planning	Minimal planning for the present or near future	Planning for the present or near future
	Leave market unfettered and eliminate need for governmentally sponsored programs	Apply obvious remedies to undesirable situations as they become intolerable	Balance allocation of resources to avoid new problems or ameliorate current ones. Improve marginal utility in the more sophisticated forms	Analyze problems as systems with subsystems and environment, design interventions, select them for effectivity as well as compatibility with larger sectoral goals, allocate resources accordingly
Present or Short-range Results	Problems will disappear	Ameliorate present problems	Alter priorities and present problems	Ameliorate present problems and future ones
Future or Long-range Results	The future will be	Haphazardly modify the future by introducing new problems as well as by reducing the future burden and sequelae of present problems	Gently balance and modify the future by avoiding obvious problems and achieving a "balanced" progress, avoiding major bottlenecks and new problems	Improve the future by eliminating problems and by reducing the future burden and sequelae from present problems
Source of Stimulus	Survival of the fittest tempered by charity	Pain and power oriented, take care of political crises	Input oriented as well as satisfying	Pain oriented, take care of social crises
Concern for Future	Nature will take its course	Only in terms of assuaging battles over given problem	Unstated, but do not want to give rise to new problems while controlling old ones	In terms of being free of given problem and of assisting to or not obstructing long-range goals

Future Time Horizon	Continuous	Very small time steps, but often under implicit normative long-range guidance	Equivalent to many small steps of undetermined time range, mostly short, continued updating	Small time steps intentionally under normative long-range guidance, continued updating
Choice of System Boundaries	Total	Concern for one system for short political peace; ignore related systems and environment	Systems respect but limited comprehension only to point of conserving resources	Systems comprehension to point of understanding causes and consequences and possible solutions of selected problems; no concern for consequences of other problems
Scope of Concern for Change	None	Secondary, limited, and relatively small changes	Takes systems and institutions that support it for granted	Considers larger systems (the environment of the problem)
Direction of Intervention	Not relevant	Alters system or its environment only inadvertently	Leave system and environment alone and optimize resources	Modifies larger systems and environment enough to control problem
Nature of Participation	None and total	Involve those vested enough to show up	Involve the groups in power	Involve groups relevant to each issue
Scope of Direct Effects	None and total	Move a few individuals, groups, or institutions as much as required	Nudge most people and institutions	Move a few individuals, groups or institutions vigorously
Concern for Side Effects	None	Little	Avoid major side effects on resources	Try to avoid undesired side effects as part of planning
Kinds of Side Effects	None	Complicated, tricky, far-reaching, not foreseen	Few major, most could be foreseen	Complicated, tricky, far-reaching, could often be foreseen
Time to Obtain Desired Effects	Not relevant	Fast	Generally fast	Moderately prompt
Cost of Obtaining Desired Effects	Not relevant	Modest	Low	Modest

Figure 2.4. COMPARISON OF PLANNING MODES, II (modified from Ritva Kaje)

	Exploitive	Explorative	Normative	Total Planning
	Planning the future	Planning towards the future	Planning from the future	Planning for all activities present and future
Planning Outlook	Foresee and make the most of trends and allocate resources so as to take advantage of what is to come	Explore the possible futures from current trends, capacities, expectations and design a desired,* feasible future; allocate resources accordingly	Decide on the future desired** and allocate resources so that trends are changed or created accordingly	Decide on the future desired and the specific goals; lay out use of all resources accordingly
Present or Short-range Results	A sense of triumphing over fate; take advantage of what is coming	A sense of choosing the best feasible destiny. Seek what could be	A sense of helping create destiny; seek what could be	A sense of controlling all destinies
Future or Long-range Results	Unbalance and modify the future by taking advantage of predicted happenings, avoiding some problems and cashing in on others without major concern for emergence of new problems	Extensively modify the future by aiming for what could be, change present outlook, predict changing goals, expectations, and particularly means	Extensively modify the future by aiming for what ought to be, change present outlook by changing values or goals, match outcomes to desires, avoid or change problems to ones easier to handle or tolerate	Extensively modify the future by aiming for what the policy makers or planners have decreed will be
Source of Stimulus	Profit oriented (suboptimizing)	Output oriented (adaptive)	Output oriented (innovative)	Output oriented (directive)
Concern for Future	Accepted as forecasted, except for a few areas to be exploited	Sought-after future in terms of forecasted capacities	Sought-after future in terms of certain major aspirations	Accepted as planned for
Future Time Horizon	All ranges including long-range continued updating	All ranges including long-	All ranges, particularly	All ranges, particularly

	Multi-systems recogni-tion and awareness	Multi-systems recogni-... good definition of system to be altered and its relationships to its environment	good definition of system to be altered and its relationships to its environment	often with more awareness for totality of plan than for system or its environment

Choice of System Boundaries	...tion and awareness	*good definition of system to be altered and its relationships to its environment*	good definition of system to be altered and its relationships to its environment	often with more awareness for totality of plan than for system or its environment
Scope of Concern for Change	Accepts system structure and manipulates system parts	Evaluates and remodels the system structures	Evaluates and remodels the system structures	Total reorganization, accepts planned system and forces actions to fit
Direction of Intervention	Modify the system or its environment to get what is wanted from separate parts or aspects of system	Change the systems or environment as consistent with goals; improve old system or fashion a new one	Change the systems or environment as consistent with goals; improve old system or fashion a new one	Force actions to fit the proposed system; may resist change or improvement of system once defined
Nature of Participation	Involve groups in power plus others specifically involved	Needs to involve all relevant systems participants to be successful	Needs to involve all relevant systems participants to be successful	Planners and technologists are (or are allied with) a numerically small group with the power
Scope of Direct Effects	Move whatever needed	Move whatever agreed to and needed, generally widespread involvement	Move whatever agreed to and needed, generally widespread involvement	Move whatever agreed to and needed, generally widespread involvement
Concern for Side Effects	Not fussy about side effects	Try to control side effects as part of plan	Try to control side effects as part of plan	Try to control side effects as part of plan
Kinds of Side Effects	Complicated, tricky, far-reaching, seldom completely expected	Complicated, tricky, far-reaching, seldom completely expected	Complicated, tricky, far-reaching, seldom completely expected.	Complicated, tricky, far-reaching; seldom completely expected
Time to Obtain Desired Effects	Generally slow	Generally very slow	Generally very slow	Moderately prompt
Cost of Obtaining Desired Effects	Low	Usually high	Usually high	Usually very high

*Usually done on a basis of current or predicted values

**Can be done on a basis of: (1) present values; (2) predicted values; (3) creating new values place, so that within certain large stipulations of, for example, safety, utility, and ecologic concerns, the market place may then provide the simplest and probably cheapest means of serving the great bulk of all consumer transactions. In health care, where competition is imperfect or nonexistent and where consumer competence is particularly low, there will have to be more planned constraints at work on the so-called market place than are needed in the simpler consumer goods market.

Disjointed Incrementalism

Defenders of the existing model of deliberate social change in the United States—well-named disjointed incrementalism—base their defense not on satisfaction with existing social conditions, but rather on the belief that the system has in general performed well, that it has shown itself capable of continual improvement, that it will continue to improve without major structural changes, and that the available alternative models are considerably inferior. The leading intellectual analyst of disjointed incrementalism is Charles E. Lindblom.[83] Lindblom argues that decision makers in a democracy like the United States use a pragmatic approach which involves making relatively small improvements, based on a comparison of a limited number of concrete program alternatives. By taking only small steps, decision makers have the opportunity to evaluate program results and test political acceptance with little more effort than it takes to cup the hand to the ear.

Comprehensiveness is provided by having a variety of government agencies at many levels. Thus, even though each agency does not have a comprehensive view, the total effect is that most problems are dealt with. Goal decisions are resolved in the pluralistic competition among private interests and the pressure they put on public decision-makers. Lindblom further argues that all the more deliberative alternative decision-making approaches call for an extreme and unavailable amount of rationality in order to design and choose among alternatives. He rightfully sees the world as an open system in which there is no end to the consequences, and he believes that men cannot compute the total good and bad effects of alternative acts because they are committed to many values which are not ordered or ranked in a way that makes computation possible.

The major arguments for the disjointed approach are:

Man's limited problem-solving capabilities.

The lack of comprehensive information.

The unlimited nature of alternatives.

The costliness of comprehensive analysis.

Inability to construct a satisfactory method for evaluating values or goals.

The openness of the systems of variables that usually have to be contended with.

Inability to evaluate intelligently the consequences of interventions.

The utility of small steps, the repercussions of which guide us.

The multiple bases from which separate small decisions are in fact made, and the inability of each base to look at more than a small area or fragment of an issue.

The multiplicity of decision-making bases provide reasonable coverage.

Much of Lindblom's criticism is sound if directed toward the strictly rational approaches used by some total planning models. But, the fact that decision makers cannot be completely rational does not mean that they cannot be more rational; the fact that they cannot consider all alternatives does not mean that they cannot consider a number of the more probable or more attractive alternatives; the fact that they cannot see perfectly into the future does not mean that they cannot try, however imperfectly, to explore the future. Etzioni points out that empirical evidence indicates that, contrary to Lindblom, decision makers have demonstrated the ability to make major long-run commitments and to lead communities rather than just respond to pressure groups.[84]

The Allocative Mode

This approach to planning depends heavily on looking ever so slightly toward the future from the narrow basis of the resources that the past has delivered for allocation. It concerns itself with the present pressures and how the immediate future can be shaped more favorably by means of balancing allocations for the coming year. It seeks to ride out many problems that can be made to diminish and avoid or overcome bottlenecks such as those that might be created by an unbalanced thrust (for example, solving the physician shortage). The allocative approach is not innovative. It depends heavily on our ability to use primarily equilibrium-maintaining type criteria as a basis for determining priorities for the distribution of skills, manpower, dollars, and other scarce resources among the various facets of our society's needs. It seeks technological and structural solutions. By careful budgetary balancing, it would prevent the inadvertent starvation of one or another sector, which now happens under our piecemeal, unplanned allocation of resources.

In some quarters the allocative approach is a much more sophisticated and somewhat future-oriented approach in that the outcomes of all expenditures or interventions are analyzed, so that marginal changes for each item or expenditure provide the same degree of gain or benefit.[85] This implies a perfectly optimal short-run strategy which, of course, is neither optimal for very long nor is likely to be considered seriously, because it fails to provide a sense of direction.

The allocative approach pays little attention to the origins or consequences of problems, to the systems in which they occur, or even to long-range goals, other than in avoiding obvious conflicts with accepted national aims. It does not mean to introduce significant or unbalanced changes, and depends for guidance on extrapolation from the past. It may use goal rhetoric in an attempt to avoid scrutiny of what it is and is not doing, but it is built around the relatively lame logic that if there is little innovation, little damage can occur.[86]

Articulated and Guided Incrementalism

The challenge of solving current or forecasted problems remains very attractive to anyone who feels that planners in our society have yet to prove their worth. To avoid the several gross defects of disjointed incrementalism, it becomes readily apparent that major differences must be introduced.

Articulation is the first difference, and speaks to the need for enough understanding of the system in which the problem is imbedded (its environment and its own subsystems) so that possible points of attack as well as all the major parties at interest are revealed. In addition to the study of the multiple options of problem control, this method also requires study of the gains and losses consequent upon each major kind of potential solution. This minimizes the unexpected and unfortunate side effects which disjointed incrementalism almost inevitably introduces.

Guidance is the second and further requirement if incrementalism is to give assurance that a solution set in motion is not in itself likely to violate higher goals, nor move away from or obstruct attainment of long-range goals. There must be enough recognition of high level goals (normative planning) so that problem solving will help us move in the direction called for by the higher goals, not away from them. In this way, long-term goals guide the planners through problem solving so that long-term major incompatibilities are not set up.

Because my planning outlook will suggest the need for guidance from the anticipated future, it must be pointed out that problem solving or incrementalism is heavily directed from the past. It tends to ameliorate in the near future painful problems now in existence. Its limitations are great. By itself, even if majestically successful, it might in a few years free us of the present problems but leave us in what could by then have become a very undesirable general state of affairs.

However, it does offer a good place to begin, to practice with the planning tools while also providing relief to those who hurt most now. In the United States, given the grudging status accorded public purpose planning, if we do not succeed in achieving some sensible solutions to current problems and rectifying some painful inadequacies, we will not be allowed to plan much of anything else. Moreover, we need the horizon-expanding practice of modern day articulated and guided problem solving, which is a far cry from the "muddling through" that has so far been typical of program planning and disjointed incrementalism, or problem solving in the health field.

The Exploitive Mode

Exploitive planning is very effective and extensively used by many large private enterprises. In the past, for example, industries have not been asked to watch out for the negative social or ecologic spillovers that have resulted from their successful and privately profitable, natural-resource-gobbling, technological or organizational breakthroughs. The exploitive approach tends to look at the future very closely, explicitly, and diversely, with the intent of cashing in on emerging wants, possibilities, or opportunities. If we can predict a parade, let us have it in our city so we can have the balloon and popcorn concession on the best corners. If big industry does this so spectacularly, why not the bigger society? A grave deficiency of this planning outlook is that we do not really ask ourselves if we like the prophesied parade. We ask only about the probability that it will occur, and if this probability is high, we will arrange our affairs to take advantage of the prophesied event. In fact, once we make up our minds to invest in this probability, we begin to implore our legislators to make sure that the parade comes off, even if everyone agrees that it is the worst possible thing that could take place.

Exploitation may be quite alert to system implications, or it may not. It generally is most cognizant of trends and prophesied changes. It is opportunistic, looking for free rides, even if it has to promote them. Its prevailing, but not inevitable, weakness is lack of concern for the welfare or futures of others than the promoters. However, exploitation need not be used in this way. It could be used to forewarn of impending breakthroughs which, for example, mean the end of certain problems, and thus spare us the cost of needlessly fighting them. Exploitive planning could forewarn of the imminent availability of more effective means toward goal achievement or toward solving particular problems, to spare expensive and needless tours de force. It could spare us the job of reinventing wheels which could be borrowed from other fields if we had an exploitive (but not exclusively so) frame of mind.

The Explorative Mode

Explorative is used in the sense of establishing a picture of the future by studying future extensions of capacities, desires, and possibilities from the viewpoint of what the present offers.[87] It represents an extension of the present, even though extensions may be bent by what is currently wanted and not presently available, so that the future is not merely an extension of the present, but an extension that the present indicates *could be*. The fact that long-term and desired goals are set up makes this mode somewhat normative. But it differs from the customary normative approach, which starts with a determination of what present or future values *would* call for, or even with a "willed future," which starts by a break with current values and postulates new values and what *ought to be* at some future point. (All the normative modes work back from the chosen goals to the changes which must be implemented today and tomorrow if those long range goals are to be reached.)

The Normative Mode

Normative is used here in the sense of desired or ideal, rather than of standards or norms. This kind of planning probably best describes how the United States came to be, or how man got on the moon. Planners who synthesize a picture of the future have three basic options regarding the panorama. (1) They may use their present value set and assume that it will remain unchanged (that their current notion of the "ideal" will hold still). (2) They may make some guesses or forecasts about the general value sets in the target year and what these values call for as the ideal of that future time. (3) They may simply cut loose and build a whole new set of values (a willed future) that *should* be operational—this is the stuff whereof the great religious and political movements come into being.[88] Planners then set about campaigning for adoption of these values and for the ideal state of affairs that they envision. If the desire is as specific as getting a man on the moon 15 years hence, and it is believed that the accomplishment will be desired 15 years from now, all that is needed is enough acquiescence to permit the assembly of the necessary resources or the invention of the missing resources needed between now and then to finish the job.

In other words, if man is to reach the moon in 15 years, planners work backward from that normative projection and determine what must be done in the fourteenth year, and before that, in the thirteenth year, and what must be accomplished in each intervening year back to today if the target is to be achieved 15 years from now. That 15-year dream was made to come to pass, and most of us were happy, or at least astounded. The fact that both exploratory and normative techniques can be used to create a normative style of planning is elaborated upon in Chapter 5 under the discussion of forecasting.

Normative planning, which is often called goal seeking, is sometimes confused with problem solving, because once a problem is attacked, the word goal is often used to describe the expected outcomes of the interventions. For example, in the attack on tuberculosis the successful skin testing of every high risk person is often called a goal (objective is the term I prefer). Problem solving is intended to bring change in what is going on without changing the value system, that is, to bring consonance between the value system and what is going on. Normative planning is intended to introduce change based on new goals derived from current values, or even from new values not presently in circulation.

Confusion between normative and problem-solving modes also arises because the means of achieving normative goals involves making incremental changes in specified time periods, from the moment the normative goal is accepted to the time it is achieved. This progression of tangible steps, or increments, to events, objectives, or subgoals along the road to normative goals is not the same as the problem solving incrementalistic outlook, which picks off one thing after another to repair without necessarily having any long-range goals in sight or mind.

Perhaps the characteristic that most clearly distinguishes normative planning from all the other kinds is its fulfillment of our sense of what *ought* to be. It provides a statement of what is particularly wanted over the long-range future, rather than of what is wanted as an immediate remedy to current ills or constraints. It is likely to involve a large-scale extension of the kinds of systems beyond those usually planned for and thus a significant invasion into the "environment."[89]

Hasan Ozbekhan[90] makes a very meaningful statement as to the significance of the version of normative which he refers to as a "willed future," and which I describe as stemming from new values. He states that the "willed" or very normative future stems from what is desirable (which qualifies both the end and the means). He uses betterment as a criterion of desirability in a broad sense of society, which includes individuals and does not limit the concept to private gains. He states further that (1) a willed future becomes more than an extension of the present for there is a change in the overall configuration of values; and (2) that only individuals initiate such value changes. He also stresses that such value changes cannot be predicted, that they have to be willed. They will occur as individual ideas, responses, or insights concerning betterment spread over the whole society. By taking Ozbekhan's criteria more explicitly, the example of how the United States came to be is a very normative or willed future; but how it put a man on the moon is not, for little change in our values was involved. He concludes with the plea for recognition that normative planning does not proceed simply from here and now to the future, but calls for modification of the here and now within our grasp, so that the intervening space is occupied by what the willed future insists we impose on the present.

Harvey Cox[91] in "The Feast of Fools" also makes an interesting contribution to the notion of how madcap escapism contributes to normative liberation from everyday notions of feasibility.

Total Planning

The total planning model is the bugaboo used to scare us away from considering any planning. Ironically, many who attack this model in its Soviet version do not hesitate to propose an essentially similar model under the guise of "let the experts do it" or "take this problem out of politics." There is every reason to be frightened of total planning, no matter how democratically designed, if absolutely nothing is left to the market. It is most to be feared if elites, of whatever background, are elected or selected to design for the rest of us.

Total planning has, in the United States, come to mean planning for unpopular or unnatural goals, planning for every last detail of human and societal activities, and planning done by a tiny minority without public participation. It has come to symbolize an aggregate of all that is undesirable. Interestingly, this apparition of total planning is often not unlike corporate planning which we admire in private enterprise and in many semi-public enterprises.

Because their ideology is so firmly set, Russians have no need to *make* a future—they already know what is to be. They are free, however, to change the means and the timing. Thus their planning is dubiously—if at all—normative in the Ozbekhan sense, even if they do firmly set up short- and long-range goals and standards of expectation as way stations on the road to their established future. Perhaps it is fairer to say that initially they were totally normative with a new ideology and a new set of values, but have since felt no great need to normatively change along the way to the goals of their originally willed future.

Other Planning Modes

Because there are several dozen other well known approaches to planning, it was tempting to introduce them here and point out in what ways they differ from one another and from what has been presented. Since, however, each of them tends to emphasize a certain feature of planning, such as advocacy or strategy or adaptivity, a comparison of them could not be undertaken on any simple set of parameters such as has been used in Figures 2.3 and 2.4. The popular modes of planning illustrate the gamut of conceivable purposes, roles, or functions of planning. For this reason it was decided to present the better known planning prescriptions (many are really just for tiny aspects of planning) in Chapter 9 for a comparison of the roles or functions to which they particularly refer and for which they have earned attention.

A DEVELOPMENTAL AND MULTI-MODE APPROACH

Normative and Articulated Guided Problem Solving as the Twin Bases

The eclectic approach to planning, concentrating particularly on a mixture of normative and articulated problem solving approaches, is the one in which I have the most faith. Normative planning seeks out the directions in which the society wishes to travel, gives them reasonable specificity, and provides the time and direction framework by which the resources of a nation or a community are allocated. Because this is a long term process, and because there are many pressing hurts that will otherwise distract public support, it usually is necessary as well as desirable to ameliorate currently bad problems at the same time. Because problem solving can eat up resources or, if done without guidance from longer range planning, can even set us on courses that preclude obtaining higher level goals or take us off in unintended new directions, it cannot be undertaken without at least an acknowledgment and spelling out of the higher level goals. These goals then serve as criteria by which to judge the suitability of solutions proposed for problems.

In the United States, the moral strengths that showed no hesitation in creating a revolution and setting up a country under very normative guidance, often seem to have ebbed away. We are now insecure about creating relevant sociopolitical goals, although we are nonchalant about firmly setting up technological ones (which inadvertently seem to determine the sociopolitical ones). For this reason, the planning duality of articulated and guided problem solving (*agps*) and normative planning are heavily weighted toward the former. In other countries, where long-range outcomes designed to change drastically a nation's status are the order of the day, normative planning is critical and *agps* is a secondary matter designed to overcome critical problems that are seen as interfering with achievement of the long-range goals. But these two modes of planning seem to make up the necessary interrelated short- and long-term aspects of planning. Etzioni recently came up with a similar configuration under the title of "Mixed Scanning,"[92] and Meyerson long ago advocated a similar approach which he referred to as the "Middle Bridge."[93]

Because I know the United States best and expect to be most widely read there, and because of the political reluctance to be meaningfully normative in the United States, it was decided to emphasize, perhaps unduly, the articulated and guided problem solving part of the proposed developmental planning. This type of problem solving requires the delineation of long-term purposes, and it provides an excellent means of portraying the various aspects of the planning processes generally.

Figure 1.2, not unlike other planning schemata,[94] tries to visualize at one time the two major ingredients of the developmental approach— the normative approach, and the articulated and guided problem-solving approach. The entire planning field is shown as embraced by values which, in essence, provide the basis for normative goal setting for the nation and the community being planned for. These normative goals (and their counterpart standards for expectations) include the health aspirations which serve as a base and provide a sense of direction for health planning. Our entire society constantly pays lip service to long-range normative goals without attempting to see what they imply or to make short-range goals conform to, assist, or at least not obstruct the long-range ones. Therefore, better quality long-range goal setting must also be carried out in earnest, and an attempt made to get the policy makers to adopt long-range goals at least in the form of general aims. Chapters 5-12 elaborate on each of the steps shown in Figure 1.2.

Contributions to the Developmental Mode from Other Modes

Exploratory forecasting and planning are needed to determine what is really going on and what is likely to be going on. They are imperative as an addition to normative planning, because they work with the forces with which the planner will actually have to contend. Achievement of the normatively designed goals is more nearly feasible with exploratory knowledge, because new forces and interventions will be meshed with the ongoing ones that exploratory planning reveals and popularizes as feasible and desirable. Planning can then come out as desired, by taking into account the resultant vector of the two sets of forces—the ongoing ones as revealed by exploration, and the newly defined ones activated by normative willing.

Allocative logic is essential to tide us over where there is a dearth of well-thought-through planning. It should avoid some disastrous bottlenecks in the future. In the United States, Medicare provided resources to buy needed care, but failed to provide more sources of care —an example of attempted problem solving without suitable allocative thinking. It led us directly to unprecedented health care inflation, which meant that Medicare probably did nearly as much harm as it did good. The allocative logic remains a standby for the great mass of policy decisions which cannot and need not be looked at on a yearly basis.

Exploitive planning, but with a keen eye for undesired secondary effects, is also much in order. Thus we can take advantage of what the future can be aided to do in bringing us at low cost some long-range goals, or in removing some current problems.

Laissez-faire, the vast capitalistic imperfect market place as we now know it, would continue as the means of making nearly all transactions. However, in contrast to the present steering of the market by innumerable and typically poorly thought-through, politically expedient forces, one would see the market guided and constrained by policies derived from the normative goals accepted for the country.

Total planning is abandoned as dangerous, unnecessary, and impractical, as well as philosophically unacceptable.

Disjointed incrementalism is discarded in favor of guided and articulated incrementalism.

Given the proposed mixture of modes involved in developmental planning, continuous planning and re-evaluation must mark its use. Rather than striving for an elaborate and detailed set of specific objectives for accomplishment at a specific time, developmental planning selects directions of long-range desirabilities and rates of accomplishment. At the same time, undesired conditions are analyzed and attacked as specifically as indicated. Observations over time may reveal that certain market (or other) forces counteract or reinforce the planned efforts. This may call for a change in intervention, a different point of application of interventions, or a change in the amount of resources for various interventions in the next planning round. The developmental approach has no intent to stop all possible counterforces by a totality of planning. Many unpredictable forces, both from inside the system of concern as well as from outside, are expected to come into play. Extensive monitoring and evaluation at all levels of community are needed continuously so that new tendencies can be spotted early and, if undesirable, altered. The developmental approach should not lead us into a heavy centralization of planning or of government.

Plans and Planning

What a planned-for future will be doing, what means it will use, and what outputs it will be delivering must be specified and organized if policy makers are to budget, agencies organize, purveyors produce and be recompensed, and consumers consume what has been produced with desired outcomes. Structured guides must emerge from the drawing boards of planning agencies. These guiding documents we will henceforth call plans, with full awareness that they do not stand for all time, that annual restudies and restatements can and will change direction as well as scope, but that they must exist if there is to be guidance to desired goals. We go into this explanation because nowadays plans are casually damned as nothing but a mass of hopelessly outmoded detail, while planning is praised in the same breath. Yet planning must deliver a utilizable product which provides tangible guidance.

If anything that takes more than one year to produce (almost any output such as trained manpower or service of consequence is likely to require a decade or more for maturing) does not have firm resource commitments and tied-in relationships along the way for its development and utilization, it is not likely to come off nor to do successfully what it was designed to achieve. The system that is to be affected must be part of what is to be changed, if the right consequences are to occur. And these changes do not often come about without extensive planning, the output of which is plans. We mean no harm by the term plans, no return to immutable once-and-for-all blueprints. We must call the output of planning bodies by some name and the word "plan" seems the most logical.

CONCLUSION

Much of normative planning and articulated-guided problem solving is hard to achieve. Democratic and deliberate are very elegant adjectives, but difficult to make tangible. But this realization does not rob planning of validity nor discredit our attempts to go further along these routes. Democracy was once a dream. Now it is a reality, but one that still needs to be pursued. The developmental planning described here seems totally in keeping with an effective pursuit.

One sizable piece of evidence that supports our belief that guidance is obtained from normatively derived general aims is presented by David.[95] He shows that in the United States a high proportion of national party platform planks are in fact carried through into relevant enabling national legislation. It is of even more interest that directions promised by both party platforms do particularly well, as do those of a single party when the president is of the controlling party. Cynical as we have been in this country about one-shot election-oriented party platforms or promises, this comes as a heartening surprise. The fact that means to carry out intent have generally been poorly planned is another matter.

I find it necessary to conclude with a warning to planners that automatic overall guidance from broad publicly held aims (one of our keys to developmental planning) may also mean that the goals thereby derived may represent the very heart of "conventional wisdom." That is, those goals may be highly acceptable and unquestioningly accepted. Yet tragic consequences from their adoption may clearly be foreseen and, if pursued, the outcomes may well prove that conventionally wise goals can be sheer folly. Throughout this book, therefore, I emphasize the need for planning bodies to converse with a wide diversity of interests in order to avoid just such unchallenged acceptance of widely held goals. (Goals of productivity, profits, efficiency, or equity, as we have already pointed out, may be in serious conflict with one another, particularly when carried to extremes.)

Can the professional planner make a significant contribution in guiding a planning body to a wiser selection of goals than conventional wisdom is likely to produce? I believe so. Perhaps the planner's unique contribution to planning may be in successfully getting planning groups, and the policy makers and electorate as well, to question all conventionally wise or freely accepted goals by means of a future or consequences-oriented analysis before they, as goal setting bodies, set down value derived goals as the commandments by which they will guide their choice making. Salk makes the point well that if we are to enjoy a reasonable level of health there is a pressing need for development of new expectations and values as life on earth passes the inflection point and enters the deaccelerating phase of the sigmoid growth curve.[96]

REFERENCES

1. Allan Blackman, "Philosophy of Planning as an Instrument of Social Change," *Health Planning 1969*, by H. L. Blum and Associates (San Francisco: Western Regional Office, American Public Health Association, 1969), Chapter 2.
2. Neil J. Smelser, "Toward a General Theory of Social Change," *Essays in Sociological Explanation*, ed. by N. J. Smelser (Englewood Cliffs, N. J.: Prentice-Hall, 1968), 232.
3. Hasan Ozbekhan, "Towards a General Theory of Planning," *Perspectives of Planning*, ed. by Erich Jantsch (Paris: Organization for Economic Co-operation and Development, 1969), 47-159.
4. John Horton, "Order and Conflict Theories of Social Problems as Competing Ideologies," *American Journal of Sociology* 71 (May 1966), 701-13.
5. Bertram M. Gross, "Planning in an Era of Social Revolution," *Public Administration Review* 31 (May/June 1971), 259-96.
6. N. J. Smelser, Ibid. No. 2, 193.
7. Everett E. Hagan, *On the Theory of Social Change* (Homewood, Illinois: The Dorsey Press, 1962), 55.
8. George M. Foster, "The Anatomy of Envy: A Study in Symbolic Behavior," *Current Anthropology* 13 (April 1972), 165-202.
9. George M. Foster, "Peasant Society and the Image of Limited Good," *American Anthropologist* 67 (April 1965), 293-315.
10. Bronislaw Malinowski, *The Dynamics of Culture Change: An Enquiry into Race Relations in Africa* ed. by Phyllis M. Kaberry (New Haven: Yale University Press, 1945), pp. 75-129.
11. E. E. Hagen, Ibid. No. 7, 99-122.
12. David C. McClelland, *The Achieving Society* (Princeton, N. J.: Van Nostrand, 1961), Chapters 1, 2, 3.
13. B. M. Gross, Ibid. No. 5.
14. Walter Buckley, *Sociology and Modern Systems Theory* (Englewood Cliffs, N. J.: Prentice-Hall, 1967), Chapter 3.
15. Adul Wichiencharoen, "Principles and Problems of Social Planning." Material distributed to WHO Senior Staff Course on National Health Planning, Bangkok, September 26, 1968, mimeographed.

16. James S. Coleman, "Conflicting Theories of Social Change," *American Behavioral Scientist* 14 (May/June 1971), 633.
17. N. J. Smelser, Ibid. No. 2, 205.
18. N. J. Smelser, Ibid. No. 2, 205.
19. S. F. Nadel, "Social Control and Self Regulation," *Social Forces* 31 (1953), 265-323.
20. Alfred J. Kahn, *Theory and Practice of Social Planning* (New York: Russell Sage Foundation, 1969), Chapter 2.
21. Alexis de Tocqueville, *Democracy in America*, Vol. 1, (New York: Knopf, A Vintage Book, 1957).
22. Gunnar Myrdal, *An American Dilemma* (New York: McGraw-Hill, 1964), Chapter 1.
23. N. J. Smelser, Ibid. No. 2, 278.
24. W. Buckley, Ibid. No. 14, 149.
25. Anselm Strauss, et al., "The Hospital and Its Negotiated Order," *The Hospital in Modern Society*, ed. by Eliot Freidson (New York: The Free Press, 1963), 147-69.
26. W. Buckley, Ibid. No. 14, 139.
27. James S. Coleman, "Collective Decisions," *Sociological Inquiry* 34 (1964), 166-80.
28. E. E. Hagen, Ibid. No. 7, 182.
29. Bronislaw Malinowski, *A Scientific Theory of Cultures and Other Essays* (New York: Oxford University Press, 1960), 57-129.
30. Abraham H. Maslow, *Motivation and Personality* (New York: Harper and Row, 1954), 80-154.
31. Amitai Etzioni, "Basic Human Needs, Alienation and Inauthenticity," *American Sociological Review* 35 (December 1968), 870-85.
32. H. M. Dunn, "Social Change and the Fundamentals of Community Organization," *Journal of Educational Sociology* 33 (May 1960), 373-83.
33. Kurt Lewin, *Field Theory in Social Science* (New York: Harper, Harper Torchbooks, 1964), 38-42. Andie M. Knutson, *The Individual Society and Health Behavior* (New York: Russell Sage Foundation, 1965), 262, 276-77, 289.
34. Robin M. Williams, Jr., "Individual and Group Values," *The Annals of the American Academy of Political and Social Sciences* 371 (May 1967), 20-38.
35. James Reston, "The Great Society—Are We Ready for It?" *John Hopkins Alumni Magazine* (March 1965), 9-11.
36. David Braybrooke and Charles Lindblom, *A Strategy for Decision* (New York: The Free Press, 1963), 29.
37. Ian H. Wilson, "How Our Values Are Changing," *Futurist* 4 (December 1970), 5-9.
38. Willis W. Harman, "Educational Alternatives for the Future." Mimeographed paper presented to a class on Forecasting at the University of California, Berkeley, April 1971.
39. Paul Davidoff and Thomas A. Reiner, "A Choice Theory of Planning," *Journal of the American Institute of Planners* 27 (May 1962), 103-15.
40. Clyde Kluckhohn, "Values and Value Orientation," *Toward a General Theory of Action*, ed. by Talcott Parsons and Edward A. Shils (Cambridge: Harvard University Press, 1951), 395-403.

41. B. F. Skinner, "Beyond Freedom and Dignity," Summa Excerpts in *Psychology Today* 5 (August 1971), 59.

42. R. M. Williams, Jr., Ibid. No. 34, 20-38.

43. Wilbert E. Moore, *Social Change* (Englewood Cliffs, N.J.: Prentice-Hall, 1963), 18. D. E. Morrison, "Some Notes Toward Theory on Relative Deprivation, Social Movements and Social Change," *American Behavioral Scientist* 19 (May/June 1971), 675-90.

44. William J. Goode, "A Theory of Role Strain," *American Sociology Review* 25 (1960), 483-96.

45. Edward C. Tolman, "Value Standards, Pattern Variables, Social Roles, Personality," *Toward a General Theory of Action*, ed. by Talcott Parsons and E. A. Shils (Cambridge: Harvard University Press, 1959), 350-51.

46. Leon Festinger, *A Theory of Cognitive Dissonance* (Palo Alto, California: Stanford University Press, 1968), Chapter 1.

47. N. J. Smelser, Ibid. No. 2, 206.

48. Lisle C. Carter, Jr., "National Purpose and the Need for Community." Mimeographed paper distributed at the 5th HEW Forum, January 31, 1968, Washington, D.C.

49. L. Festinger, Ibid. No. 46, Chapters 5 and 7.

50. B. Malinowski, Ibid. No. 29, 57-129.

51. L. Festinger, Ibid. No. 46, 1-47.

52. Lester R. Brown, *Seeds of Change: The Green Revolution and Development in the 1970's* (New York: Praeger, 1970).

53. Norman Beckman, "Legislative Review 1970: Development of National Urban Growth Policy," *Journal of the American Institute of Planners* 37 (May 1971), 146-61; and 38 (July 1972), 231-49. Sheldon J. Plager, "Judicial Review 1970: Policy, Planning and the Courts," *Journal of the American Institute of Planners* 37 (May 1971), 174-91.

54. Robert Chin and Kenneth D. Benne, "General Strategies for Effecting Changes," *The Planning of Change*, ed. by Warren G. Bennis, Kenneth D. Benne and Robert Chin (New York: Holt, Rinehart and Winston, 1969), 32-59.

55. Ritchie P. Lowry, "Power to the People—Political Evolution or Revolution," *Urban and Social Change Review* 3 (Spring 1970), 2-6.

56. Peter Menke-Glukert, "Mankind in the World of Tomorrow: The Changing Environment," *Technological Forecasting and Social Change* 2:3/4 (1971), 231-35.

57. Peter F. Drucker, *The Age of Discontinuity* (New York: Harper and Row, 1969).

58. Jonas Salk. *The Survival of the Wisest* (New York, Harper and Row, 1973) Kenneth E. Boulding, *Economics As A Science* (New York: McGraw-Hill, 1970), 139-57.

59. Harvey Brooks and Raymond Bowers, "The Assessment of Technology," *Scientific American*, (February 1970), 13-21.

60. A. Blackman, Ibid. No. 1, Chapter 2.

61. Leonard J. Duhl and Janice Volkman, "Participant Democracy: Networks as a Strategy for Change," *Urban and Social Change Review* 3 (Spring 1970), 11-14.

62. A. Blackman, Ibid. No. 1, Chapter 2.

63. For a brief review of some of the evidence in this area, see Martin Rein,

"Social Science and the Elimination of Poverty," *Journal of the American Institute of Planners* 33 (May 1967), 146-63. For a more general discussion of means-ends problems in planning see "Environment and Behavior," *American Behavioral Scientist* (September 1966).

64. A. Blackman, Ibid. No. 1, Chapter 2.
65. H. Ozbekhan, Ibid. No. 3, 64.
66. A. J. Kahn, Ibid. No. 20, Chapter 2.
67. Allan Blackman, "Definitions of Planning." Mimeographed material dated October 1, 1970, Association of University Programs in Hospital Administration, 1424 Washington Heights, School of Public Health, University of Michigan, Ann Arbor.
68. P. Davidoff and T. A. Reiner, Ibid. No. 39, 103-15.
69. John W. Dyckman, "The Practical Uses of Planning Theory," *Journal of the American Institute of Planners* 35 (September 1969), 298-301. John W. Dyckman, "Planning and Decision Theory," *Journal of the American Institute of Planners* 27 (November 1961), 335-45.
70. Gunnar Myrdal, "The Necessity and Difficulty of Planning the Future Society." Address to the National Consultation on the Future Environment of a Democracy, Washington, D.C., October 3, 1967.
71. John Friedmann, "A Conceptual Model for the Analysis of Planning Behavior," *Administrative Science Quarterly* 12 (September 1967), 225-52.
72. William Petersen, "On Some Meanings of 'Planning'," *Journal of the American Institute of Planners* 32 (May 1966), 130-42.
73. Paul Davidoff, "Advocacy and Pluralism in Planning," *Taming Megalopolis*, Vol. 2, ed. by E. Wentworth (New York: Doubleday, 1967).
74. Russell L. Ackoff, *A Concept of Corporate Planning* (New York: Wiley-Interscience, 1970), 1-22.
75. Jan Tinbergen, *Central Planning* (New Haven & London: Yale University Press, 1964), Chapter 3.
76. Gunnar Myrdal, *The Challenge of World Poverty* (New York: Pantheon, 1970), 414.
77. Vicente Navarro, "Methodology on Regional Planning of Personal Health Services," *Medical Care* 8 (September/October 1970), 386-94.
78. John K. Galbraith, *The New Industrial State* (New York: Signet, 1967), 37.
79. Mary Arnold, "Use of Management Tools for Health Planning," *Public Health Reports* 83 (October 1968), 820-26.
80. C. Jencks, "Who Should Control Education," *Dissent* (March 1966), 145-63.
81. A. Blackman, Ibid. No. 1, Chapter 2.
82. John W. Dyckman, "Social Planning, Social Planners and Planned Societies," *Journal of the American Institute of Planners* 32 (March 1966), 66-76.
83. Charles E. Lindblom, "The Science of Muddling Through," *Public Administration Review* 19 (Spring 1959), 79-88. D. Braybrooke and C. E. Lindblom, Ibid. No. 36, 1-57.
84. Amitai Etzioni, "On the Process of Making Decisions," *Science* 152 (May 6, 1966), 746-47.
85. J. Friedmann, Ibid. No. 71, 225-52.

86. A. O. Hirschman and Charles E. Lindblom, "Economic Development, Research and Development, Policy Making: Some Converging Views," *Behavioral Science* 7 (April 1962), 211-22.

87. Erich Jantsch, *Technological Forecasting in Perspective* (Paris: Organisation for Economic Cooperation and Development, 1967), Chapters 1, 2.

88. E. Jantsch, Ibid. No. 87, Chapters 1, 2.

89. H. Ozbekhan, Ibid. No. 3, 100-102.

90. H. Ozbekhan, Ibid. No. 3, 88-96.

91. Harvey Cox, *The Feast of Fools* (Cambridge: Harvard University Press, 1969).

92. Amitai Etzioni, The Active Society (New York: The Free Press, 1968) Chapter 12.

93. Martin Meyerson, "Building the Middle-Range Bridge for Comprehensive Planning," *Journal of the American Institute of Planners* 22 (May 1956), 58-64.

94. Carl E. Taylor, "Stages of the Planning Process," *Health Planning*, ed. by Wm. A. Reinke (Baltimore: Waverly Press, 1972), 20-34. H.E. Hilleboe, "Mass Health Examinations as a Public Health Tool," *Mass Health Examinations: Public Health Paper No. 45.* (Geneva: World Health Organization, 1971), 28-39.

95. P. T. David, "Party Platforms as National Plans," (Special issue: "Changing Styles of Planning") *Public Administration Review* 31 (May/June 1971), 303-15.

96. Jonas Salk, Ibid. No. 58.

3. A Working Definition of Health for Planning: A Multifaceted Concept

The inability of the various health services practitioners to formulate any suitable or working definition of health attests to the difficulties our society has with this concept. Health planning bodies almost take for granted that there will be significant differences of willingness among board members to undertake studies of health problems that go beyond obvious physical, mental or emotional health deficits. They can also reasonably expect serious disagreements about how far to pursue various environmental and behavioral factors that are clearly the precursors, if not the actual causes, of health deficits.

This chapter seeks to clarify the reasons that the concept of "health" embraces such different levels of concern among different persons. It does so by tracing the points of view about health from value and belief systems. Each value-belief system has sufficient credibility and is of sufficient popular concern to be high in the consciousness of one or another of the participants at the planning table, thereby defining his belief about what health is and therefore, what health planning bodies should be doing.

Awareness of these legitimate forces at work enables planners to acknowledge the underlying value-belief systems by putting them in the form of criteria by which goals, problems, or solutions can be given preference (see Chapter 6). Awareness of these widely disparate value streams allows the discussion of specific planning undertakings to be guided by the recognition of the social validity, as well as the political feasibility, of each value position. The forces deriving from values are thereby harnessed for positive purposes and are no longer disruptive issues to be unsuccessfully swept under non-existent policy rugs. They provide the makings of policy.

Rogers[1] tells us that the word health has an Anglo-Saxon origin denoting wholeness, a state in which all organs function in harmony and create total well-being, not merely the absence of disease or infirmity. The same concept of wholeness appears in the New Testament and in the writings of Pindar, *circa* 500 B.C., where it is applied to people and things and is meant to reflect a state of "sane happiness." With a

76

sense of wholeness, let us then pursue the analysis of the value systems on which people base their definitions of health. Some of the value systems have been effectively operative for only a few years, such as the ecological point of view; others, such as the humanitarian view, have had socially significant roles of varying intensity for thousands of years. Although we might like to restrict ourselves to the state or degree of health of individuals, society creates the forces that define health, and some definitions have social connotations (that is, for the health of society). Therefore, the social aspect of health cannot (and should not) be ignored. We must understand that each position, narrow or broad, recent or of long standing, is part of a series of historical, legitimate, and meaningful perceptions of health that in the aggregate make up our broadening and socially useful present-day concept of health or wholeness.

THE MAINSTREAMS OF SOCIAL CONCERNS THAT CONTRIBUTE TO OUR PRESENT-DAY CONFUSED VIEWS ABOUT HEALTH

The Medical View

For perhaps 17 centuries, physicians carried from culture to culture the dwindling handful of empirically satisfying health-restoring procedures which had survived from the Graeco-Roman golden era and held their own against the endless offering of mystically derived incantations and potions. With the coming of the Renaissance, there were few men who could resist applying their new found knowledge to the ills of man. With each step into the biological world, speculative minds could see the significance of the health practices that had successfully survived. The first new wave of Renaissance scientific revelations provided evidence that disease or illness was either a superimposition of some malignant force upon man or, on occasion, was a deprivation of a necessary item of intake. Clearly, the logic of the medical model meant that the cure should consist of the removal or neutralizing of some superimposed noxious substance or parasite or the addition of certain required life-maintaining substances.

Illness came to be perceived as an untoward state of feeling bad, of poor performance, or of unusual behavior observable by others even if not noticed by the victim himself. *Disease* came to be recognized as specific abnormal or pathological states due either to the presence or the deprivation of specific foreign substances, living or inanimate. Disease might exist without illness or with subliminal levels of illness, but illness could not occur without disease. When it appeared to do so, it was only because the nature of the disease had not yet been elucidated. The causes of disease were sometimes expressed in terms of the nature of the deprivation, of the excess, or of the foreign invading substances. Sometimes diseases were described in terms of the gross or microscopic or metabolic distortions present. Sometimes they were described in terms of the organ, body part or function that was disturbed.

In every case, health was seen as the pristine state pre-existing disorder or disease, or as the newly achieved state resulting from the eradication of the superimposed disorder. There has been a general understanding that the state predating disease is usually a healthier one than that following recovery from a disease, with a few interesting exceptions where recovery from a mild version of the disease seemed to confer protection against encounters with more virulent forms of the same or related disease.

Not unlike the traditional or prescientific society, the medical model sees disease as essentially something superimposed upon man, and therefore essentially removable, even by replacement therapy. Health is, then, freedom from superimposed or unnatural influences.

The goals for health were accordingly placed in the hands of medical leadership for definitions. They have turned out to be primarily the prolongation of life and the minimization of departures from derived norms, consistent with age and sex, of the physiologic and bodily functions.

What Have Been the Failures of the Medical Viewpoint?

Verification of the validity or quality of medical innovation and intervention has not been made in terms of the influence on recipients of care, or on society, but rather on the technological accomplishment itself. It also can be argued that the medical view almost has antihumanitarian aspects. In the achievement of medical miracles, people have been kept alive at crushing—even bankrupting—cost, often in chronic agony, and not infrequently against their own desires. It can truly be said that for too many people dying, not living, has been prolonged. Furthermore, with the exception of the great contagions, little interest has been shown in the prevention of disease occurrence or reoccurrence, or for the functional restoration of persons damaged by disease.

The Preventive or Public Health View

Very slowly, and ever in the shadow of the medical model, public health promoted prevention, early perception of illness and disease, and avoidance of premature death (prolongation of life). Health in this outlook became identified as a state of affairs in which avoidable hazards have been:

Padded against (prophylaxis for malaria, etc.).
and unavoidable hazards have been:

Found early before symptomatic and disposed of (cancer of the cervix).

Found as soon as possible, treated and damage minimized (tuberculosis).

Found, treated, and functional restoration pursued as far as possible (diabetes).

In this, the public health way of looking at things, we see that the last two proposals are identical with those of the medical view, although couched in terms of minimization of the effects of disease. Also, disease is seen as resulting when man is pitted against the various elements of the environment about him or is deprived of certain essential nutrients. This viewpoint is more cognizant than the medical of man as an internal system interacting with the external system about him, but it still focuses on specific causes of disease, and on disease as something thrust upon man or something denied him.

What Have Been the Successes of the Public Health Outlook?

Control of the great deficiency diseases and of contagious disease plagues, massive environmental upgradings, and the new era of epidemiologic sleuthing against the still unsolved mystery of many of man's diseases, are all attributable to this outlook. It is of interest that, in England, on the basis of recorded law and intent, local government and planning are said to have arisen directly from public health concerns, which led to need for control of housing, and thus to city planning and thence to regional planning, in order to prescribe for more healthful living conditions.[2] It would be my guess that public health was a politically more saleable euphemism for various humanitarian concerns to be discussed shortly.

What Have Been the Failures of the Public Health Approach?

Public health has failed to appreciate the forces at work beyond the interactions of man and some disease vector in the immediate environment. By focusing primarily on mechanical and biologic forces, the overall environment has been given a limited or static place when it might better have been considered as a composite of forces, including at least the more important social ones. As a result of ignoring overpowering background or ecologic forces, few of even the well understood deficiency diseases are really under control, and similarly, many preventable contagions remain unprevented. Overpopulation and malnutrition are major threats resulting in great part from preventive measures which were technically successful, but whose social consequences were not considered.

The Humanitarian or Well-Being View

Humanitarian concerns often predated and then grew apace with the post-Renaissance medical discoveries. They have led to a series of postulations about what human beings should and should not endure as they make their way through life. A society is seen as suitably wise and healthy if man is at the center of its concerns. Paramount among its criteria of a healthy society are:

The survival of infants.

The survival of their mothers.

Freedom from hunger.

Freedom from inhumane treatment or punishment.

Reasonably available care or succor for those in illness, pain or distress of any kind.

A safe and pleasurable environment.

Man, the object, is seen at the center of the contending forces of the social and physical environment that endlessly swirl around him, and only the mutual help of man to man can keep him well.

What Have Been the Successes of the Humanitarian Outlook?

The humanitarian viewpoint gave impetus to various movements which have had broad effects on society:

The social welfare movement led to: feeding the hungry; institutions or funds to care for the homeless, destitute, disturbed, diseased, and demented; removal of chains from the mentally ill; attempts to provide decent and safe jails which do not brutalize the inmates; opportunities for day-to-day recreation; provision of "upward guidance" (as through settlement houses); and establishment, in western countries, of concepts and practices of social justice as a way of life (most recently manifested in the United States by attempted advances in political democracy, economic and other opportunities, desegregation, Medicare, and so on).

The education movement grew rapidly, for education was seen as the way out of most problems and the way up for most individuals. Health education became the fair share of the educational burden allocated to the public health agencies, both official and voluntary.

The clean and sanitary environment movement became the mainspring for public health and its sanitation control functions. As a result of these basic concerns with filth and unsafe environment, and with the development of knowledge about the spread of contagious diseases, funds, authority, and "real life" were pumped into the official public health agencies—not a few of which have added little more to their activities in the 20th century.

The maternal and infant welfare movement was firmed up, and the vague and often contradictory feelings about the welfare of infants turned into a very positive posture that accepted making the world safe for innocent children as an obligation of society. This led to a concern for the health of mothers who, after all, were the most important influences in the lives of infants and children. This concern led to another of the mainstay functions of the official health agencies. The U.S. Children's Bureau, almost unconquerable even in its recent anachronistic isolation, was the national symbol of the pre-eminence of children in the hierarchy of values to which we give lip service.

City beautiful concerns were a direct consequence of man's growing concern for his fellow man, and were expressed quite promptly by schemes for improving the enjoyability as well as the safety of the artificial living environment of the new, industrially induced cities. Architects and landscape architects began once more to concern themselves with environments for communities of people, and city planning became an honored and widely pursued civic function. Some of the extension of interest in conservation, such as recreational concerns, the creation of national parks, or the preservation of wilderness areas, is probably also based on humanitarian values.

What Have Been the Failures of the Humanitarian Outlook?

The humanitarian view led to significant oversights: Provision of resources for valued causes has been made in a most uncritical manner. The humanitarian view has contributed to the uncritical achievement of prolongation of dying as much as of living. It has substituted charity for justice, and has tended to obscure issues of equity by use of philanthropy. In the United States, it taught us to hide our social failures by means of massive philanthropy and governmental welfare, which allowed us to overlook the kind of adulthood we assigned to the "adorable little ones" that we saved with ostentatiously presented, but to this day, niggardly funded measures. Legislation has been passed under the rubric of humanitarianism, popularly entitled to appear to satisfy such values. But all evaluatory concern for relevancy, adequacy or effectiveness has been sidestepped. Examples abound. Aid to Families of Dependent Children was one of the first. It has been followed by insincere posturing, such as the pathetic attempts to feed our starving children.

Now that agedness is more common and fewer extended families remain to care comfortably for their elders, the votes generated by the aged and their children have led to massive attempts to have an impersonal and more provident hand care for our mothers and fathers in their old age. As a result, we now undertake to care for the health needs of our aged by substantially financed programs. But many aged have been pushed into nursing homes (unscrutinized, ghastly holes for a century, although much better now to be sure), because our insufficient concerns really did not lead us to offer other significant options. For a while, we even helped push old people into beds in the nursing homes by paying bonuses for those kept in bed.

The Economic View

Freedom from disability, incapacity, and premature death express well the economic outlook on the meaning of health—another legacy from the Great Enlightenment and the Industrial Revolution. This view concerned itself with those factors that might:
Prevent entry into the work force.
Cause the loss of effective workers or homemakers, temporarily or permanently.
Prevent educability.
Cause partial losses resulting from sick workers performing below capacity.
Affect cost-benefit ratios of health or social interactions by virtue of their effects on productivity, and thus on the GNP (which in many quarters is taken as the critical measure of national success).
Divert resources to the care of the sick or the unproductive.
In the 20th century, no less than previously, the logic of micro-economics led us to perceive health care as a consumption of private goods, and thus confusedly related to issues of a free market, which essentially had never existed in medical care by any customary market criteria. At the same time, the welfare and macroeconomic views, tied to the dream of an ever-increasing GNP and the necessary increase in worker productivity, found health to be a social necessity, and health care to be a right, an investment, and a public good. Overall, the micro and macro levels of economics, different in vintage, could probably agree that man is a rational producer and should be a rational consumer. But they could not agree on how this healthy state of affairs could best be helped to take place.

What Have Been the Successes of the Economic Viewpoints?

Vital statistics were utilized early to determine what was happening to the labor force and the potential labor force. Counting the dead was necessary in order to plan for replacements. The economic views led to concern about unnecessary disease, illness, and above all, disability. And it later led to concerns about absenteeism and loss of expensively trained labor. The goals of expanded productivity justified the expenditure of greater amounts of resources to protect the health of workers and future workers, and the attainment of productivity goals provided the means.

Better education, desired for reasons of productivity, also created more citizen understanding of health and health care. The economic views led to better understanding of decision making and to an extension of concepts of rationality in planning, producing and operating all production activities. These are now finally being applied to the activities of the health care sector.

What Failures Have Been Encouraged by the Economic Views?

They led to concentration on equal opportunity, to get the vote, and on political rather than economic democracy—a remarkable feat, in retrospect. The well-being of man was overlooked in favor of such criteria as evidence of his aggregate production. While the overall GNP was observably soaring, Appalachia was allowed to "die." We were taught to ignore values of well-being in our pursuit of growth. Devices, such as discounting to convert future costs and gains to present value, helped to obscure the nature of decisions relevant to future generations.

We learned that it might be wise to concentrate on the best producer (WASP, age 21, college, male), because the returns would be greater if he were spared illness. Cost-benefit and PPBS methods were uncritically applied to health decisions. Inadvertently, productivity as measured in terms of dollars was usually the largest dollar item, and it, therefore, became the dominant criterion by which success was to be judged. The half-digested, conflicting, economic logics left unreconciled our studied attempts to keep the size of the labor force down and diminish production by prolonged schooling and enforced early retirement, while measuring diseases and control measures in terms of their effect on increasing productivity.

If carried just a bit further, this view opens the way to extermination (calculated neglect) of poor risks and poor producers. However, the frustrations produced by its majestic shortcomings are now becoming a major force in promoting a more holistic view of man and his well-being. They are sparking a search for new criteria that will be of more use in determining what well-being is, and how we can tell when we are improving it, and for new economic criteria, such as the price people would be willing to pay for good health.[3] (See Chapter 7.)

The Super Biologic Systems View of Health and Disease

Here disease is seen as a natural phenomenon, and health as adaptation to the environmental demands to the degree to which the individual is capable.

The super biologic outlook calls for an ideal of:
    Normal growth.
    Normal development.
    Normal anatomic achievement.
    Normal physiologic functioning.
    Normal psychologic functioning.
    Normal sociologic functioning.

It acknowledges that from the beginning of life *in utero* there are genetic "short-changes" and that there are harmful environmental impacts on the infant from the mother and from the environment, even if mediated by her life processes.

In this viewpoint man clearly remains at the center of the universe of concerns. He radiates and receives impingements which shape him and which shape his world. This viewpoint comes close to an ecological outlook in the sense that man is seen as containing a series of systems and as being part of a larger system. Largely technological, it does not adequately take into account values, social forces, and man's goal-seeking behavior, nor the philosophical issues of the interrelatedness of man's well-being with that of appropriate ecological balance among all living things.

What Have Been the Successes of the Super Biologic View?

Genetic, cellular, enzymatic, and molecular discoveries ricochet from great laboratories and great minds into the world of applied medicine. Diagnosis, therapy, replacement, and even sensory substitution are becoming commonplace. From a practical standpoint the super biologic view acts mostly as an extension of the medical. Concern for the future forces us into an awareness of what such an outlook is doing and what it might do. For example, might it be directed to changing the thoughts in our conscious mind, or changing our protoplasm through interventions in our genes? This influence has provided basic support for new research into the behavioral sciences—for example, it relates psychological and organizational concepts to political, molecular and other systems theories. It has finally helped bring into focus the scientist's responsibility to society for his activities.

What Have Been the Failures of the Super Biologic Model?

This view has so far not provided any new sense of direction for our biologic researches, even while it tampers with life as though tampering with something so precious as to make such activities sacred. True, tampering is called science, and we are often reminded that freedom of scientific pursuit must go unchallenged even if we are totally unprepared for the consequences. Proposals at any cost are called for to research further into man's diseases, even those which cluster about him as he reaches senescence. Such priorities ignore the reality that even a 50% reduction in heart disease, cancer and stroke would add but little to life or life's span in the United States. The overwhelming scientific commitment (usually where the funds are) to the control of diseases of advancing age reduces the means to conquer diseases of childhood and young adulthood, where losses to family and society are maximal. It also ignores the inhumanity of prolonging any kind of life, regardless of level of cost.

The Philosophical View of Health

The philosophical view, which may well be synonymous with the mental health view, can best be stated as the pursuit of the maximal capacity for self-realization or self-fulfillment. Thus is posed the meshing of an individual's internal systemic relations with those of his external environment, so that self-realization must take into account the ability of his available capacities to cope with the challenges he has to meet. Obviously, many issues arise.

How far do we want to alter the environment? If we alter it for some persons, such as infants or the aged, will it be suitable for others? In what ways do we want to alter environments? Should we remove psychosocial distresses? If we are successful, will we do away with future Mozarts and Michelangelos? Can a man achieve a sense of self-realization if others moderate the challenges posed by his environment? Can environments be modified suitably overall, given the variations between the needs and capacities of individuals for overcoming obstacles? Yes, we know that polio can be removed, accidents minimized, and risk-taking behavior modified, but at what point do we trade self-realization for security, at one extreme, or pleasure seeking, at another?

The issues further multiply with the awareness that self-realization as a value may also polarize us in regard to other values, such as individual liberty to do what we wish, against concern for infringement on the rights of others. Should we tolerate and support able but non-working persons? What about the happy criminal who gets his kicks from robbing a bank (hurting others), or the one who smokes pot (hurting no one else directly)? What should we do about the white-collar criminal who is productive and honored for his capability, but who callously exploits legal technicalities to sell dangerous or inferior products? What can we say about those great leaders (or misleaders) like Napoleon, Hitler, Stalin and a few others closer to home? We also get into the problems of birth control, abortion, population control, and lebensraum, all related to some aspects of self-fulfillment of individuals, tribes or nations.

What Have Been the Successes of the Philosophic Viewpoint?

The concepts of values, goals, standards, deviancy, social behavior, organization, social change, and culture differences have all been made more coherent as man is seen as a goal-seeking, self-fulfilling being. In this area we are particularly beholden to Parsons for major insights.[4] The role of education to enable people to live more satisfying lives has vied with the notion of training to produce the workers necessary for our society and its industries, and has raised our sights from "labor to survive" to "labor to enjoy." The ideas of social justice have reinforced the ideal that man must be given reasonable equality of opportunity if he is ever to be more than an animal seeking to exist from day to day. The more philosophical approach has led to many formulations about the purposes of life, to opportunities for self-fulfillment, and to a more ecological or overall environmental focus, with the expectation that man may be able to reach new levels of self-realization.

What Have Been the Failures of the Philosophic Viewpoint?

Rampant individualism as proof of self-fulfillment, heedless use of natural resources for purposes of individual aggrandizement, and wars as a means of enforcing fulfillment of ambitions may all seem like peculiar side products of what we call the philosophical outlook. However, they have been justified under every conceivable kind of world and political outlook, suggesting that exaggerated views of self-realization are probably no more than low-level rationalizations for continuing ancient modes of behavior. In any case, the self-realization outlook has not apparently led to the unbroken stream of improvements it would seem to call for.

Either as a result of appearing unrealistic or because it is incomprehensible to a majority of people, only the more selfish interpretations of the philosophic view predominate. They have generally been the means by which improvements in general welfare have been thwarted, and they have supported vicious social practices, such as the ones arising from the dogma that the well-to-do should not have their initiative impaired by heavy taxes to support the "incompetent." Similarly, as scientists began to pluck off society's highest awards, the pursuit of science has been divorced from concern about the consequences of its discoveries. However, the very horrendous nature of the failures of the philosophical viewpoint—which often resulted from unwise application of brilliant technologic breakthroughs, such as atomic energy—has forced an awareness of ecology that might not have occurred if the new heights of folly had been achieved more gradually.

The Ecological View (Survival of Our Species)

We have discovered that man may well be master of the universe, but his immediate welfare cannot be the sole guiding force by which he makes decisions that affect all things around him. Man is surely not the "center" or the *raison d'être* of the universe. The only way he can maintain this pretense is to make sure that he does not so disrupt his environment as to affect other things that will shortly affect him adversely. Because the changes that man induces are regarded as great improvements by some and as disasters by others, it is worth recalling that ecology does not refer to some never-ending state of homeostasis or equilibrium. Ecology refers to the interrelationships of all things. These interrelationships continue to shift with man's interference as well as with natural changes, such as earthquakes, lightning-set forest fires, floods, or volcanic eruptions. As man learns the significance of his own strength, he finds that he can move the world toward the extinction of a bearable life, even to the extinction of most life. Alternatively, he can change his activities so that his environment becomes safer and more pleasant. That is, ecological understanding allows shifts that are more favorable in the long run for many or all species as well as for man. However, certain short-run gains for man may have to be foregone if long-term gains are to be achieved. The ecological view is often limited to the advocacy of the "survival of our species" in practical or man-centered terms.

Our actions based on the failures or limitations of all the other outlooks about man's well-being have probably driven us to "discover" the ecological view, which had really been partially understood for many, many years in our culture, and in cultures that flourished before ours. But the breadth of ecologic ramifications has rarely been well enough understood to forestall the withering of the great earlier cultures and may not be sufficiently comprehended in time to extend the survival of ours.

What are the Successes of the Ecologic Viewpoint?

We cannot as yet be sure whether apparent early successes are in fact only a longer fuse to bigger and better disasters, because we are at present unable to comprehend fully the complex inter-relationships we have undertaken to influence. However, in conjunction with one strand of the humanitarian view, the maintenance and improvement of our environment, the ecological viewpoint has become effective in mobilizing support for more than creation and preservation of great natural areas. It has led to major concern and some dubious controls of land poisoning and scarring operations, stream and ocean pollution, and intentional or unintentional disposal of wastes into the air. Of

equal importance has been the growing understanding of the significance of overpopulation, combined with the world-wide mania for affluence. The effects of these are perhaps most meaningfully measured
in terms of energy and food consumption and their pollutant by-
products.

Tremendous research operations have been put into motion to il-
luminate the interrelationships among all living species and things.
They have forced awareness of the scope and unexpectedness of the
unintended effects of technological discoveries and applications,
enough perhaps to insist that all significant breakthroughs be submitted to pilot applications so that unexpected consequences of their
use can be observed and evaluated.

The ecological view has created a new awareness that natural resources may after all not be the property of individuals but of all peoples, and that their exploitation falls into the realm of public concern.
Resources deserve public protection not only because their use may
produce unpleasant side effects, but also because the earth's resources
may be irreplaceable or damageable beyond further use. The ecological view has also brought new meaning to the concept of cost-benefit
evaluations of the application of innovations, which in all morality
must now be calculated in terms of damage or benefit to all species and
all resources over a long time span.

What are the Potential Failures of the Ecological Viewpoint?

This viewpoint has not been operative long enough to get a handle
on its weaknesses, but some can be anticipated. Overreaction to the
possibilities of ecological imbalances may lead to a short-run protection of the status quo that would eliminate the possibility of long-run
gains. Also, premature applications of the little that is known, may
lead to worse messes than the ones against which the correctives will be
directed.

Ecology obviously lends itself to exploitation, and many ventures
will be urged in the name of ecology. The obvious industrial bonanza
resulting from the development, promotion, and sale of antidotes to
control environmentally poisonous influences could at first blush only
be seen as an improvement. But these well-promoted advertising campaigns should be regarded as a warning against applying technologic
antidotes or substitutes on a massive scale without reasonable prior
ecological study. Moreover, such campaigns create a magnificent diversion away from the real issue, which is whether ecologic mischief
should be permitted to continue.

Ecology must not become man-centered. If it does, its practitioners
will not be clever enough to foresee the long-term effects on men of
planned neglect or damage to most other species and resources. It is

equally important that the ecologically powered fund of national energy not be focused on absolutely maintaining the status quo among species. Nature has continuously altered species balance, and man can undoubtedly continue to do so within wide limits derived from stringently applied forethought and experiments.

Similarly, it is important that ecology not lead us to insistence on the status quo of existing energy and food consumption relationships between countries, thereby dooming some to perpetual near starvation and deprivation while others continue to live in affluence beyond comparison or toleration. Excesses committed in the cause of ecological balance or status quo maintenance become glaring violations of values, such as equity, arising from that other great mainstream to our concept of health, humanitarianism.

The Third World View (Survival of "Victims")

A student review of this material, in a seminar, under the faculty leadership of Laura Anderson and George Keranen, produced a viewpoint of health from a sub-group, that of the domestic "Third World."[5] Purportedly this is the view held by a significant proportion of our minority populations. The students' position specifies the following parameters:

> We implicitly limit our discussion to the Third World population of the continental United States. But in our quest to delineate a set of shared belief systems about health, it is possible that our determinations will be proven to have a quality of universality. . . . This class is comprised of the people disenfranchised from the mainstream of their country's social structure for one reason or another. . . . Social scientists continue to debate the dynamics of this group, but all seem to agree that the manifest behavior and underlying thought processes exhibit a real degree of intra-commonality and differ enough from the norms of the larger society to justify special consideration.

The group saw the Third World as reactive rather than active or goal-oriented, and as placing much emphasis on maintaining the status quo, as a result of the extremely limited number of opportunities made available to it by the majority or ruling class. Persons in this underprivileged class do react when their meager status quo is threatened. The Third World is also seen as having a "tempo of life metered at the survival level. . . . and the Darwinian theory of natural selection can still be seen in unrestricted operation. Health is viewed as the natural state, God-given and neutral to enhancement by the human element. As a result, three major themes come into focus. There is an emphasis on *productivity, reproductivity,* and *mysticism.*"

These three keys, each having a major bearing on health outlooks and health practices were described by the students as follows:

Productivity.

Productivity is very important in the Third World. Self-survival and the survival of the family constellation is dependent upon it. Welfare practices in this country, in recent years, have distorted the scientific and lay view; but, suffice it to say that the dollar amount which actually reaches the needy could not sustain them without the productive input generated from within the Third World community. The extended family is significantly more prevalent at this level than in the population at large. Subjectively, the absence of health (the inability to produce) is shameful. Quite often a person will avoid treatment of a condition or completely deny the existence of a health problem until it is too late for corrective procedures. Motivated by the basic need to be productive and reinforced by the fear of being unable to—death is the only solution. Ironically, there is a great deal of compassion for and tolerance of the apparent lack of health in others.

Reproductivity.

Reproductivity is basic to the Third World life style. Birth control is a hot issue. Children are viewed as an extension of self. This is the one way to guarantee a future. It is often said that "life has been hard for me but my children will have it better". . . . This means that a major community concern will be for the well-being of the children.

Mysticism.

Finally, metaphysical elements play an important role in the health views of the Third World. Two components merge to provide impetus for this third theme. First, mysticism and theological exercise act as a buffer against the psychological characteristics born of oppression. Feelings of fallibility, vulnerability, impotence, helplessness, ignorance and predestination are handled by ascribing the responsibility for control over life and death to the "Higher Authority," a deity or a collection of deities. All health matters are more or less viewed as "God's will be done." There is a strong reliance on folk medicine to solve the day-to-day community health needs; persons presumably gifted with the power to heal and the knowledge of the ages are looked upon as a valuable community resource. The religious healer, witchdoctor, midwife or local L.V.N. is constantly called upon to dispense medical advice, medicinal potions, and other remedies to the ill. In addition, they administer aid and comfort to the involved families through friendship and counseling.

We are inclined to agree, as this class has stated, that there is a "quality of universality" about these points for groups which are "disen-

franchised from the mainstream of their country's social structure."
The two common factors seem to be the element of struggle for survival (either as individuals in terms of hard, physical labor, or as a group in terms of reproduction), and the preference for the metaphysical over the scientific, whether in the form of magic, folk medicine, or mysticism. We must, as planners, be aware that conditions we call bad may not seem so to sub-groups, and what we call good may be of little concern to them, given the pressure of their needs which allows little room for fanciful flights of imagination about new patterns of living.

This Third World viewpoint surely is a dominant one for those tens of millions involved, while the preceding sets of viewpoints tend to be diffused among the entire population, with relatively few people totally entangled with just one of those viewpoints. This further sets apart this significantly sized group. It is one that has few resources, a particular set of viewpoints that is not understood by the dominant group, and an excess of illness. It also is one that often displays easily visible personal differences that have for long been associated with a disrespected status and with latent, if not active, discrimination. How do we, the beholders, describe what is good and what is bad, what is strong and what is weak of such a viewpoint? As usual, we use our middle class standards and pass judgments accordingly.

What Are the Strengths of the Third World Viewpoint?

The ability to survive under minimal living conditions, the capacity to retain extensive familial and extended group interpersonal relations, the search for mutual survival, the fortitude to carry on in spite of illness, an evident sense of compassion and an ability to express concern meaningfully and to help others in illness and trouble, a sense of loyalty that often supersedes right and wrong, have all been commented on as the "happier" concomitants of the Third World outlook. The major thrust of this outlook is ostensibly survival, although as we shall discuss shortly and document in Chapter 4, this is survival at a measurable sacrifice of health and longevity.

What Are the Weaknesses of the Third World Viewpoint?

The fortitude associated with the need to produce is a threat to recognition of early or even advanced illness. Feelings about reproduction may further tax those already failing, and deny everyone in a family a better standard of living or health care (even for the essentials of survival). The reliance on mysticism and the so-called fatalism about individual survival augur poorly for concern about habits or practices which pertain to or protect health, or to the use of relevant health care early or late.

The student group saw as the major disadvantage to the holders of this viewpoint their resistance to change. Whether this is immutable or would change if doors to opportunity were thrown open is another matter. It does suggest that planning for social change with this group, under its current living circumstances, is probably going to have to move each of the four determinants of social change in order to get significant alterations in the behavior of those holding the Third World's viewpoint. This resistance to change also casts doubt on the possibility that the health of the Third World citizenry is likely to be affected significantly by what the health care sector alone does or does not do.

The most important point to be deduced is the need for sub-group (Third World) participation in planning. We all know about the resultant difficulties, but they are often handmade by the controlling majority, and can and have been surmounted with modest planning acumen. We label disadvantaged people as "victims" throughout this book, and insist that they must be gotten to the planning table, as a minimum, whenever their needs are under consideration. Tuberculosis "victims" are needed to consider the problem of tuberculosis. Third World "victims" must be present for discussions of all situations which cause excessive casualties to their members (just about every disease from hypertension to hernia, and just about every condition from lack of care to lack of understanding about every aspect of health).

A WORKING DEFINITION OF HEALTH FOR PLANNERS: CONVERSION OF THE CONCEPTS OF HEALTH INTO MEASURABLE ENTITIES

The critical ingredients of a definition of health can be garnered from each of the major value-belief systems and reconciled into a working definition. No single sentence can capture all of these aspects of health, although some come close to providing a conceptual picture.

Definitions

The World Health Organization defines health as "a state of complete physical, mental and social well-being, and not merely the absence of disease or infirmity." This is obviously an ideal state of affairs that few of us approach even at birth. It is not of any practical use as a standard against which to measure health or as a goal to try to achieve. However, it is significant, for it takes into account most of the factors that we now can agree are important.

According to Romano, "health consists in the capacity of the organism to maintain a balance in which it may be reasonably free of undue pain, discomfort, disability or limitation of action including social capacity."[6] A more complete view might state that: health consists of (1) the capacity of the organism to maintain a balance appropriate to its age and social needs, in which it is reasonably free of gross dissatisfaction, discomfort, disease, or disability; and (2) to behave in ways which promote the survival of the species as well as the self-fulfillment or enjoyment of the individual. If this concept were harshly condensed it might conclude that: health is a state of being in which the individual does the best with the capacities he has, and acts in ways that maximize his capacities.

Aspects of Health Needing Measurement

The multifaceted concept of health that is emerging must be given tangibility if planning bodies and health purveyors are to be able to give rational consideration to what health means to various members of society. This train of thought must be carried to the stage where it defines the nature of goals and measurements that need to be used by a planning body if it is to accord to health the multiplicity of meanings that society anticipates. In an excellent review, Goldsmith traces the span of definitions or concepts of health over into the derivation of indicators which can be used for purposes of measurement.[7] In the process he has gathered and analyzed many major definitions. His analysis lends support to our purpose, as have the more advanced Fanshel and Bush formulations.[8]

No less than eight separate scales must be used to measure the health of individuals. The scales are reasonably distinct. Several of the value-belief systems discussed contribute to each of the derived indices. The behavior which seeks "survival of species" is probably not really measurable, for it seems to be more of a group attribute than that of an individual, and is not the sum of any as yet easily measurable individual characteristics. The eight aspects of the state of health (or lack of it) that call for measurement and consideration are: (1) *prematurity of death,* (2) *disease* or departures from physiologic or functional norms appropriate to age and sex, (3) *discomfort* or illness, (4) *disability or incapacity,* (5) *internal satisfaction* (joy of living, self-realization), (6) *external satisfaction,* (7) *positive health,* and (8) *capacity to participate.*

In Chapter 5, these eight health scales are converted into indicators for assessing health status. The nature of goals that might be established for health could be phrased in terms of these eight rubrics, and the conversion of the concepts of health into measurable goals would be thereby completed.

THE SCOPE OF HEALTH CONCERNS

Inputs to Well-Being

The major inputs to health fall under the rubrics of environment, behavior, genetics, and health services (see Figure 1.1). These not only affect health but also interact with one another in such innumerable and intricate ways that I have found it desirable to tie them together in one systemic whole. However, to make the issues clearer, the four inputs will be briefly considered as though they were independent entities.

Environment

Social, cultural, political, educational, economic, and physical environments all need to be considered here. Their relationship to health and well-being is overwhelmingly well documented,[9] even though it is hard to estimate the exact contribution of each. Deprivation, frequently in all of these spheres, is the lot of a significant proportion of our citizenry, and its relationship to deficiencies in all kinds of well-being is readily observable. The effects of density on survival and mental illness[10] are not always clear, but the effects of education and to a lesser degree, those of income are clearly health correlated.[11] Vast health improvements and fantastically increased survival rates have been made solely through changes in the physical environment (insect, waste, and water control), with or without significant individual participation. In fact, we have helped to create a world population crisis by this onesided environmental manipulation. McHale provides a brief review and bibliography of man in the biosphere.[12]

Behavior

Personal behavior and habits are major influences on our well-being and our survival (consider smoking, drinking, dangerous driving, overeating, neglect of personal hygiene, delay in seeking medical care, etc.). These influences can be visualized as the incorporation of prior environmental influences into the makeup of each individual. Whether he has acquired his habit patterns from his parents, his peers, his teachers, or from mass media or advertising, his behavior reflects the way in which he reacts to environmental influences. The actual availability of health services might also be listed among these habit-shaping factors.

Heredity

Adverse genetic constitution (which may be confused with deleterious in-utero environmental influences) makes up another major determinant of well-being capacity.[13] Effects of heredity can be modified primarily through applications by the health services of genetic studies and counseling. The in-utero effects of the environment will be avoided through environmental control and health services. The possibilities for confusing effects of heredity and environment after birth have been the subject of many studies.[14] A brief review of genetic and congenitally acquired abnormalities and their effects throughout life has been provided by Kilbourne and Smillie.[15]

Health Care Services

Undoubtedly a significant factor in overcoming or avoiding illness, disability, and death, health care services nevertheless cannot continue to dominate our perception of how man stays healthy. Planning for health will involve altering each of the above listed inputs, not just the traditionally emphasized health (illness) care services. Increasing the health care input is not the only way, or necessarily the most economical or socially intelligent way, to remedy a situation where many influences are increasing the level of need. Finding other solutions to the problem may lessen the urgency for application of health care that often comes too late to avert serious disability or death. Witness auto accidents caused by defective cars or highways, malaria caused by uncontrolled mosquitoes, tuberculosis spread in the circumstances of poverty.

Manipulating inputs to attain a desired end is a complicated affair. Presumably, removing the financial barriers to medical care, which can be described either as a removal of an environmental obstacle or as the extension of accessibility of health services, would result in some improvements. Yet there is evidence that the differences in perinatal mortality among the various socioeconomic classes persisted for years in England, despite changes which equalized the availability of services. Differences in relative availability, and variations in patterns of utilization persisted even with almost total eligibility for care.[16] Koos[17] presents evidence of basic differences in health practices and attitudes towards health services among the various socioeconomic groups in the community. These manifestations represent corroborations of the "Third World" viewpoint and the difficulties it implies.

Aspects of Health: Vistas of Potential Achievements

A review of each of the facets we have used to describe health reveals that plenty of work is left to be done.

Prolongation of Life

The reasonable prolongation of life through prevention of premature death is still high, if not the highest, among health concerns. We can postulate, therefore, that although all gradations of concern are to be considered, planners will have to seek out goals that are within reach and that do not overlook the loss of relatively easy-to-save lives.

Minimization of Departures from Physiologic or Functional Norms Consistent with Age and Sex (Disease)

This level of health concerns introduces a high degree of complexity, focusing attention on the precursors of illness, such as genetic distortions, latent or incipient illness, sex-related or age-related physical conditions, and so on. Not only are we confronted with the problems of finding out about a person's health status before he becomes personally concerned, but also we are at the mercy of the psychosocial pressures and habit patterns which may result in unpredictable somatic problems.[18] Technically, we are still unprepared to provide norms for individuals (sex and chronological age are insufficient as markers) by which one can give biologically relevant examinations and health-relevant advice.

Minimization of Discomfort (Illness)

Some pains may be as obvious as the ugly physical wounds causing them. Others may be deep within the psyche—the terror, for example, of hallucination, or the agonies of being rejected by individuals or society. Humanitarian approaches may not tell which of these pains can be properly assigned to the health sector and which to other sectors. One pain may turn into another with frightening rapidity and overwhelming consequences. It may lead to incapacity, even death, either for the victim or for others in his environment.

Minimization of Disability (Incapacity)

From the point of view of loss in productivity, incapacity is presumably at least as serious to society as the loss due to premature deaths. Moreover, much incapacity, whether due to illness or incarceration, involves cost aspects well beyond the measurable loss of production. If the father of a family is incapacitated, the mother and children suffer losses which are difficult to define; incapacity of the mother also creates costs for the father and children. The incapacitated individual may become a burden to himself (or others) because he resents his dependent status or because he is no longer able to carry on a desired manner of existence. He may also become a high-cost burden to society, through hospitalization and medical care. Neither the significance nor the origins of incapacity are clear. Some persons are incapacitated by the loss of a limb or by a chronic source of pain. Some are deterred from activity by fears of failure, others by the image they have of themselves as a result of poor education, lack of clothing, or physical characteristics such as skin color.

Promotion of High Level Wellness or Self-Fulfillment (Internal Satisfaction)

Dunn calls for concern with a high level of "wellness," which may be described as "an integrated method of functioning which is oriented towards maximizing the potential of which the individual is capable within the environment where he is functioning."[19] No optimum level is delineated. Direction is set toward a higher potential of functioning, with no ceiling on what successive generations may aim for. This goal includes all of the health levels considered so far and adds one more, "maximizing potential," something which is also called for under the banners of self-fulfillment, self-expression, satisfaction, or desire to live.[20]

Self-fulfillment might be divided into three elements: a desire to survive; a desire to perpetuate one's species; and a highly personal sense of gratification related to social participation, the creation of outputs valued by one's society, recognition, love, the satisfaction of one's own desires, and the achievement of dignity.[21] Etzioni supports the idea of a universal set of *basic* human needs which are not determined by social structure, cultural patterns or socialization processes: *affection* and *recognition*.[22] Goal attainment can provide a man with dignity, recognition, and other forms of gratification. In some cases, the individual's purposes relate to gratification of desires on a relatively primitive level. Although this form of gratification has been socially controversial in America, it is becoming less so, and in many countries is accepted as a basic form of self-fulfillment. Gratification must therefore be considered in its cultural context. Self-fulfillment also seems to be closely related to a never ending succession of fresh perceptions of new ends, even new values, and attempts to achieve them. For many, self-fulfillment includes extending opportunities to others. But how many professionals in the health field would agree that health embraces high-level wellness or self-fulfillment?

A few problems arise. Self-fulfillment may, under conditions of stress and open conflict, lead a person (or a group such as the "Third World") to actions which are relevant to himself (or to the small group) but which are generally anti-social. How far do we support action such as cop-baiting or cop-killing, which will seem to some as despicable acts of lawlessness, while our hypothetical individual may view them as action toward "bringing down the tyrant?" We suspect that cop-killings or Boston Tea Parties occur with frequency only at times of tyranny, when radical change is called for. When social inequities are obviously being resolved, self-fulfillment will only occasionally pose a real threat for the larger society.

If self-fulfillment is generally an acceptable ideal, is it also useful? Clearly, fulfillment must be something different for each person, and perhaps must depend on how far up his ladder of aspiration and accomplishment he has come. How then can self-fulfillment ever be engaged by planners as an achievable goal? The answer is fairly clear. It need not be; it need only be a direction to be kept in mind as we doggedly work to free those whose life and well-being are threatened by gross hazards. At the same time, those further up the ladder can continue their climb more easily if we have not, intentionally or otherwise, imposed barriers at the higher levels. Obstruction or limitation at the higher steps of self-fulfillment undoubtedly leads to repercussions just as violent as obstructions further down the ladder. Since self-fulfillment for many individuals involves service and social participation, the very concentration of effort to encourage those at the lowest rungs of the ladder toward the limits of their capabilities should provide undreamed of levels of opportunity for self-fulfillment for persons in all walks of life who wish to lend a hand. The discussion of goal-setting and values in Chapter 2 bears on this point.

Promotion of a High Level of Satisfaction with the Environment (External Satisfaction)

This area is, of course, dependent on more than one set of forces. A person who is himself low on internal satisfactions may receive little satisfaction from what goes on around him, no matter how satisfying others may find it. At the same time, a person with a reasonable level of internal satisfaction may well find his environment limited. No doubt the internal and external satisfactions affect one another. One can even postulate that high internal and low external satisfaction in one person or group might set up the necessary dissonance, as well as provide inner strengths, with which to overcome external tribulations, and therefore forge a powerful influence for change. Bradburn and Caplovitz utilize both the internal and external satisfactions in their attempts to measure changes in feeling states of a population due to social, economic and political changes about them.[23]

Extension of Resistance to Ill Health and Creation of Reserve Capacity (Positive Health)

This aspect of health is still to be explored. It would seem to be a desirable approach which could be undertaken at a not unreasonable cost. When a physician intentionally provokes stress in a patient by a challenge or stressor test so as to watch its effect on glucose metabolism, kidney function, heart output, and so on, he is using the principle of provocation to look for evidence of potential failure not revealed by customary demands or tests. Obviously, the test is searching for a latent or incipient condition which, if discovered, could better be brought under control at this early stage. Guiding such a patient to a life style that would avoid acts likely to overstress him in relation to his Achilles' heel, creates one kind of resistance to ill health.

In a more general way, might it not be wise to look periodically for evidence of an unreasonable decline in the reserve of general vigor relative to age and sex? For example, can a person work or play all night and recover promptly to carry on the following day? Evidence of prematurely declining reserve might spark an investigation that would direct an individual to more appropriate work, recreation, and other living habits, and might prevent the development of illnesses.[24]

Cutting out tobacco is often accompanied by feelings of "boisterous health" on the part of those who never thought they were ill in the first place. A study of this phenomenon could be the source of clues about the real meaning of reserves of general well-being. Immunization to build up defenses against some disease could also be considered as a reserve measure. Similarly, particular habit patterns create, conserve or diminish reserves against various diseases.

Adaptable as man is to his environment, it should be noted that he has changed very little genetically over thousands of years.[25] His genetic constitution is the basis of his biological capabilities, which are activated by stimuli from the environment. To a degree at least, genes determine responses to stimuli and in this sense may be considered traits. Not all genes are active; some will be activated only under certain influences. Investigation of potentially adverse response-points in the individual's biological makeup could suggest habits that avoid the stimulation of adverse reactions and maintain reserve. The appropriate use or avoidance of exercise might be one such example.

Increasing Capacity to Participate in Health Matters

This facet takes note of those who are chronically victimized by society, most particularly those of the "Third World" who suffer from poverty and ignorance and who are easily, traditionally, and actively discriminated against. They have no trust for the system and, therefore, little or none for its health-promoting services. When they are cajoled or, in desperation, driven to use health services, they do not know for what purpose information is requested nor where records are sent. They may have had skirmishes with the law, welfare, bill collectors, schools—what do they dare reveal to the system which may, and sometimes joyously does, squeal on them? Sub-groups, in turn, often have a bad reputation with the system for accuracy, veracity, comprehension, even intelligence, and may soon be made aware of their presumed low estate by discourtesies, lack of consideration, and blatantly tactless and distressing discussions about them held in their presence.[26]

In addition, these people have neither the cost-free time, if they are marginally employed, nor the means to get to or pay for care. When care is accessible financially, its costs in transportation and time may still be prohibitive. The victims often cannot better themselves financially or environmentally without losing their health care eligibility because of financial or residence requirements which will not follow them. Thus, a marginal general improvement may mean a loss of health care coverage, and upward mobility can occur at a cost that is excessive, if not dangerous.

These same groups may have a shortage of faith in science and health care, and of education which could give them access to new ideas and information, thus bettering their options for health or health care. They also have a way of life that is remarkably hazardous from conception to death, and would seem to require more, rather than less, health support. Obviously, increasing capacity to participate includes mobilization of the full environmental set of forces, all the behavioral ones, and much of health care. It is astounding how closely the plight of poor people, so bounded by their very poverty that every move they make seems likely to risk health or well-being and further poverty, parallels the kinds of constraints that poverty creates for nations.[27]

Deviancy as a Useful Concept

Thurlow[28] suggests that psychosocial causes are indeed important sources of illness (at least in some persons). Typically, these illnesses break through at some point, taking the form of bacterial, metabolic, traumatic, or emotional diseases. In addition, psychosocial forces probably determine an individual's willingness to "give in" and accept the sick role. Such a person receives more medical care and his illnesses are more frequently diagnosed, adding to the total number and variety of somatic episodes credited to him.

These kinds of concerns indicate the need for a unifying or holistic, even multifaceted, concept of health and disease in place of a collection of innumerable, specific, isolated and unrelated causes for departures from health. Before attempting to outline this more nearly total approach, some of the terms to be used must be defined so as to explain how they relate to the concept of deviancy. The concept of deviancy is very useful to the planner as he sets about contributing to well-being. Once we have seen how to take man apart for purposes of measurement of health, it helps us put him back together again.

Deviancy is the disruption or alteration of a person's ability or desire to carry out his self-assigned and/or socially assigned roles, whether resulting from internal or external influences. Deviance may be observed or imputed. A person labeled deviant may be encouraged or forced into a clearcut deviant role. For example, a normal child mistakenly labeled as a rheumatic heart disease victim becomes or acts out the role of a cardiac cripple. (For a classic discussion of "roles" see Parsons.[29]) Deviancy may also embrace important new or creative roles which are atypical or unacceptable to the times.

Disability and *incapacity* also represent the disruption of a person's ability or capacity to carry out one or more of his normally accepted roles. In common parlance, these terms, although equivalent in meaning to deviancy, rarely carry the pejorative flavor which clings to the term deviancy in lay usage.

Illness or lack of well-being is the manifestation of a disease or condition which may or may not progress to the extent of causing any disability or disruption of role function.

Disease or disordered functioning, although not necessarily carrying the ultimate threat of illness or disability to the person suffering from it, becomes a deviancy once its presence is acknowledged, and particularly if it becomes the object of medical care or surveillance.

Good Health or well-being, as we have already indicated, is a personally and societally relevant set of optimal relationships between one's states of physical, emotional and social functioning, not solely the absence of illness, disability or disease. Good health is only one among many descriptors of a person's ability to function in the midst of a great variety of biological and social goals and desires. It is subject to myriad variables. Most obviously, capacities normally change with age and with exposure to social and physical environments. What is a normal expectation of physical performance for a young laborer might be life-threatening to a middle-aged scholar. Good health is basically the capacity for those tasks for which a man has been socialized and trained. It is different for every walk of life and varies for each individual with the shifting assignment of family or professional duties, of recreational and social activities. These differing role assignments are not regarded as deviant. However, it is difficult to accept as non-deviant infirmities brought on by old age. In fact, it would even seem that in our society old age per se is basically regarded as a deviant state.

We have focused on the aspects of deviancy which bring an individual to society's remedial attentions because he has not been carrying out his roles. But this does not mean that deviancy has only negative connotations. Improper role playing may also be the most distinctive identifier of creativity. Persons perceived as being antisocial—they avoid currently accepted role norms—may, with or without persecution (attempts at reformation), also be perceived as gifted artists, artisans, or innovators. Even persons with manifestly deviant psychological or somatic attributes may be sought out for special and often well-rewarded roles as performers, basketball players, wrestlers, and so on.

Depending, then, on the culture, deviancy may be a badge of honor and well-rewarded, or a stigma, such as the one often attached to the ailing, who can either be treated or punished. Of course, once the deviant is allowed to proceed in his new roles, only semantics decides whether he remains a deviant or becomes socially acceptable, unconventional though his role may be.

The concept of deviancy is a most suitable framework within which to consider departures from well-being. To make the point sharper, we are saying that the significant health and social problems are, or generally soon become, interrelated and often indistinguishable. Their manifestations change and interchange; they cluster and show up in many forms in the same individual, so that often one cannot be guided toward the resolution of a well-being problem by an exclusively medical outlook. The "battered child" occupies the obvious no-man's-land between physical and psychological ill health in a family, but so do alcoholism, addiction, peptic ulcer, asthma or hypertension in an individual.[30]

The promotion of the concept of deviancy in health circles is, of course, intended to be a permanent reminder of the impact of social forces, imperative if intelligent consideration is to be given to altering the inputs that affect health. Deviancy concepts are concerned with both transitory (primary) and way-of-life or career (secondary) forms of deviancy (the latter sometimes arising out of innumerable transitory phenomena).[31] Society reacts to deviancy in accordance with whether it presents itself in acceptable form and leads to acceptable actions (for example, "respectable" psychosomatic illness which takes one to the doctor), or in an unacceptable form (such as latent homosexuality, which might lead to another unacceptable form, the excessive use of alcohol). Sometimes, the manifestation is acceptable, but not the action to which it leads; sometimes the reverse is true. Patients showing acceptable deviant behavior are distinguished from nonpatients by their sickness behavior, not by their sickness—another way of illustrating the dichotomy between need (professionally defined) and demand (consumer defined). This issue has been elaborated by K. E. Boulding, an economist, in a most effective way.[32] The dichotomy points out, however, that it is difficult to know the size of health problems and when or how to intervene. Moreover, if sickness behavior violates other social norms, it becomes "criminal" or "insane" behavior. Obviously, society's institutions act in these instances on quite different etiologic and therapeutic principles, and the whole matter of care for the deviant is confused by society's needs for protection against strange (unacceptable) behavior.

In other words, society's reaction to a deviancy helps to establish the nature of the deviancy. From a medical standpoint, this complicates the matter, for typhoid is typhoid, or so we would like to think.[33] We must learn to separate the deviancy from the behavior grafted on to individuals by society's reaction to the kinds of people who most frequently display that particular deviancy. If the causes of a particular deviance are obscure and the felt illness vague, the person may be forced into accepting the posture of the neurotic, because, as a rule, only traditional somatic sources of illness are dealt with by physicians. A neurotic soon perceives what he is free to describe and what he must conceal. He may even be taught to proceed according to values inimical to acknowledgment and exposure of the forces which create his deviancy (illness). The definition of the sick role by Parsons[34] and a review of the concept of deviancy as a departure from well-being by Freidson[35] are landmarks in the comprehension of illness and illness behavior.

Waitzkin summarizes another stream of concern. Deviancy or the sick role as expressed by illness brings the individual to medical type care. The sick role provides a controllable form of deviance which mitigates potentially disruptive conflicts between the needs of one's personality and the role demands made on him by his social system.[36] This in no way changes our plea for suitable services for an illness or for a personality role mismatch, but it does not seem necessary or wise to penalize the medical care sector with providing care for all such mismatches. Claiming physical illness may provide good excuses to "the boss," but we would do better to have the deviant reach a service which would help resolve conflicts in a positive way, rather than temporizing with irrelevant pills, services or excuses from work.

If indicators are to be of practical use in determining the level of well-being and in categorizing the departures therefrom, they must not focus solely on the etiology of supposedly isolated disease causes. Indicators should serve as a reminder of all the manifestations that make up ill health or lack of well-being. Thus, deviancy terms are very useful in characterizing departures from well-being.

Labels and Treatment Assignments: Interrelationships of Deviancies and Multiplicity of Treatment Sources

The scope of what must be scanned by planners at the outset is awesomely broad. Figure 3.1 provides only a sampling and at the same time indicates, at least in a crude way, the contributions to care or control made by several professional fields or social institutions in each deviancy area sampled.

The following are some of the implications that come to mind in examining Figure 3.1. The words *disability* and *deviancy* are now used

FIGURE 3.1
SAMPLING OF DEPARTURES FROM WELL-BEING (DEVIANCY) AND ESTIMATE OF CURRENT
EXTENT OF ROLE RESTORING ASSIGNMENTS* MADE BY SOCIETY TO VARIOUS OF ITS AGENTS

SAMPLING OF DEVIANCY LABELS

Society's Agents	crimi-nality	delin-quency	addic-tion	alco-holism	unem-ployed jobless	drop-out	suicide	mental illness	ulcers	acci-dents	measles	URI	aged-ness	cancer
Education														
Religion														
Economics														
Law Enforcement														
Social Work														
Mental Health														
Physical Health														

*Assignment may include all or part of prevention, diagnosis, treatment and rehabilitation.

Arrow indicates current tendency to increase or decrease extent of assignment.

Height of shaded area in each box indicates relative extent the society's agent plays in each deviancy.

interchangeably to indicate an inability to function fully in one or more roles which are either societally or self-assigned.

The nature of a deviance is assumed to be variable, and interveners may play a key role in shifting its nature or appearance. Therefore:
The deviance label in great part depends on which resource accepts it, and by which of these resources its holder is willing to be processed. And so, the name and nature of the deviancy is truly a treacherous entity for the planner who wishes to intervene intelligently. This state of affairs suggests that many alternative interventions might be useful in assisting a given deviant.

More than one "label" per person is common, and any person having significant problems in one area of disability or deviancy may be expected to have them in others. Persons frequently shift from area to area. Moreover, through intervention in one area of disability, a person may be moved to another.

Smaller, even if significant, problems, initially obscured by massive or threatening pathology, become visible when the latter are favorably acted upon.

Emotional problems may change into somatic or social problems, and vice versa.

The interveners push the deviant from one deviancy area to the next according to the service they believe his stage of disability requires. For example, the acute asthmatic will come into emergency care, his long-range therapy may take him to allergy and psychiatric services, and needs unearthed there may shift him to services provided by welfare for housing and employment.

Inappropriate interventions create new problems. For example, the "don't work" advice often given in error to a peptic ulcer or post-coronary victim creates dependency and thus disease-provoking, unnecessary anxiety about unmet responsibilities.

Individual deviancies have been viewed from many etiologic, functional, and therapeutic modality positions and may be serviced accordingly. For example:
Society's assignments of responsibility for helping any one kind of disability are typically shared. Most persons who seriously need help require the services of more than one set of institutionalized skills, such as those of a doctor, nurse, and a dietitian, as well as help from more than one sector, such as clergy, medicine, and economic assistance. Preventive aspects of control customarily come from one social agent, treatment from others, rehabilitation from still others. "Crisis" rescue may be separated from all other health intervention points; witness the major police and fire department roles with suicide, mental illness, and disaster victims. Categories of

services and assignments are changed as new concepts of etiology occur in an area of deviance, or even when new diagnostic tools are introduced. Because such changes do not occur uniformly, different communities or even different institutions in a single community will be working in various ways. A clergyman does in one situation what a psychiatrist, public health nurse, social worker, or psychologist does in others. Deviancy labels may be changed as new skills are created or as different skills enter the picture to care for a condition.

No two communities necessarily make the same assignments for care. A single category of deviancy may be perceived in terms of its danger to others, its etiology, or the skill most ready, able, or available to service the problem at the time it gets community notice. Where and how a problem is to be cared for in a community may be determined by political maneuvering, the availability of new resources, or reactions to particular agencies and modes of operation. (Health Department versus Mental Health for care of alcoholics in California; constraint and punishment of rioters vs. the alleviation of underlying causes in Watts.) Society also shifts labels by legislation or court interpretation. The old social agent may be carried along under a new banner or may relinquish the client to a new social agent. For example, alcoholics are now being sent to medical care instead of penal care in some communities as a result of court decisions.

Available assistance on behalf of one type of deviancy may unintentionally open the door for persons to use this more easily available service for the wrong kind of problem. The lonely person who comes to the clinic waiting room loses his *lonely* label and gets an *illness* label. The person who is too *poor* to purchase 25 cents worth of fuel comes to the clinic to keep warm and thereby gets 25 dollars worth of medical attention for his *illness*.

The agent who first receives the client may cement him to a special "type" of deviancy. Working in one area and understanding one set of problems, the helping and helpful agent tries to fit people into his brand of clientele and teaches them the appropriate behavior. The kind of service used in considering departures from well-being not only has a tremendous impact on how a problem is looked at but may determine how intensively it will be attacked.

Deviancy has complex origins. It can be assumed that just as there are four interrelated streams of inputs that affect health (Figure 1.1), so deviancy of any consequence has complex origins. Not only are there multiple sources of inputs or etiological or contributory factors, but many deviancies arise from others. For example, because individuals are often part of a larger pattern of deviance, their families may be a better unit to study when interventions are contemplated. (Remember the wife who becomes alcoholic as her husband is sobered up, and the family who cannot surrender a schizophrenic child to care without cracking up.) In Chapter 7, the systems analysis approach to problem solving and goal achievement elaborates on complex origins of problems.

APPLYING THE CONCEPT OF DEVIANCY TO PLANNING FOR WELL BEING

Use of the deviancy or role disability concept appears to have practical advantages in the initial planning stage of assessment and priority setting for problems to be studied. If the medically-oriented morbidity and mortality-labeling approach is used exclusively, even when aided by the best diagnostics available, a different kind of casualty figure is obtained. Such figures cannot be compared between one condition and the next for extent or significance of disability, and they do not allow comparisons of the relative burdens imposed on individuals or society. There are major problems as to what constitutes a medical diagnosis that will be useful to planners. For example, when is diabetes a diagnosis? When it is a gene in a predictable carrier? A latent disease in a predictably potential victim? A clinical entity with symptoms? A clinical entity with disabling complications? When deviancy characteristics are used, results at least indicate the numbers of the currently accepted types or degrees of disabilities, even though initially the etiological considerations may be unrevealed.

By taking cognizance of the deviancy labels, the community can participate in the assessment of its ills. Once the source of distress is identified, and analysis begins to focus on the cause of the problem and what can be done about it, use can be made of more technical information, such as bodily processes or genetics which can be contributed by physicians, behavioral responses by social scientists, or responses to other aspects of the environment by scientists from the appropriate disciplines. True, many situations, such as high incidence of tuberculosis, seem clearly defined because of the single underlying identical characteristic of all cases—the presence of a particular organism. But it does not arise solely from medically-controllable conditions. It is overwhelmingly associated with poverty, ignorance, overcrowding, malnutrition, somewhat with genetics, and but minimally with health care or with the reservoir of health care personnel. In areas of high incidence, it may be reasonably effectively immunized against by lay personnel at a low cost in dollars or expertise.

Once the issues of origins and consequences of a health problem or deviancy are made clear (not obscured by professional proprietorship as might be the case in adhering to medical nomenclature), there is ample opportunity to determine which factors contribute to the deviancy. Then responsibility for action can be placed on the sector with the most relevant or most feasible set of preventives or remedies at its disposal. More typically, many preventive or treatment modalities must be combined even for such a simple thing as control of tuberculosis—for example, medication, appropriate work and family support, appropriate rest and diet, counseling, or even major assistance with habits or personality disintegration, particularly when they threaten the capacity to carry out required modalities of therapy.

For purposes of rational planning we conclude that:

There are several measurable and meaningful aspects of health (eight are developed as providing adequate comprehensiveness).

We will continue to be concerned with multiple inputs to each aspect of health as well as to all of health.

The concept of deviancies is useful in getting public testimony about health problems and as a reminder that the manifestations of deviancy are constantly changing and are heavily socially determined.

We must remember that society regards problems, irrespective of origins, in terms of their affect on society, and that control or care of deviancies may therefore be assigned to many institutions and sectors other than those labeled health or those guided by medically-oriented skills and interests, even when the problems have a component of what has traditionally been called ill health.

All of the relevant societal agents must be represented at the planning table.

REFERENCES

1. Edward S. Rogers, *Human Ecology and Health* (New York: Macmillan, 1960), 267-76.
2. Great Britain, *Report of Royal Commission on Local Government in Great London, 1957-60* (London: Her Majesty's Stationery Office), Chapter 7.
3. Vincent Taylor, *How Much is Good Health Worth?* (Santa Monica, California: The Rand Corporation, P-3945, 1969).
4. Talcott Parsons, *The Social System* (Glencoe, Illinois: Free Press, 1958).
5. Jimmie E. Armstrong, et al., "Another Value-Belief System: The Third World Concept of Health," School of Public Health, University of California, Berkeley, August 1971, mimeographed.
6. John Romano, "Basic Orientation and Education of the Medical Student," *Journal of the American Medical Association* 143 (June 3, 1950), 411.
7. Seth B. Goldsmith, "The Status of Health Status Indicators," Department of Health Services Administration, School of Public Health and Tropical Medicine, Tulane University, New Orleans, July 1971, mimeographed.

8. S. Fanshel and J. W. Bush, "A Health-Status Index and Its Application to Health-Services Outcomes," *Operation Research* 18 (November/December 1970), 1021-66.

9. U.S. Department of Health, Education, and Welfare, Division of Research and Welfare Administration, "Low Income Life Styles," by L. M. Irelan, 1966.
   Charles T. Stewart, Jr. "Allocation of Resources to Health," *The Journal of Human Resources* 6,1 (Spring, 1971), pp. 103-22.
   Richard Auster, Irving Leveson, Deborah Sarachek. "The Production of Health, an Exploratory Study," *The Journal of Human Resources* 4, 4 (Fall, 1969), pp. 411-36.
   Robert J. Haggerty. "The Boundaries of Health Care," *The Pharos,* (July, 1972), 106-11.
   Warren Winkelstein. "Epidemiological Considerations Underlying the Allocation of Health and Disease Care Resources," *International Journal of Epidemiology* 1, 1 (Spring, 1972), pp. 69-74.

10. Anthony J. Marsella, Manuel Escudero, and Paul Gordon, "The Effects of Dwelling Density in Filipino Men," *Journal of Health and Social Behavior* 11 (December 1970), 288-94. Edward T. Hall, *The Hidden Dimension* (Garden City, New York: Doubleday, 1966). Robert E. Mitchell, "Some Social Implications of High Density Housing," *American Sociological Review* 36 (February 1971), 18-29.

11. Evelyn M. Kitagawa, "Social and Economic Differentials in Mortality in the United States, 1960." Mimeographed paper distributed at the Session on Socio-economic Differentials in Mortality, General Assembly and Conference of International Union of Scientific Study of Population, London, September 3-11, 1969.

12. John McHale, *The Ecological Context* (New York: Braziller, 1970).

13. V. A. McKusick, "Ethnic Distribution of Disease," *The Journal of Chronic Disease* 20 (March 1967), 115-18.

14. Jan Howard and Barbara L. Holman, "The Effects of Race and Occupation on Hypertension Mortality," *Milbank Memorial Fund Quarterly* 48 (July 1970), 263-96.

15. Edwin D. Kilbourne and Wilson G. Smillie, *Human Ecology and Public Health,* 4th ed. (New York: Macmillan, 1969), 29-78.

16. Richard M. Titmuss, "The Role of Distribution in Social Policy," *Social Security Bulletin* 28 (June 1965), 11-20.

17. Earl L. Koos, *The Health of Regionville* (New York: Columbia University Press, 1954).

18. B. P. Dohrenwend, "Social Status, Stress and Psychological Symptoms," *American Journal of Public Health* 57 (April 1967), 625-32.

19. Halbert L. Dunn, "What High Level Wellness Means," *Canadian Journal of Public Health* 50 (November 1959), 447-57. Halbert L. Dunn, *High Level Wellness* (Arlington, Virginia: R. W. Beatty, 1961).

20. L. C. Ford, M. Cobb, and M. Taylor, "Community Health Nursing," Western Interstate Commission for Higher Education (WICHE), East Campus, University of Colorado, Boulder, February 1967, 13-37.

21. Abraham H. Maslow, *Motivation and Personality* (New York: Harper & Row, 1954), Chapter 5.

22. Amitai Etzioni, "Basic Human Needs, Alienation and Inauthenticity," *American Sociological Review* 33 (December 1968), 870-85.

23. Norman M. Bradburn and David Caplovitz, *Reports on Happiness* (Chicago: Aldine Publishing Co., 1965), 1-21.
24. H. John Thurlow, "General Susceptibility to Illness: A Selective Review," *The Canadian Medical Association Journal* 97 (December 2, 1967), 1-8.
25. Pan American Health Organization (WHO), "Man and His Environment: Biomedical Knowledge and Social Action," by Rene Dubos (*Scientific Publication* No. 131), March 1966.
26. Anselm L. Strauss, "Medical Ghettos," *Trans-Action* (May 1967), 7-15.
27. Naomi Caiden and Aaron Wildavsky, *Planning and Budgeting in Low Income Countries,* forthcoming, (New York: John Wiley & Sons, Spring, 1974), Chapter 2.
28. H. J. Thurlow, Ibid. No. 24, 1-8.
29. T. Parsons et al. *Toward a General Theory of Action,* (Cambridge, Harvard University Press, 1951).
30. Thomas H. Holmes and Minoru Masuda, "Psychosomatic Syndrome." *Psychology Today* (April 1972), 71-72, 106. Peter Sedgwick "Illness-Mental and otherwise." The Hastings Center Studies 1 (1973) 19-40. Alan Sheldon "Toward a General Theory of Disease and Medical Care" in *Systems and Medical Care* edited by Alan Sheldon, Frank Baker and Curtis P. McLaughlin, (Cambridge, M.I.T. press 1970), 84-125. Howard Brody, "The Systems View of Man: Implications for Medicine, Science, and Ethics." Perspectives in Biology and Medicine (Autumn 1973) 71-92.
31. David Mechanic, "The Sociology of Medicine: Viewpoints and Perspectives," *Journal of Health and Human Behavior* 7 (1966), 237-48.
32. Kenneth E. Boulding, "The Concept of Need for Health Services," *Milbank Memorial Fund Quarterly* 44, Part 2 (October 1966), 202-23.
33. Manfred Pflanz and Johann Juergen Phode, "Illness: Deviant Behavior or Conformity," *Social Science and Medicine* 4 (December 1970), 645-55.
34. T. Parsons, Ibid No. 4.
35. Eliot Freidson, "Disability as Social Deviance," *Sociology and Rehabilitation,* ed. by M. B. Sussman (Washington, D.C.: American Society of Sociologists, December 15, 1965), 71-99. Eliot Freidson, *Profession of Medicine* (New York: Dodd Mead, 1970), 205-44.
36. H. Waitzkin, "Latent Functions of the Sick Role in Various Institutional Settings," *Social Science and Medicine* 5 (1971), 45-75.

4. Comprehensive Planning for Health: Concepts, Contrasting Points of View, Importance, Limitations

It is time to relate what has been said about planning and about health. Because in the United States Public Law 89-749 set the precedent of including the word "comprehensive" with health planning, I will also pursue what seems implied by that term as applied to health planning.

PLANNING FOR HEALTH AND COMPREHENSIVENESS

A Working Understanding of Planning

In Chapter 2 we explored our interest in matters of public concern and in democratically undertaking deliberate attempts at social change. Planning is seen as having the purposes of:

Specifying what is wanted.

Attaining what is wanted by means of designing plans and strategy for accomplishment.

Measuring the degree of success in attaining what was desired.

Planning, therefore, can also be described in everyday parlance as a marriage broker for politics and technology.

A Working Understanding of Health

Experience tells us that it is customary in all health circles to repeatedly and compulsively confuse health care services with health. Therefore, you are referred to Figure 1.1, and the related discussion in Chapter 3, which says, in summary, that:

The major influences determining degrees of individual health will include a great deal more than health care services.

Health is a relative matter.

Psychic or somatic well-being is commonly judged to be absent only because we observe disordered social functioning.

The need to consider not only manifestations of health but all inputs to it is stated pungently by Seliger in reference to the comparable but larger and overriding problems of the mindless use of resources and burgeoning population:

111

> To argue that there is still room in many other places for our present rate of expansion is like ignoring a cancer because the rest of the body is still healthy. So, we blithely go about picking up tin cans, putting better filters on our smoke stacks, and setting water quality standards for our rivers and bays. In the terminal cancer ward this is called making the patient comfortable. But in the terminal cancer ward nobody fools himself—not the doctors, not even the victims. . . . And so we busy ourselves by concentrating on the symptoms of this malignancy.[1]

We need to consider not only all departures from health, but at the same time all the inputs, both those that contribute to ill health and those that avoid or overcome it. Because resources are limited, we must consider how to spend them wisely. An excellent study by Burgess, Cotton and Peterson[2] compares death rates from various major causes in three countries, and points out clearly when attacks might profitably be made on illness, when on the triggering or background factors. A similar study is available for infant deaths in the United States and Sweden.[3]

Figure 4.1 charts the three general areas for intervention in behalf of health: existing problems, predisposing factors, and background factors, and compares the three in terms of security of cause-and-effect knowledge, satisfaction to be derived, effectivity, ability to evaluate effects, and costs. To quote Elizabeth Jolly:

> The limitation of health planner concern to interventions first at the level of morbidity and then to its immediate predisposing factors has been a natural consequence of the fact that interventions at the level of the basic background require implementation by non-health sectors. However, on the wide-angle screen which the politically mandated concept of "comprehensiveness" now requires us to use, it is becoming increasingly clear that health planners can no longer avoid the background inputs to health if they are to protect the investment of their efforts at the level of morbidity and, equally important, if they are to exert any control over the kinds and quality of morbidity with which they will be confronted.[4]

This in no way means that we are required to do all things at one time. It does mean, however, that we should look at all health conditions and consider which call for the most urgent attention, which for most profitable or feasible attacks (see Chapter 6 for criteria for deciding on priorities), and the point at which attack should be centered (see Chapter 7 for problem analysis). On just this basis, Jean Mayer makes an incisive critique of the "De Bakey Report" (heart, cancer, and stroke), for its futile recommendations.[5]

We must assemble an overall viewpoint about what is worth heading for, so that in our haste to remedy undesirable situations we do not

Figure 4.1 INTERVENTIONS AGAINST THREE ZONES OF HEALTH FACTORS (Modified from Elizabeth Jolly)

Health Problems (Psycho-socio-somatic)	Adverse Triggering, Intermediary or Predisposing Inputs	Background Factors of Well-Being
● Heart Disease, Accidents, Mental Illness, Cancer, Etc.	● Environmental: e.g. smog, starvation ● Fetal: e.g. infection, metabolic deprivation ● Emotional: e.g. stress ● Intellectual: e.g. intellectual deprivation ● Health Services: e.g. unavailability, unobtainability, low quality ● Behavior: e.g. bad habits ● Heredity: e.g. adverse genes, etc.	● Population Characteristics: e.g. size, gene pool, growth rate, etc. ● Physical Environment: e.g. resource quality, quantity, ecologic balance ● Social Systems: e.g. societal behavior, health care system ● Individual Characteristics: e.g. health, happiness, intellectual functioning, adaptability
If Attack Here: ● Cause and effect validity can be kept high. ● Can provide some general satisfaction from "easy" to obtain good quality health care services and from some gains in health that will result. ● Will cut a few health burdens and create new ones. Will not prevent many occurrences, not even too many reoccurrences. Some specific preventions good, e.g. polio. ● Effects are those primarily of repair, often too little, too late. Non-self-maintaining except insofar as immunizations, therapy and rehabilitation "last." ● Effects will be rapidly observable over weeks to a year. ● Effects are fairly easy to measure. ● Costs will be moderate overall, but majestically high per unit of gain. They will be never-ending.	*If Attack Here:* ● Cause and effect validity is fair. ● Can provide some general satisfaction from easier to obtain specific services and possibly from some improvement in health that will result. ● Will cut some health burdens and need for health care; will minimize occurrences and reoccurrences of many kinds of ill health. ● Effects will be maintained mostly as long as specific efforts or programs are enforced. Some self-reinforcing of improvements is possible. ● Effects will be observable over months to years. ● Effects will be hard to measure relative to a given intervention when many other factors are at work. ● Costs will be high, probably midway between the other two per unit of effects.	*If Attack Here:* ● Cause and effect validity often low. ● Can provide much general satisfaction as through 　—employment 　—recreation 　—housing 　—food 　—education 　—safe, cheery surroundings. ● Will cut per capita health burdens and need for health care services in each age group. Will minimize occurrences and reoccurrences of ill health of all kinds. ● Effects will be well-maintained, even self-reinforcing of improvements. ● Effects will be slow to set in, from one to many years. ● Effects will be hard to measure in relation to any one intervention. ● Costs will be very high, long-term, but in all probability much the best investment because of the broad scope of effects.

113

overlook long-range welfare. We do not quarrel with the high probability that cause-and-effect validity is likely to be maximal for the most immediate zone of interventions (direct attack on health problems) and that it may be less close or hinge upon longer chains of causality if we employ interventions effective at the intermediary or triggering inputs to ill health. Cause-and-effect may be even more speculative as we come to the interventions to be used against background factors of well-being.[6] Some of the attempts to shed light on human ecology are beginning to provide the means of increasing our validity.[7]

The Meaning of Comprehensiveness in Health Planning

Although Public Law 89-749 has given us the impetus to pursue comprehensive health planning, there is no intent in any part of this presentation to be limited by the content of that law or by its omissions. We in the United States now have the concern that the law imparted, and we anticipate that it has given rise to much more than could have been understood at the time the legislation was drafted.

If planning for health is to be comprehensive, all aspects of health problems, all health-related aspects of social problems, and all services directed toward the prevention or amelioration of problems or consequences are the beginning of what must be taken into account. The health activities which are aided, promoted, funded, or carried out by public agencies at all levels of government are only one of the planner's concerns. Health activities initiated by voluntary agencies, professional or citizen groups, and those carried out for private and personal gain are equally a concern of comprehensive health planning. Anyone or anything affected by health-related matters or participating in them can expect his interests to be part of comprehensive health planning.

Concern with All Manifestations and Consequences of Departures from Health and All the Inputs to Health

Concern for health has traditionally been limited to concerns with morbidity and mortality and thus with the so-called direct causes of each type of sickness episode. Health is now seen more broadly and in many, if not most, of the aspects described in Chapter 3. We will not repeat those here except to say that departures from health have further consequences for individuals and society. The inputs to any degree of good or bad health have multiple and complex origins (Figure 1.1), and these, too, must be the basis of any earlier interceptive or preventive interventions. The case is getting stronger for a better understanding of etiology, and this must modify the choice of interventions.[8]

Concern with All Parties Involved, the Partnership for Health

Establishing the nature of the victims of a situation and identifying the people who stand to gain or lose from corrections addressed to it are primary considerations. Such knowledge is part of planning democratically. Moreover, it is a basic element of strategy, for without concern for who gains or who loses, a very small amount of implementation can ever be expected. In Chapter 7 we explore the means of searching out and drawing into the planning those who will be involved, including those who must serve, those who must administer, those who must approve, and those who must cooperate in utilizing the services. In Chapter 11 we further explore how people are brought into participating in the implementation of what they have already helped to shape. A review of mental health services for urban Mexican-Americans points up the inescapable necessity of gaining consumer involvement in planning and operation, without which little utility can be expected.[9]

It is evident that health planning must involve extensive collaboration; Public Law 89-749 somehow captured this realization even if little else about the law seems reassuring. Many possibilities have been expressed about the nature of the partnership referred to in Public Law 89-749. The following have all been accepted as reasonable and, in fact, very important interpretations:

Joint action among the major levels of government; federal, state, metropolitan, and local. This idea remains one of the key interpretations, even though six years after the law was enacted no national level health planning body had yet been established with which the lower levels of government might partner. All that is available at the national level for this purpose is a part of the Public Health Service that has neither the authority nor the capacity to do planning. The PHS remains a very peculiar partner, one with authority over how its partners behave, but with no particular ability to create a national sense of direction, or even to measure the nature of the nation's drift and probable path. In a series of articles around this topic in the *Bulletin of the New York Academy of Medicine*, released three years after the law was passed, only one contributor thought to raise this issue.[10]

Joint venturing between the public, semi-public, and private medical interests. This interpretation has been among the most meaningful and profitable. As a result of the bitter public-private battles over P. L. 89-97 (Medicare) and P.L. 89-239 (Regional Medical Programs), a feeling emerged among health interests that decentralized get-togethers might go a long way towards resolving future issues in a less openly antagonistic and destructive way.

Progress on this front has been noteworthy. Participation in planning by the private medical sector, denounced for so long by its more conservative segments, has gone on remarkably well under the leadership, pressures, and education of the medical societies. By contrast, the middle-class, community-oriented, semi-public, voluntary health agencies have a checkered history of participation to date. The old line disease or organ agencies have mostly viewed with alarm and not understood the possibilities. The so-called planning types, both those for facilities and those for health and welfare, ultimately fought vigorously for the opportunity to serve as the comprehensive health planning agency (CHP), and between them have given birth to a high percentage of all CHPs. It is also very interesting that the public health departments as the representatives of the official agencies have as frequently as not inherited the CHP mantle at the state level. However, at the local and metropolitan levels they are not much in evidence. In a few cases they have captured CHP, sometimes letting others in and sometimes not.

Joint venturing of the professional and purveyor with the health layman and consumer. Consumer-professional partnership is an area of great posturing built upon Office of Economic Opportunity and Model Cities breakthroughs of "maximal feasible participation." Although the original legislative concerns with consumerism were fuzzy enough, their significance was not to be sidetracked, and they were written into P.L. 89-749 as a requirement for at least 51% consumer participation on the CHP boards. However, observations made around the country indicate that consumers do not typically become the leaders, nor are they a dominant force on boards. Moreover, the disadvantaged or victim types are few and far between. On key committees, consumers of any kind are usually in such a minority that they do not participate effectively.[11] They are often made to feel very unknowledgeable because everything worth a decision is handled, in the traditional medical manner, as being purely a professional issue, much like writing a prescription. The classic professional reaction to consumer participation in decision making has been: "How would you like a committee of consumers to fly your plane?" What is being suggested by consumer-professional partnership is a committee type approach in which, with a majority of consumers, the itinerary is selected, as are options for schedules, amenities, and price. No one is suggesting consumer operation of the technical machinery.

Joint venturing between the various subsectors of the health world. This activity has fortunately been taken for granted,[12] but the area is not actually clearly understood. Even as knowledgeable a group as the American Hospital Association, which put together Ameriplan, suggests that the standards for each profession and type of activity be set by the appropriate national professional body. Obviously, it is just these splendidly isolated and heavily fence-guarding standards that are so destructive to effective or efficient health care delivery. What is needed to hatch new kinds of performance criteria which do not constrain each worker and institution is joint venturing of these groups at every planning level. The same Ameriplan document proposes that the operating health care corporations be held responsible for competency, efficiency, and effectivity, yet precludes this possibility by assigning standard setting to other nationwide professional bodies. Lack of joint planning between health subsectors is regarded as so grave by knowledgeable persons that the then Surgeon General, William Stewart, devoted a significant amount of his testimony before the Congress to this one area as justifying P.L. 89-749.[13]

The marriage of technology and politics. Probably the most important element of partnering is the process of planning which, through the preceding partnerships (all of which must be seriously implemented), sets the stage for the key partnership, the marriage of technology and politics. Planning that has taken into account what is desirable, what is feasible, and what is affordable, that has made the problem clear to the community and described the nature and advantages of the major options, has already begun the decision-making process, particularly if it has involved the policy makers along the way.

Concern with All Aspects of Health Care

Today, comprehensive health planning will not be allowed to look the other way when health care is being fashioned. No matter how dirty the politics or how limited the actual contribution health care makes to health itself, no health planning body will be allowed to move on to bigger problems until the situation of inequitable, unacceptable, fragmented, and expensive care is significantly improved. Thus, all issues of financing, manpower, technology, and facilities must be woven into a reasonable organizational structure (or structures) capable of making all aspects of health care and related services available to all types of people, as needed for whatever health complaints or concerns they have. Surely all persons, all services from prevention to rehabilitation, and all aspects of delivery are the intimate and pressing concerns of comprehensive health planning.

Concern for All Aspects of the Planning Process Including Learning Better how to Plan

"Comprehensive" might appear a vague or an overwhelming modifier, but it is useful to remind planners that the term is also meant to tighten up their thinking about planning. The steps of the process, shown in Figure 1.2, from assessment to evaluation are essential parts of planning. Even when minimally scrutinized, the consideration of what is involved prevents planning agencies from spending two years exclusively on organization, or from devoting their energies to five-year data collection programs—not uncommon events in comprehensive health planning circles.

Comprehensiveness as applied to planning also includes the idea of making conscious choices among the modes of planning and among the roles and functions open to a planning body once it understands what alternatives are available and what these options offer to the community. Caiden and Wildavsky describe "comprehensive" in the same terms they use for "macro planning."[14] Briefly stated, an effort is made to understand how the major parts of a society or an economy interact, so that the effects of any policy can then be traced in advance, offering the means of obtaining desired outcomes. To do this, all public and private production and consumption, all income and expenditures, demands and attitudes of consequence must be reasonably well understood. The level and relationships among major variables must be known in the present and be anticipated for the future. And the policies and actions to be taken must stay in general accord with a given accepted set of general aims. If not, the comprehensive approach is abandoned.

Concern with Planning at All levels

Anyone who has seriously undertaken the selection and analysis of a problem with an eye to significant intervention knows how soon potential interventions segregate themselves into those which can only be reasonably handled at the state level, at the national level, at the metropolitan level, or at the neighborhood level. As has long been noted there are levels at which problems arise and levels from which the best interventions can be mounted. Without first-class operant relationships between levels of planning, and without planning activities at each level, meaningful comprehensive planning cannot be accomplished (see Chapter 10).

Concern for Guidance of a Complex Social System rather than a Totality of Planning

I decry the attempts made to draw majestic or detailed blueprints for health, or for the provision of health care. In the very open system in which we are living, even with truly comprehensive planning, no blueprint can be of much guidance for long. We are concerned with guiding a vast open system dynamically and heavily interrelated with all the other sectors of our life. Therefore, criteria of goodness which could be revised every few years, would provide a much better kind of open blueprint, for values change fairly slowly. At the same time, technologically based activities could and should change frequently to cope with what is unwanted in a manner that is wanted. Some criteria can serve as reminders of how to judge specifics as to benefits, costs, acceptability. Other criteria are needed for checking the compatibility of specific programs with general aims that are in accord with our major values (a social cost-utility reckoning). Without a suitable list of criteria, we will continue to have unwanted programs, or those which are mixed blessings. Clearly, "comprehensive" is not a fully suitable word when applied to health planning, because health planning is at best sectoral. Nevertheless, the reaching out to make health planning more relevant to what else is going on probably justifies the retention of the term "comprehensive."

WHOSE VIEWPOINTS WILL BE BROUGHT TO BEAR ON HEALTH PLANNING?

The point of view from which one looks at health in great part determines the issues seen to be at stake. It therefore determines who will become involved and the criteria he will use to check out whether all is going well and by which he will make decisions. It seems worthwhile to study the issue from a more tangible base than the eight general, and now merging, viewpoints about the meaning of health which were presented in Chapter 3. Let us therefore use the broad area of health and health care delivery as the basis for analyzing any territories which might be examined in a systems way to discern if any logic can be formulated as to who "should" make the decisions in the health care sector (or societal subsystem) and in its own internal subsystems. (See Ozbekhan for a description of a system.)[15]

The work of Agnes Rovnanek has been invaluable in providing the insights necessary to develop a means of fixing the location and criteria used for decision making in the health care sector, both in practice and in theory.[16] Willy DeGeyndt has similarly opened up ways of looking at health and health care by means of examining what quality of care means from different viewpoints.[17]

Because every major sector of our society's concerns has a profound impact on health status, there is no pure health sector. The only one that can be identified clearly is that of the health care interests. It is because of preoccupations with health care that the medical nucleus of that sector has been given a free hand in the sector's affairs, with the consequent obliviousness to health and planning for health.

Figure 4.2 tries to portray some of the major subsystems at work in the issues of health and health care. The overlap of the health care sector with the educational sector is important because they share many significant tasks. The educational sector provides the potential manpower resources for the health sector and is further involved in the major effort of shaping and polishing these resources into some 300 kinds of health technicians. In addition, the educational sector has the major hand, shared somewhat with the advertising sector and others, in determining the capacities of citizens to participate in the offerings of the health care sector. (Naturally, both the health and education sectors have similar overlappings with other sectors which we have not attempted to show in this kind of diagram.)

The health care system has at its center a sizable medical nucleus which interrelates and overlaps in part with the university nucleus at the center of the educational sector. The medical nucleus also interrelates with the planning ribbon, which is mostly non-operative outside

FIGURE 4.2
THE HEALTH CARE SECTOR AS A SUBSYSTEM OF SOCIETY
(WITH THE EDUCATION SECTOR SHOWN AS A PARALLEL
AND OVERLAPPING SUBSYSTEM)

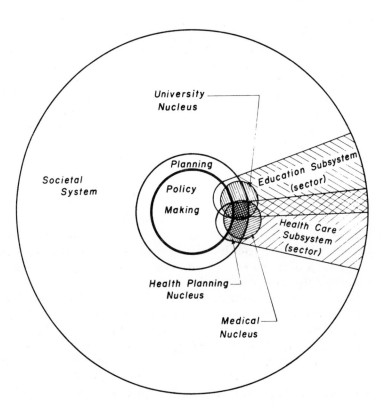

of the health care sector. It also reacts with the policy making center which is surrounded by the planning ribbon. (This diagram does not mean to imply that there is necessarily or desirably a centralized focus of policy and planning—for example, solely at the national level.)

Let us examine each piece or subsystem that is of special interest.

The Medical (Purveyor) Subsystem Outlook

The medical subsystem of the health care subsystem has a delicate shadow built around it known as the public health subsystem. It is also generally guided by M.D.'s and takes its cues, willingly or unwillingly, primarily from the medical subsystem. The medical subsystem is relatively small, comprising some 300,000 physicians. This group is at the heart of the larger health care subsystem. Because of its high prestige and the well paid nature of its work, this medical cadre has been tightly welded into a system of organizations with a homogeneous value orientation for their work of directing and providing health care and for generally conservative precepts of what constitutes the good life. Several splinter groups of modest importance have divergent beliefs, but they have never overcome the central medical viewpoints about medical care.

Because members of the dominant medical nucleus can also be seen as among the last of the individual entrepreneurs, it is interesting to note how their orientation fits in with the medical view of health to produce the guiding criteria for the medical world known as GOOD MEDICINE. (This viewpoint is supported generally by the public health and super biologic worlds as well.)

When the lesser criteria that enter into making up this symbol of medicine's views are analyzed, GOOD MEDICINE tends to signify:

Good medical technology.

Good medical practices or expertise.

Good clinical results.

Doctors can and should make all relevant decisions for health care (currently they have added: "by a system of peer review") that would encompass such issues as:

(1) Doctors practice as they see fit in relation to others in the health care machinery.

(2) Doctors practice where they see fit.

(3) Doctors are paid as they see fit.

(4) Doctors conduct research as they see fit.

(5) Doctors decide how money is obtained and dispensed in behalf of health care, manpower training, research, and so on.

A good environment for M.D.'s and their supporting cast at work will mean good care for all (this is giving way to some sense of reality).

Good care for all will secure good health for all (this is giving way to some sense of reality, too).

The major cast of decision-making characters to date in planning medical care activities, are:

Physicians.

Related professionals.

Related scientists.

Key purveyors of services, such as hospitals.

Key purveyors to health services, such as drug suppliers.

The Health Care Subsystem or Health Sector Outlook

The health care subsystem in the United States includes at least three million workers. By including the direct purveyors to the health care subsystem, there may be as many as another two million persons whom we would tend to identify closely with the health care system. This subsystem (with its medical nucleus) now directly accounts for over 7% of our national expenditures. It has been guided by the medical nucleus, which is heavily oriented to societal laissez faire, but rigidly organized in its internal medical affairs. As a result of the confused belief that, if physicians maintain a tight control, health care will run itself, the health care subsystem is very nearly a galaxy of public and private medically controlled fiefdoms held together only by the mutuality of interests of the dominant central core of physicians. Although occasionally competing, the hospitals, insurance companies, and the major vendors to the sector, such as the drug industry, have until recently generally given heavy support to the doctors' philosophy that the goodness or quality of medicine combined with laissez faire in serving consumers creates the best health care.

The guiding criterion about how this system should function is indubitably GOOD CARE. Unfortunately, because of the makeup of the health sector leadership, it is still thought that GOOD MEDICINE suffices to create GOOD CARE. Let us be a little more rational and see what the health sector must provide to foster good health care for society. Inevitably this would include additional health concerns oriented beyond the tools of the trade, which so obscure the vision of the medical, public health, and super biologic views. The humanitarian, philosophic, and Third World viewpoints mentioned in Chapter 3 clearly have contributions to make. GOOD CARE includes at least:

GOOD MEDICINE.

Available entry to all, for all conditions, for all services at all facilities where best carried out.

Removal of financial barriers or fears of catastrophic costs.

Removal of eligibility barriers.

Overcoming geographical barriers.

Overcoming significant time barriers for necessary care.

Removal of lost-wage barriers to participation.

Improved acceptability:

(1) Patient is made to feel welcome.

(2) Patient can be understood and be enabled or assisted to understand.

(3) Patient can trust the care system to look after his best interests and the system can trust the patient to participate.

(4) Reasonable choice.

(5) Consumer participation in evaluating, planning, deciding.

Improved relevance: what is most suitable for the patient:

(1) Socially.

(2) Functionally.

(3) Cosmetically.

Relevance adds up to the idea that individuals receive the care they need in a meaningful way at the most appropriate time—care which is designed to give them the best functional results to be expected. Magraw says: "What must be done must be arrived at by considering the patient's life situation as a whole."[18] Bjorn and Cross say: "This means one must include at least the patient's age, family structure, economic status, and life goals and that whatever is done is done only in the context of the patient's complete problem list . . . and that we have attempted to avoid the disasters that may occur if single problems are treated out of consequence . . . ."[19] Anselm Strauss[20] cites requirements for serving the lower income groups:

Speed up initial visit for care.

Improve experiences in medical facilities.

Improve communication given and received about regimens.

Improve likelihood that regimens will be carried out at home.

Increase likelihood of revisits.

Decrease time between revisits.

Relevancy or good health might also have been placed under the societal system to follow, but because it is so directly tied to delivery, we have placed it here.

The Societal System Outlook

For many citizens well-being for the people of our country is health writ large, but I prefer to think of society in terms of the general well-being, not only of today's people, but of those who will live here in the future. The societal system is obviously an endless galaxy of subsystems subdivided not only by the major sectors or networks, such as health or education, but also in terms of political entities, age groups, social groups, and so on.

What might society's criteria for good health consist of? The overarching one could probably be GOOD (SATISFYING) LIVING. Aided by further concepts from the ecological, economic and Third World viewpoints discussed in Chapter 3, the previous concepts of the subsystems are illuminated by the following subcategories of criteria (probably in the reverse order of how they are presently valued):

> GOOD CARE, including good medical technology and expertise.
>
> Good general education.
>
> Employment and reasonable distribution of affluence.
>
> Special care for groups with special needs.
>
> Pleasant environment.
>
> Freedom, liberty, mobility and broad choice options.
>
> Reconciliation of major viewpoints.
>
> Justice and equity, as exemplified by provision of care in accordance with nature of needs, raising money fairly, and so on.

These criteria add up to the notion that the aggregate of men as well as the individuals in our society must progress in all ways, not just in terms of health. For example, expenditures for the health sector may come at prices that will harm other major societal concerns—even survival may be prejudiced—and thus, some health sector plans may not be to the overall advantage of society.

The Health Planning Subsystem Outlook

Although ultimately an intimate part of the entire planning band, the health planning nucleus shown in Figure 4.2 is at present usually most closely identified with the health care sector, and even the medical subsector. The 51% consumer planning board requirement might crossrelate the sector in a feeble way with society at large. However, the appelation of "consumer" really undercuts such an interpretation and causes the present consumer members to see themselves as a consumer segment of the health care system, rather than as representatives of a concerned society.

What is of more consequence, however, is the viewpoint likely to be generated by this new and relatively tiny planning group that may come to have crucial importance for the entire direction taken by the health care sector. This sector is very likely to determine what is critical in terms of what is good for planning technology and planners, rather than in terms of what is good for society, the health care sector, or the medical subsystem. At the moment, the planning nucleus is highly co-opted by the medical nucleus in many areas. But with more sophistication in planning this position may be altered, perhaps into a highly technical or professional view of what planning for health should be, in somewhat the same way that medicine has substituted technologic views as guidance for the health care sector.

The planning sector viewpoint can be expected to consist of GOOD PLANNING, which would call for:

Good planning technology.

Good practitioner expertise.

Results occurring as planned for.

Planners making all relevant proposals and designs for all health and health-related issues.

Conformance to overall plans.

Good planning balance.

Good image of planners, planning body, planning process.

Good environment for planners.

Figure 4.2 does not show the health planning nucleus as bottled up inside the medical nucleus, but in practice this has been the case until very recently.

From our analysis, it is apparent that the traditional view that good medicine is the sole source of direction for good health care is pathetic as a source of planning guidelines by which to deliver care to people. There is no concern for anyone's interests but the purveyors', and few who are independent of those interests participate in the limited planning or in the policy making. This provides a straightforward explanation of why our health care services serve least well those with the most care needs.

Which viewpoints and biases must be involved in planning or policy making for health care services? Clearly we must hasten to add people from all sectors to the planning table. Until the planning nuclei for all sectors are in operation, we should be striving for a system in the health care sector in which a widely representative health planning nucleus replaces the medical nucleus in the policy-shaping role.

Planning for Health Cannot be Limited to Planning for Health Services

Health is seen (Figure 1.1) as inevitably affected by four major influences: genetics, environment, personal habits, and health services. I am not at all sure that the last is the most important of the four in determining the health or well-being level of our society. I would repeat, therefore, that health planning cannot be described as comprehensive if it is directed solely to health care services.

For example, the poor have higher prevalence rates of physical and mental illnesses as presently defined and recognized.[21] They generally possess less accurate health information. Illness is perceived differently by the poor and by the rich. The poor take fewer preventive measures, participate less in community health programs, delay longer in seeking health care, and when they do seek care, are more likely to use lesser qualified healers. When using professionals, the poor often turn to the more marginal, or those denied hospital privileges and educational up-dating. The poor as patients are apt to be treated differently, if not less well, than the more affluent patient.

In attempts to improve health, must not each health condition and delivery system be analyzed to see what kinds of interventions should be made to improve health, and at what points they should be made? Conceivably, even probably, each of the additional $5-7 billion chunks of health-funding—the annual and rising escalation rate for health care in the United States—might better be spent on jobs or on education, if levels of health are to be improved. More efforts should be directed at changing our destructive personal habits and into research that will reveal how to convert health knowledge into behavior change. None of these thoughts, of course, is intended to imply that everyone should not have the opportunity to use first class health care services.

The reasons for undertaking comprehensive planning can be summed up in a series of observations. We wish to intervene to achieve a different set of outcomes from those which we foresee. We must carefully assign the resources available. Because resources are limited, an unwise attempt to save lives in one area may mean the loss of as many or more in another. The consumer as purchaser is rarely effective in bending the health system toward what he wants; nor, indeed, is he by himself necessarily a good judge of what will be most useful to him. At the same time, each health professional is biased toward the area he knows, and that is often the only area in which he will perceive deficiencies.

Life-saving technologies change rapidly, are often expensive to invent, and compete for funds. They may call for massive changes in delivery systems, often requiring national interest and support which are not always readily obtainable. In other cases, technology alone does the planning, usually by luring public and political concentration on services which have been publicized as exciting breakthroughs and which may or may not justify high priority. Professionalism, licensure, and traditional means of delivery also have affected the dispersion of new techniques, and unrealistic "merit badge" requirements have indirectly resulted in making health services at any level unavailable in various parts of our country. We have what comes dangerously close to being a "let them eat cake or starve" philosophy.

Modern man sees life as a series of alternatives, with living itself a continuous choice. At one extreme, the objective is to raise the human state to its highest potential, at the other, to provide here-and-now satisfactions, regardless of the outcomes. Alternatives are based on variable mixes of objectives somewhere between these two extremes. Thus, we need ways to compare alternatives in terms of net benefits. The economists' use of the dollar as a common denominator is not valid for all problems of health benefits and their costs, at least, not without knowledge of the major assumptions and deficiencies of such calculation. It is apparent that the humane goal of prolonging the life of the disabled and incurably ill offers dubious benefits to a relatively few persons, while imposing large and prolonged costs on others. Health professionals must be prepared to see health objectives and their associated costs carefully weighed against other forms of well-being support. Planning cannot be comprehensive unless planners come to understand man in his total context.

Although it is an unattainable ideal, planners must strive to be the brokers for the marriage between technology and politics. We must approach the level of social planning that will do significantly more good than harm, be conducive to change, be based on broad public participation and be educational in nature. Comprehensive health planning can suggest basic, change-oriented approaches designed to remove the cause of ills, rather than to cover them up or treat them symptomatically. Perhaps in the long run we will end up not with plans, but with a better set of guides and processes with which to expand the probabilities that these decisions and actions for change will be accepted more rationally.

The Need for Joint Planning by Major Sectors of Our Economy

Do the current assignments to the health sector give us any clues to the joint nature of the health planning task? Presently, in which areas of deviancy from well-being do health interests have the major responsibility for amelioration? In which areas must others help? In which areas must health interests help other agencies carry out their responsibility? Figure 1.1 suggests that a list of major areas involving health services can be formulated, and that a decision will have to be reached at each planning level as to which of these areas will be given attention by the health planners. A decision has to be made simultaneously about which other social agents must be invited to assist in the planning.

Health controlled resources which are typically adjunctive to such social agencies as schools, employment services, or law enforcement operations must also be scrutinized to see if valid use is being made of health resources. This evaluation will stimulate planning in other fields, and health interests will have to make themselves available to help in the consideration of how health resources are to be used in such fields.

To many in the United States, it may seem ridiculous to call for comprehensive planning for health when such major health care areas as mental health, mental retardation, and general improvement in the technical quality of the delivery of health care (such as were found in the Regional Medical Programs), for the most part, are unrelated to CHP. It must seem impossible to consider planning for health, on any more than a general patchwork basis, if no comparable activity is being undertaken in those areas or sectors from which our main health failures arise. Governmentally acknowledged planning is being done in the environmental sector on a piecemeal basis; similarly, nothing is being done in education, employment, or housing that can be called either sincere or competent planning. And these are among the major determinants of health.

Perhaps we in the health sector might constrict our concept of comprehensiveness in health planning in such a way as to ignore the precursors of health, and simply dedicate ourselves to coping with what other sectors expectedly and unexpectedly thrust on us. This approach may be practical but surely then, as a simultaneous step, the health sector must 'focus the attention of the country on health destroying activities now permitted in other sectors. Otherwise these will continue to result in conditions which must be handled by the health sector at outrageous costs not attributed to the sectors causing them. The health sector cannot be held accountable for every societal folly perpetrated under the guise of private profit, saving the world from "isms," or acquiring better foreign markets. It can be asked to patch up the messes, but it should then not be blamed for our poor health and survival record. When society finally looks at whether specific activities are good or bad for the country's survival, it must also have some idea of the probable health consequences. To tolerate lead poisoning in infants from bad housing or in adults from leaded fuels seems irrational, particularly since we know that medical care cannot undo all the damage once it occurs. The health sector, whether asked or not, has the obligation to impress on other vital sectors what planning they need to do if health is to be spared.

We have stressed how the encompassing or societal system affects the health system by heedlessly creating unnecessary work and by providing means—in some areas excessive and in others deficient, but always uncoordinated—with which to do an unplanned job of taking care of health. Only recently have the costly antics of the health care subsystem forced the larger system to demand of it some logical sense of direction. Accordingly, the subsystem will now have to ask the larger societal system for cooperation in establishing a sense of direction for itself, for its health subsystem, and for the other subsystems which are also proceeding without plans—generating casualties, preventing them, or blindly helping the health sector to care for the unavoidable casualties. When this happens, then we will have social planning.

If the multiple levels of systems in the United States are to work happily in mutually profitable relationships, we will have to change some historically sanctioned relationships. We will have to ask the largest of the systems to provide new leadership by updating the preamble to the Constitution and by clearly stating a set of descriptions of a fit state of affairs for the nation. Congress and the President will then have to validate these prescriptions by allocating the necessary resources. Political planning at the national level, too, must be activated, so that national actions coincide with professed intents.

From this, the largest system base, it does become possible to plan, allocate, and design in the health sector so that health care is delivered according to prescriptions that are relevant. Yet by late 1973, for example, not a single national legislative or allocational response (proposed health legislation) to our so-called national concerns for the health sector is capable of doing the job. Interestingly, the major deficiency now is organizational rather than a shortage of financial or manpower resources. Considering what they buy, money and manpower are currently being madly squandered in the health sector. However, within a reasonable and attainable set of health subsystem or network goals, based upon national goals and aims, the needs and relationships of the health sector could be worked out.

C. W. Churchman calls our attention to the fact that we have entered another arena where the values of "individualism" compete with those of the "ethics of whole systems."[22] Similarly, values of a "sector" compete with values of the "large scale system." I have sided heavily with the ethic of the social system over that of the sector, and supported the sector over subsectors or special interest groups. In terms of the issue of health, it seems hard to abandon our concern for well-being on a national scale which, we believe, would be better achieved by following goals of the larger social system, rather than goals of a subsector fully controlling its own affairs through its medical nucleus. The medical nucleus has had, if you will, peer review of all the happenings of the health sector and has brought it to the present unwholesome mess, in great part due to medical disinterest in health and in health care. I assume that society has contributed to the situation by accepting the belief that GOOD MEDICINE is really the only factor producing good health.

The preceding considerations force us to recognize the hopelessness of depending solely on the physician or his customary health associates to do the community planning required to improve overall health status, or at a lesser level, even to provide suitable health care delivery machinery. The physician is intellectually bound by parameters of illness categorized by his discipline. Constraints, both material and professional, may reward him for staying within an area and penalize him for straying beyond it. His fame more often stems from new techniques than from social perceptions. He is also aware of the limited means available to him with which to treat the patients who have the greatest number and grossest kinds of deficiencies. He has had bitter experiences caring for the most afflicted, who seem to need non-medical assistance he has never been able to muster on their behalf. Popular demand may force him to work in areas in which he does not believe (annual physicals) or to give therapy which he would not prescribe for himself (penicillin for colds).

The physician, constrained by an ethical tradition that opposes advertising and gross competition, is prohibited from reaching out to catch the patients who need him most. He is often unable to identify or even to hear about such people. Public and voluntary agencies sometimes try to do this for him and often affront him in the process of referring persons who fit their notion of high risk suspects. The physician is unable to concentrate on preventing illness, because his work is concerned for the most part with prevention of disability and death. Heroic measures, beyond any conceivable reason, are expected of him (or at least so he feels), often to the detriment of those patients who are relatively healthy.

The physician is best able to deal with individual medical problems, although in this area he is driven by social, economic, professional and self-fulfillment factors that are more relevant to him than to the patient. Clearly, for planning, the physician needs a great deal of technical assistance to extend his horizons and capabilities. He also needs the experience of popular participation so that he can learn about what people want and at the same time disabuse them of fallacious notions about many of their wants.

Strauss, in his attempts to define problems of delivery of care to the poor, indicated partial willingness to settle for a study of the interface of professional delivery and client acceptance.[23] Such a study is a significant beginning, but it does not enable us to look at all the inputs to health. It still focuses on a better match of health care inputs with client capacities. Improved insights by one profession about its clients, even if carried through a systems type of analysis, will be dubiously adequate if designed by that one profession alone. Let us consider the problem of child abuse. A medically oriented systems analysis would suggest many relevant inputs which probably would include fewer than half of the truly important factors. Each relevant relationship that is discerned, immediately suggests interventions which in turn lead to new sets of problems. For example, shall we intervene only when the child asks for help; or shall we wait for a signal from the parent, some well-meaning bystander, or an officially appointed agent? Or are so many of us ultimately hurt by the failure to intervene that we want interventions that are activated on the least suspicion of neglect?

If an intervention is to take place, on what grounds will it be based: that the person to be intervened against is likely to be hurt, might hurt himself, might hurt others, is very likely to hurt others, has hurt others already? If the intervention is to be set in motion, shall it be in the form of education, remonstrance, persuasion, enforced participation, total restraint, or even the threat of death if necessary to enforce restraint?

Questions such as these are manifestly part of the scope of social planning, not just of health planning. They cannot go unanswered, nor can answers be determined for all of society by a group of like-minded producers with a professionally limited culture. If a single group does take the initiative but fails to include all other relevant groups in the planning, another special group will come along sooner or later to plan independently. More ineffectual remedies will result; plans will be directed only to one aspect of a problem; the present partial servicing will continue. As a consequence, a person may qualify for service through a variety of characteristics: address, age, sex, occupation, economic status, race, category of deviancy (disease category) or by the type of person he has offended. He may never be aided on any of these bases, except by happenstance, because each agency or program tends to serve only particular needs, in highly specific ways, at times and places convenient to the agency and the staff delivering services.

A REVIEW OF THE NEEDS FOR HEALTH PLANNING

One might question the wisdom of presenting a parade of reasons for health planning. Presumably, opponents of the planning process base their adversary position on values that have little direct relationship to the situations that we believe cry out for planning; proponents, no doubt, are well-convinced and need no reinforcement. Notwithstanding, the decision was made to review the health areas requiring assistance from planning.

Health Needs Change

Lest we become too comfortable once a few of our problems are laid to rest, it is worth remembering that after even a very few years without planning scrutiny, we will again be seriously out of whack, not because our initial plans were so bad but because so many changes in health-promoting and health-hindering conditions will have been introduced. These enter the scene from many directions.

Environmental Changes

Our health needs are changing with new environmental forces. The ubiquitous presence of herbicides and pesticides, of organic and metallic residues and wastes in our air, water, and food represents an example of the needs for new substitutive, preventive, and therapeutic services. These vary with the location and the threat of poisoning. We need to plan for a safe environment, one that can also safely maintain a volume of harvested natural resources commensurate with needs.

Attitudinal and Behavioral Changes

A very obvious area of change is the increasing use of new drugs on a prescription (legal) basis and the spectacular increase of drug use on a nonprescription (illegal) basis. The anti-establishment bias of the flower children is also being manifested by many who renounce traditional or scientific medicine, even to the point of demanding "organic" penicillin for therapy of syphilis (if there is to be specific therapy). Where such people live in significant numbers, these views must be taken into account, and planning requirements here are no less complicated than they are for other minority groups.

Population Differences and Changes

The increasing numbers of the elderly, the substitution (or addition) of one ethnic group for another in a community can make differences not only in terms of the actual health deficits to be countered, but in the nature of demands and attitudes that must be comprehended if needs are to be met.

Key Social Attributes and Changes in Them

Poverty: The poor (some 20% of the population) have more than their share of illness, particularly chronic forms (see Figure 4.3). The poor have more than their share of disability but less than their share of doctoring, except for the more expensive hospitalizations (see Figure 4.4). Paradoxically, the poor spend a higher proportion of their income for medical care than do people at other economic levels.[24] The situation has been altered by Medicare and Medicaid, but it has not changed entirely.

Affluence and our overall environment: The findings described in Figure 4.5 are in part also explained by the ability of 70% of us to afford the kinds of accidents, diets and recreational hazards that help us to account for the bad health record we maintain. And 100% of us also reap the harvest of life-endangering environmental pollution that goes hand in hand with our present ways of creating affluence.

Education: Highly associated with affluence and inversely correlated with poverty, education makes its own specific contribution to health.[25]

Overall incidence of specified conditions continues to change: Figure 4.6 summarizes examples of some major and minor changes that have occurred over the years. There is no reason to think that future changes will be less frequent or less impressive.

FIGURE 4.3
NUMBER OF CONDITIONS CAUSING ACTIVITY LIMITATION
PER 1,000 POPULATION, BY SELECTED CONDITION
CATEGORIES AND FAMILY INCOME

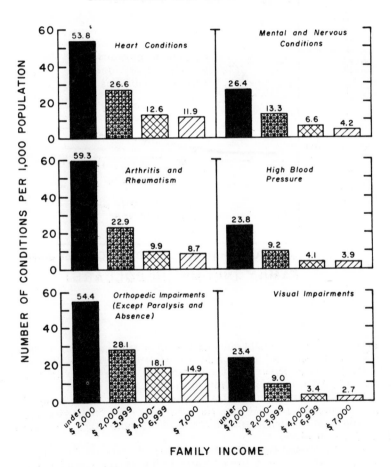

Source: Medical Care, Health Status and Family Income, VHS Series 10, Number 9, May 1964, p. 60, DHEW, PHS, National Center for Health Statistics.

FIGURE 4.4
RELATIVE NUMBER OF PHYSICIAN VISITS, OF PERSONS
WITH LIMITED ACTIVITY, AND OF BED DISABILITY
DAYS, BY FAMILY INCOME (U.S.A., VARIOUS YEARS)

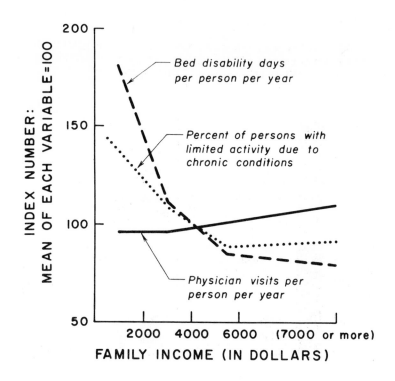

Sources: (1) U.S. National Center for Health Statistics, *Volume of Physician Visits by Place and Type of Service, United States, July 1963-June 1964,* Public Health Service Publication No. 1000, Series 10, No. 18, Washington, D.C., 1965, Table 7, p. 19, (Mean = 4.5).

(2) U.S. National Center for Health Statistics, *Chronic Conditions and Activity Limitation, United States, July 1961-June 1963,* Public Health Service Publication No. 1000, Series 10, No. 17, Washington, D.C., 1965, Table 15, p. 26, (Mean = 3.4%).

(3) U.S. National Center for Health Statistics, *Medical Care, Health Status, and Family Income, United States,* Public Health Service Publication No. 1000, Series 10, No. 9, Washington, D.C., 1964, Table 1, p. 71, (Mean = 6.6).

Copied from: University of Michigan, School of Public Health, Bureau of Public Health Economics, *Medical Care Chart Book,* Ann Arbor, 1968, p. 31.

Health Care System Imbalances and Deficiencies

The Relationship of the Level of Health Care Services to Health Care Needs

The health care paradoxes described by Glazer are nowhere more evident than in this area.[26] What has been the nature of endeavors to bring medical care to bear on improving the situation? The ratios of health care personnel (although, not of practicing physicians or dentists), of beds, dollars, percent of Gross National Product spent on health have risen in comparison to the growth in population and to available dollars. Moreover, the GNP can hardly be said to be declining on a per capita base. Why then is the health record in the United States so poor considering the current unprecedented level of investment in the health services?

If mounting expenditures have not produced any significant proportional improvements over the decades, would matters have been much worse without this high-cost care? Will more health care really improve this record without a concomitant attack on poverty, ignorance, and discrimination which affect the deprived 20% of our population? Will new massive infusions of health services directed to the 50% of the population who are truly affluent bring about any improvement unless there are concomitant changes in living patterns? These are questions planners must ask and seek to answer.

In the last 50 years other countries have progressed more rapidly with significantly less expenditures. Is this due to a more healthful environment or to a different development of health care resources? For example, for the years 1956-58 the annual number of hospital admissions per 1,000 population in Great Britian averaged 88, as compared with 130 in the United States. Physician visits per person per year were 3 in Sweden and 5 in the United States. Days per hospital admission, however, were 15 in both Sweden and Great Britian and 8 in the United States.[27] Yet, the expenditures of health and medical care expressed as a percentage of the GNP are 8% in the United States, and they are less than 4% in Great Britian.[28] The level of health care in the Netherlands, Denmark, Sweden, and Finland is generally considered high, but these countries have far more people per physician than we have in the United States.[29] Fry provided information on the U.S., Great Britain and Russia.[30]

Figures 4.7 and 4.8 give some idea as to what the past has held and what the future seems to indicate for manpower needs and prices for health care if the traditional modes of distribution, skill distinction, and methods of application are adhered to. On the basis of this kind of evidence, should we continue to stock more of everything in supermarket style? Had we not better plan, not how to create more health

FIGURE 4.5
COUNTRIES EXCEEDING THE UNITED STATES IN AVERAGE REMAINING LIFETIME AT BIRTH, 10 YEARS OR 20 YEARS, ARRANGED IN ORDER OF RANK AT BIRTH FOR MALES[1]

Rank	Country	Date of data	Males			Females			Difference, females minus males— At birth
			At birth	At 10 years	At 20 years	At birth	At 10 years	At 20 years	
1	Netherlands	1956—60	71.4	63.4	58.7	74.8	66.5	56.7	3.4
2	Sweden	1962	71.32	63.05	53.40	75.39	66.76	56.96	4.07
3	Norway	1951—55	71.11	63.65	54.11	74.70	66.72	56.96	3.59
4	Israel[2]	1962	70.78	63.52	53.93	(72.80)	(65.21)	(53.35)	2.02
5	Iceland	1951—60	70.7	62.8	53.3	75.0	66.8	57.0	4.3
6	Denmark	1956—60	70.38	62.77	53.12	73.76	(65.60)	(55.79)	3.38
7	Switzerland	1959—61	69.5	[3]61.9	52.3	74.8	[2]66.7	56.8	5.3
8	Canada	1960—62	68.35	61.02	51.51	74.17	66.41	56.65	5.82
9	New Zealand[4]	1955—57	68.20	60.77	51.29	(73.00)	(65.09)	(55.40)	4.8
10	United Kingdom (England and Wales)	1960—62	68.0	60.2	50.6	74.0	65.7	55.0	6.0
11	Northern Ireland	1960—62	67.64	60.21	50.53	(72.40)	(64.59)	(54.76)	4.76
12	Greece	1960—62	67.46	62.53	52.90	(70.70)	(65.48)	(55.76)	3.24

13	Spain	1960	67.32	60.96	51.41	(71.90)	(65.03)	(55.31)	4.58
14	East Germany	1960—61	67.31	60.62	51.09	(72.18)	(64.89)	(55.11)	4.87
15	Japan	1963	67.21	59.70	50.10	(72.34)	(64.45)	(54.70)	5.13
16	Czechoslovakia	1962	67.21	59.49	49.92	(72.83)	(64.72)	(54.93)	5.62
17	France	1963	67.2	59.3	49.7	74.1	65.9	56.1	6.9
18	Puerto Rico	1959—61	67.14	61.66	52.20	(71.88)	66.02	56.37	4.74
19	Australia	1953—55	67.14	59.53	50.10	(72.75)	(64.78)	(55.06)	5.61
20	Malta and Gozo	1960—62	67.01	59.95	50.26	(70.70)	(63.37)	(53.56)	3.69
21	United States	1964	66.9	59.2	49.7	73.7	65.7	55.9	6.8
22	West Germany	1959—60	(66.69)	59.92	50.38	(71.94)	(64.65)	(54.89)	5.25
23	Italy	1954—57	(65.75)	60.53	51.04	(70.02)	(64.37)	(54.68)	4.27
24	Hungary	1959—60	(65.18)	59.67	50.16	(69.57)	(63.52)	(53.79)	4.39
25	Poland	1960—61	(64.8)	59.7	50.1	(70.5)	(64.7)	(55.0)	5.7
26	Bulgaria	1956—57	(64.17)	61.29	51.85	(67.65)	(64.09)	(54.47)	3.48
27	Albania	1960—61	(63.69)	62.27	52.82	(66.00)	66.19	56.66	2.31
28	Cyprus	1948—50	(63.6)	60.3	50.9	(68.8)	(65.4)	(55.8)	5.2
29	Yugoslavia	1960—61	(62.18)	59.83	50.31	(65.27)	(62.82)	(53.21)	3.09
30	Portugal	1959—62	(60.73)	59.33	49.88	(66.35)	(64.48)	(54.85)	5.62
31	Ceylon	1954	(60.3)	60.2	51.0	(59.4)	(59.3)	(50.3)	—0.9

[1] Figures in parentheses below are corresponding figures for United States. [2] Jewish population only. [3] Values interpolated. [4] Maoris excluded.

Source: From Report of the National Advisory Commission on Health Manpower, Volume I, Appendix 1, Table 6, November 1967, U.S. Government Printing Office, November, 1967.

FIGURE 4.6
AGE-ADJUSTED DEATH RATES FOR SELECTED DISEASES, U.S. 1950-1964 RATE PER 100,000 POPULATION

AGE-ADJUSTED DEATH RATES FOR SELECTED DISEASES, U.S. 1950-1964.
RATE PER 100,000 POPULATION

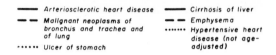

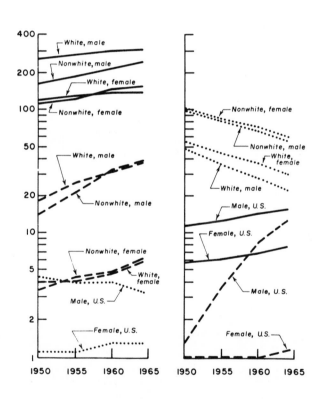

Source: National Center for Health Statistics, "Mortality from Diseases Associated with Smoking 1950-1964," Vital and Health Statistics Series 20, No. 4, HEW, PHS, Washington, 1966.

FIGURE 4.7

ESTIMATED MANPOWER NEEDS IN SELECTED HEALTH OCCUPATIONS RESULTING FROM GROWTH OF EMPLOYMENT REQUIREMENTS AND NET REPLACEMENTS, 1966-75

Occupation	Employment 1966	Employment requirements, projected 1975	Growth and net replacements	Manpower needs 1966-75 for	
				Growth	Net replacements[1]
Medical "professions"					
Physicians[2]	295,000	390,000	145,000	95,000	50,000
Dentists	97,500	125,000	45,000	27,500	17,500
Optometrists	17,000	20,000	6,100	3,000	3,100
Podiatrists	8,000	9,600	3,000	1,600	1,400
Nursing					
Aids, orderlies, and attendants	700,000	1,080,000	690,000	380,000	310,000
Professional nurses	620,000	860,000	390,000	240,000	150,000
Licensed practical nurses	300,000	465,000	290,000	165,000	125,000
Other professional and technical					
Pharmacists	120,000	126,000	38,000	6,000	32,000
Medical X-ray technicians	72,000	100,000	51,000	28,000	23,000
Medical laboratory assistants	50,000	100,000	70,000	50,000	20,000
Medical technologists[3]	40,000	75,000	50,000	35,000	15,000
Physical therapists	12,500	27,000	19,500	14,500	5,000
Medical record librarians	12,000	18,000	10,000	6,000	4,000
Occupational therapists	6,500	16,500	13,000	10,000	3,000
Dietitians	30,000	38,000	17,000	8,000	9,000

[1] Net replacements include separations from the labor force because of deaths, retirements, family responsibilities, or other reasons, minus workers qualified in the occupation returning to the labor force.

[2] Includes Doctors of Medicine (M.D.) and Doctors of Osteopathy (D.O.).

[3] Includes workers who require 4 years of post-secondary training or the equivalent in experience.

Source: U.S. Department of Labor, Bureau of Labor Statistics, "Health Manpower 1966-75, *A Study of Requirements and Supply*," Report No. 323, June 1967, p. 40.

services, but how to analyze current conditions so that future investments will be made where they will do the most good? Even though
health care is not the key item in obtaining improved levels of health,
the health care system should be scrutinized for opportunities to save
moneys and to improve distribution of care for reasons of economy
and equity. The use of multiphasic testing has been advocated particularly on these grounds.[31]

Financial Barriers and Fears of Bankrupting Costs Continue

All health care costs, and hospital costs especially, have risen spectacularly, largely from inflation evident in the industry. Another urgent question for planners is: "What could happen to cost and availability of services if we changed our ways of attacking the problems of
ill health, or of supplying health care, or of meeting its costs in a more
comprehensive way, using the knowledge which is available?" A number of clues are to be had from the data at hand.

The percentage of persons with hospital insurance coverage is high

FIGURE 4.8
RAPID INFLATION IN COSTS . . .

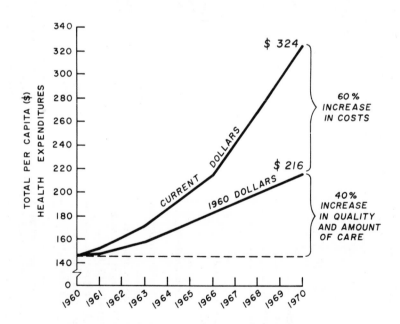

From "The National Health Partnership: A Comprehensive Health Policy for the '70's," Department of Health, Education, and Welfare, February,
1971.

FIGURE 4.9
FINANCIAL BARRIERS TO CARE
(by income)

Percentage of People
Under 65 Without
Hospital Insurance

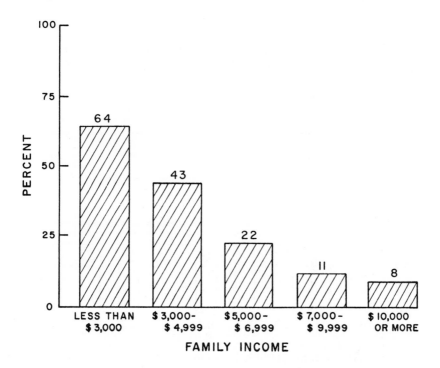

From "The National Health Partnership: A Comprehensive Health Policy for the '70's," Department of Health, Education, and Welfare, February, 1971.

in all high income groups, whatever the size of the family, but in lower income groups the larger families have less coverage than smaller families.[32]

By 1965, having increased significantly over the preceding decade, 81% of the total civilian population had some form of health insurance; about 9% had additional surgical insurance and nearly 72% regular medical insurance.[33] The percentage of consumer expenditure for medical care met by voluntary health insurance has risen considerably (although far from adequately) in recent years; for all medical care the total was 10% in 1949, rising to 30% in 1963, and 35% in 1968. Insurance met 30% of all hospital care costs in 1949, and about 67% in

1963. For physicians' services the respective figures were 9% and 36%.[34] Figure 4.9 brings us up to 1970 for hospital insurance coverage. Figure 4.10 shows how poorly we were covered as a nation in 1970. One cannot blandly accept assumptions about how cost control might be instituted by offering more ambulatory coverage, if this is done without control over inpatient usage.[35]

FIGURE 4.10
PERCENT OF CONSUMER HEALTH EXPENDITURES MET BY
HEALTH INSURANCE, 1958-68

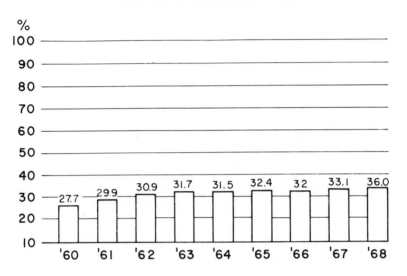

Source: Department of Health, Education, and Welfare.

THE GAPS IN NATIONAL HEALTH INSURANCE

Of the 177 million non-institutional civilians in the United States in 1968 under 65:

20.5%*	36.3	million	had no hospital insurance.
21.9%*	38.8	million	had no surgical insurance.
34.5%	61	million	had no in-the-hospital medical expense insurance.
50 %	89	million	had no insurance to cover X-ray and laboratory examinations when not in the hospital.
57.5%	102	million	had no insurance for visits to doctors' offices or doctor visits to their homes.
61 %	108	million	had no insurance against the cost of prescribed drugs.
97.5%	173	million	had no insurance against dental expenses.

*Source: National Center for Health Statistics, Department of Health, Education, and Welfare.

Manpower Deficiencies

There is grave question whether current proposals are either necessary or sufficient (planning is a fairly unknown activity in this area). Many so-called studies evidently have been oblivious of the possibilities of attacking much of the unwise demand, so that what is available could be better distributed.[36] And the idea of enforced location of each new medical practitioner for a certain number of years, as well as new kinds of training, so that practitioners could practice in presently underserved areas, has apparently never been considered as a way to end distribution-caused manpower shortages. Many planners have conjectured that, just as we now have a surplus of general surgeons and an excess of nurses, we may in not too many years have a glut of all kinds of physicians, unless they are trained differently and required to serve in underserved areas.

Health Facilities and Technologies Misused

There are lessons to be learned from thriving outpatient surgery units, and remedies to be approached through the more intelligent use of insurance, so that laboratory procedures are not used as a device to extend hospital utilization. During the 1972-1973 facility debacle in the city of San Francisco, some hospitals were on the verge of enlarging or rebuilding while 40% of the beds remained empty. Yet no one was dying in the streets, nor was there apparent postponement of serious care needs. This paradox resulted in part from utilization review, and because tight money discouraged needless procedures (actually, only a small percentage of people in San Francisco lost their health insurance coverage by becoming unemployed). The experience speaks to a critical need for a new kind of planning with particular reference to needless procedures in times of affluence.[37] (See Figure 4.11.)

Consumer Education Deficiencies

Although we accept the lack of general education among consumers as a highly specific cause of poor health comprehension, we rarely realize how important education is. We have already been assured by Kitagawa that survival correlates best with education.[38] We can also expect that wise use of care to contribute to improved health is tied as closely to education as it is to economics. In one study on utilization of care during pregnancy the percentage of mothers receiving adequate amounts was checked against both education and income.[39] Thirty-six percent of low education-low income, 69% of high education-low income, 74% of low education-high income, and 79% of high education-high income, mothers were regarded as obtaining suitable services. This suggests that education is always a factor in utilization, and a particularly potent one in the presence of other adverse factors, such as low income. At the same time that we would improve the education of those with highest morbidity and mortality rates we might seriously consider dampening the needless demands which we have been witless-

FIGURE 4.11
NEEDLESS PROCEDURES

Number of justified and criticized operations on uterus, ovary, and tubes that resulted in castration or sterilization (one hospital, U.S.A., circa 1954)

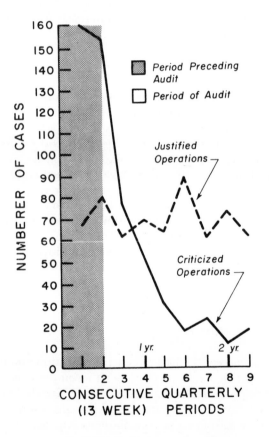

Source: P.A. Lembcke, "Medical Auditing by Scientific Methods," *Journal of the American Medical Association,* Oct. 13, 1956, Vol. 162. pp. 646-655.
Copied from: University of Michigan, School of Public Health, Bureau of Public Health Economics, *Medical Care Chart Book.* Ann Arbor, Michigan, 1964. Chart G18.

ly promoting for 20 years. We need to teach more about helping one-self[40] and about the virtues of self-denial in medications and procedures. There is, for example, perhaps as much as 100% more surgery in the United States than in Britain.[41]

Organizational Failures: Universal Access to Acceptable Care

Eligibility requirements are another barrier of significance for great numbers of persons. In many parts of the country the only first rate, or even the sole, facility may be maintained by the armed forces, the Public Health Services, or the Veterans Administration. Only by special action and recent directives have other populations been permitted occasional use of the potentially available and excellent care in these institutions—care that is not always utilized to capacity by the special eligible clientele for whom the services were established. Until there is a national scheme of financing so that services can be bought in behalf of all persons in all health care facilities, eligibility remains a serious issue.

Physical access to care remains another area of concern. Granted, not every person should feel free to settle anywhere in the country and still expect to be within 30 minutes of superlative care. However, such special circumstances are an exaggeration of the situation confronting many rural as well as big city neighborhoods. If lack of transportation were the only aspect to this problem, it probably would have been solved. The issue is complicated by such factors as attrition (older doctors retreat from isolated or less pleasant surroundings) and the unsuitable training of new doctors, who need heavy equipment and shoulder-to-shoulder specialists in order to feel capable of rendering good service. Figure 4.12 describes one aspect of geographic maldistribution in 1970.

The needs for other kinds of physicians, assistant physicians, medical aides, and the issues of their relationships, responsibility, insurance, payment, and the substitution for them in part by new communications technology are clearly in the forefront of manpower distribution and patient access problems now before health planners.

Consumer understanding and acceptance present another set of access issues which have been addressed by National Consumers Health Committee activities.[42] Although the issues remain far from solved, important lower income and minority consumer oriented literature is available to planners for guidance. Persons who point out that not all consumers are poor or minority have a valid point, but the overwhelming delivery failures and the dismal health and survival records still occur among the poor. This is true even when they have direct physical access, eligibility, and financial coverage to some of the technically best medical centers in the world.

FIGURE 4.12
RATIO OF PHYSICIANS TO POPULATION

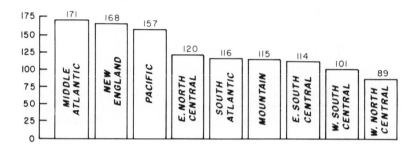

From "The National Health Partnership: A Comprehensive Health Policy for the '70's," Department of Health, Education, and Welfare, February, 1971.

Quality and Relevance Considerations of Health Care

The concept of quality includes avoidance of needless life-risking procedures. A study of the patients in seven New York hospitals shows that 14.3% were judged not to require hospital care. Of these, 17% needed no services, 37% needed ambulatory service, 21% needed some type of organized home care, 12% needed nursing home care, and 10% needed long-term institutional care.[43] Similar studies made in each area that delivers hospital services could be the basis for planning the kinds of services needed, considering both the well-being of the patient and the utilization of health facilities and manpower.

What could happen to the costs of care and to the health status of the population if relevantly planned changes were introduced in rendering services, in control of the quality of services, and in the means used to measure the results? The following studies suggest some answers. In Baltimore, a study was conducted in two university and three community hospitals to determine what percentage of the appendectomies performed could be classified as unnecessary or doubtful, according to patient pay status. In the university hospitals, the percentage was about 35% throughout, but in the other hospitals it was 40% for patients on welfare and private pay, and more than 50% for patients with insurance coverage (close to 60% for those with Blue Cross coverage).[44] In the New York area, another study concerned with quality of hospital care showed that according to expert clinical judgment, 79% of the patients received care rated as excellent or good in hospitals affiliated with medical schools; 60% received care rated as excellent or good in hospitals approved for residency and/or internship; 42% in other accredited hospitals, and only 34% in nonaccredited hospitals were rated as excellent or good.[45] Figure 4.11 shows results of an older study which we hope are no longer true. But its message was vigorously denied in those times, until the figures were brought out. Figure 4.13 shows more current information, as does the report by Perrott.[46] The New York area study also gives the following figures for quality of care rendered by physicians certified by American Specialty Boards: in hospitals affiliated with a medical school, excellent or good 79%, and poor 13%; in nonaffiliated but approved hospitals, excellent or good 67%, and poor 15%; and in nonaffiliated and not approved hospitals, excellent or good 41%.[47] Expert clinical judgment of care received in 406 hospital admissions, according to both the qualifications of the attending physician and the hospital auspices, showed that in voluntary and government hospitals, excellent or good care was given in 71% of admissions by specialty board members, and 54% by nondiplomate physicians. In proprietary hospitals, excellent or good care was given in 38% of admissions by specialty board physicians, and 39% by nondiplomate physicians.[48]

The problems of quality service delivery are compounded by disagreements about what constitutes quality,[49] and about its relationships to inequity, misdirection, maldistribution, poor organization, inadequate financing and ineffective controls. The complexity of these problems and their underlying interrelationships suggests that health

FIGURE 4.13
SURGICAL PROCEDURES PER 1000 PERSONS COVERED, 1966

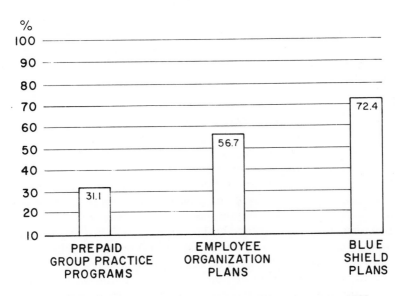

Source: Report of Federal Employees Health Benefits Program, 1966.

professionals working alone should be wary of introducing revolutionary overall changes in the delivery of services or in training new skills before making a survey of all the production factors with the assistance of many other interests. The revolution must come first in our thinking and in our approach to planning.

Demands on Scarce Resources by Competing Needs

In 1969, Allan Blackman described the "reasonable" growth outlook made by the radiologists in terms of keeping abreast of the growing demands for their services.[50] Clearly, all other branches of medicine are under similar pressures. This kind of thinking, exemplified in many studies such as the Carnegie Report,[51] inevitably makes massive demands on all other sectors in behalf of medicine. Other fields can be expected to rationalize similar demands. From where will the resources come to train these new armies? Will there be a political tug of war, filling one gap now, withdrawing resources (as has been done to medical schools, whose so-called research grants have been withdrawn at the height of their training crisis) in order to bestow a dollop on some other need? It would be better to plan, to evaluate the work that needs doing, cut back on parts that provide little well-being (irrespective of professional satisfaction) and substitute skills appropriate to the functions (rather than indiscriminately using the most highly trained cadre society can imagine). Might it be wiser to go outside the health system to cope with problems that are clearly coming to medical care from failure of concern at their source, or to alter malpractice laws and insurance practices which supposedly require unnecessary procedures such as film taking?

Reliance on Governmental Regulations
as a Substitute for Positive Approaches to Change

The growth of red tape is in great part the result of the absence of positive (planned) inducements that would encourage individuals and groups to follow generally desired patterns of actions. Lack of planning finds citizens demanding control over particular practices.[52] These demands may result only in erecting a series of sanctions and negative inducements to desired behavior and become a substitute for planning. Influences that need be applied only at a few key key spots represent the substitution of planning-type intelligence for detailed regulations that try to force everyone to do everything in a prescribed way.[53]

Waste and Conflict Introduced by Legislative
Short Term Political Goals and
Unverified Assumptions about Popular Goals

For lack of informed planning, the United States, through Public Law 89-97, was saddled with a nearly incomprehensible set of rules that represented a series of politically acceptable but practically irreconcilable pieces of a plan. Eveline Burns points out that Title 18 and Title 19 of the Medicare-Medicaid law take on the form of a policy enigma that squares with no sense of direction. The law utilizes:

The social insurance principle (18) vs. the means test (19).

Health (18) vs. welfare (19) as the government intermediary.

The private (18) vs. the public (19) middleman.

The item (18) vs. the comprehensive (19) approach.

The federal (18) vs. state (19) position of dominant control.[54]

In short order the same Congress then went on to P.L. 89-237 and 89-749, which competed for the same resources, the same interests and planning talents, and both specified that no changes be introduced into medical practice.

A rather different level of problem arises when the shortage of medical care in a ghetto is attacked by locating an OEO or HEW neighborhood health center there. Those who are responsible for delivering these centers sometimes act as though the primary concern of the ghetto or minority group is for quality care. Experience does not bear this out. What the ghetto and minority groups typically want are the jobs associated with locally placed health care operations and, secondarily, the financial coverage for needed care. They may very well laugh at the middle class goals for health care as irrelevant to their problems of survival. This does not mean that they want second rate care; it simply says that quality of care does not have top priority. Failure to undertake the requisite planning studies has produced health care institutions that hit no particular mark, because the goals held by people were never clarified, and the false assumptions drawn about these goals led to unwanted results. Another example of nonplanning directed from on high was the spate of rehabilitation centers spawned by HEW around 1960, with the popularization of the concepts of rehabilitation. Many of these centers collapsed for lack of use; of those remaining, many are still badly underutilized. Neither financing nor suitable incentives to uninformed practitioners were arranged; without both, rehabilitation centers could not be intelligently utilized.

Confusion of Growth with Development

The growth of the nation's population has led to innumerable inadequate projections of the need for manpower and facilities. But growth implies merely an increase in size. The critical issue is that increasing size has also been accompanied by changes in relationships, new concentrations of population, new and more specialized technical, medical, and other activities, and new means of communication. These all constitute development, and development is more relevant to what is needed and possible in the way of health care than is growth.

Impacts of Technology

In America, technological advances are prized for themselves, and this spur encourages a growing avalanche of technological changes. Although each successful innovation has its own specific utility, many also have significant impacts on our social, political, and economic life. Whether the technological advance is for health (replacing a heart) or more general (the SST), the cost alone may preclude more relevant well-being activities.

In addition to the economic considerations, the heart transplant or the artificial heart have significant social and political ramifications. The ten-year old (and growing) program of artificial and transplant kidneys raises issues of selective victim neglect which we have not even begun to face. Shall we do reasonably comprehensive planning,[55] or shall we continue to permit place of residence, publicity, ability to pay, or desire to experiment decide selective survival, merely because these criteria emerged initially when an unplanned technical breakthrough was thrust upon us? Opportunities that must be foregone because no money remains available, represents another aspect of selective victim neglect.

Failure to Relate Proposed Services to Desired Ends

On occasion, assumptions are substituted for planning and are accepted without validation. Services predicated on these assumptions often, with the best of intentions, have little if any relation to actual needs. A classic example is the myth that group practice cuts costs of care. Except for armchair logic and the support of the president of the United States, the only information on the subject casts serious doubt on the economies of scale envisioned; in fact, studies produce the opposite conclusions.[56]

Program "Feast or Famine"

Measures created in response to misunderstood or unresolved difficulties produce an excessive variety of programs in some areas, and a dearth in others. By way of example, the home-care dollar has been the center of competition between community based and institutionally based home care agencies. Each approach can be justified; each has its obvious deficiencies. The institutional agencies send out workers who overlap one another's territories and create high costs in travel and travel time. The community agencies do not relate well to the doctors or to their hospitalized patients, in spite of many devices to overcome this problem. Lack of planning study saddles communities with expensive and often failing agencies, as well as with splintered competitive services. In some smaller outlying communities, no home care services at all are available, because the dollar provided may be utilized only by certain specified types of organizations.

Failure to Obtain Views from Above, Below, and Around

An obvious and satisfactory means of accomplishing an objective at one level of our society may fail at other levels and may even create increased difficulties.

Raising standards of infant and maternity unit personnel for no specific purposes at a metropolitan center may call for more nurses. The resulting new job opportunities, coupled with the desirability of urban work and living, may further deplete adjacent rural areas, where operations are already only marginally safe because of lack of personnel. Another example is the state by state revision of licensing and training requirements for assistant physicians. This has been done without seeking a national approach. Training centers will discover that their new kinds of graduates can only work in some states and can only obtain further training under very special circumstances.

The Consequences of Failing to Consciously Plan: The Health Sector Disorganized, Democracy Discredited

A brief quote from Finch and Egeberg will suffice to sum up the needs for health planning:

> Our overtaxed health resources are being wastefully utilized, and we are not adding to them fast enough to keep pace with rising demand. Our health priorities are critically out of balance. Our incentive systems all lead to over use of high-cost, acute care facilities, while the need increasingly is for low-cost alternatives. We emphasize spectacular achievements in the healing arts, but have given too little attention to the prevention and early care of illness, which must be the first line of attack on our health problems.[57]

Not only are lives lost and disabilities created or prolonged, but families are broken and incalculable costs are inflicted on individuals and society. The wastefully financed and incompetent delivery system brings discredit to the entire health care sector, as though it were willfully carrying out a subversive campaign of sabotage on the nation's health and wealth. Lack of planning has made our health care sector the best financed in the world and one of the least effective, considering its capacities. This is almost entirely the result of total lack of organization. It is hard for outsiders to perceive that the health care sector, with its tight and well-phrased cliches, is not simply either a stupidly organized system, or a clever one conducted by the purveyors for purposes of maximum take home pay. No matter how erroneous the perception, the realities of the problems—major maldistribution of manpower and services, uncontrolled cost, lack of guarantee against catastrophic cost, and unacceptable forms of delivery—have gone a long way to discredit the health care sector and our democracy as well.

Doubt is raised in the minds of citizens who are denied adequate or acceptable care, and of those who must pay exorbitant costs for piecemeal care. And every health-conscious visitor to this country begins to wonder whether our democratic process can be trusted to assure citizens of the wealthiest society in the world something as basic to security and happiness as health care services. Uneasiness over an ailing democracy is further aroused when we realize that no planning or other significant attention is expressed in any meaningful way for the major inputs to health, in spite of an annual 5-7 billion dollar increment for the health sector.

The concept of developmental planning is offered here with the intent of steering a course between the hidden rocks of ineffectual remedial patchwork, euphemistically known as social programming, and the truly uncharted *mare incognitum* of comprehensive planning,[58] toward goals on which there is not yet agreement and about which perhaps little more than a guess can be ventured. What are the difficulties developmental planning will face?

DIFFICULTIES TO BE ANTICIPATED IN COMPREHENSIVE HEALTH PLANNING IN THE U.S.A.

Having aroused awareness of the desperate needs for health planning, is there any importance to reminding would-be planners that planning may be hard to achieve, and that once achieved, need not be an unmixed blessing? Perhaps forewarning about limitations or even dangers may help us achieve the maximum of what is desirable from planning without blind risk taking.

The difficulties foreseeable around comprehensive planning for health are many and varied, occurring on the philosophical as well as at the technical operational levels. Some difficulties will derive from opposition engendered by beliefs and attitudes; others can be expected from technical limitations of the process; and some will arise from operational difficulties that will beset the health planning and delivery agencies as they are blown about in the air of controversy, desires, and incompetencies.

An attempt was made to categorize the problems, but it soon became clear that the problems do not stay in neat classifications. What begins either as an attitudinal or technological problem may, depending on the viewpoint of the beholder, soon be seen as the other, or even as operational. Naturally, all the difficulties have been exaggerated by those who fear comprehensive planning and who interpret it to mean a totally planned society (see Figure 2.4). But the threat of totalitarian planning is not an excuse for the total avoidance of planning. Experiments in planning on a large scale are necessary and inevitable, so we had best face the opposition, the limitations, and the dangers.[59]

There are many and real obstacles to good planning. Wildavsky's analysis of the influence exerted by the economics of the planning approach on decision making and Caiden and Wildavsky's impressions of comprehensive planning have already been referred to and deserve wide reading.[60] Kraemer and Elling also provide a helpful panorama of planning theory and practice, with glimpses of the future tucked in along with the realities and limitations of present planning endeavors.[61]

The projected hazards have not been conjured up as part of some Orwellian future; they already exist as painful problems of our society, generally predating the advent of modern planning concepts. Their existence has brought them to mind. Planning would probably minimize existing unsavory and non-utilitarian activities, even if it failed to get rid of them. Planning would also open a new door to familiar abuses, unless planners and others remain constantly on the alert and make serious efforts to build them out. We conclude that being forewarned is being forearmed, that many of the limitations and hazards are real enough, but that, in fact, they come to mind primarily because they are already prevalent problems which planning efforts must try to overcome or build out.

REFERENCES

1. Howard H. Seliger, "Making the Patient Comfortable," *BioScience* 20 (October 1, 1970), 1041.
2. Alex M. Burgess, Theodore Cotton, and Osler L. Peterson, "Categorical Programs for Heart Disease, Cancer and Stroke," *New England Journal of Medicine* 273 (September 2, 1965), 533-37.
3. Gunnar Geijerstam, "Low Birth Weight and Perinatal Mortality," *Public Health Reports* 84 (November 1969), 939-48.
4. Elizabeth Jolly, "A Model to Put Comprehensiveness into Health Plan-

ning and Health into Comprehensive Planning." Mimeographed, School of Public Health, University of California, Berkeley. 1970.

5. Jean Mayer, "The Doctor's First Job—Preventing Sickness," *New York Times Magazine*, November 28, 1965.

6. Warren L. Ilchman and Norman T. Uphoff, *The Political Economy of Change* (Berkeley & Los Angeles: The University of California Press, 1969), 260-73. Bernard Benjamin, *Social and Economic Factors Affecting Mortality* (New York: Humanities Press, 1965).

7. Edward S. Rogers and Harley B. Messinger, "Human Ecology: Toward a Holistic Method," *Milbank Memorial Fund Quarterly* 45, Part 1 (January 1967), 25-42.

8. Warren Winkelstein, Jr., "Epidemiological Considerations Underlying the Allocation of Health and Disease Care Resources," *International Journal of Epidemiology*, 1:1 (1972), 69-74. Greer Williams, "Needed: A New Strategy for Health Promotion," *New England Journal of Medicine* 279 (November 7, 1968), 1031-35. Herbert Pollack and Donald R. Sheldon, "The Factor of Disease in the World Food Problems," *Journal of the American Medical Association* 212 (April 27, 1970), 598-603.

9. E. Fuller Torrey, "Mental Health Services: How Relevant for Urban Mexican-Americans," *Stanford M.D.* 9 (Fall 1970), 2-7.

10. Bernard Bucove, "Public-Private Partnership: Its Influence upon Official and Non-official Health Agencies," *Bulletin of the New York Academy of Medicine* 45 (November 1969), 1227-30.

11. Daniel P. Moynihan, *Maximum Feasible Misunderstanding* (New York: Free Press, 1969).

12. California Medical Association, Advertisement: "You're suffering from an ailment doctors cannot cure." *Newsweek* California edition, April 19, 1971.

13. James Menger, "Intent and Implications of the Congress in the Enactment of P.L. 89-749." Report for American Hospital Association Invitational Conference on Comprehensive Health Planning, Chicago, 1969, 3-49.

14. Naomi Caiden and Aaron Wildavsky, *Planning and Budgeting in Low Income Countries*, forthcoming. John Wiley and Sons, New York, 1974.

15. Hasan Ozbekhan, "Towards a General Theory of Planning," *Perspectives of Planning*, ed. by Erich Jantsch (Paris: Organisation for Economic Co-operation and Development, 1969), 105-18.

16. Agnes Rovnanek, Dr. P. H. thesis, under way, 1973.

17. Willie DeGeyndt, "Five Approaches for Assessing the Quality of Care," *Hospital Administration* 5 (Winter 1970), 21-41.

18. Richard M. Magraw, *Ferment in Medicine* (Philadelphia: Saunders, 1966), 1-84.

19. John C. Bjorn and H. P. Cross, *The Problem Oriented Private Practice of Medicine* (Chicago: Modern Hospital Press, 1970), Chapter 10.

20. Anselm L. Strauss, "Medical Organization, Medical Care and Lower Income Groups," *Social Science and Medicine* 3 (1969), 143-77.

21. U.S Department of Health, Education, and Welfare, Division of Research and Welfare Administration, "Low Income Life Styles," by L. M. Irelan, 1966.

22. C. West Churchman, *Challenge to Reason* (New York: McGraw-Hill, 1968).

23. A. Strauss, Ibid. No. 20, 143-77.
24. O. W. Anderson, P. Collette, and J. J. Feldman, "Family Expenditure Patterns for Personal Health Services, 1953 and 1958," *Research Series* No. 14, Nationwide Surveys Health Information Foundation, New York, N. Y., 1960, Chart D19, 29.
25. Evelyn M. Kitagawa, "Social and Economic Differentials in Mortality in the United States, 1960." Mimeographed paper distributed at the Session on Socio-economic Differentials in Mortality, General Assembly and Conference of International Union of Scientific Study of Population, London, September 3-11, 1969.
26. Nathan Glazer, "Paradoxes of Health Care," *The Public Interest* (Winter 1971), 62-77.
27. A. Donabedian, S. J. Axelrod, and Judith Agard, eds., *Medical Care Chart Book*, 3rd ed., rev., Bureau of Public Health Economics, School of Public Health, University of Michigan, Ann Arbor, January 1968, 49.
28. A. Donabedian, S. J. Axelrod, and J. Agard, Ibid. no. 27, 75.
29. A. Donabedian, S. J. Axelrod, and J. Agard, Ibid. no. 27, 105.
30. John Fry, *Medicine in Three Societies* (New York: American Elsevier, 1970).
31. S. R. Garfield, "Multiphasic Health Testing and Medical Care as a Right," *New England Journal of Medicine* 283 (November 12, 1971), 1087-89.
32. U. S. Department of Health, Education, and Welfare, Public Health Service, Health Services and Mental Health Administration, National Center for Health Statistics, Vital and Health Statistics-Series 10-No. 9, PHS Pub. No. 1000, *Medical Care, Health Status and Family Income*, May 1964, 7.
33. Health Insurance Institute, *1966 Source Book of Health Insurance*, New York, 10-11.
34. New York Academy of Medicine, Report of the 1965 Health Conference: "Closing the Gaps in the Availability and Accessibility of Health Services," *Bulletin of the New York Academy of Medicine* 41 (December 1965), 1298.
35. Charles E. Lewis and Harold W. Keairnes, "Controlling Costs of Medical Care by Expanding Insurance Coverage," *New England Journal of Medicine* 282 (June 18, 1970), 1405-12.
36. Carnegie Commission on Higher Education, "Higher Education and the Nation's Health," Report, October 1970.
37. R. P. Bolande, "Ritualistic Surgery—Circumcision and Tonsillectomy," *New England Journal of Medicine* 280 (March 13, 1969), 591-96.
38. E. M. Kitagawa, Ibid. no. 25.
39. A. Donabedian and L. S. Rosenfeld, "Some Factors Influencing Prenatal Care," *New England Journal of Medicine* 265 (July 6, 1961), 1-6.
40. O. C. Stine, "Mother's Intended Actions for Childhood Symptoms," *American Journal of Public Health* 59 (November 1969), 2037-44.
41. J. P. Bunker, "Surgical Manpower: A Comparison of Operations and Surgeons in the United States and England and Wales," *New England Journal of Medicine* 282 (January 15, 1970), 135-44.
42. Alberta W. Parker, "The Consumer as Policy-Maker—Issues of Training," *American Journal of Public Health* 60 (November 1970), 2139-53.

Rudolph V. Seller, "The Black Health Worker and the Black Health Consumer—New Roles for Both," *American Journal of Public Health* 60 (November 1970), 2154-70.

43. *Medical Care Chart Book*, 2nd ed., Bureau of Public Health Economics, School of Public Health, University of Michigan, Ann Arbor, 1964, F-13.

44. A. Donabedian, S. J. Axelrod, and J. Agard, Ibid. no. 27, 190.

45. *Medical Care Chart Book*, Ibid. no. 43, G-14.

46. G. S. Perrott, "The Federal Employees Health Benefits Program," *HSMHA Reports* 86 (May 1971).

47. *Medical Care Chart Book*, Ibid. no. 43, G-15.

48. *Medical Care Chart Book*, Ibid. no. 43, G-16.

49. W. DeGeyndt, Ibid. no. 17, 21-41.

50. Allan Blackman, "An Example of Non-Planning," *Health Planning 1969*, by H. L. Blum and Associates (San Francisco: Western Regional Office, American Public Health Association, 1969), Chapter 1.

51. Carnegie Commission on Higher Education, Ibid. no. 36.

52. Gunnar Myrdal, "The Necessity and Difficulty of Planning the Future Society." Address to the National Consultation on the Future Environment of a Democracy, Washington, D. C., October 3, 1967. Andrew Shonfield, *Modern Capitalism: The Changing Balance of Public and Private Power* (New York: Oxford University Press, 1965), Chapters 13, 14.

53. Robert A. Levine, "Rethinking Our Social Strategies," *The Public Interest*, Winter 1968, 86-96.

54. Eveline M. Burns, "Some Major Policy Decisions Facing the United States in the Financing and Organization of Health Care," *Bulletin of the New York Academy of Medicine* 42 (December 1966), 1072-88.

55. Herbert E. Klarman, J. O'S. Francis and G. D. Rosenthal, "Cost Effectiveness Analysis Applied to the Treatment of Chronic Renal Disease," *Medical Care* 6 (January/February 1968), 48-54. Mark S. Blumberg, *Artificial Heart Devices: A Conceptual Phase Study* (Menlo Park, California: Stanford Research Institute, January 1966).

56. Richard M. Bailey, "A Comparison of Internists in Solo and Fee for Service Group Practices in the San Francisco Bay Area," *Bulletin of the New York Academy of Medicine* 44 (November 1968), 1293-1303. Joseph B. Newhouse, *The Economics of Group Practice* (Santa Monica, California: The Rand Corporation, October 1970). Vincent C. Taylor and Joseph P. Newhouse, *Ambulatory Care in the Good Samaritan Medical Center* (Santa Monica, California: The Rand Corporation, November 1970).

57. Robert H. Finch and Roger O. Egeberg, "The Health of the Nation's Health Care System," *California Medicine* 111 (September 1969), 217-19.

58. N. Caiden and A. Wildavsky, Ibid. no. 14.

59. Charles E. Lindblom, *The Intelligence of Democracy* (New York: Free Press, 1965), 169. James Q. Wilson, "An Overview of the Theories of Planned Change," *Centrally Planned Change. Prospects and Concepts*, ed. by Robert Morris (New York: National Association of Social Workers, 1964), 12-40. N. E. Long, "The Local Community as an Ecology of Games." *American Journal of Sociology* 63 (November 1958), 251-61. Ida R. Hoos, "Systems Analysis, Information, Handling and the Research Function: Implications of the California Experience," Internal Working

Paper No. 68, Space Sciences Laboratory, University of California, Berkeley, November 1967. Bertram M. Gross, "National Planning, Findings and Fallacies," *Public Administration Review* 25 (December 1965), 269. Aaron Wildavsky, "The Political Economy of Efficiency: Cost-Benefit Analysis, Systems Analysis, and Program Budgeting," *Public Administration Review* 26 (December 1966), 292-311. Henrik L. Blum and Alvin R. Leonard, *Public Administration: A Public Health Viewpoint* (New York: Macmillan, 1963), 195, 232-36. Richard S. Bolan, "Emerging Views of Planning," *Journal of the American Institute of Planners* 33 (July 1967), 233-45. Cyril Roseman, "The California State Development Plan—Issues Related to Social Organization and Interaction." Paper given at the California Chapter of the American Institute of Planners Conference on "Growth and Quality of Life in California," September 30-October 1, 1966, Monterey, California. Mimeographed. C. N. Aldrich and E. Mendkoff, "Relocation of the Aged and Disabled: A Mortality Study," *Journal of the American Geriatrics Society* 40 (March 1963), 185-94. Outlook Section: "New Blueprint Emerges for Air Pollution Controls," *Environmental Science and Technology* 5 (February 1971), 106-08. Roger M. Battistela, "The Course of Regional Health Planning: Review and Assessment of Recent Federal Legislation," *Medical Care* 5 (May/June 1967), 149-59.

60. N. Caiden and A. Wildavsky, Ibid. no. 14. K. L. S. Kraemer, "Book Reviews and Notes," *Public Administration Review* 28 (July/August 1968), 382-99.

61. Ray H. Elling, "Health Planning in International Perspective," *Medical Care* 9 (May/June 1971), 214-34. John R. Seeley, "Central Planning: Prologue to a Critique," *Centrally Planned Change*, ed. by Robert Morris (New York: National Association of Social Workers, 1963), 41-68.

Part III

PLANNING TO DETERMINE WHAT IMPROVEMENTS ARE WANTED

5. Assessment: Measurement, Projection, and Forecasting

In assessment I visualize, first, the application of a measuring tool to an overall situation and, second, the application of a judgment to the evidence accumulated. As a result of this process, a picture emerges enabling us to weigh the overall situation and draw broad conclusions. I tend to give the term assessment a fairly wide area of relevance which is best described by the several purposes which it encompasses.

This chapter considers the aspect of assessment best described as the attempt to measure the nature of the situation—the application of the measuring tool. The aspect of assessment seen as the attempt to draw conclusions about the situation from the measurement phase—the application of long range judgment—follows in Chapter 6.

Evaluation is not included in this discussion of assessment. I use the term "evaluation" to refer to the process of checking the actual output of a deliberately designed intervention against the desired output. Ascertaining the extent of activity and the efficiency, effectivity, or relevance of current programs are also included in evaluation.

Because the work of this chapter constantly refers to extensions into the future, several definitions are provided about "Future Mapping," or visualizing the future.

Although I continue to use the term "forecasting" in a generic way to describe what we do when we try to "future map"—that is, learn about the future or describe it—there are several specifically defined ways of looking into the future that convey highly specific meanings. The only well worked out schema of definitions about forecasting is that of Jantsch, who focused on Technological Forecasting.[1] Although our concerns are primarily social, they do, of course, embrace technological ones which, as shown, often create the social situations and goals, even if inadvertently. Because I find it hard to use Jantsch's scheme inviolate I am going to "misapply" some of his definitions from operational level forecasting. In very general terms, they make distinctions that are useful in discussion of assessment, with which aspects of forecasting are so closely bound.

The specific terminology to which I shall try to adhere is as follows: A *forecast* is a probabilistic statement about the future made on a relatively high and defined confidence level. Probabilistic refers to the explicit probabilities of the forecasted events falling within the range described for the forecast. Forecasting can be further subdivided into *exploratory* and *normative* types, as already indicated in our discussion of planning modes. *Exploratory* forecasting speaks of what the future will force us to contend with, and the options that might lie before us. It starts from today's assured basis of knowledge and projects forward both externally to and inside the system of concern. *Normative* forecasting first assesses or defines future goals or desires and works backward to the present, both inside the system and in its environment.

A *prediction* is an apodictic or nonprobabilistic statement about the future on an absolute confidence level. Such a statement expresses a complete confidence, but no attempt is made to establish the confidence. There is little to choose from among predictions because they are not burdened with probabilities.

An *anticipation* is a logically constructed model of a possible future on a confidence level as yet undefined. It is a sequence of postulated happenings each depending on and flowing from the preceding. It may also utilize any of the forms of forecasting and provides possible models of the future. Anticipations are no stronger than their weakest link and are the outputs of the Weltanschauung that organized them. Forecasts give the greatest security. However, probabilities are not easy to come by and often depend on anticipation. Anticipations, therefore, are probably the most commonly used of the foretelling devices and may resemble explained guesstimates.

THE PLANNING MODE UTILIZED DETERMINES THE TYPE OF ASSESSMENT NEEDED

Because the developmental approach to planning to which I subscribe includes a composite of several more definitive modes of planning, assessment needs must be viewed from the requirements of the particular planning mode involved. Figure 5.1 shows the type of data called for by each mode of planning whose use I suggest.

Problem Control

The two incremental modes of planning dedicated to problem solving—the disjointed (which shall be ignored) and the articulated and guided—involve an appraisal of those conditions currently regarded as health problems. This requires sufficient assessment to identify significant departures from current health and health care goals. The necessary data is usually available from generally recommended health-type statistics, although unserviced health needs and deficient services may be unrecorded anywhere and may only be elicited by a carefully designed public inquiry (discussed below). This data is called health "flak" because of its diverse, and often nonspecific, and confusing abundances and shortages of valid health information.

The problem-solving or incremental-improvement approach to planning, however, soon leads us to the need for an early warning kind of mind-set that requires data beyond that needed for identification and dimension setting for present problems. So that conditions present or anticipated but not yet disclosed by customary data collection can be brought to the attention of planners, strong, continuous inputs from members of the public are needed.

However, the problem-centered incremental demands on data do not stop here. In the hands of an intelligent planning body, collections of simple data and publicly expressed apprehensions, either singly or to-

FIGURE 5.1
DATA NEEDS FOR ASSESSMENT
ACCORDING TO PLANNING MODE

Planning Mode	Assessment Data
Problem Control (Articulated and Guided Incrementalism)	1. Usual "Health Flak"-Health Data —departures from good health —available health care resources —utilization of health care resources —unserviced health needs —deficiencies in service 2. Publicly voiced apprehensions 3. Future Mapping (primarily anticipations) 4. Scoreboard
Allocative Guidance	1. Scoreboard—set of selective comparative indices 2. Future Mapping (primarily anticipations)
Exploitive Guidance	1. Future Mapping (anticipations and exploratory forecasting)
Construction of a Desired Future	1. Future Mapping (exploratory and normative forecasting which include publicly desired goals)
Special Tasks or Combinations Often normative for broad, national or diffuse concerns and allocative for community planning	According to the appropriate planning mode

gether, will point to *possible* future problems or suggest that some of the present small problems are on the way to becoming first-class public headaches. Demands for the kind of perception that will allow us to act in time or preventively against anticipated future problems call for totally different approach to assessment from anything suggested so far. This process of perception is labeled "anticipating."

Although unintended for problem control, the scoreboard approach sometimes does produce evidence of problems in an unequivocal way. However, discussion of the use of selected indicators in the scoreboard will be placed under the allocative planning approach for which it was designed.

Data needs related to problem control, therefore, fall under four headings:

Health flak—to assess current problems demonstrable by typical currently available data on health and sickness, health care resources and their utilization, and on unserviced health needs.

Publicly voiced apprehensions—to assess potential or current problems not revealed by presently collected data.

Anticipating—to reveal anticipated future health problems.

The scoreboard—to reveal specific problem areas which the selected scoreboard indicators indentify.

Allocative Guidance

The allocative mode of planning suggests maintaining continuous overview of the health of the community under study so that its current status can be compared with that of other places and with that of its own past. Allocative logic suggests not making an excessive resource allocation for any one area of social concern, such as health, unless absolutely necessary. An ongoing comparative health *scoreboard* based on a handful of well-chosen indices can tell us whether we are in any remarkably serious trouble, either in terms of well-being or in terms of an equitable and accessible distribution of the available health resources. This is a somewhat limited but important part of assessment. If the scoreboard shows that a community is getting along reasonably well compared with other communities, significant changes in health activities need not be contemplated, and perhaps more resources can be devoted to sectors where things do not look so rosy. Although allocative guidance is clearly a short-range approach, I think it deserves a firm, even if not primary, place in planning activities. It is probably most valuable where there is a dearth of any of the more future-oriented planning outputs.

In allocative guidance, as in problem solving, there is need for early warning, and thus for anticipations of what cannot easily be seen without the forecasting approach.

Allocative guidance, then, requires assessment data in the form of:

A Scoreboard—a set of selected, health indices to compare departures from health, availability of health care resources and their utilization.

Anticipating—to reveal the most probable models of the future.

Harnessing Exploitable Opportunities that Might Be Revealed by Forecasting

Exploitation may enable us to avoid current efforts in behalf of adverse situations that are about to go away by themselves. It may enable us to take advantage of forecastable situations in a way that allows goals to be reached at a level of cost that would not otherwise be possible. The possibilities for exploitation are revealed only by forecasting about the environment around our health system with the intent to exploit opportunities foreseen as coming with a high degree of probability. Potentially rich, both in promise and in hazards that are discussed elsewhere, exploitation is one more significant reason for the use of forecasting. It utilizes a mixture of anticipating and exploratory forecasting.

Construction of a Desired Future (The Normative Approach)

This process is based entirely on *forecasting*. Not only do we intend to come closer to our current goals, but we have every intention of trying to anticipate the goals we are likely to treasure in the future, so that we do not burst onto a future scene with the then-desired values and goals receding from grasp because we failed to anticipate them.

We can begin by using the apparently more conservative *exploratory* stance to speculate about what the future will force us to contend with and to want (what could be). Or we can begin by choosing the more daring and idealistic *normative* approach to create a desired future (what ought to be). For either approach we need to begin with data-offered clues. These include extensions or projections of many of the same types of data needed for problem-solving and allocative decisions. But a much wider spectrum of concerns is covered because the environment of our system must be thoroughly scouted, and directions selected. Because exploratory and normative forecasting are really inseparable parts of a mutual feedback relationship of what might be and what ought to be, they are both used. Anticipation using any and all forecasting modes is also likely to be involved.

Selection of the Means of Assessment in Accordance with Special Tasks Before a Planning Group

Figure 5.1 contains an implied element of guidance for choice of methodology in accordance with the type of planning to be undertaken. However, some planning tasks seem not to fall in any one category of planning. Two examples can be used to indicate when one approach is more meaningful than another.

A new manpower approach, or the contributions to be made to it by an innovative medical school, should undoubtedly be designed on the basis of exploratory forecasting about the condition of the country. Such forecasting would provide information about the health conditions likely to be encountered, the resources available, and the attitudes prevalent about promoting health and caring for illness. The planning should probably also be normative about what will be desirable in the way of manpower. In addition, it could call for a first-rate center so designed as to contribute of itself new directions and make a significant impact on what the future of health services and health care could and should be. That is, the new institution, as the result of normative planning for manpower, could by intent become a source of further normative inspiration.

By contrast, new construction or design of new programs or alterations of old ones in a community might be guided by the scoreboard indices shown under allocative guidance. They would give any community an indication of whether it or any of its subsectors is in a bad way or is getting along adequately. Combining this information with the available health flak and public participation should reveal special areas needing special programs, even though the overall situation might be adequate.

METHODS OF ASSESSMENT

Assessment commences with measuring and enumerating the various phenomena and entities which might affect the health of the populace under consideration, or which are themselves quantitative expressions of various states of health. Assessment goes on to postulate the significance of the measured state of health affairs, identifying those that have succumbed and those that are at risk. In fact, by combining knowledge of present health conditions with those of the past, assessment helps us make deductions about the future. Furthermore, by examining the history of current major social parameters influential in determining levels of health, and then forecasting where these are going, a description of a future environment begins to emerge. Forecasts of the probable state of health under those future circumstances are then possible. Because the specific uses to which assessment is put also call for specific kinds of data, we adhere primarily to the description of assessment tools shown in Figure 5.1 and discuss each kind of assessing tool in the context of the planning purpose served.

As multifaceted as our definition of health has become (Chapter 3), indicators directed only to health (our system of concern) are not enough and must be matched by batteries of indicators useful in the nonhealth sectors of our society (the environment around our health system). These indicators emphasize other aspects of social or economic well-being, and often suggest goal conflicts with the health sector. Goal conflicts, as manifested by choice of indices in different sectors, are discussed by McGranahan,[2] and may be as obvious as those posed by "the proportion of productive to nonproductive persons" versus "the proportion of health needs served." Seth Goldsmith's paper on "The Status of Health Status-Indicators" gives one pause before rushing on to suggest the use of whole batteries of indicators, many as yet untried.[3] However, suggestions must be made towards correlating indicators with significant aspects of health, and I have made such suggestions.

Health Flak: Health and Health-Care Related Data

The usual health and health-care related data are useful primarily for problem identification and, to some degree, for the measurement of subsequent control. Some of these same health data are also necessary for filling in past and present health markers in the "future-mapping" process of forecasting or in the "scoreboard" used for allocative planning, to be described later.

Quick and Suggestive Indices

For a "quick and dirty" determination of the effect of the composite of life influences (including available health services) on a community, infant mortality and prematurity rates are probably among the most easily obtained and most meaningful data.[4] If these rates are high, the community almost surely has an adverse or life-threatening environment, usually observable also in such concomitants as low educational level, low employment, and inaccessible or unacceptable health services. Dropout and crime rates, quality of housing, and income, all cross-correlate highly with one another and with health status, so that any of these can be used to find trouble spots. With such indices, real differences may be concealed if figures are aggregated for large populations. If they are kept for small units, differences may be spurious. Census tracts or combinations of two or three tracts, or cumulations over several years for small areas seem to provide a suitable base for determining rates of infrequent events. Mechanistic statistical surveys without public testimony may overlook key problem groups which do not conform to geographical or other census utilized markers.

As good as the comprehension of statistical problems involved in the national census is, and as carefully as census procedures have been designed to provide a baseline of critically important information, the mechanical deficiencies in census data may also be important to local communities—the most notable such deficiency in recent years has been the undercounting of poor, nonwhite, adult males.[5] Thus, inadequate or erroneously small denominators provide falsely high rates for well-counted conditions, which are the numerators.

Measurements for All Aspects of Individual Health

The collection of customary and proposed measures of the various aspects of health presents an array of concerns. We will now proceed to discuss the possible measurements for each aspect of health, as set forth in the multifaceted definition presented in Chapter 3.

1. Enumeration of deaths (and births). The first great public health pressures for assessment were created by the need to control epidemics which always carried the potential of social and economic paralysis. The enumeration of deaths from specified causes was followed by the tally of deaths from all causes and then by the measurement of births which might be looked upon as replacement for those lost. These figures remain the cornerstone of health projections.

The concept of the delay of death also has Renaissance origins and has been expressed in death rates or span of survival. It was always casually assumed that this use of death information spoke of the quality as well as the duration of life, and, in fact, common observation as well as statistics still tells us that the relationship between longevity and "the good life" is a reasonably solid one. However, changes in our beliefs as to what constitutes the good life (more than duration or adequate food and shelter) make it appear that prolongation of life may now be so effective that many are kept alive, but with an ever increasing level of impairment. As a result, a "well served and saved" population conceivably can be one that has a high incidence of all kinds of ill health[6] and, therefore, may superficially be confused statistically with a "poorly served and seldom saved" population that has many neglected disabilities.

Deaths. Reasonably well reported as events, deaths are poorly reported by cause.[7] Multiple causes of death further confuse the data.[8] Few health departments investigate any but the most incredible entries under cause. Analyses by cause and breakdown by age groupings and other classifications are still not done uniformly, except nationally.

Mortality also places emphasis on conservation of life at any age for any person. That is, it forms one kind of equity measurement in that all deaths are regarded as equally important. In the United States, major health indices are generally based on death—for example, infant, perinatal, maternal and other age-adjusted rates. Both crude rates and expectation of life at each age are used. In recent years there has been only a very modest decline in death rates. Either our use of death rates is a poor choice for telling us about our health, or we have failed to improve health. We also know that new causes of death have replaced former ones, and people saved from death by one cause must die ultimately of another.

Disease-specific mortality rates suggest only the hazards facing groups, not the health status of the living; nor do they relate too well to morbidity or disability. However, the United States still gets ample clues from the nonspecific infant death rate, particularly when analyzed by economic status, race and location. The listed causes as well as the totals tell us that there must be gross and in some cases comparatively growing deprivations of basic living needs for various segments of the population. Good indices for broad comparisons between countries where data are minimal are: expectation of life at birth; expectation of life at one year; and proportionate mortality ratios, such as percentage of deaths age 50 and over out of total deaths.

We should continue to use and improve our mortality studies, for they are still the most reliable indices we have. They provide a ready means of measuring prematurity of death and man-years lost, that is, the major part of the wasted opportunities or loss of productivity and consumption factors necessary for economic analysis.[9] When measuring losses from premature deaths, the standard to be used in comparison must be justified. Should that standard be our national average, that of some other leading nation, the current average of the victims' cohorts, or an ideal survival goal? It should also be remembered that lowering mortality will show up in part as additional morbidity, much of it probably chronic.

Births. Although the health significance of the birth count might once have been the portrayal of the capacity for reproduction, it is hardly of use in that capacity any more. Birth rates are mentioned here because of their utility for composing certain death rates, for the reports of infants found damaged at birth, and as a contribution to our knowledge of the total population base. Reporting of births is still not complete, and complications are inadequately and even dishonestly reported. Reallocations are tedious, age breaks of parents are kept according to different systems in each state or county, and few modern data handling schemes are used. A prematurity and perinatal set of indices seems useful, both as specific problem indicators and as general health indicators.

2. Measurement of disease. Disease refers to identified entities or types of departures from health. But the motivation to seek care, and thus have a condition diagnosed in terms of the disease present, usually results from the feelings of malaise or discomfort which we call illness, or from the perceptions that a bodily attribute is changing, or from the inability to carry on a role, which we call disability. On occasion, screening programs bring persons with incipient diseases to care without illness or disability.

The goal of minimization of disease uses for criteria the incidence and prevalence of various identifiable conditions, as well as symptom complexes or syndromes which may not have an etiologic or causal type of diagnosis but which have a well-defined place in the medical repertoire of diagnoses.

Prolongation of life is inevitably associated with a higher proportion of those living who have manifest hereditary defects, acquired defects, and increasing degeneration of the bodily mechanisms. Superimposed on the real increased incidence of diseases that our life-saving permits, there are many spurious evidences of an increase in disease due to improvement in diagnosis, to diagnosis of less advanced conditions, to false diagnoses associated with expanded use of health technology, to desire for early diagnoses, and to the increased numbers of diagnoses resulting from greater use of health care by growing numbers of the less affluent and the elderly, whose health needs we expect will be more frequently met in the coming years.

The following aspects of disease measurement need to be considered. Unfortunately, they introduce not only considerations of prognosis or threat to life but also such issues as disability and discomfort—issues we are trying to keep separate in order to create a useful scheme of measuring health. It would be my preference to utilize the terms "major" or "minor" morbidity to describe the degree of threat of life. For the time being there are no widely accepted standards, and the devisers of the analyses will have to define their own terms.

Reporting. Routine reporting is currently confined to a varying list of contagions, a scattering of malignancies, and some compensable conditions with build-in biases. Even if carried out on an etiologic base, when is tuberculosis, for example, a diagnosis? For an excellent summary of all the deficiencies, possibilities, and advantages of various measuring and reporting schemes, see Sullivan.[10] Few diseases are now reportable. Moreover, not all sick persons pay attention to their health or are motivated to seek medical care; many illnesses do not come to anyone's attention; not everyone receives a diagnosis; disease may never be reported even if a reporting scheme exists; disease may be undiagnosed even when treated.

Numbers of cases have little meaning unless segregated by specific causality, degree of frequency or duration, and degree of severity. The last leads us to other indices, such as: extent of impairment of bodily function; extent of resultant disability for work, family, recreational, and other roles. The effects of disability may vary widely from person to person—an aging laborer, for example, ordinarily needs less vision than an aging professional. To prevent spread or to control many serious contagious diseases, knowledge is also needed about the stage of the disease.

Even if more satisfactory patterns could be worked out, disease reporting remains difficult. Doctors resist reporting because of patient confidentiality, costs, resentment of reporting requirements, and failure of recipient agencies to use reports meaningfully. However, doctors might accept reporting if it were done on a rotating sample basis and if they could be reimbursed for time spent. Under medical care via third party and other current devices for payment, labeling of what is treated is often required. As a result, we may some day get 90% plus reporting, if reports from the care agency or the financial agent can be efficiently transmitted. Unfortunately, such reports may not be fully trustworthy because the physician often is forced by programs using illadvised control devices on expenditures to exclude specified conditions from care, or use specified disease labels in order to be reimbursed. Doctors are also often unfamiliar with roles and health norms and could not report on such descriptions; moreover, doctors do not always agree on diagnoses, limitations, or prognoses even for rather straightforward entities. And finally, of course, doctors and their assistants will continue to err.

Use of reporting by medical institutions would necessitate interpretation of their indigenously devised criteria for admission. The frequency or duration of hospitalization may occur more as a result of economics, culture, bed supply, insurance practices, or rurality than because of actual illness. Changes in usage may, therefore, occur abruptly and must be watched constantly to uncover the effects of new influences that have little to do with health status. The use of health insurance and other inexpensive data sources must be considered in terms of vagaries introduced as a result of the varying sources and purposes of insurance (to pay for lost time, to get good care, to repay for costs of care, to prevent illness and get people back to work, to make money, or as political pap). Also, much insurance reporting is by medical care procedure and not by diagnosis or health status, because often the only information desired is relative to the amount owed the producer.

School and industry absences, whether labeled by cause or not, are potentially inexpensive data sources. But health excuses using traditional causology labels can be coverups for pleasure absences and for social symptoms (weekend binges and Monday absenteeism). Self-carried versus purchased insurance, and the desire for good insurance ratings introduce hard-to-compare variations from industry to industry. The records of industries with strong preventive and safety programs, when compared with industries that have poor programs, reveal differences, but the data is not representative of their workers and surely not of communities from which the workers come. Economics, culture, sex, and family responsibilities determine usage of care. Sickleave is based not solely on the health of the worker, but also on that of his family, which may keep the worker at home to care for children or the sick. The sickleave practices of employers have a bearing on these rates. Whether the school or company provides medical services, pays for them, does or does not discriminate against sick persons, are also major factors in the extent of usage, and thus of apparent illness and disease rates. Types of insurance bought, limitation of services to particular vendors, limited coverages which exclude first visits or previously existing conditions, and so on, are reflected in usage. Even such issues as whether an employer or the government has access to employees' records, the union's role in worker's rights, and who actually pays insurance money to vendors are probably reflected in usage for many conditions. A new scheme for deriving "at death" rates for specific diseases may help fill some gaps.[11]

Surveys. The intent of a survey generally is to learn about everyone in a population, focusing on evidences of disease, illness (and/or disability) from whatever cause (s)—physical, emotional, social, contagious, degenerative, and so on. Because of the costs of what must be extensive examinations, this can only be done on special population samples chosen in a number of ways.[12] Sampling must be rotated throughout the year to minimize effects of such factors as climate, diet, or employment. Doing an entire sample at one time may not be a fair comparative device for some populations—for example, those with chronic respiratory deficiencies may appear to be in better health when winter is avoided; those with allergies may appear better off in summer or winter; poverty groups may appear better off during a brief employment season. The survey techniques most commonly used are described in the paragraphs that follow.

History taking. Taking a history, a critical part of most surveys, is complicated by such problems as memory time span for various levels of discomfort of illness, different group levels of verbalization and recall. Incidence for two weeks does give ample information, and longer recall periods can be used for more serious episodes involving change of role, use of hospitals, medicine, doctors, etc. However, these very items are predetermined in part by cultural and socioeconomic factors. One report on utilization of three survey instruments points out the inconsistencies between them as well as over time, and provides a good summary of the literature.[13] Surveys often ask interviewees for ascribed cause or nature of illness (disease); inaccurate replies may reflect the doctor's failure to explain to the patient, the patient's reluctance or inability to understand or relate, the patient's unwillingness to comprehend or to face implications of his illness, or the doctor's error.

Examination for perceived or nonperceived conditions. Extensive individual examinations are required to go beyond clues picked up in the history. Examinations include such procedures as a physical examination, various physiological and performance tests, and laboratory tests of bodily contents and excretions. This data is likely to mesh with the well-defined terms of a diagnosis by etiology or altered function and provide a prognosis by deduction. It requires an absolutely uniform set of procedures and diagnostic and performance standards, preferably administered by standardized teams. The National Health Survey in this country has worked the method out well, but because such expensive procedures can only be used on a large sampling base they only provide information on large population groups.[14]

Special single or multiple disease surveys. Surveys for syphilis, tuberculosis, glaucoma, diabetes, carcinoma of the cervix, singly and compositely, have now become rather elaborate affairs (for example, the multiphasic health checkups that were first offered routinely by some of the Kaiser Permanente organizations). This technique approaches the National Health Survey sampling device, except that information about massive samples of specific local populations is produced. When such surveys are organized into comprehensive health care plans they can be done at reasonable cost. Except in a controlled experiment, these surveys suffer from the problem of a selected population, and further depend on which individuals present themselves for the test. At present, multiphasic checkups are often restricted to employed groups who are probably more "well" than some other population groups or the population at large. Results also cannot be compared because of lack of uniformity in standards for test referrals, diagnosis, and other procedures from one testing center to the next.

3. Measurement of discomfort (illness). Because discomfort or illness is one of the major reasons that people seek care, and because it is one of the better recognized departures from normalcy, illness is heavily bound up with identification of disease. Much of what was said about the measurement of disease is, therefore, valid for the issues of recognition of discomfort or illness. Measurement of selected symptom conditions by sample survey, either as a specific tool or combined with queries about disability, can serve well for some of the more common and better recognized conditions such as sore throat, hernia, and others, and can offer various points for specific comparative measures between populations. Simple controls, such as inability to read newsprint by age level, give clues as to whether the responses about symptoms are being influenced by social factors rather than disordered physiologic functioning.[15]

4. Measurement of disability.   The concepts of rehabilitation and amelioration of disability are relatively new, apparent for the most part since World War II. In combination with concerns about loss of productivity, these have led to increased attention to levels of functional capacity. Accurate measurement of disability, as of other departures from health, is complicated by personal, employment or economic, and social forces. Individuals respond to injury or disease with widely varying degrees of discomfort, disability, and immobility. Suffering from the identical condition, one person may continue to work with relative effectiveness, another stay at home, and yet another go to bed. Medical care will be utilized according to still other considerations, such as insurance, cultural beliefs, and availability of transportation. Among the employed, standards for a day off (disability) may be influenced by the availability of sickleave. The selfemployed or the professional will have other standards. All the issues raised under insurance, social, economic and cultural pressures affecting acknowledged illness or disease affect the measurement of disability, except that ratings are not cluttered by the issue of diagnosis. Confusion between social, mental, and physcal origins of disability is inescapable. In the light of the difficulties described above, personal interviews about disability for recent short periods of recall seem the preferred tool for measurement, and interviews are best done on a survey sampling basis.

Various techniques have been developed to handle data. A composite of many schemes, such as utilizing samples of all persons in the home, at school, at work, in institutions, and in the armed services, can give an overall picture of disability within a community. Such data can then be broken down for the major population subgroups, by age, employment, school status, race, educational level, income level, ethnicity, and neighborhood. Measurements of the degrees of disability and their duration (using an estimate from briefer recall periods for the noninstitutionalized sick) can be used to compare populations. It is possible to estimate the level of disability, weight the various levels numerically, and multiply the weighting by the days per year at each level of disability. If the total levels of disability are aggregated, an overall rough index is obtained as to the well-being of the population. Agreement has yet to be reached on a weighting system.

Some refinements needed in disability measurements are totally obscured by these crude counts and by composite indices. Disability which remains as the residuum for a life-sparing procedure does not have the same societal significance as a needlessly occurring or uncared for disability. Institutionalization, interestingly enough, may be a better or less limited (disabled) life situation for some than living outside; in fact, some people might be productive in the institutionalized situation and nonproductive otherwise. Although the truly chronic disability can be separated from the evanescent, the total harm from both is relevant for the overall picture of well-being. One refinement could be

effected through the establishment of ratios between the stages of severity for a disability which results from selected symptom-conditions.
This would bring into focus the sociocultural or other factors that
cause variations from one population group to the next in basic responses to dysfunction and distress.

Fanshel and Bush,[16] in an excellently documented article, have accomplished various quantitative definitions of disability states, prognosis (transitional probability of a change in functional state with
time), population health status, and so on. On a function/dysfunction
axis, they break disability down into: disability, minor; disability, major; disabled; confined; confined, bedridden. They indicate further
worsening states: isolated, coma, death; and several states toward the
functioning end of the scale: discomfort, dissatisfaction and, finally,
well-being. I was pleased to see essentially all of the aspects of health
described in Chapter 3 picked up by this scheme, and several new areas
of measurement elaborated. Obviously, we do not all use the terminology of function or dysfunction in the same ways, but Fanshel and Bush
have made the most useful applications of which I am aware. They
arbitrarily weight the different departures from health in accordance
with their interpretation of social consequences. They also look ahead
to the prognosis in terms of duration at each stage of a condition and
of the nature and level of departures from health correlated with it, so
that types of loss calculations can be applied to the measurement of
disease problems. By the same token, improvement achievable in a disease problem can be estimated in these terms, and cost-benefit calculations can be made and compared for various interventions against a
disease.

Although disability ratings may provide only a simplistic measurement of health problems and an inadequate guide to health status, role
dysfunction probably provides the major impetus for wanting to retain or regain physical, mental, or social health. Therefore, measurement of disability does seem to be a reasonable, if not preferred, way of
compositing the ability to carry out roles and estimating amounts and
levels of dysfunction.

Direct interview techniques on a survey sample basis can be applied
to collect evidence of levels of social malfunctioning below that of
gross disability. However, data indicating malfunction tell little about
cause or appropriate intervention, even though they suggest areas for
in-depth exploration.

Evidence of social malfunctioning falls into two classes: factors *observable by a trained interviewer* and those which can be *elicited by an
interviewer.* For example, such matters as home tidiness and cleanli-
ness, personal appearance and grooming, and certain intrafamilial relationships can be observed. Information can be obtained by interview
about relationships between adults in the family, adults and children,

neighbors, worker-to-worker and worker-to-supervisor; participation in organizations, institutions, and voting; feelings about accomplishment or failure at home and work; feelings about children's accomplishments or failures in school or out.[17]

These questions need to be developed, as has been done by the U.S. National Health Survey, to avoid unknown artifacts produced by procedures or approaches. It would seem suitable to acquire useful data by asking questions in such a way that responses are given on a scale from very poor to very good. Queries would cover both personal expectations and what the interviewee believes that others seem to be experiencing. For example, for marital happiness:

My marriage has turned out to be: much more happy [   ], a little happier [   ], about as happy, [   ], less happy [   ], very much unhappier [   ] than I had expected.

I believe our marriage has been: much happier [   ], probably happier [   ], about as happy [   ], less happy [   ], much less happy [   ] than most marriages I am familiar with.

Comparable personal and familial function scales have been used in mail, telephone, and personal interviews although the major areas of utility have yet to be worked out.[18] (This type of material might also be considered as part of measurement of internal and external satisfactions.)

5. Measurement of productivity.   Because productivity is an aspect of disability which the economists have popularized, it is at this point treated apart from disability per se. Loss of productivity might be regarded as an extension of the concepts of disability or incapacity, but it includes, in addition, loss of production from premature death. Concern for maintained productivity grew along with belief in the GNP as a national guide and in the role of the Federal Government as an instrument for promoting the general welfare.[19] Prematurely disrupted or limited work capacity and the undesired diversion of resources to care for the needlessly sick became meaningful as cost-benefit analysis and Planning-Programming—Budgeting Systems (PPBS) came on the scene. To be noted in considering the concern with loss of productivity from illness or injury are unanswered contradictory practices such as compulsory early retirement and the desired increasingly delayed entry of youth into the work force. Furthermore, if we were consistent in our demand for productivity, the present low-productivity groups of the nonwhites could be brought to current levels of white education and earnings. This would have made the GNP of 1965 27 billion dollars higher, and by the year 2000 would add and accumulate an additional 1.5 trillion dollars.[20] Examples of how to proceed in dollar accounting for production are presented in two papers by Rice.[21] The pros and cons of this approach are discussed in Chapter 8.

Productivity need not be measured in dollars; in fact, a non-dollar set of measures for loss of potential productivity seems more useful at this time. Such a set would include the following major categories (all of which have on occasion been used as the basis for dollar calculations of loss:

Premature death.

Major role disability.

Partial interference with efficiency or output in major role.

Interference with efficiency or output in other roles.

6. Measurement of internal satisfactions. Internal satisfaction is equated with a sense of self-realization and is marked by feelings that life should be lived, that one should "do his thing" or "try to leave his mark." A sense of destiny, a striving for self-fulfillment and above all, an expression of joy about living are the relevant criteria. An individual who has many interests and enjoys pursuing them rates high on this scale; the person who finds life "a drag," who feels helpless or doesn't care, rates low. This aspect of enhanced well-being brings us to further questions. How do these measures relate to conditions such as freedom from pain or from limitations of a physical, social, or economic nature? Need these all be related to the dollar values we place on production of marketable services? Since men set new goals at each stage of life,[22] and rarely agree with one another about satisfactions despite supposedly common value systems, must we accept the subjective measure of well-being or are there more adequate and objective evidences of its presence? Will self-gratification be taken for self-realization? Do they differ? The presence of affluence and the gluttonous and surfeiting uses to which it is put—uses which probably tear down our physical well-being and our reserves—could perhaps show up as false measures of enhanced well-being. (More food and more automobiles per capita are currently used as markers of well-being, even though beyond some level they contribute to disability and death.)

Saftisfaction with one's own life can be determined in the form of questions such as: Do you feel that life is worth living? Excitingly so [   ], generally look forward to each day [   ], don't always feel it's worth pursuing [   ], usually feel it's a bore [   ], dread facing another day [   ]. These are very specific questions about how one feels about his own life. A paper by Berkman provides recent experience in surveying with an eight-item "Index of Psychological Well-Being" that is relevant to this area,[23] as is the book by Bradburn and Caplovitz[24] and Phillip's study relating mental health status and participation to happiness.[25]

7. *Measurement of external satisfactions.* External satisfactions can be measured by expressions of feelings on half a dozen parameters such as jobs, opportunities for education for oneself or children, living conditions, and recreation. Both current feelings and expectations may be asked about. These measurements would have to measure the areas of satisfaction and the intensity of satisfaction. Someone who finds most of the questioned areas very satisfactory would rate high, while someone who finds few areas even slightly satisfying would rate low. Figure 5.2 shows a set of areas for inquiry which explore how an individual feels about the life he sees around him, his sense of satisfaction with various aspects of life, the discomforts he is subjected to, the social rebuffs he may receive from each of several quarters. The means of inquiring about each area is portrayed using a ratable scale, so that from a list of 10 to 20 questions about satisfaction with the various major aspects of the environment, an overall rating can be derived.

FIGURE 5.2
SAMPLE OF SCOPE AND NATURE OF QUESTIONS* TO
ELICIT INDIVIDUAL SENSE OF SATISFACTION WITH THE
STATUS OF HIS ENVIRONMENT

1. Relationships with other workers
   A. I get along with fellow workers:
      Very Well _____ Fairly Well _____ Adequately _____
      Poorly _____ Badly _____
   B. Compared to other people, I get along with fellow workers:
      Much better _____ Better _____ Average _____ Less Well
      _____ Much less well _____
2. Relationships with supervisors at work
3. Participation with neighbors and/or friends
4. Participation in politics
5. Participation in voting
6. Participation with organizations
7. Social participation with spouse
8. Participation with children
9. Employment level at present
10. Employment level desired
11. Education attained
12. Education desired
13. Education desired for children
14. Transport needs met
15. Health services needs met
16. Recreation needs met
17. Housing needs met
18. Schooling needs met
19. Neighborhood needs met
20. Social and counseling needs met
21. Police, security, protection needs met
22. etc.

*Each of the 21 subjects shown would be asked about in the two-part manner shown in the first question.

There is some potential overlap in searching for external satisfactions and for evidences of social disability, discussed previously. It is interesting to speculate about the relationship of the internal to the external scales of satisfaction, and what this relationship might mean in terms of willingness to accept change.

8. Measurement of "positive" health. We have so far discussed the deviations from well-being toward the negative side of a function/dysfunction scale. There are also measures that have been devised for determining how far we have come along the paths of prevention of disease and disability toward some more firm or stable state of health. Focusing on enhanced well-being introduces a new level of sophistication.[26] Evident as a concept of reserve strength in the Peckham study,[27] the suggestion is made that we look for a set of measures dedicated to describing reserve as a capacity to carry on successfully through an unexpected demand or crisis. Areas of study which might produce data to measure reserve are described in the paragraphs that follow.

Levels of stamina or reserve. We can estimate the reserve in specific areas, for example, can a person stay up all night on an emergency job without being exhausted the following day? An evaluation of a person's knowledge and attitudes about the warning signs of certain conditions, such as skin cancer, tells us of a potential reserve that he possesses in the form of behavior guidance. Level of fertility once was a measure of another aspect of reserve, but is no longer valid because of increasing desire for intervention directed against conception. This concept gets bound up with the toll taken by stressful events and how they might be enumerated and weighted in an attempt to determine the degree of depletion of reserves.[28] Immunization level is a relevant measure of community reserve. Immunization efforts are measures of a population's desire to act in certain areas, and are relevant to health status. Surveying for population immunization levels may be done directly and also, in some communities, through health department, industrial, or medical records. Resistance to the economic and social ravages of disease represents a form of reserve and can be estimated by interviewing for the level of insurance or social security coverage for health care. Industrial or traffic safety programs are other measurable aspects of concern for the prevention of disability in a community. Correction of congenital and other defects and care of dental disease may offer estimates of a population's will to act (or willingness to be trapped into action). These two examples are dubiously a measurement of positive health per se, but speak to correction of defects.

Health knowledge and attitudes. Although knowledge and attitude toward health may represent an individual reserve, survey sample interviews for levels of general and specific knowledge or information about health and health services do not necessarily reflect the actual status of anyone's health. However, data on levels of information might cast light on why some members of a population group have better health or are at lower risk from various kinds of diseases than are others. Good data about attitudes might be more revealing, because attitude, more than knowledge, is believed to be the basis for motivation and action.

Health practices and habits. Standing in a somewhat more causal relationship to levels of health and illness are certain practices and habits which could be expected to influence the occurrence of conditions, such as dental caries or cirrhosis. Just as studies of cigarette smoking first shed light on lung cancer and then on coronary artery and other diseases, data on these practices and habits might be useful as prognosticators of future types of illness and disability. Immunization, mentioned earlier as a form of reserve, is nowadays usually the result of health practices.

Utilization of medical care. Special surveys of utilization of inpatient and outpatient facilities might define the reserve of wisdom about the use of care, but will only rarely provide data representative of a given population. The figures on utilization from one facility are probably not comparable to those for any other user or general population group, or with those from another facility supposedly serving the same population. Whether reported by the patient or family respondent or by medical or institutional sources, the errors inherent in data on use of care to measure health attitudes and knowledge or health status have already been discussed in several other contexts. Data, such as the month in which pregnant women seek care, the number of prenatal visits, or the use of annual physical examinations, can be very useful as health indicators even though their specific significance may be misleading and may vary from place to place. The use of care may be related to means, social class, knowledge, access, or acceptability of care. Evidence of a stepped-up rate of using services may not necessarily mean that disadvantaged persons are better off in terms of health—just poorer if they pay for more care. The positive effects of many medical services on health status simply have not been convincingly proved.

9. Measurement of capacity to participate. Capacity to participate, discussed in Chapter 3, has been covered in part by different aspects of some of the preceding measurements. Community levels of participation are of greatest concern. Just as under measurement of positive health, we seek levels of immunization, levels of insurance coverage, and levels of correction of congenital defects. Data on health knowledge, attitudes, practices, and habits tell whether a community has the capacity to participate, and information about utilization of medical care firms up the evidence as to whether a community can and does actually get health services. Probable capacity might be revealed by some of the information derived from the measurement of external satisfactions, such as how well individual health needs are met. Once neighborhoods are discovered to have low capacity or low utilization or both, a more specific search will probably be necessary to establish the actual nature of the key failures of capacity to participate.

Measurement of Health and Well-Being Status of Communities: The Aggregated Status of Individuals Contrasted with the Community Itself as an Entity

Aggregates of individual health status.   Provision of a picture of one phase of a community's health status depends on the individual health assessment devices already described. Data for individuals can be aggregated for the communities in which they reside. Additions to national and state health survey instruments to achieve a suitable picture of a given locality are determined by local acceptability and the financial resources available to carry out an assessment in greater depth than the nation or state would undertake. The foreseeable use of the information collected by each segment of the assessment instrument determines what additions are made. Ordinarily in-depth assessment need only be done on a sampling basis, using the block, neighborhood, census tract, community, or political jurisdiction as a data base. The sum of the individual assessments give the picture for the entire sample and for whatever identifiable subsamples were defined when the sample was chosen. The sample in turn tells the aggregate and average health status of the individuals of the population unit sampled. The most tangible or objective aspect of evaluation, physical health status, might be achieved by something like the formulation of White, et al.[29]

Some aggregate or proxy shortcuts have been devised which essentially lump together all aspects of individual health status. One such method studies two areas: (1) evidences of *chronic* conditions in terms of continuous use of medication for one month or more, and number of chronic conditions indicated on a check list; (2) evidences of *acute* conditions over a given time period in terms of nonobstetrical days in a hospital, and number of episodes of acute illness indicated on a check list.[30] These techniques are neither functionally nor socially oriented, but for just this reason they may be an important part of a tool for individual and community aggregate assessment.

A combination of the symptom complex,[31] National Health Survey,[32] and the more subjective material in Figure 5.2 could provide long-desired data. Such combined information might be put to community uses such as:

Measurement of levels of various conditions, knowledge, beliefs, behavior, accessibility to care, aspiration levels relevant thereto, satisfaction with prevailing services, etc.

Comparisons among various subgroupings within the community,[33] and with neighboring areas, the state, other states, the nation and other nations.

Evaluation and periodic re-evaluation to study any effects from education, planning, participation or services applied. This does not guarantee or even suggest the utility of such a survey device in evaluation of specific programs or interventions. Evaluation of a six-year project directed at improving individual and community well-being by using somewhat similar measuring approaches was able to demonstrate changes in the experimental over the control community.[34]

Status of the community as an entity unto itself. Because the bulk of changes that might improve health are actions that only communities can stimulate or, often, activities that only communities can provide, it is important to get an idea of how healthy a community is in a second sense: intrinsic community-level capacity to introduce changes which will favorably affect, first, the individuals residing there and, second, its own capacity as a health-producing community.

The well-being aspects or characteristics of the community which are different from the sum of the individual well-being statuses are enlarged upon in Figure 5.3. Much of the data desired can be determined from available institutional data sources. Parts can come from the sample surveys of individuals already described, parts from questions, not yet formulated, to be asked of the sample of individuals. The averaged sum of responses reveals community sets of perceived and unperceived gaps, barriers, frustrations, and so on.

Both the aggregated individual and the community assessments may disclose that health and health services are not high on the community's list of concerns, nor on the list of its capabilities. The individual's perception of his own well-being status, the actual condition of his well-being status, his belief about the possibilities of care for his condition, and his belief about the availability or utility of facilities may be quite unrelated to what the community does or provides, except that ultimately the community outlook may determine whether needed services are offered or denied.

Measurement of Health Resources and Utilization

Every community needs a count of health resources, although even the largest cities do not stand alone, for they serve others, and the smaller towns depend on their larger neighbors. The Nation also needs a measure of resources which must be compiled on a state-by-state base

FIGURE 5.3
A COMMUNITY WELL-BEING SUMMARY SHEET

SOCIO ECONOMIC	Rate 1-5
—occupational diversity	1 = very homogeneous, 5 = very heterogeneous
—degree of income spread	
—proportion earning over $15,000	Give in %
—proportion earning under $3,000	
SOCIO CULTURAL	Rate 1-5
—religious diversity	1 = very homogeneous, 5 = very heterogeneous
—ethnic diversity	
NATURAL RESOURCES	Rate 1-5, 1 = very low, 5 = very high
—available	
—utilized	
SELF-FULFILLMENT	Rate 1-5, 1 = very low, 5 = very high
—future oriented	
—pride in place	
—amenities	
—growth	
—degree to which everyone is included in goals	
INDUSTRIAL RESOURCES	Rate 1-5, 1 = very low, 5 = very high
—present	
—future	
FINANCIAL RESOURCES	Rate 1-5, 1 = very low, 5 = very high
—present	
—future	
HEALTH STATUS	Rate 1-5, 1 = very low, 5 = very high
HEALTH SERVICES	Rate 1-5, 1 = very low, 5 = very high
—*geographic accessibility	*consider hours of using, time, distance, etc.
—**acceptability	**belief in efficacy, relevancy, cleanliness, courtesy, etc.
—***financial accessibility	***absence of financial barriers
—****scope of coverage	****necessary services available and connected
HEALTH MANPOWER	Rate 1-5, 1 = very low, 5 = very high
—quality	
—quantity	
EDUCATION 0-12 GRADES	Rate 1-5, 1 = very low, 5 = very high
—quality	
—availability	
—utilization	
EDUCATION 13+ GRADES	Rate 1-5, 1= very low, 5 = very high
—quality	
—availability	
—utilization	

to reveal the distribution and permit comparisons between states and regions. The following categories of health resources are important:

Health manpower, trained, shown by numbers of the major professional categories such as physicians, nurses, dentists, etc.

Manpower, untrained but potentially available for indicated categories shown by probable degree of potential skills.

Health facilities, both general and special.

Educational resources for the various major categories of health skills, for example, size of entering classes and graduating classes, and capacity for change or growth.

Tax and dollar resources and the portion spent for each of the above purposes.

Organizational structures providing the means to put the preceding elements together in a usable and available form.

Planners and the community also need to know about the pattern of utilization. Unused resources are not only a luxury—their maintenance robs services from other needs. Surveys of use demonstrate some basic principles of utilization.[35]

In concluding this section on measurement, it is worth commenting that just as we recommend separate tables by race and sex, we might be better off keeping two sets of accounts to make sure that we do not aggregate the status of the poor with that of the affluent. The accounts for the poor will indicate the harmful effects of deprivation and ignorance on health reserve, life span, and disability. The accounts for the well-to-do will demonstrate the effects of surfeit-manufactured hazards in spite of a comparatively prolonged survival. Whenever we use such general gross indicators as length of survival, we may lose sight of the fact that the intermediary ill effects spawned by deprivation are not the same as those caused by affluence. For the socioeconomically lower 25% of our population, infant deaths, prematurity and life span would tell us most directly of progress. For the relatively affluent 75%, the life expectancy at age 20 as well as total life span might be more revealing. The more refined indices, determined by age and by classes of prominent causes, can tell more about the quality of life than we can learn from its duration.

Measurement of Sources of Authority

There is validity in having some understanding about those institutions and persons that have a history of involvement or control in health issues. In problem solving, discussed in Chapter 7, identification of the parties at interest in each issue is a key purpose of the problem analysis. And in Chapter 11 we will examine the many aspects of authority. Nevertheless, it is timely here to make a few general comments and observations on authority figures, and to list briefly some worthwhile data inputs.

In every walk of life we can expect to find individuals with authority among their own groups. We can also anticipate finding some whose authority is so great that it transcends many other authorities for some types of issue. Unfortunately, figures who have earned authority in an outside area such as baseball, may somehow become involved in health issues, and the extent of their influence can no more be anticipated than their entry into the issue.

The seat of authority for different kinds of health issues among groups and communities is not always easy to determine on a cursory scrutiny. A reasonable search in at least three areas is called for:

> The political parties.
> The major ethnic groups.
> The major activity systems, including institutions and their agencies.

Groups within these areas should be examined individually for a history of involvement in health issues and for general posture and capacity. The following concerns are worth cataloging for each of the major groups within the three areas:

> Evidence of interest in health issue, and which kinds.
> Positions generally taken on such issues.
> Access to resources.
> Level and extent of citizen participation.
> Ability to get voter turnout.
> Integrity.
> Alignments and obligations, machines.
> Organizational capacity.
> Identified leaders.
> General gatekeepers.
> Health issue gatekeepers.

Measurement of Values

I am not impressed with the importance or feasibility of formally measuring values themselves, whether to provide a guide for planners or for the community itself. However, one might assess the value configuration in terms of attitudes and goals. Davidoff and Reiner feel that at least five elements are required:

> How widely key values are held.
> The intensity with which each value is held.
> Presence of individual belief that he can influence the achievement of desired goals.
> Variations in individually held values and hierarchies from those generally held.

Divergences of individual goals from stated values.
In order to get this information, several methods are suggested:

Assigning exchange prices to several goals.

Posing alternatives, analyzing ramifications, and disseminating information to assist effective bargaining between proponents of opposing values.

Rendering value meanings explicit to provide common grounds for appraisal.[36]

It would be my guess that what people choose as being most important from large lists of issues would come closer to providing a sense of what individuals value. Because values are operant in so many ways (see Chapter 2), maintaining a high level of public participation in hearings and committee work is much more useful than surveys in making the community's values apparent. In broad public participation the values held have a free range. Unless, as suggested by Davidoff and Reiner, well-known, specific issues or goals are utilized as the basis of a survey tool for values, a survey will encounter the usual cultural and language differences, and the formidable task of working through artificial examples will, in all probability, produce not evidence of values, but rather evidence of feelings of the moment.

The Public Voice as an Assessment Tool to Help Reveal Problems

Although a markedly different data-gathering device from the methods already described, the public voice may well be the most effective way to overcome the data gaps on subjects over which no agency seems to have jurisdiction or about which few of our middle-class-dominated communities have previously expressed great concern. Public participation may not only cut through the value biases which allow society to conveniently forget to measure certain of its problems, it may call attention to the peculiar ways in which we now count certain aberrations or deficiencies. The unbelievably high level of apparently retarded Spanish-speaking children in San Francisco was not well accepted by the Spanish-speaking public in 1970. Their resistance led to the "discovery" that Spanish-speaking children were being tested by English I.Q. tests. Thus emerged a new kind of problem—the cognitively retarded status of the white middle-class educators, rather than that of the Spanish-speaking children.

If voices are to emerge from the public, the major conclusions being drawn from available data must be portrayed in simple formats, publicized and presented at meetings to which all and sundry are invited, but particularly those who might suffer from or be related to the problem in one way or another. From these encounters, new problems and revisions of old ones will emerge, and support will materialize for analyzing the nature and origins of those problems to which the public draws particular attention. These sessions also begin to provide some notion of the priority ratings the public is giving the problems being unearthed. A highly developed schema by which excellent problem awareness has been elicited from large groups in a matter of hours has been presented by Delbecq and his associates as the nominal group technique.[37]

Future Mapping (Forecasting)

In the words of Dr. Elizabeth Jolly:

> If planning is to achieve the best of possible results—if planning is even to achieve results that, given an adverse turn of events, are not self-defeating—it must anticipate the future. In the sense that the future is never more than a breath away, that the present is only an interface between the future and the past, planning, of course, is anticipation. But I am talking about futures that are five, ten, twenty, and more years away. And the point I am making is that the planner is not doing his planning best if he does not consider the various kinds of futures that, by default and otherwise, are available to him. In short, he simply cannot work with his nose so close to the grindstone of the present that, in that myopic stance, he perceives none of its transiency and none of what lies beyond. Perhaps there is a better example of this kind of reasoning in the reverse approach: in what situations can planning possibly succeed without a perspective of the future.[38]

Forecasting is done to improve policy making,[39] and because planning bodies have the same mission for society, they will utilize forecasting. I see forecasting required to varying degrees in the problem-solving, allocative, exploitive, and future-building modes of planning, and although I will appear to have, in the words of Dror,[40] "operationalized and concretized" a bit too much, there is no real disagreement with the notion that the uses and modes of future mapping blend one into the other.

Methods Used in Exploratory Forecasting

Exploratory forecasting is a good place to begin an examination of forecasting techniques because it provides one of the most tangible places from which to start our probes into the future. In addition, it provides much of the data on which anticipations are built.

The areas of measurement reviewed so far were essentially in terms of the present or near past. Often, data are available from regular intervals into the further past which give an idea of the stages through which phenomena have passed to arrive at the present. These figures provide an opportunity to review the paths followed and to speculate where they might be leading (trend extrapolating). Trending and observing changes in trends call for data from more than one point in time, as can be seen from a listing of the ways in which future probes are made.[41]

Persistence. Tomorrow will be the same as today.

Trajectory. Tomorrow will be on an extension of the line from previous days to today.

Cycle. Tomorrow will be on an extension of the cyclic trajectory which we have been on.

Association. Tomorrow can be determined by watching certain associated phenomena or "social indicators" which, in the past, have had a high correlation with the phenomena under observation.

Analogous. Tomorrow will hold for us what was held for *x* in what is believed to be an analogous situation or in passing through a like situation. A recent article explains how analogies can be utilized and made more trustworthy.[42]

Correlation. Tomorrow will find us in a situation created by a multitude of trends and cycles. Contextual mapping fits here, and variations of describing the options open in complex futures may take on more explicit formats, such as morphological research or analysis.[43]

Experimentation or simulation. All the factors thought to have a major bearing on the subject being trended are defined mathematically and entered into an overall systemic equation. Generally only feasible by means of computerization, each and all of these factors can be altered experimentally or in accordance with the trends anticipated for each, and the net effects (possible futures) observed on the model of the system being simulated. This is an experimental type of extension based on the idea of correlating. A similar approach may be made nonmathematically, and various forms of games or gaming are meant to be system simulations.

The best guess approach. For lack of capacity to harness current information, intuition or wisdom is relied on in some techniques. In the Delphi, for example, the best judgment of "expert" individuals becomes the data about specified issues or outcomes and is then accepted as anticipation.[44]

Anticipations. Many fleshed-out versions of the future of a given subject, situation, or community can be assembled by utilizing any or all of the foregoing devices. These can be rated in terms of most to least probable.

In the terminology of Abt,[45] the first three devices are primarily *extrapolative,* the next three primarily *speculative,* the seventh *analytic,* and the eighth *judgmental*. Abt provides a brief and lucid description of these four underlying approaches.

The ninth device, anticipations, can be based on a composite of any of the preceding. If one wanted to stretch this definition it could include cross-impact types of analyses and resolutions, harmonizations of spatial and temporal interdependencies, even going on to scenario writing. Scenario writing is not so much directed at forecasting as at utilizing forecasts. Associated with the name of Herman Kahn, it tries to deal with several aspects of a problem more or less simultaneously. The scenarist starts from a situation and thinks forward a short stretch to apparently important "decision nodes." From each of these many possible courses of action branch out. Each in turn can be followed to its next important decision nodes.[46]

The relevance tree, systems analysis, networks, and the Delphi as well are applicable techniques.[47] Intuitive thinking contributes to all forms of forecasting. In addition to the exploratory methods (opportunity oriented) and anticipations are the normative forecasting (needs and desires) opportunities and techniques. These are newer and less tangible, as well as more characteristic of the capacities of a goal-setting society than of a laissez-faire system. The classic text describing these and all other modes of forecasting and their applications is that of Eric Jantsch.[48]

The overall contextual map of forecasting records the present and past scores on each of the contours of contexts thought relevant enough to be worth describing. In addition to serving as the baseline against which measurements in future years are to be compared, the map provides the means to extrapolate or to project the future. For example, if changes appear in the infant death rate and we can conclude that they seem to have resulted from new or accelerated long-term factors which have modified the overall situation, we are able to anticipate the future picture from extensions of the whole contextual map.

A very easy-to-follow set of guidelines as to which future mapping (forecasting) technique should be used for a given problem has been derived for the business world by Chambers, Mullick, and Smith, and my observation indicates that their method may have similar applicability for public purposes generally.[49]

Multisectoral Future Maps and the Need to
Square Them with One Another
by Means of Repeated Rounds of Projecting

Future mapping, of course, takes us much further than has been implied so far. The better alternative estimates should be extended ten and twenty years for each of the subjects of measurement. When the markers for all contours or contexts in each sector are extended over such a time span it soon becomes clear that each sector must affect the others. Improved and prolonged education will surely have an impact on our economic condition, and both will have an effect on our health. At the same time, forecasted changes in health status will have effects on productivity, employment, or longevity, and consequently on overall productivity or on burdens to society.

Since changes in any one sector suggest inevitable modifications in other sectors, a first round of isolated sectoral future maps must be followed by a second, wherein the predicted alterations of each sector are now checked for their effect on each of the other sectors. Any resulting changes in the sectors inevitably will call for another round of speculation on what each of these subsequent sectoral changes will further do to the others. This is essentially a type of futures-feedback *(ff)* from the hypothesized futures, known to the followers of Geoffrey Vickers as "forward feedback."[50]

How far can one go on with these rounds of conjectures and keep his sanity, let alone come up with clever forecasts on each parameter? For those capable of generating a set of mathematical formulae and using a computer, repeated rounds need not be an impossible task. We who are not yet computerized may be able to settle for as little as a second round of forecasts in the major sectors and the resultant forecasted health status trends, because our primary interests are health status and (in these times as a result of political demand) availability of health care services.

Since health probably correlates more directly with level of education, environmental factors and affluence than with health care, it is a little difficult to limit oneself intelligently to forecasts or anticipations of society's ability to produce health care resources—about all that is usually asked of health planners. Comparing forecasts of health status or level of needs with the forecasted availability of resources for health care services does give us the nature of anticipated gaps. The demand factor, which may be right on target with needs, above it, or below it, obviously requires a separate forecast.

How Much of the Environment Surrounding the System of Our Concern Must be Future Mapped?

Forecasting promises some highly rewarding insights into the future, but clearly to use the more sophisticated of the trend-producing methods such as correlation and simulation is not easy. The scope of the system (or to be more exact, some specified portion of the system's environment as well as the system itself) to be simulated determines the number of relevant factors to be included and the number to be disregarded. Forrester, in his simulation work on urban places, probably did us no particular favor when he assumed that a city can be safely looked at as an isolated citadel.[51] He concluded, in part, that the city can be isolated for certain parts of its policy-making (self support and a growing economic base) and get away with it and, in fact, can improve its future by so doing. Yet at the same time he concludes that the city cannot be isolated when it forecasts and deduces other policies (such as housing the poor), because it will become inundated with problems from the outside, which its isolation-spawned policies inadvertently invited. These he calls surprises. It seems safer to conclude that Forrester's simulations of suboptimizing at the city level which calls for excluding the poor from any given city will have some other disastrous effects on society and thus on the cities as well. In part, of course, Forrester is contrasting short versus long-range outcomes and small versus large system outcomes. (Intuitive thinking that is "right" for the very short run often comes out "wrong" for the long run.)

However, when Forrester applied the same systems logic to a more complete system, our earth, he is able to assume finite (world) boundaries. Then his simulations lead to what is for many of us expected rather than to unexpected long-range information.[52] It is also heartening that he finds only a handful of variables key to our well-being, with most other variables having minimal effects. Again, the key variables are really the expected ones. Perhaps this happy phenomenon is simply the result of the exhausted state of our intellectual vitality which on the next round of interchanges will reveal that our hope for a limited number of vital variables is indefensible. And, in fact, this is just the stance taken by many of Forrester's critics.

Since health and general well-being are so intertwined and so heavily dependent on other factors, it is important to repeat that we need the forecasts of the non-health sectors most; from these we deduce the nature and extent of health needs and demands. The critical nature of this information brings up another issue—where does this information come from? Clearly, we must have national-level future maps within which we can build our state-level counterparts. We need state anticipations within which to build metro, metro to build county or city, and city to build neighborhood projections. We must be aware that the direction of higher-level projections cannot be taken as equivalent to the direction of local ones, for any local projection may have a special course of its own, even though that course may be caused entirely by the higher level ones. Overall national-level future mapping might indicate a depletion of certain resources which could create another Appalachia, yet it might not call attention to the particular area that is about to be wiped out. However, planners at lower levels can utilize national-level future maps to determine that certain of their localities may face special problems. For example:

Their resources will no longer be needed or will rapidly be exploited, or they will be reduced to a slag or shale mound.

A new kind of activity can or will be generated in their area.

A new population distribution or a new kind of settler will be coming to join them.

A new kind of hazard will face them.

Unfortunately, the idea of an earth-world system also makes clear that no significant national contextual mapping for twenty years into the future can be done without a world-wide or international set of maps. (The Club of Rome may be pointing the way, and the techniques of Forrester find their appropriate utilization in this effort.)[53]

How Small Are the Subsystem Elements for Which We Need Future Maps?

Just as national-level, multi-sectoral future maps are needed to create local general and health forecasts, local level future maps are useful in guiding forecasts made at higher levels. The larger system and the contained subsystems must be examined at the same time, so that each can be advised by the other. Disruption which many small communities foresee from local or state future mapping could well be the source of ensuing major state and even national disruption. Such disruptions could be invisible at higher levels except as revealed to them by local-level forecasting.

Recapitulation of the Benefits and Hazards of Future Mapping

A most readable statement on the state of the art of forecasting is that of Otis Dudley Duncan.[54] It also contains an excellent bibliography. Duncan makes us feel the necessity to recapitulate what has been adduced or implied about the benefits of future mapping.

Benefits.   Forecasting clues us in as to what is going to happen— what, when, where, and why—with probabilities of occurrence, time, place, extent. Therefore, we may learn:

The fate of problems that now worry us (for example, they will go away by themselves, they will grow).

The degree of danger from new problems to our well-being in such areas as personal satisfaction, comfort, illness, general work capacity, life itself.

The likelihood of alterations in value systems and their probable nature (for example, acceptable future goals, future problems, future needs, future demands, modes of governance).

The future availability of such resources as dollars, trained manpower, education capacities, facilities, organizational and governmental capabilities.

The possibility (on the basis of exploration or of normative forecasting) of creating alternative futures, that is, other than the one that seems most likely to occur unless intervened against and altered, and the losses and gains to be anticipated from achieving any of the alternatives as compared to the expected future.

Alternative ways to reach other futures, and the losses and gains to be anticipated along each of these routes.

Clearly, forecasting is at the heart of planning, perhaps an indistinguishable part that goes on in one form or another no matter how hard we try to separate it semantically from planning.

Hazards.   Forecasting can never be more than a set of deductions based on particular assumptions. Therefore, we should realize that:

—In the compiling of probabilities, as Alonso has pointed out, errors may grow startlingly as a result of multiplying or adding errors.[55]

—Partial comprehension or failure to appreciate the full significance or ramifications may cause us to lose our way.

Furthermore, in the utilization of anticipations—small missteps in logic, the uses of conventional or intuitive or short range wisdoms (which Forrester claims are almost inevitably in error over the long-range), the suboptimal or too small system base, the extension of too short a time span—all may produce consequences which give one pause.[56] Of course, this is rather typically a hazard of our present day, nonforecasting, nonplanning approaches as well.

—Political impacts on the legitimacy of forecasts, such as the imminence of presidential, gubernatorial or mayoral bids, may have a bearing on the quality of future maps released at each level of government.

Assuredly, we have to date had our fill of forecasts that are either wishful thinking or the materials from which credibility gaps are built. However, it remains our hope that bona fide planning bodies at each level will be able to release bona fide future maps, and that the planning bodies are structured and financed in a way that is reasonably free of immediate political pressures.

—Distortion caused by the approach of the forecaster is another hazard.

Some forecasts are labeled exploratory in the sense that they are basically projected from the present. They then tend to limit the horizons of the future to what the past and present seem to hold feasible (what could be). In sharp contrast are forecasts that openly or surreptitiously are normative—the person making them wants to have a particular future come to pass and his forecasts lead in that direction (what he thinks ought to be). The wide discrepancies in advice given to our government in all its foreign policy, and much of its domestic policy as well, seem to stem not from sloppy methods of forecasting nor from the data at hand, but rather from the Weltanschauung of the forecaster[57] or the state of his politics.

The March, 1971 issue of the *Annals of the American Academy of Political and Social Science* is partly devoted to these issues under the rubric of scientists advising government. Several references are made as to how personal values, beliefs, and politics distort the advice given. Most of this advice is based on forecasts (the forecaster's belief) of what will happen if we act in one way as compared to what will happen if we act in another.[58]

Choosing between exploratory and normative styles of forecasting is not simple, but fortunately, it is not necessary. As Ritva Kaje so clearly demonstrates, the two styles are complementary.[59] The exploratory technique works forward in many small normative steps, while the normative takes one large step forward, but this step is really built on small exploratory blocks which in turn are built on tiny normative steps. In other words, exploratory refers to forecasts derived from searches ahead, while normative refers to forecasts which are goal oriented and which work backward from ends by searching for alternative routes to lead to the goals.

It is important for the users of future maps or forecasts made elsewhere to receive, as part of the package, some statement about the general world outlook or value position of the forecasters. It must be known for example whether they are optimistic or pessimistic about the general concern of industrialists for ecologic considerations over profits; whether they believe peace or war to be the natural state of affairs; or if they believe that economic growth and increasing affluence is a good thing. Of course, the forecasts might make the positions of the forecaster clear to a well-informed person. Forecasts that put things in an unbelievable outlook demand fuller explanation. Where forecasts are done normatively and so stated, one knows the desires of the forecaster. However, his judgment about underlying assumptions or the adequacy or practicability of the means to achieve his stated goals is still open to question.

— Distortion is also caused by the style or methodology used.
There are many styles of forecasting, and the methodologies used may have a remarkable effect on the value of the forecasts. The Delphi technique, so useful for tapping the innovative and critical faculties of expert observers in areas where other means of forecasting are not easily available, has some specific plusses and minuses. The technique is good in that it avoids the possibility of dominant personalities overpowering others, as might occur if the prophesiers were gathered at a meeting to probe the future. However, because the Delphi technique

usually utilizes multiple rounds of exchange (wherein reasons advanced by proponents for defending their particular forecasts are made known to the forecasters before each succeeding round) the net effect is slowly to eliminate the extreme positions by forcing their holders to the median. Sometimes extreme positions are simply dropped, in order to produce a single forecast or one reasonable range of forecasts of events. This aspect of the Delphi technique is worrisome, for it would have effectively eliminated detection of the most important and generally unsuspected, far-out, but nevertheless later verified forecasts, inventions, discoveries, or extreme positions offered by scientists and others in years gone by. It is possible to order the Delphi technique in such a way that polarization of views is encouraged when a broader spectrum of ideas is desired.

　—There may be a tendency to self-fulfillment of a highly publicized future.

If an anticipation, a prediction, or a truly probabilistic forecast is used widely in planning circles, it may gain credibility simply through visibility as an established and to-be-awaited certainty. Tolerance of even a most unpleasant prophesied future may develop as it is awaited. Worse, some persons may see how to exploit the forecasted future, and although aware of how bad it is, may promote it because they are developing a way to profit personally from the eventuality.

　The foregoing considerations lead up to the potential dangers of (1) misdirection, (2) loss of resources, (3) mismatch of the goals we will be wanting in the future with our achievements at that time, and (4) possible monstrous side effects because consequences of the forecast and planned-for-results were not intelligently scrutinized and broadcast in time. Donald Michael wisely questions whether society should determine which areas of technology ought to be explored, since technology does change society.[60] Ozbekhan raises the whole level of discussion of planning to the need for normative planning,[61] and thus for massive participation to make planning normative for all, not just for the elites.

　Do these admonitions indicate that we cannot use forecasting and, therefore, that we must abandon long-range planning? Lindblom says something like this,[62] and so do Caiden and Wildavsky.[63] Other planners say that more of a sense of what we want, of direction, of on-paper trials of what will happen on one or another route to our goals, could not possibly create a worse situation than the one in which we now find ourselves. Duncan points out that a wrong forecast is not necessarily a bad one if it is thoughtfully done and serves to focus attention on areas needing change.[64]

　What we claim to want is in part guided by what we have and do not like, in part by what we hope for and do not have. Future mapping should help us overcome both deficiencies. It gives us clues as to what is in store for us, it gives us an idea of other possible futures and their consequences, and it suggests alternative routes to each future with price tags attached. Obviously, once forecasting is begun it cannot be stopped. Like planning, of which it is the critical ingredient, forecasting must constantly reassess the newly current situation, both to determine the results and, thus the validity of prior future mapping, and to identify other forces and events that have surreptitiously introduced themselves (our forecast and analytic failures) and must now be reckoned with as forces shaping the future.

Future Mapping: A Proposed Procedure

Future mapping is designed with the understanding that all the non-health sectors have a much larger aggregate effect on health needs than the health sector, essentially that they dictate the state of health. At the same time it is acknowledged that the health sector must respond to all the manifest health needs and that its capacity to do so is determined primarily by the non-health sectors, and only secondarily by the size of health needs, met or unmet. Thus, a forecast will also have to be made about the nature of general social objectives over a period such as the next 20 years, and about the implications of those objectives for the place of health and health care among the national priorities.

To make the procedure more tangible, a series of anticipations was created by which a two-county community in the state of California (which will be called here the East Bay) might be able to guide itself in planning for its future contributions to health. Appendix A shows much of the detail of the contextual logic used to create this series of anticipations. The tables have the same headings as the discussion in the text.

In keeping with Ackoff's[65] advice, several projections were considered: (1) a *reference projection* of what was expected to come about as things now seem to be going; (2) a *modified reference projection* to take into account what might happen if some of the more recent glimmers actually took over and changed old trends; (3) a *wishful projection* (normative), the one we would want to come to pass; and (4) a *planning projection*, the estimate of how far toward our goals the plans could probably take us. The reference projection is purely anticipatory while the "modified reference" projection has some exploratory elements. The wishful projection is purely normative, and the planning projection is a combined normative and exploratory outlook of what the planners feel they can come up with as a significantly improved future.

I suggest using either the reference or the modified reference projection initially, to get an idea of what is likely to happen for the non-health sectors and national population distribution and health aims. However, until there is comprehensive planning inclusive of health and non-health concerns at the national level, the construction of "wishful" or "planning" projections for those concerns sounds like a hollow exercise at any level of society. It is possible to do wishful and planning type normative projections at the state and local levels for health needs, well-being needs, and distribution of resources, for these can in part be shaped at levels below the national one. However, national level health sector planning could surely eliminate much heroic and ultimately wasted or suboptimal state and local efforts.

Distribution of People

The demographic attributes of the population are the first data needed. Without a population baseline, we do not know for whom to anticipate, nor can we build estimates of the numbers of departures from health, such as morbidity and mortality. Starting with their rates, classes of events can be given reasonable perspective. Working with numbers of events allows estimates to be made of actual loads and numbers to be faced. The characteristics to be tallied and made available at least every ten years by means of the census, are kept at a minimum; they include population numbers in terms of major ethnicity, further subdivided by sex, age groupings, educational attainment, income, type of housing, rural/urban distribution, and nature of employment. Ideally, the data would allow any kind of cross tabulation among these groupings and, with other factors and the original data, would be kept intact for future calculations that might be indicated. Built on these measurements and extended by anticipations about other issues such as migrations, changes in educational and other attainments, changes in sources and levels of income and disparity between haves and have nots, the proportions of various population groupings can be pursued into the future.

Distribution of the Capacities and Outputs of the Non-Health Sectors

From forecasts about the state of these non-health sectors we can anticipate how healthy we will be in the future (what health needs we will have), and at the same time we can anticipate the kinds of resources that can be allocated to care for these needs. The non-health sectors may be subdivided in many ways. The measurements for the divisions we suggest are not as yet always easily come by. Fortunately, estimates expressed in percent of change up or down over 10-year periods may be of as much or more use than specific numbers for each desired period.

Educational status. The level of education has already appeared under demographic data. Indicators from this sector, such as level of education, proportions with higher or lower amounts of education, and the relationship of sex, social, ethnic and rural attributes to the level of education are important. Evidence of increases or decreases in educational disparities between groups is vital because of the relationships of social mobility, territorial mobility, employment, and utilization of health services to educational level. These in turn are the basis for forecasts and many conclusions about the well-being of the population.

Educational capacity. Information about the product educational institutions are capable of delivering, such as the quality of their offerings, their current output by regions, training or subject matter, and so on is basic to understanding what can be done or is likely to occur to popular health understanding, to professional manpower and to various support segments of the economy, including the general level of affluence. To train unutilizable manpower just to achieve a higher level of education can be a disaster in terms of wasted resources and the mounting dissatisfaction of educated persons who are irrelevant to the employment market. The 1971 revolt in Ceylon is a testimonial to this truism.

Distribution of physical environmental attributes. Because so much of man's well-being depends on his environmental exposure, an assessment of this situation is in order. The environment, for assessment purposes, can be split into two areas, natural and man-made. Obviously the two are sometimes hard to separate, but the purity of these health-relevant categories may not be critical. Adequacy of housing might show up here or under the demographic section, nature of employment might show up under well-being, economics, or occupational environment. The quality of the air, water, and soil, safety, and any threatening practices such as lack of basic controls of effluents into any of these media all need to be forecast. Estimates need to be made of the adequacy and acceptability of such necessities as transportation, recreation, safety, and enforcement of related laws (which in the aggregate also takes into account the special needs of the various age groups in the population).

Natural resources. Although the health hazards of pollution of air, water, and soil have already been included, other issues are involved here. Natural resources may be destroyed as well as used up. The disappearance of resources such as some of our best soils, certain minerals, our forests, and our oil and coal reserves has implications not only at the national level but for each community. Because survival or economic welfare often depends on a community's climate and available natural resources, the dissipation, exhaustion, contamination, or destruction of these resources may spell the end of a community's general well-being. Populations may have to change from one source of livelihood to another, and one can anticipate emigrations of workers whose skills are no longer needed, of the unemployed, and of hopeless youth.

Problems similar to exhaustion of resources arise where pollution has destroyed the economic value of sea life or of forests or has altered the air so that certain crops can no longer be grown. Irrigation practices may have similar adverse effects on soils over a prolonged period of time. Alterations of climate and moisture conditions may directly affect the incidence of certain diseases. At a minimum, the nature of the populace, with their concomitant health needs and their capacity to produce resources, is likely to be altered and will have a significant health impact. Issues such as recycling are part of both the natural resources aspect of our lives and of the next category, the state of our technology. A set of forecasts at this interface has recently become available.[66]

The state of technology generally. Although often put out of mind by planners working below the national level, the outputs and state of technology cannot be overlooked when assessing the state of affairs that will have an impact on health and well-being status. Facets of possible concern are:

Level of productivity.

Nature of technological promises, such as the economic availability of desalinated water; threats or misuses of technology as exemplified by the internal combustion engine.

The ability to replace or overcome the lack of certain scarce natural resources.

The ability to increase the supplies of specific foods or suitable substitutes.

Demands that technology makes on people may well become excessive, leading to boredom, alienation or anxiety, depending on how different individuals react to the increasing variety, intensity or subtlety of the demands, resulting from technological alterations in every aspect of home, work, and social life.

Transport and urban living. Although dependent on technology, these factors have such a massive impact on our well-being that several pertinent indices must be sought. A basic consideration is adequacy of public transportation so that excessive demands are not made on more and more persons in their attempts to get to and from work or to other activities of living. A spillover from this problem is its effect on air pollution. Housing policies which create low-density suburbs and abandoned central cities might be taken into account. The degree of urban living, density levels, degree of geographic mobility, effects of proposed freeways, and levels of congestion and noise are all tangible matters. Some anticipations of disproportions between needs related to family size, education, dwelling space, health and resources such as transport, communications, recreation, and housing can be made. Although no clear evidence of what is health threatening seems to exist,[67] this area should be kept in mind.

Economics. Employment, earnings, inflation, areas of expenditure, savings, job security and skill renewals are critical areas. Again, the national economic picture overshadows local tendencies, although long before national changes are visible, some local ones can be anticipated. The death of certain industries, declining need for unskilled agricultural workers, enlarging size of farms, security of local employment may all be decisive factors in a community's health status, as well as in its ability to procure health resources.

Politics, government and authority. The issue of how well people are served by their government is acute at this time. Assessment might study different groups, looking at geographic, ethnic, age and social differences, and at the kinds of participation and response to government and institutions that are occurring among these groups. Evidence of participation will not only provide clues when it comes time to seek plan implementation, but it may also be a critical factor in any attempt to give a voice or power to those previously not heard from. Phenomena that deserve forecasts are:

The level of popular participation in community affairs, parent activities, voting, and disturbances.

The capacity of political parties to be reached and to respond to significant needs of individuals and neighborhoods.

The capacity of government to be reached and to respond to significant needs.

Levels of government that seem to be able to reach citizens effectively.

Government willingness or unwillingness to formalize local community participation, as measured by the level of reaction at open hearings, extent of membership on advisory boards, actual delegation of decision-making power to local areas, and contracting out or authorizing service distribution by neighborhood entities.

Governmental activity and capacity as producer of services.

Governmental capacity to effectively specify and purchase services from producers of services.

Scope and Direction of Widely Accepted Societal General Aims

These aims represent the tangible social and political expressions of our national credo and values, and forecasts are needed to prepare ourselves for changes among them. Aims are, of course, of top-level importance when they are nationwide in scope and forcefully espoused by national leaders. They can be identified from political rhetoric, and currently include such issues as consumer protection, the right to health care, ecological watchfulness, full employment, and non-discrimination. State and local aims may add such items as restraint of population growth, encouragement of industry, or clearing the bay, and these may have to be seen as top-priority items in those communities. In addition to professed priorities, heed must be paid to the forecast of actual standards of performance required for each issue, because these standards, rather than the nature of the issue, may be the critical variables that will change.

Scope and Direction of Widely Accepted Societal Health Aims and How Health Will Be Perceived

Generally reflections or derivations from the preceding group of societal general aims, societal health aims may be, or forecastably become, independent societal goals (such as available health care for everyone) or implied health goals carried in other societal aims (such as special health services for the aged, with national or local priority given to every facet of the needs of the aged). The issues of birth control and abortion are examples of shifts in mores which create significant health sector tasks, and forecasts here would be of tremendous value. This set should presumably be dependent on projections made in all the preceding sectors.

The set of forecasts on how health will be perceived is also important. It is worth considering what aspects of health, or what new ways of looking at health, are likely to emerge over the years. Just as many views now exist (see Chapter 3), new ones can be anticipated and some of the present views may well collapse. It is possible that economic productivity (the main concern behind disability) as a health concern can be put in the category of has-beens within five years. It is also a good guess that well-being of the "spirit" will be of serious importance 20 years from now.

Health Needs, Distribution of Traditional Physical and Mental Health Afflictions

The preceding sets of anticipations are the basis of estimates in this area. We still are obliged to measure departures from desired states of health. In general, numbers of deaths and illness by several major causes, shown by the same future demographic distributions already described, allow us to forecast rates by which we can intelligently contrast the health state of various groups and communities over time. Emotional well-being, as distinguished from loss or absence of intellectual capacity, such as retardation, senility, or toxic states, may be placed in this category or in the following one.

Well-Being Needs, Distribution of Health Capacity, Social Spiritual Dissatisfactions

The sets of forecasts from the preceding areas are the basis for making estimates in this area. Traditional health indicators need to be supplemented by more modern concepts of well-being to provide some concept of spiritual or social well-being capacity. Not all of the desired measurements are always available, and surveys of the type already described may be indicated. Measurement of internal and external satisfaction, or of spiritual and social well-being, inevitably concerns matters that are regarded as the territory of social workers, recreationists, law-and-order personnel and others in whose hands most of this data now resides. In spite of all their weaknesses, useful surrogate measurements are currently available. (They appear in the tables in Appendix A.) These might include age, race, and sex rates of specified crimes, family breakdown as expressed by child abuse and abandonment, divorce and separation, delinquency, truancy, and drug utilization, employment-dependency status, and so on. Data on health knowledge, misinformation, attitudes, and behavior also help clarify anticipations about health capacity.

Distribution of Resources for Traditional Health Needs and Well-Being

These anticipations are dependent on the forecasts preceding, in terms of the levels and natures of health interests and the dominance these are given among our national and more local aspirations, and of the pressures for services that will probably arise from perceived health needs. Although the items to be measured will not be spelled out here, we must keep in mind the scope of these concerns: the presence and utilization of the gamut of health manpower, the variety of facilities and technical equipment, the financial, service-enabling, underpinnings necessary to allow use of the services, and the organizational machinery and consumer relationships needed to make health care into a tangible, accessible, acceptable, and comprehensive reality.

In addition, this forecast extends to patrol of the physical environment to keep it acceptably safe, to health education, and to the role played by nonscientific healers. Diverging from the traditional, we need to assess the availability of social and emotional counselling services; adequate assistance for those in need; the acceptable solicitude of agencies capable and interested in serving the threatened suicides, persons caught up in marital and family discords, alienated children, and the unemployed capable of employment. In many small communities and pockets of large cities recreational opportunities are lacking or access to them is difficult; poor transportation keeps people from de-

sirable human contacts, such as church activities or continuing education lectures and films, where these are available. People lack information about employment opportunities and vocational counselling
about new careers or upgrading current status. Yet, agencies able to
assist realistically or even to provide comprehensible information are
conspicuous by their absence in most communities.

Discrepancies between Distribution of Health and
Well-Being Needs and the Resources

These anticipations represent the differences between the reference
projections or anticipations for health and well-being needs and the
distribution of resources. They are the resultant consequences of the
interactions of the preceding sets of anticipations. They give us an idea
of how the gaps between needs and resources will develop. Even if we
just wish to cope with what the future threatens to bring, this is an
important set of determinations.

If we had made our normative or wishful projections seriously and
emerged with tangible planning projections for health and well-being
needs and resources, this set of discrepancies should be diminishing
and not of critical concern to us now, except as ammunition to warn
ourselves about what would be happening if we had not proposed to
forcibly attack them. It is not, therefore, necessary to bog down in the
differences of meaning implied by need (what technologists know exists in the way of adverse states which can be effectively serviced), popular demand (what people claim to want), potential demand (what
people would want if they knew what they could get, could get it, and
had no limitations of any kind interposed), and effective or economic
demand (what people can and do purchase with their resources).

How to Proceed

Each of the various sets of anticipations must be checked for its effects on the others, and a round or two of revisions is inevitable. (The
absence of any national or state guidance at this time makes the forecasting effort for a locality no small chore and does reduce it to a guessing game, but one that is quite rewarding because of its eye-opening
visions of possible futures.)

Given the anticipated futures in the nation, state, region, and our
own locality, and the inability of our own locality to build its future
independently, our local health planning body can probably only be
significantly wishful (normative) in the limited areas of health and
well-being needs and health resources. Even this is realistically limited
in the United States.

There is no coordinated planning of consequence for the non-health sectors of a given locality to which the health planners can relate. Yet, I have already shown that the state of health and well-being is most affected by what goes on in these non-health sectors. So we can only be guided by our anticipations for these sectors without seeing any particular way to significantly influence their outputs, except by public appeals to the innumerable public and private actors and policy makers acting in the non-health sectors.

However, based on the anticipations for national general aims and health aims, there is significant opportunity to make extensive wishful and planning projections for our locality and to anticipate a significant outpouring of health care resources and some environmental control resources. For these concerns, the planning links between the locality, the region and the state are growing. Although the implementing authorities are still quite independent of one another, anticipations indicate improvement on this score. The missing planning link is the national one. This is particularly important because implementing capacity at the national level is high and the nation could, in its unplanned way, overlook or upset the planned-for interests of our locality.

If, for their own guidance, localities and states in the United States attempt first to create national projections and then more local ones, what they find in the way of health outlooks will not be reassuring. Nonetheless, these projections may stimulate concern for intelligent and planned-for futures on the part of legislators elected from their areas to the Congress, as well as among local legislators and the many citizens' groups which do not currently understand what is to be gained from future mapping. The tremendous growth of interest in the United States for the ecologic aspects of future mapping suggests that arousal of interest in future mapping for the health sector may well be the means of creating awareness of what the non-health sectors are about to do, and the ways these sectors affect our health and general well-being.

With the general academic interest in national social accounts, as well as occasional legislative and executive interests, it is not too hard to visualize that pressures generated by local and state health planning efforts for future mapping may provide the impetus to create an adequate national futures intelligence scheme. Even if such a scheme does not actively guide the creation of that future, it will at least help us to cope with health care in the future.

Future mapping is more easily undertaken in countries where extensive overall planning is underway. Such nations usually have normatively guided planned projections for each non-health sector. Occasionally they have similar projections for the health sector, although these are usually restricted to coping with anticipated health care needs. However, because of the confused belief in almost every country

that the level of health care services somehow determines the level of
health, the future mapping for the non-health sectors is rarely utilized
to point out the nature of the state of health that they will generate and
the nature of the health needs that will consequently arise.

Even in rather well planned economies, health plans commonly
consist entirely of projections of health care needs and resources. These
are based on past and present documented needs, and are converted
into future projections primarily on the basis of demographic projections, the overall availability of resources, and what political promises
suggest can or must be diverted into health care.

Activities in other sectors, such as industry and agriculture, are part
of the planning behind vast water, power, and fertilizer plans. Yet they
are often not considered in the light of their effects on the lives or
health status of great masses of people. The creation of massive enteric
and insect-borne disease exposures are among the terribly obvious failures which go unanticipated, but which will swamp the health care
services with endless, needless, life-threatening and expensive illnesses
caused by "successfully" achieved plans in the non-health sectors.

We are entitled to be ironic when we describe such plans as "successful." Well though they may have been planned, and well though
cost-benefit approaches may have been utilized to get the most for
available money, the costs in ill health, even if measured only in terms
of the extra unplanned-for burdens placed on the health sector, may
more than offset anticipated gains. In fact, had these secondary effects
been taken into account, markedly different development plans might
well have emerged, plans which would not peril the health of great
numbers of people or the solvency of the health care system—events
which might well topple expensive plans as well as governments.

With appropriate future mapping involving all sectors, the effects of
the planned projections for each sector would be tried out against
those for each other sector. With the active participation of knowledgeable health and social planners, forecasts would not only point
out the areas where extensive health changes are likely to be introduced, but also where health needs and plans are likely to affect other
sectors in turn. These exchanges will begin with such obvious but often neglected matters as spread of contagious disease. And then they
will go well beyond, into areas of major life habits affecting, for example, nutrition and education, attitudes about services, capacity and desire to work vigorously, housing and adequate income. Even ease of
transport or changes in educational methods or curriculum may completely alter the use of neighborhood health services and the utilization
of lesser skilled health workers, as differently educated people are able
to rapidly and inexpensively bypass outlying services for what they
perceive as more complete, elegant, and desirable centralized services.

The educational pattern, including the determination of languages to be taught (not an uncommon issue in newer countries), may make obsolete certain kinds of medical practice or important groups of practitioners, unless there is extensive retraining or use of teams capable of handling any language or custom barriers.

Without future mapping which involves equally the health and non-health sectors, it is unlikely that good overall planning can emerge. Even though certain sectors may seem to be doing excellent projections in splendid isolation, that work is likely to be so suboptimizing that disaster may be inevitable. I am aware of the arguments for intentionally unbalanced planning.[68] But I do not equate unbalanced planning with blindfolding oneself to the realities of unintended adverse consequences of what is planned. The availability of appropriate future mapping data is now being promulgated by the United Nations as well as other internationally involved agencies.[69]

An Annual Scoreboard: The Use of Selected Indices to Provide an Assessment Tool Primarily for Use in Allocative Considerations and to Point Out Problem Communities or Groups

The Logic of the Scoreboard

In addition to the health flak and to the forecasts, another kind of marker is needed for year-in and year-out use for measuring in a general way, the current state of health affairs. These markers or health indices would point out improvement or deterioration of certain selected, but very representative, key health conditions among different groups, and would provide the means of checking how well health anticipations are keeping on schedule. The scoreboard's key use is to make comparisons over time, from group to group, and particularly to tell where an unusual number of conditions are out of line. From such observations, one learns of the need to allocate more planning attention, if not more resources generally, to communities or groups that are in trouble on many fronts. This approach identifies problem or sick communities particularly and in that way helps to reorient allocations.

Annually recalculated data, along the selected markers, reflect the general level of health progress and can also be of use in keeping annual track of certain major current problems (the logic of the choice of many specific markers). One could, of course, use all the customary age, sex, race, disease morbidity, and mortality data to compare groups from year to year. But the usual health flak, as we have called it, is much too voluminous to serve as an easily comprehensible overall community scoreboard. We are, therefore, suggesting use of a carefully selected handful of individually important indicators to provide an adequately wide-ranging scoreboard that will inexpensively clarify the entire well-being situation. So that no major population segment goes without scrutiny, indicators must be selected which, as a minimum, tell about the current most health-sensitive areas of both sexes, about each of the "seven ages" of man, and about the major ethnic groups.

Because the scoreboard approach is used to detect differences between specific age, race and sex population groups living under different circumstances, a basic set of items of data collected nationally or internationally might also be enlightening as a base for comparisons. However, state, metro, county, and neighborhood or census-tract-level data are needed to clarify the differential nature of the hazards suffered by the seven ages and two sexes of the major ethnic groups from locality to locality. In addition, various localities will need a few other indicators of particular significance to them, especially if they are more normatively minded than allocative, and wish to ferret out discrepancies between neighborhoods or groups which are probably more distinctive to their area than to a state or a nation as a whole.

One planning agency in each state, preferably at the state level, should be chosen, by agreement of all state planning agencies involved, to collect and distribute data for all units in the state. For the national-level concerns, a national-level entity is necessary to receive, composite, and distribute interstate comparisons. Without interstate data uniformity, there will be no useful comparisons—one more compelling reason for a national health-planning body. One of the first duties of the national body would be to develop nationwide consensus on the choice of health-relevant indicators and a practical, simple means to display the material for general planning and public consumption.

The scoreboard is a comparative tool which makes no attempt to describe each aspect of the well being of a community. Its utility is to point out presently sicker communities or groups in a community by focusing on a few sensitive indicators for each major well-being parameter. Only a few of these indicators were among those utilized in future mapping, and there is no reason why they should be identical. Future mapping is particularly normative as well as exploratory, while the scoreboard is essentially problem finding and allocative in outlook. The scoreboard is not used to provide normative or reference (exploratory) projections, indicate tradeoffs, or assist with future feedback, all aspects of future mapping. However, by looking back ten years it does allow a sense of trending, important to anyone who has to pass judgment on how sick a community is and whether it is currently more or less sick than it has been. From the results of the future-mapping effort already described it will not be hard to anticipate what the next ten years will hold for the scoreboard items of the communities under study, if one wishes to carry the scoreboard ahead for that period of time.

Possible Indicators

By judiciously selecting the health indices from among:
  traditional physical-mental health areas;
  newer social well-being/health-habits areas;
  well being services and social environment; and
  physical environmental areas
a fairly wide and meaningful check on health progress can be kept at a
low cost, community by community. Choice of indices will vary somewhat with the population under study as well as over time, since markers are useless for conditions which are unlikely to occur. Some conditions presently provide particularly good markers, in that they are potentially labile and will tell fairly rapidly whether health as defined by
them as improving or worsening. Leprosy seems to be a poor marker
in most of the United States because few meaningful changes can be
expected. But tuberculosis is still a fair marker, and coronary artery
disease and lead poisoning seem very relevant subjects for comparisons
between groups and over time.

The list of suggested indices in Appendix B includes several where
data are presently partially available, and a few for which there is not
direct traditional measurement. Rate of alcoholism, for example,
might be expressed in prevalence figures as estimated from the Jellinek
formula; or, in some communities, active treatment services might
yield data in terms of the numbers coming under treatment. However,
what is really needed here are some more trustworthy prevalence rates
by age.

Suggested Tabulations

Possible prototypes for intergroup and intercommunity comparisons are given in Appendix B. We would go further and suggest
that a set of data for 1960 and another for 1970 be developed to provide the base against which future annual compilations could be contrasted. Hopefully, before the 1980 census we will have annual or biannual sampling techniques, so that census data will always be kept
up to date. We hope also that the particular handful of presently unavailable indicators felt to be most desirable for our national to neighborhood health scoreboard will be included in the census-taking machinery. The purposes they are to serve are as critical to our national
well-being and to our "big business" health sector as are the markers
so willingly inserted into the census on behalf of commercial and industrial interests.

If suitable indicators were selected and made part of the national
census and sampling survey procedures, it would be relatively simple
to provide all communities—neighborhoods or the nation—with annual or biannual comparisons. Each smaller community could then

develop its own ten-year scoreboard projections, with guidance from larger encompassing communities. At the national level, data should include international and state comparisons; at the state level, data should show the national as well as metro and county-level data. Metro level data should show data for the state as well as for the counties or major communities the level encompasses. At the county or big-city level, data from the metro, adjacent comparable units and its own neighborhoods should be shown. Neighborhoods might be conglomerates of contiguous and relatively similar census tracts. In some cases use of data from individual census tracts might be justified, although census tract rates are generally open to too wide a variation for all but a few indicators, because of the scarcity of the indicator events arising from such a small population base.

Possible Graphic Presentations

Graphic presentations would facilitate public or planning use of the comparative data for the various geopolitical communities. These could be done in color by quintiles for each of the indicators at the various levels: the first, national; the second, comparison among the states; a third, comparing planning metros of each state; a fourth, comparison among the major local planning sub-units of each planning region; and the fifth, a comparison among the neighborhoods in each local planning unit. At the top of each list would be shown the total population in the unit, to give some notion of its overall import. These sets, one at each of the five geopolitical levels, would avoid both the hazards of obscuring critical "bad" places by lumping them into excessively large aggregates, and the obverse hazards of failing to see big pictures by concentrating solely on small units.

DATA AND MEASUREMENT ISSUES

What Needs Measurement

Planning and analytic approaches eventually will either distinguish or reconcile technically perceived needs and felt needs (wants). But what is most often measured is the effective or currently met demands, and these, for many reasons, may be less than either technically perceived needs or felt needs.[70] As evidence is put on record of who and how many are ill, disabled, or prematurely dead, along with evidence that relevant action can be taken, the needs revealed will be translated into wants. But problems in correlating needs with wants will continue unless planning leads both the haves and the have-nots to compare their values in open discussion. From this mutual exposure, planners should discover which data are wanted, as well as shed light on controversial issues such as over-demand and artificially stimulated utilization.

Another important consideration is the reciprocal relation that the choice of certain service indicators may have on priority awards. Just specifying the services that are to be measured favors services whose goal achievements can be measured. Other outputs which are difficult to measure may either look poorly justified or go unmeasured and remain less known and be seen as less deserving of further allocations. The so-called preventive services provided by public health departments forever fall in this category of hard-to-measure and are thus ignored routinely.

The circumstances under which data are being acquired may not match those from which the underlying concepts emerged to shape the data model in use. There may be semantic confusion and dubious linkages; comparisons from one set of circumstances to another need careful scrutiny.

The use of trend lines for projections must take into account the frequency of data points in the past. A trend may have been up or down between infrequent points and really be the reverse or more extreme than would be indicated by a line drawn between two widely separated points in the past. What is implied in the way of effects of other current trends such as age composition, political environment, or wars cannot be overlooked.

The negative and the positive aspects of phenomena both need scrutiny. The negative side of employment (unemployment) is not the whole story, although it is the "pathology," "pressure" or "panic" indicator for priorities in planning, because it is couched in terms of human distress. Notwithstanding, we must know what employment is doing when unemployment goes up; employment too may be going up as fast or faster, or it may be dropping. This combination of information is critical for planning. The positive side of social indicators is more "physiologic" and often more relevant for long-term planning. When referring to people in distress, rates should not be substituted for numbers because rates obscure the size of the group in trouble (our use of unemployment rates is a case in point). Attention must be given to both absolute numbers and rates.

How gain or loss is expressed needs careful interpretation. A change in the proportion of persons over 65 may be expressed in percent of increase in that group. For example, going from 5% to 6% of total population looks trifling for national welfare, but in terms of the needs of the elderly this is a 20% increase. The very same matter may be expressed as a change in the non-aged from 95% to 94%, a truly insignificant affair. Planning often requires that such matters be seen both as the proportion of change in those who are at risk, and the proportion of change in those who are not at risk from the concern at hand.

A preliminary look for "sick communities" is an approach often recommended to those initiating planning. The search is relatively simple, directed to looking for troubled areas which will arouse concern. By using the scoreboard approach already described, a few easily obtained local averages can be compared with state or national averages in the fields of education, employment, mortality, or availability of services. Professionally advocated standards may be used for comparisons. Much as the use of generally accepted standards for definitive planning is derided, they may be used in looking for troubled communities which then must be studied in relevant depth. Needs that might be serviced are considered in the light of levels or standards that represent local decisions on how much is to be done. These may be influenced or even determined by state and national requirements or advocated minima.

One ubiquitously available indicator that transcends the utility of all others with which we are familiar, is the infant death rate, because it is so heavily correlated with every kind of social failure. In depth studies indicate that in one city it is not as sharp an indicator as the prematurity rate and the level of prenatal care received.[71] No exercise of genius is required to take any one or several of these social indices, such as education level, overcrowding, unemployment, or income level, and thereby pick out the sections of the community with a disproportionate share of life-threatening problems.[72] This quick look tells which neighborhoods are out of health and social control. It does not necessarily tell which individuals are at the greatest risk, nor what galaxy of underlying causes is creating the perilous life situation. This kind of quick assessment bears out once again that many areas of input, other than the application of health services, must be scrutinized if health deficiencies are to be planned against and minimized.

Differing Data Needs and Uses at Local, State, and National Levels

Much of the national-level concern with any disease should justifiably be created by the loss of production occasioned by disability or premature death. National comparisons between diseases would then be heavily weighted in favor of giving priorities to diseases which entail such loss. Local comparisons between diseases are equally important but less likely to give highest weighting to production losses. Local-level analysis of a disease is often done from the standpoint of its actual demands for care, personnel, facilities, available dollars, as well as issues of equity in receiving care.

States have in the past looked at health problems much as local areas do, but may now begin to be concerned with production losses too, because their involvement with PPBS keeps reminding them of productivity. (Chapter 6 is heavily devoted to these issues of priority rating.) Clearly, an aging population exerts great local pressure because of the needs for prolonged or repeated care, while auto accident fatalities among young people may get low local priority since usually only inexpensive burials are required. Yet from a national position, the death of youngsters signifies a higher loss to the GNP. Of course, such PPBS administrative outlooks are heavily counter-balanced politically by the votes tied to the care of the aged.

For still other reasons, national bookkeeping differs from state and local. A local community must always question nationally-set disease expenditure priorities for new dollars. The community may already be spending at high enough levels, and local expenditures already may be falling into the low payoff range; the condition may be absent or declining naturally in the community; the condition may be at a much lower payoff level than others to which the same dollars could be applied locally; or the need for research may be justified nationally while another particular activity or service is justified locally.

In a condition such as tuberculosis, the level of expenditure indicated at the national level may be unrelated to what is needed in a state or locality which is already spending heavily on wise programs. More dollars there might buy very little more control, because of high marginal costs. In other communities, poor programs or low levels of anti-tuberculosis activity may call for a much higher level of activity or new kinds of activity because new anti-tuberculosis dollars still have a high payoff. Yet the latter community is likely to be one that needs outside assistance. Again, a combination of local, state, and national assessments is needed to tell where money and activity should be shifted, and against which diseases.

At the national level there must be a predominant concern with health status and with well being as well as for health care services. To generalize, at the national level there is need for data which will allow:

Comparisons to be made of national benefits or gains which might result from investments made in (1) satisfying needs inside the nation versus demands on behalf of international commitments, (2) the health sector versus other sectors, (3) health improvement versus health care, (4) one area of health care versus others, (5) one region versus other regions, (6) one group versus services to all (primarily, correction of inequities).

Priorities to be set for allocations for research and development by subject and by state.

Guidelines to be set up for allocations to pay for direct services, training, and back-up services.

At the state level, some of the same considerations apply, but the major concerns in the past have paralleled those evident at the local level. If planning becomes more popular, the states may shift their posture toward the kinds of concerns suggested for the national level. At the local level, the data needs are in the direction of satisfying the unserved, remedying inequities, and, particularly, facing the problem of how to create accessible services of a generally acceptable nature.

Current gaps or surplusages in each of the major resources in states or localities can be indicated by departures from national averages. The use of more normative standards than national averages is justified by common consent and will be imperative in many states, once they begin to determine their own needs patterns.

Required Uniformities and Conjoint Data Collecting

No attempt is made to outline what is involved in the way of formal data-collection machinery. Fortunately, some thinking has taken place on this subject in the United States, and it strongly puts the finger on a federal-level health agency to provide the basic underpinning, as well as to initiate the approaches for local and state levels.[73] Federal-state-local partnerships are now being seriously envisaged.[74] An excellent series of Bureau of Census publications specifically addresses itself to how to do health assessment. The series provides, in addition, every detail of an assessment done for one community, showing how multiple data sources were put together to get the job done.[75] Other sources show how multiple studies can be coordinated.[76]

A new and very good so-called environmental survey tool has been developed by the U.S. Public Health Service and is available in a package called "NEEDS." This tool not only provides neighborhood and housing data but elicits demographic health status, mobility and satisfactions data. It is apparently inexpensive to apply and simple to conduct and utilize.[77] Another survey tool recently used in Yolo County, California, does some comparable and some different measurements, and also looks valuable.[78] A general review is available.[79]

In every case, only by a firm relationship to the census and to the national health survey can the same kinds of information be available throughout the country. There is no reason that localities should not have a richer statistical program. But unless such a program is built onto a nationally uniform base, there will be little chance to make comparisons with other groups or jurisdictions—an inevitable key function of all health assessments. The limitations to the assessment process—technical, conceptual, and interpretive—are discussed at the end of Chapter 6.

REFERENCES

1. Erich Jantsch, *Technological Forecasting in Perspective* (Paris: Organisation for Economic Cooperation and Development, 1967). Erich Jantsch, *Technological Planning and Social Futures* (London: ABP/Cassell, 1972), 54-59.

2. Donald W. McGranahan, "Analysis of Socio-Economic Development Through a System of Indicators," *Annals of the American Academy of Political and Social Science* 393 (January 1971), 65-81.

3. Seth B. Goldsmith, "The Status of Health Status Indicators," *Health Services Reports* 82 (March 1972), 212-21.

4. H. Wallace, et al., "Availability and Usefulness of Select Health and Socio-Economic Data for Community Planning," *American Journal of Public Health* 57 (May 1967), 762-72.

5. D. M. Heer, ed., *Social Statistics and the City: Report of a Conference held in Washington, D.C., June 22-23, 1967* (Cambridge: Joint Center for Urban Studies of the Massachusetts Institute of Technology and Harvard University, 1968). "The Census—What's Wrong with It? What can be Done?" (A Staff Report), *Trans-Action* 6 (May 1968), 49-57.

6. Barkev S. Sanders, "Measuring Community Health Levels," *American Journal of Public Health* 54 (July 1964), 1063-70.

7. U.S., Department of Health, Education and Welfare, Public Health Service, Publication no. 719, Revised Edition, "International Classification of Diseases, Adapted," December 1962; reprinted March 1965.

8. Lillian Guralnick, "Some Problems in the Use of Multiple Causes of Death," *Journal of Chronic Diseases* 19 (September 1966), 979-90.

9. U.S. Department of Health Education and Welfare, Public Health Service, Health Services and Mental Health Administration, National Center for Health Statistics, Vital and Health Statistics Ser. 2, no. 17, PHS Pub. No. 1000, *Conceptual Problems in Developing an Index of Health*, by D.F. Sullivan, May 1966. U.S., Department of Health, Education and Welfare, Public Health Service, Health Economics Ser. no. 6, PHS Pub. No. 947-6, *Estimating the Cost of Illness*, by D. P. Rice, May 1966. D. P. Rice and B. S. Cooper, "The Economic Value of Human Life," *American Journal of Public Health* 57 (November 1967), 1954-66. James D. Hennes, "Measurement of Health" Medical Care Abstracts 29 (Dec. 1972), 1268-88.

10. U.S., Department of Health, Education and Welfare, *Conceptual Problems* (See no. 9).

11. R. E. Markush and D. C. Seigel, "Prevalence of Death, A New Method for Reviewing Death Rates for Specific Diseases," *American Journal of Public Health* 58 (March 1968), 544-52.

12. U.S., Department of Health, Education and Welfare, *Conceptual Problems* (see no. 9). U.S., Department of Health, Education and Welfare, Public Health Service, Health Services and Mental Health Administration, National Center for Health Statistics, Vital and Health Statistics Ser. 1, no. 1, PHS Pub. No. 1000, *Origin, Program and Operation of the U.S. National Health Survey*, August 1963. U.S., Department of Health, Education and Welfare, Public Health Service, Health Services and Mental Health Administration, National Center for Health Statistics, Vital and Health Statistics Ser. 1, no. 1, PHS Pub. No. 1000, *Health Survey Procedures, Concepts, Questionnaires*, etc., May 1964.

13. John Kosa, Joel L. Alpert, Robert J. Haggerty, "On the Reliability of Family Health Information," *Social Science and Medicine* 1 (July 1967), 165-81.

14. U. S., Department of Health, Education and Welfare, Public Health Ser-

vice, Health Services and Mental Health Administration, National Center for Health Statistics, Vital and Health Statistics Ser. 1, nos. 1-10, *U. S. National Health Survey: Origins, Programs, Operation, Findings in Vital and Health Statistics*, 1963 on.

15. Kerr L. White, et al., "International Comparisons of Medical Care Utilization," *New England Journal of Medicine* 277 (September 7, 1967), 516-22.

16. S. Fanshel and J. W. Bush, "A Health Status Index and Its Application to Health Services Outcomes," *Operations Research* 18 (November/December 1970), 1021-66.

17. D. L. Phillips, "Mental Health Status, Social Participation and Happiness," *Journal of Health and Social Behavior* 8 (December 1967), 258-91. Norman M. Bradburn and David Caplovitz, *Reports on Happiness* (Chicago: Aldine Publishing Co., 1965).

18. State of California, Department of Public Health, "Health and Ways of Living." A questionnaire prepared by J. R. Hochstim. J. R. Hochstim and D. A. Athanasopoulos, "Personal Follow-up in a Mail Survey: Its Contribution and Cost," *Public Opinion Quarterly* 34 (Spring 1970), 69-81.

19. Andrew Shonfield, *Modern Capitalism: The Changing Balance of Public and Private Power* (London: Oxford University Press, 1965), Chapters 13 and 14. Leon Keyserling, "The New Health Care Economy: Forces Reshaping General Policy, Structure, Financing and Quality of Care," *Bulletin of the New York Academy of Medicine* 42 (December 1966), 1157-77.

20. L. C. Fitch, "National Development and National Policy," *Environment and Policy: The Next Fifty Years*, ed. by William R. Ewald, Jr. (Bloomington, University of Indiana Press, 1968).

21. U.S., Department of Health, Education and Welfare, Public Health Service, Health Economics Ser. no. 6. PHS Pub. No. 947-6, *Estimating the Cost of Illness* by D. P. Rice May 1966.

22. Erik H. Erikson, *Childhood and Society* (New York: Norton, 1950), 247-69.

23. Paul L. Berkman, "Life Stress and Psychological Well-Being: A Replication of Langner's Analysis in the Midtown Manhattan Study," *Journal of Health and Social Behavior* 12 (March 1971), 35-45.

24. N. M. Bradburn and D. Caplovitz, *Reports on Happiness* (see no. 17).

25. D. L. Phillips, "Mental Health Status, Social Participation and Happiness," *Journal of Health and Social Behavior* 8 (December 1967), 285-91.

26. Edward S. Rogers, *Human Ecology and Health* (New York: Macmillan, 1960), 155-78.

27. I. N. Pearse and L. A. Crocker, *The Peckham Experiment* (New Haven: Yale University Press, 1946).

28. T. H. Holmes and M. Masuda, "Psychosomatic Syndrome," *Psychology Today* (April 1972), 71-72, 106.

29. K. L. White, et al., Ibid no. 15.

30. Arnold I. Kisch and Joel W. Kovner, "The Relationship between Health Status and Utilization of Outpatient Health Care Services," *Archives of Environmental Health* 18 (May 1969), 820-33. Also, C. O. Carlton and R. Miller, "Kisch's Health Status Proxy: Two Suggested Improvements," *Health Services Research* 6 (Summer 1971), 184-86.

31. K. L. White et al., Ibid no. 15.

32. U. S., Department of Health, Education and Welfare, Ibid no. 14.

33. State of Hawaii, Department of Public Health, "Ethnic Differences in the Prevalence of Selected Chronic Conditions," by C. G. Bennett, *Chronic Disease Newsletter*, March 1968.

34. T. Miyasaka, "An Evaluation of a Six-Year Demonstration Project in Community Health in a Rural Area in Japan: Chiyoda-Mura Health Project," *Journal of Social Science and Medicine* 5 (October 1971), 425-40.

35. David G. Berger and Elmer A. Gardner, "Use of Community Surveys in Mental Health Planning," *American Journal of Public Health* 61 (January 1971), 110-18. R. M. Andersen et al, "Health Service Use: National Trends and Variations—1953-1971" U.S. Department of Health, Education and Welfare, National Center for Health Services, Research and Development, HSM Publication 73-3004 Washington 1972.

36. Paul Davidoff and Thomas Reiner, "A Choice Theory of Planning," *Journal of the American Institute of Planners* 27 (May 1962), 103-09.

37. Andre L. Delbecq and Andrew VandeVen, "A Group Process Model for Problem Identification and Program Planning," *Journal of Applied Behavioral Science* 7 (July/August 1971), 466-92.

38. Elizabeth Jolly, "Forecasting: A Health Planning Tool," School of Public Health, University of California, Berkeley. Mimeographed. 1971.

39. "Toward the Year 2000: Work in Progress," *Daedalus* 96 (Summer 1967). Herman Kahn and Anthony J. Wiener, *The Year 2000: A Framework for Speculation on the Next Thirty-Three Years* (New York: Macmillan, 1970), 398-409. Bertrand de Jouvenel, *The Art of Conjecture* (New York: Basic Books, 1967). Roy C. Amara and Gerald R. Solancik, "Forecasting: From Conjectural Art Toward Science," *Technological Forecasting and Social Change* 3 (1972), 415-26.

40. Yehezkel Dror, "A Policy Sciences View of Future Studies," *Technological Forecasting and Social Change* 2:1 (1970), 3-16.

41. Irwin D. Bross, *Design for Decision* (New York: Free Press, 1953), 33-38.

42. Thomas J. O'Connor, "A Methodology for Analogies," *Technological Forecasting and Social Change* 2:3/4 (1971), 289-309.

43. E. Jantsch, *Technological Forecasting* (see no. 1). Olaf Helmer, "On the Future State of the Union," Institute for the Future, Report R-27 Menlo Park, (May 1972).

44. Olaf Helmer, *Social Technology* (New York: Basic Books, 1966).

45. Clark C. Abt, "An Approach to Methods of Combined Socio-Technological Forecasting," *Technological Forecasting and Social Change* 2:1 (1970), 17-22.

46. E. Jantsch, *Technological Planning* (see no. 1), 171, 174.

47. E. Jantsch, Ibid., 116-32.

48. E. Jantsch, *Technological Forecasting* (see no. 1), 116-32.

49. John C. Chambers, Satinder K. Mullick, and Donald D. Smith, "How To Choose the Right Forecasting Technique," *Harvard Business Review* 71 (July/August 1971), 45-74.

50. Geoffrey Vickers, *Freedom in a Rocking Boat* (London: Allen Lane, The Penguin Press, 1970).

51. Jay W. Forrester, *Urban Dynamics* (Cambridge: Massachusetts Institute of Technology Press, 1969).

52. U. S., Congress, House of Representatives, Committee on Banking and Currency, Subcommittee on Urban Growth, "Counterintuitive Behavior of Social Systems," testimony by Jay W. Forrester. Jay W. Forrester, *World Dynamics* (Cambridge: Wright Allen Press, 1971).

53. Donella H. Meadows, et al., *The Limits to Growth* (New York: The Universe Press, 1972).

54. Otis Dudley Duncan, "Social Forecasting—the State of the Art," *The Public Interest* (Fall 1969), 88-118.

55. W. Alonso, "Predicting Best with Imperfect Data," *Journal of the American Institute of Planners* 34 (July 1968), 248-55.

56. J. W. Forrester, Ibid no. 51.

57. C. West Churchman, "The Design of Inquiring Systems," Internal Working Paper no. 107, Space Sciences Laboratory, University of California, Berkeley, September 1969, 225-39.

58. *Annals of the American Academy of Political and Social Science* 394 (March 1971).

59. Ritva Kaje, "Methods of Inquiring for Planning: Social versus Technological Forecasting." Master's thesis, University of California, Berkeley, June 1970.

60. Donald N. Michael, *The Unprepared Society* (New York: Basic Books, 1968).

61. Hasan Ozbekhan, "Towards a General Theory of Planning," *Perspectives of Planning*, ed. by Erich Jantsch (Paris: Organisation for Economic Co-operation and Development, 1969), 47-159.

62. Charles E. Lindblom, *The Policy-Making Process* (Englewood Cliffs, N. J.: Prentice-Hall, 1968).

63. Naomi Caiden and Aaron Wildavsky, *Planning and Budgeting in Low Income Countries*, (New York, John Wiley and Sons, 1974).

64. O. D. Duncan, Ibid. no. 54.

65. Russell L. Ackoff, *A Concept of Corporate Planning* (New York: Wiley Interscience, 1970), 23.

66. Alfred J. Van Tassel, "A Seminar Exercise in Forecasting Ecological Changes: Pollution from Rising Industrial Output," *Technological Forecasting and Social Change* 2:3/4 (1971), 237-45.

67. Robert E. Mitchell, "Some Social Implications of High Density Housing," *American Sociological Review* 36 (February 1971), 18-29.

68. A. O. Hirschman and C. E. Lindblom, "Economic Development, Research and Development, Policy Making: Some Converging Views," *Behavioral Science* 7 (April 1962), 211-22.

69. United Nations, Economic and Social Council, "Second Development Decade: A System of Overall Review and Appraisal of the Objectives and Policies of the International Strategy," May 1971.

70. National Commission on Community Health Services, *A Self-Study Guide for Community Health Action Planning*, Vol. 1 (New York: The American Public Health Association, 1967). W. C. Richardson and D. Neuhauser, "The First Question in Health Planning: Does the Public Know What It Wants or Not?" *Modern Hospital* 110 (May 1968), 115-17.

71. H. Wallace, et al., Ibid no. 4.

72. E. M. Kitagawa and P. M. Hauser, "Education Differentials in Mortality

by Cause of Death, U.S.A. 1960," *Demography* 5 (January 1968). M. J. Lefcowitz, "Poverty and Health: A Re-examination," *Inquiry* 10 (March 1973), 3-1.

73. American Rehabilitation Foundation, *Project 759: A Study of Methods of Implementation of Public Law 89-749* (Minneapolis, Minnesota: American Rehabilitation Foundation, February 1967), Chapter 4 and attached appendices. U. S., Department of Health, Education and Welfare, Public Health Service, Health Services and Mental Health Administration, Document No. 26, "A State Center for Health Statistics," revised October 1969.

74. "Closing the Health Opportunity Gap," The 1970 Meeting of the Public Health Conference on Records and Statistics, *HSMHA Health Reports* 86 (February 1971), 145-48. Health Statistics Today and Tomorrow, The Report of the Committee to Evaluate the National Center for Health Statistics, Amer. Journal of Public Health 63 (1973) 890-910.

75. U. S., Department of Commerce, Bureau of the Census, Publications Distribution Section, "Census Use Study Documentation Reports 1-15 [particularly no. 12, "Census Use Study, Health Information System-II"], 1970-1971.

76. D. M. Heer, Ibid. no. 6.

77. U. S., Department of Health, Education and Welfare, Public Health Service, Environmental Health Service, Bureau of Community, "Neighborhood Environmental Evaluation and Decision System: NEEDS, A Manual with Survey Tools, 1970."

78. "Yolo County Health Survey," Department of Community Health, School of Medicine, University of California, Davis, 1971.

79. Robert L. Berg, editor, *Health Status Indexes*, (Chicago Hospital Research and Educational Trust, 1973).

6. Assessment: Interpretation, Problem and Goal Selection

In Chapter 5, I strongly suggested that each community use several kinds of assessment. One method outlined, the scoreboard, is a basic set of health indices on which the community could be compared with neighboring communities, the encompassing region, the state, other states, the nation, and with its own past. Its general health status picture would be made reasonably clear in that manner. To delineate specifics which are out of line, the usually available health data can be combined with well-publicized hearings which are used to elicit citizen views on special problems—problems that a general scoreboard of 25 or even 2500 indices might not suggest.[1] In addition to data, these assessment activities would reveal general and health aims and value positions. It was strongly urged that future mapping be undertaken by more sophisticated health planning agencies to yield an idea of what goal or value shifts and non-health sector situations lie ahead that might be major determinants of future health and well-being status, and how the health sector would have to respond.

By matching indices, opinions, and forecasts for health goals and health problems (evidences of resource shortages without supporting evidence that they are hurting someone do not count as real problems) with the value systems which enjoy community support, planners will point out the locally desired goals as well as the unacceptable nonconforming situations. An actively thinking and planning health sector may of itself bring to pass general value changes and subsequent cultural and institutional changes.

ASSESSMENT AS A SIGNAL SYSTEM

Assessment provides the basic information from which come the early warning signals of current deficits, surplusages, use and misuse of health resources; the extent to which various conditions (at various stages) go unattended or unprevented; the extent and nature of the losses incurred by these service deficiencies; and the inequities in delivery of service.

Assessment offers clues, suggests interventions and, ultimately, helps to develop means of verifying the etiology, and the predisposing and aggravating factors in various conditions which need to be subjected to medical and ecological research.

By assembling intergroup, community, and national comparisons of health status, assessment uncovers discrepancies which signal failures of prediction or of reasoning about the influences acting on well-being. Such discrepancies may also warn of suspected or unsuspected correlations between well-being and various modes of distribution of resources, of care, of access to services, and poverty.[2] Comparisons with immediate neighbors may point up the early stages of a crisis situation. The least well-off unit in a prosperous metro, for instance, may require emergency measures to correct an inequity, even though its level of services and well-being are not below average for the state or nation.

Assessment provides early warning. It also assists with long term strategies by identifying the boundaries which are relevant for successful attack on a given condition. Assessment clarifies geological, climatological, and other natural ecological boundary phenomena, as well as political, legal, economic and special interest factors that also help determine the base from which an effective attack can be mounted (see Chapter 7).

As a basis for determining strategy, assessment can provide information about community value systems, and about political, social and economic outlooks. Planning bodies need such information to decide where to start health planning and when conditions are ripe for action; how to get started on important matters which may have been hidden or withheld from consideration; how best to pursue each issue so that it has a chance for fair consideration and implementation; and how to set priorities among a welter of needs.

The broadest possible range of information enables a community to look at itself and at other communities, insuring that issues do not remain obscure but are seen in terms of their reality and their proportional importance. Public opinion can then be alerted and appropriate pressures exerted where special interest groups or legislators have remained indifferent or ignorant of the hazards,[3] delaying or blocking action. The populations involved in a problem will be enabled to see their plight more clearly. The service groups will be able to compare the magnitude or the nature of the problem with the interventions they are offering.

Enumerations are, of course, conceptually premeditated and thereby produce so-called facts. These facts are believed to identify conditions or situations. What is perceived is a condition which is not necessarily good or bad per se. The identical situation may be seen as good by those whose value expectations are met, and bad by those whose values are not; those whose values are unrelated, or who do not connect the condition to values, may not perceive the condition at all, or view it as a neutral state of affairs. The situation may be seen as different things by those who hold different concepts of the system of which it is a part.[4] An earthquake fault may be a problem to a city planner, but, ordinarily, only when property or lives are lost by an earthquake jolt does the condition become a problem for inhabitants, or become widely perceived by the community at large. Even then, some groups might see the condition only as a source of reconstruction jobs and never regard it as a problem, unless rebuilding were prohibited.

SELECTION OF GOALS OR LONG-RANGE DIRECTIONS

From the main streams of social concerns (presented in Chapter 2) that created our present-day attitudes about health, a planning body can derive a set of generally valued goals and health aims toward which it believes the community would like its planners to direct its health activities. From the viewpoints of the four sets of interests discussed in Chapter 4—the medical subsystem, the health care sector, the societal outlook and the planning outlook, all of which are represented on the planning body—planners can further derive some guidance about which health goals stand high.

From the assessments conducted of our community, as discussed in Chapter 5, should come up-to-date evidence about the general concerns that health planners must support while they attempt to obtain the more particular health goals that have emerged. By combining the information collected in these diverse ways, an operating set of goals for the health areas can be attained. The more general types of interests that society holds dear, like efficiency or equity, are placed on the list of goals which are also to be conformed to. Sometimes these general goals are clearly higher in value and override health goals, and they must be so acknowledged.

To illustrate how to select problems for priority consideration, later in this chapter, I pick out a sampling of likely criteria; among them are assembled goals that are very highly valued in the United States. And I arbitrarily weight them by my own preferences. These goals are not only the endpoints toward which our plans will strive (the normative aspects of developmental planning) but serve also as a means of assigning priority of attention to the long lists of problems which communities also want solved (the problem-solving portion of developmental planning). In Chapter 7, the same list of criteria, including the goals, is again used to weigh the suitability of proposed solutions (interventions) to problems.

ESTABLISHMENT OF GOALS AND STANDARDS OF EXPECTATIONS DETERMINES THE DISCOVERY OF PROBLEMS

The concept of a problem, and therefore demands for change, originates in human values. The more that individuals share attributes—age, social, ethnic, economic, or geographical—the more likely they are to hold common values and to put problems in comparable priority rankings. Values operate to set goals, and simultaneously set standards of expectations to measure accomplishment toward those goals. Goals lead to behavior, and thus to particular results or accomplishments. Evaluation by value-set standards shows up any discrepancies between the goals and the accomplishment. Figure 2.2 tries to make explicit how values dictate both long-range goals and standards of expectations, and thus set the stage for the discovery of gaps between achievement and expectations, better known as problems. This in no way denies the reality of alterations in standards of expectation, goals, or values themselves, as was elaborated in Chapter 2.

Who Is Looking Determines Which Values (Goals and Standards of Expectations) Will Rank Highest

Chapter 4 pointed out that the medical view of good health is more concerned with good medicine and technical quality than with adequacy of delivery; as long as physicians make the major decisions about health care services, little attention will be paid to availability, accessibility, or acceptability. Whether patients are made functionally better as a result of medical care has also not been of much concern to physicians. It took World War II and a charismatic medical leader, Howard Rusk, to make rehabilitation concepts acceptable, although to this day needed rehabilitation services are poorly prescribed or supported. Certainly then, what the health sector and citizens generally see as major problems has never necessarily been of much concern to organized medicine (even though many individual physicians have made tremendous sacrifices to call attention to health care shortcomings).

Similarly, the health sector takes for granted tremendous wastes of resources for some activities, such as transplantations. Yet it does nothing about such problems as infant starvation at a time when the nation's food surpluses caused acreage cutbacks or storage problems. This suggests that the larger society, if informed, might see different health problems than those seen by the health sector. (It is, of course, heartening that areas of the health sector now provide the leadership to publicize their discovery of health-destroying situations.[5])

The activities and traditions of any group tend to determine their value hierarchy. And their values determine not only what is worth seeking (goals) but the amount of accomplishment which will satisfy the value holder (standards of expectations). These standards are quite different from those generally professionally promulgated and utilized, even though both originate in values, albeit values of different walks of life. It is of some interest to examine the kinds of widely utilized standards promulgated by various groups and their relevancy for interpreting "facts" and finding evidence of problems.

Use of Generally Promulgated Standards as a Substitute for Value-Derived Standards of Expectations

The average community has been compared not once, but hundreds of times, against so-called national standards which usually represent some professional group's idea of the norms they would like to see met everywhere in the country. Need we say more? Perhaps not, but it does seem pertinent to extend the discussion of what generally promulgated standards really mean in practice and why they are useful, although caution is required. We are indebted to Allan Blackman for assembling these thoughts.

There have been many great standard-setting and standard-using documents in the field of health. Among the most famous are "Local Health Units for the Nation" by Haven Emerson, "Planning the Neighborhood," by the American Public Health Association Committee on the Hygiene of Housing, the Hill-Burton Act and its implementing regulations, the "Guide to a Community Health Study" also by the American Public Health Association, and most recent, "Health is a Community Affair," by the National Commission on Community Health Services.

National standards in the field of health deal with an amazing variety of subjects. There are standards for bed/population ratios; health personnel/population ratios; the size and content of hospitals; qualifications for personnel and programs for public health departments; facilities and services for cities and neighborhoods; the design, both detailed and general, of hospitals, homes and communities; the organization of health services; per capita expenditures for health services, and more. Within this diversity, there appear to be three meanings to the term "standard." (1) A standard may be a uniform measuring unit.[6] The Hill-Burton regulations suggest a standard width for hospital doors. While there may be some reason related to human scale or traditions of hosptal design for choosing a particular door width, what is important about this type of standard is that it is an agreed-upon convention. (Hospital furniture manufacturers need a standard door width in order not to make their products too wide.) (2) A standard may be a prevailing practice or average level of attainment. We talk about the standard test for a disease or the standard number of procedures performed daily by a technician, and we are simply making a descriptive statement about the average existing condition. (3) A standard may be a goal or a statement about what ought to be. Most of the standards proposed by the American Public Health Association and by the National Commission on Community Health Services have this meaning.[7]

Utility of Generally Promulgated Standards

Generally promulgated standards have utility for planners and others who do not have any codified way to know the actual levels of performance called for by prevailing goals. They obviously are intended as a substitute for closely value-related standards of expectations which would vary widely from place to place and from time to time, and would be hard to specify. Moreover, without some rather tragic experiences, such as casualties in hospital and nursing home fires, the value machinery and standards of expectations would be gravely deficient. Collective values and the collected experiences under which they were shaped are aggregated for larger communities, states, or nations and put forth in the form of generally promulgated standards. They are meant to avoid the consequences of fire in hospitals, of untrained doctors, of untested medicines and appliances, and so on. They represent a sort of collective, even if not too distinguishing, means of guaranteeing a reasonable minimum of performance or achievement. Their most unfortunate side effect is the stifling of more specifically needed standards and even the prevention of reaching for higher levels of performance, because they often do not allow variations in any direction.

—Standards do, then, provide a quick reference as to what is regarded as adequate to meet values (usually unspecified) and their norms. Most standards try to give firm measures, even if at multiple levels.

—When standards are matched to local conditions, any local areas which fall significantly short of desired levels stand out, and thus gaps or problems become visible.

—By comparing multiple gaps revealed by standards, a community is able to see which of many gaps are proportionately worse and might deserve higher priorities.

—Development of a set of local standards does not seem practical for several reasons. It will probably go beyond the budget and, conceivably, the capacity of the local expert or technologist. And it should lead to essentially the same kind of guidance provided by national standards, because the local expert shares the value orientation of the group to which he belongs and from which he is willing to take guidance. Communities presumably cannot each have a different set of standards, a situation which would emerge if locally designed standards were actually the product of the personality and circumstances of its author as well as of his community. Moreover, a locally composed set of standards for problem recognition often does not carry as much influence as a nationally devised set. Locals are too often inclined to close their eyes to long standing problems, and only national comparisons are presumed capable of shocking them into meaningful comparisons of what is versus what could or should be.

—Standards also provide an opportunity to compare one community with another, with, of course, as much opportunity for doing harm as good. When well done, comparisons of standards to measure health status enable communities to see what can be accomplished. When utilized to compare levels or types of resource expenditures, comparisons beg the issue of what is needed or useful in such matters as levels of beds provided or dollars spent per person for care or for educational qualifications of personnel.

—Standards are most valuable at the operational levels for such matters as man-machine safety, building and highway construction and repetitious mechanical tasks where reassessment or justification for the standard is needed infrequently. Periodic reassessment of the standards can be built in, to take into account new knowledge, new techniques, and new needs. The reference handbooks used by the various kinds of engineers, and particularly those which become uniform building, plumbing, or electrical codes are supposedly reassessed periodically, but usually at the hands of vested interests.

Hazards of Generally Promulgated Standards

Almost every use of generally promulgated standards involves reservations, but awareness of the reservations allows salvage of the good.

—The most critical issue is the tragic acceptance of widely promulgated standards, as though they were themselves the goals wanted locally. Norms of some group they certainly are, and presumably goal oriented. But these standards cannot be blindly accepted in lieu of local goals.

Yes, accreditation for a community's hospital may force compliance with a professional set of standards. But in truth, these may violate or contradict other goals of that community in major ways. Sources of standards for communities, such as *Health is a Community Affair*[8] by the National Commission on Community Health Services, and re-released by the American Public Health Association,[9] call for certain personnel and activities which have not always worked out too well where they are used, and for which there is often little justification in areas where they have not yet been instituted.

Are these standards to become goals by adoption? If so, what purpose could planning serve except to get these mass-produced goals adopted? I have urged planning first as a means of defining the improvements wanted. But these generally promulgated standards typically confuse means with ends; they tell us that if we create in sufficient number or quality according to standards, we will become healthier. Yet, usually, they neither name the goals nor guarantee that the standardized means will bring them any closer. Perhaps such standards are best used as reminders of implied goals, which we may wish to reconsider for ourselves.

—Blackman points out that standards are promulgated as technological or biological requirements, but that the very values or goals which they are supposed to help us reach are often hidden from sight.[10]

Standards often are not real requirements in that what they are supposed to achieve does not really depend on them. Rather, standards are designed in response to some other value held by their designer. Design standards for crowding are repeatedly presented in the cause of health, when in fact given the evidence at hand, they should more realistically be presented in the cause of equity, comfort, or esthetics.[11]

Setting standards for means on the basis of fallacious notions about what the means can or will accomplish, can be an even greater hazard than not bringing us closer to our goals; meeting such standards may actually deplete our resources. The annual medical checkup probably comes close to being one such standard. Even worse, many medically inspired bed and physician levels are patently inflated figures, and many societies with much better health records happily use fewer of each (see Chapter 4). Seemingly, standards too often plug for the most expensive or tangible but less useful means and divert attention away from the truly practical.

—Another great failing of standards is their inability to priority order gaps except by the "proportionate degree of failure" approach. All gaps cannot be tackled at the same time. An approach which does no more than identify supposed gaps is not a healthy instrument by which to promote citizen motivation for change in the presence of unlimited numbers of problems and limited assets.

How shall the community allocate its badly overdrawn resources when everything comes up looking like a problem (with implied, expensive, standardized solutions)? The contrast between the standards approach to planning and the priorities approach is clarified by comparing the maternal recommendations of the APHA's "Guide to a Community Health Study"[12] with the proposals by Ruth and Edward Brecher.[13]

Again, most standards have been created by operational level planners, usually in conjunction with purveyor or specialist groups. Sometimes broader sponsorship results when several planning, specialists, and purveyor groups have gotten together to avoid multiple standards or levels advised for the same situation. On occasion, the standard-making agency has a significant non-purveyor element. But even then, such organizations as public health, and more particularly the one-organ or one-disease health associations, are likely to act as though there were no other concerns than the ones they represent, and for which they promulgate outlandishly high and therefore expensive standards to apply. When such standards are stated in an authoritative way, they may even obscure the relationships of what is being advocated to what is desired in the way of outcomes.

—Standards tend to promote a single view of how to do business, build a hospital, and so on. Although they should be stated as minimal criteria to be met, they often are so specific as to bar substitution or improvement which might be at lower cost as well. Not only does this inflexibility hinder innovation, but it precludes responding to local conditions, contexts, and demands which might elicit more practicable means than what the standards call for.[14]

In my experience, hospitals that are most innovative and less expensive to operate, some of which draw visitors from all over the world, often have difficulty meeting standards which were inevitably designed for the more general place which, of course, never quite exists. Requirements for a hospital should also vary according to the relation of its location to other hospitals and health facilities.[15]

—Further attention is focused on means instead of results by standards which present quantified elements or quality judgments based on licensure or advanced degrees, themselves merely measures of input. Moreover, quality may easily be sidetracked by concern for quantity and merit badges. In this way, standards are antievaluatory, and, as previously noted, antiplanning as well.

—Standards, of necessity, ignore supply factors. Yet many communities, by substituting one kind of service or skill for another, find it quite feasible to cope with the needs. The failure to count midwives as part of the medical equivalent explains in part why the physician-population ratios in some European countries are low compared to those in the United States.

—Standards similarly ignore demographic differences which have a tremendous impact on what kinds of beds are needed, for example, long-term or maternity. Moreover, during a relatively brief period of time even the same community may change from an aged to a very young community (as happens when new ghettos replace old neighborhoods) and completely confound standards by new demands.[16]

—Finally, standards already tend to be fairly traditional or sclerosed and they further inhibit innovative practices built on newer values and the newer standards that would arise from them.

The promulgation of generalized standards probably has one major use: it gives planners and community a notion of what a significant number of purveyors or one-cause types have thought is required in a given set of endeavors. Because such standards are more easily framed in simple terms than in outcomes, they are usually input rather than output oriented. Input standards must be taken with a sizable pinch of salt, but they do provide a reference point for checking whether one's planned use of inputs falls in any approved ball park. However, if estimates fall exactly on widely accepted standards, one should be suspicious that local conditions and thinking have had little to do with the planning. Let us close with a quote from Blackman about generally promulgated standards:

> Despite any virtues, we do not think standards serve well the purposes of a technologically complex, pluralistic society. The simplicity of standards is an evasion. The hidden supplier-goals around "standards" are increasingly rejected by the public as has been demonstrated by "revolts" against highway departments, redevelopment agencies and welfare departments. The technical difficulties of the new planning approaches that might help us avoid dependency on standards have been over-rated, we believe. The essential goals of these techniques often can be accomplished without technical sophistication or computer hardware. The major job of those doing planning should be (1) to focus on defining community goals; (2) to assess the nature of the goals as the basis for choosing programs; (3) to assess the nature of the community as a basis for designing programs; (4) to use community goals as the basic criteria for evaluation of the efficacy and desirability of programs.[17]

Measurements Define Situations and Attitudes Convert Situations into Problems

Even though a community may not have clearly vocalized its goals nor their related standards of expectations, it is very apparent that communities do find excessive discrepancies or gaps between what they want and what they find occurring. Of course, communities may misjudge discrepancies—some gaps seem over-publicized (usually those which violate high priority value goals), and some gaps are never noticed (usually those violating values not held widely or those which are gaps only to technologists who know from experience or experiment that certain events need not occur).

The discrepancy between what is technologically feasible and what is in fact being accomplished is a technological gap. Technologists who know that certain conditions need not exist may persuade communities to change their values and thus come to see long established and accepted conditions as gaps or problems. Advertising the gap may well lead to community development of new values or the reordering of old ones, so that a technical gap becomes identified as a new value gap. (An example is the priority now extended to utilization of artificial kidneys.) A problem then can be defined as a condition sufficiently distressing that relief is sought or desired, that is, an effort will be made to bring behavior and achievement into line with expectations or norms.

Relevant statistics may not be available or even reasonably procurable for every serious problem. Even worse, no one may come forward to point out that a particularly bad and well-known situation is a problem, for where problems occur, they may be accepted as "the way things are." Perhaps no one understands that there is a remedy, or no one is capable of speaking out to draw awareness to the situation. Terrible emergency care, for example, has been more typical than atypical in the United States.

The plea was made long ago in the United States that public health departments become the advocate for those in need and for those whose problems attract no attention.[18] In practice, this advocacy has not worked well. We have known for decades that infants get lead poisoning from eating lead wall paints. Yet only in the late 1960's did any agencies bestir themselves, and only in 1971 has the problem been perceived as sufficiently significant to reduce lead in paint. Even that is more of a gesture for the future than a remedy for infants being poisoned now, for this is a problem of neglected children whose quarters get little new paint. In other words, even those professionally trained and paid to search out problems of health may not see problems of certain types of people as worth fighting about. Obviously then, a problem lies in the eyes of the beholder. In the field of health, given the spread of involved actors, even selection of the kinds of problem appropriate for consideration by health planning bodies is a major issue.

Because values may conflict and goals be divergent, discrepancies between sets of values must be understood. But with understanding, decisions become more complex, particularly if society tries to offer a "little something" for each of the competing value holders. In theory, by focusing on long-term goals, divergent value holders may find agreement less difficult. But not all disagreeing value holders are likely to accept long-range planning, particularly not those who have been regularly shortchanged in the past. For these and many other reasons, we do not predict that setting priorities among problems to determine order or magnitude of attack will be an easy task for planning bodies.

SELECTION OF PROBLEMS FOR STUDY

In this welter of problems, divergent goals, conflicting values, and varied viewpoints, can any order be imposed to aid judgment without doing violence to the importance of minority or unpopular value systems or submitting to the dangers of oversimplification? The situation is similar to the attempt to measure subjective feelings, that is, to quantify qualifying factors. The method I propose for applying the judgment tool of assessment is to set priorities for problem selection by means of criteria. The criteria which the planning body adopts are, for the most part, applicable restatements of the general goals and of the health aims which the community (at whatever level) has already selected as the ends toward which the normative aspects of its developmental planning will be working. In the same way that the criteria were selected they are weighted to show their relative preference as envisioned by the community or its representatives on the planning body. The problems are rated for relevance and importance according to each of the criteria. Thus significance levels can be compiled and a priority list set up.

Categorizing Problems to Facilitate Application of Criteria

I do not subscribe to the logic that all problems can be pressed into the format whereby size or importance is measured solely in terms of dollars lost. I also do not think it is sensible to try to reduce all problems to person-days-of-disability, person-days-of-work-lost, or person-days-of-good-health-lost (see Chapter 8). Reducing all problems to terms of person-year-of-life-lost by premature death is even less meaningful. Deaths, disabilities (illnesses), or discomforts are not the obvious outcomes of many problems nor the only reasons that many problems worry us.

Different criteria are therefore needed for application to different types of problems. Although problems may appear to be diverse, examination will usually reveal that they cluster around certain main groupings for which criteria can be chosen. For day-to-day work we have found the five categories listed below of practical use. These five kinds of problems are significantly different from one another, and each category would best be measured by a different battery of criteria. In addition to making comparisons more rational, the five problem categories will make decision making among the mass of proposals easier when it is done for one category at a time on the first round of selection.

Disorders (diseases, morbid conditions as identifiable by medically trained persons).

Physical environmental threats to well being. Although these are not different conceptually from disorders, they often require involvement of very different interests, information, and participation, and so they justify a separate category. These failures may be one of the causative factors underlying disorders.

Failing communities (those that have many health and well-being problems of all kinds).

Inequities in receiving health-promoting opportunities or health care services. These problems can be part of any of the other problem categories, particularly that of the failing community.

Health care delivery system failures (such as lack of organization, lack of articulation of services or deficient consumer participation). We would also include here such lesser delivery system management failures as inefficiency and ineffectiveness.

Other categories of problems are frequently noted. They are often important in the long-term considerations of what needs to be done but are not likely to rouse keen community interest, for they are more planning process-oriented than immediate or hurt-removing matters. These include:

Resource inadequacy, such as lack of financing for health care for the poor.

Inadequate planning machinery or capacities, planning failures.

Planning process problems, such as lack of citizen participation by victims, vested interests, consumers at large, and so on.

Knowledge shortage.

Inane or misdirected policies with which planning or operating systems must comply.

The first five categories are health sector problems per se. The next five are more in the nature of constraints pressing on planning and operations machinery. A hundred significant other, comparable types of problems, which often are contributory or causative factors but not health problems per se might also be listed here. In Chapter 7 we show how these can be identified in the process of analyzing any given health problem. However, if a community so desires, any issue believed to have an impact on well-being may be regarded as a significant problem, provided that it is ultimately correctly identified by analysis in terms of its causes and consequences.

This categorization of problems is not offered as an ideal list. Any planning body could and should make up its own categories. The point is that, for convenience in making decisions, similar problems should be grouped to establish order of attention and to facilitate elimination of the less important ones in each class, presuming that not all problems can be acted upon initially, if ever.

Selecting Criteria to Rate Problems Competing for Priority Consideration

In the deliberations and decisions of a planning body, this process of priority setting can provide a means to quantify many qualifying factors, and will prove to be equally relevant whether used to resolve the difficulties of choosing problems to study, selecting causes of problems to be attacked, or choosing among interventions directed at causes or consequences of a problem. Priority setting may also be needed as a means to justify decisions. In this chapter attention is directed primarily to the choice of problems to be studied.

Braybrooke and Lindblom point out the weakness or indefensibility of the criteria approach, but offer an unsatisfying substitute which really boils down to continuing much as is done now without attempts to improve rationality.[19] We can persist undeterred but forewarned of the limitations sensed in utilizing criteria.

Correspondence of Criteria to Highly Preferred Goals

Criteria to be utilized and the weights to be given are pure value judgments. Rating would be simpler if there were a continuity of national criteria, that is, if general aims which brought leadership into office were adopted as policy and made manifest, not just in rhetoric but in legislation and public investment. Many criteria could then be derived from the general aims of the national, state, and local levels of government which affect a given planning jurisdiction. If a planning body chooses major criteria consistent with generally held values and goals, it then need have little fear that its criteria are irrelevant or meaningless to its constituents.

In some countries these goals are not hard to determine nor is there any question of their predominance. Unfortunately, in the United States, goals differ widely among cultures, regions, and levels of government; they are rarely stated well nor are they clearly mandated, as by legislation with adequate funding. For example, in the past several years national housing concerns were superseded by a push toward ethnic goals, ethnic concerns by urban problems, urban problems by unemployment and poverty, poverty by hunger, hunger by peace and peace by inflation. For a time, inflationary concerns were nudged over by those of ecology, and ecology felt the hot breath of health care services.

Reality testing shows that in relation to their size, little was accomplished about most of these concerns, and that we were led from one dance to another without any concern for concluding the preceding one. It is not psychologically easy to develop criteria for a planning body from these dubiously sincere expressions of goals which shift priority according to the most recently politicized problems. However, the adoption of significant legislation relevant to goals expressed in party platforms, and the increased likelihood of passage of such legislation if both parties manifest the same goals, or if the president comes from the same party expressing the platform goal, does tell us that nationally perceived goals are meaningful.[20] Some of the failure of such legislation to result in desired improvements might be attributed to insincerity which produced legislation that was meant to be ineffective. But I am of the belief that failure to understand the systems involved and the rudiments of planning has more to do with the fact that legislation does not produce the desired effects in spite of heavy allocation of resources. The health planning legislation in the United States provides substantial evidence of the ineffectualness of our planning for planning.[21]

The question might be raised: "How important is it that major criteria coincide with national concerns, if the latter are so evanescent?" Obviously, planning bodies must be guided by their perception of what people want. As poorly as nationally expressed wants seem to have been supported, the panoply of recent, so-called national aims is probably still a useful reminder list, since support of these issues gets politicians elected.

As a first theorem we are prepared to state that all criteria must be sensibly chosen to ensure that health planners do not run counter to significantly powerful general aims, either intentionally or inadvertently. For example, if full employment were a major guiding national aim, health planners could not rationally come up with schemes to save labor by substituting equipment. Of course, this choice based on employment goals might run headlong into another less critical national aim, promotion of the greatest health care efficiency. But a decision cannot be made irrespective of its effect on the higher valued goal of full employment. Similarly, if adequate distribution of health care services is or becomes a major national concern, a planning body may not leave equity out of its key criteria.

Criteria Are Often in Conflict with One Another

Many highly held values, and their goals which are to be used as criteria, are in unintended conflict or, at least, in competition with one another. Our desire to reduce deaths may find us producing more prolonged disablement, another undesired outcome. Our desire for a "best buy" may result in automation and more underemployment for unskilled persons, violating our desire for employment and equity. The approach to be described which uses averaged ratings of weighted criteria is intended to minimize this dilemma.

Preparation of Lists of Criteria

Criteria might best be placed in four batteries, one for each of the four major aspects of each proposal: (1) technologic concerns; (2) health status goals; (3) overall social goals or concerns; (4) health planning concerns. Health status concerns correspond in part to the medical viewpoint described in Chapter 4, and in part to the health care sector viewpoint. Overall social concerns correspond to the societal viewpoint. Health planning concerns, another minute yet important set of viewpoints, correspond to the outlook of those engrossed in planning in the health planning nucleus shown in Figure 4.2.

The choice of criteria should be made before problems have been placed on the agenda. If this is not done, a planning body will find that criteria and weightings are likely to be excessively shaped by the problems placed before it. Without a previously agreed-upon list (always open to change), development of criteria, as well as their weighting and rating, is likely to become an exercise in partisanship or one-upmanship, as various board members find means to favor problems dear to their hearts.

Criteria lists should be prepared by the combined efforts of staff and the planning board (with its consumer, victim, purveyor, political, and professional expertise) reviewing possible criteria obtained from various listings, from their sensing of community concerns, and from their own hurts. It would seem necessary that the citizen board finally vote on each criterion. A truly diverse council membership should, of course, come up with a more useful slate of criteria, even though they may have to work harder to get agreement.

The overall planning board might decide to insist that a general list of criteria be applied to every type of problem, while each of its task forces or committees might best use a special list for each class of problem. The need for new criteria, as well as for periodic reweighting, will keep criteria current with new knowledge or value changes among the board and the constituency.

Setting Priorities by Significance Levels

Four steps are involved: weighting, rating, compiling significance levels, and setting up priority lists.

Weighting

The idea of establishing a significance level by use of weighting in accordance with the relative importance of various criteria to society (I suggest a one to five scale) was supported by the work of Gordon and

Kurz and the State Environmental Health Task Force of New Mexico in their January 1970 report to the New Mexico Comprehensive Health Planning Council.[22] In the New Mexico technique, the planning board—combining consumer, purveyor and technical expertise—discussed the selected criteria and then individually weighted them, adopting the averaged weighting. They concerned themselves with a single class of problems, those of the environment, and were able to develop a neat and concise set of factors. There is nothing about their technique that cannot be extended to a much wider range of concerns.

Rating

Rating the problem under consideration for relevancy and importance according to each criterion is the next step. By rating the value of the problem on a -10 to +10 scale for each criterion, each planning body member expresses his feeling about that specific aspect of the problem. The average of the individual ratings is utilized. Only occasionally will it be necessary to rate problems on the negative side of zero.

Obtaining Significance Levels

For each criterion the averaged rating is multiplied by the accepted (averaged) weighting. The product provides a significance level. Adding the positive significance levels and subtracting the negative gives a total of significance points. The total should be divided by the number of applicable criteria, because not every problem is measured against all the criteria. The result is the averaged significance level for the problem. The significance level is intentionally skewed by dividing by the number of criteria applied rather than by the sum of the weights involved. The problems in each category can then be arranged in a priority sequence according to these significance levels.

Setting Priorities

The entire rationale for the process just outlined is built on the assumption that board members will be unable, without an analytic tool, to come to agreement on complex decision issues. However, by considering problems in the light of relevant value factors (weighted criteria) and then rating to provide significance levels for each problem, the board or council members could come up with reasonably satisfying group decisions. (The issues of how public choices and public decisions are made are presented in Chapter 11.)

The problems receiving the highest significance level on each of the four batteries of criteria are easily visible and can be given major consideration promptly. The lowest rated problems are also very visible and can easily be excluded. The issues in the middle range may be postponed or opened to further scrutiny or hearings to determine if they have some peculiar hidden significances not yet revealed. The planning body may select some of the modestly rated problems for analysis, particularly where such problems would help remove an imbalance in the council's work.

The critical question remains: Will minority value holders ever get their day, or will they be outvoted on every issue? If so, the old scheme of tossing them an occasional bone just to keep them quiet may have to be reinstituted. At that point, criteria, weighting, rating, and significance levels could all be dispensed with since the major issue of equity would seem to have been outmaneuvered by the numbers game.

It is important to note that rating problems, criterion by criterion, to establish their relative importance is not always feasible until the more complex problems have had at least a superficial analysis for their significance, their consequences and the nature of their precursors, as described in Chapter 7.

Uses of Priority Setting

Assignment of priorities has many meanings. Generally it does not imply exclusive concern with the highest priority item, nor does it necessitate waiting to control that one problem before going on to the item second on the priority list. Fortunately, rank ordering usually produces a series of high ranking items and does not preclude taking action on many, particularly where problems are not all in competition for the same limited resources or for the resources allocated to a major area. For example, services for children do not necessarily compete for the same interests or funding as those for environmental control.

Priority setting may be used with the following intentions:

Indicate which items in each category are to be implemented first.

Indicate which items in each category are to receive no further consideration.

Indicate which items in each category are to receive the major share of resources.

Indicate whether the activities called for by the high priority items in each category are to be firmly established before others are to be embarked upon.

Indicate which among the high ranking items in all the categories are to get the go-ahead, on what time table, and with what proportion of the resources.

Choosing one group of criteria to do a task, such as *selection* of problems to be acted on, and another group of criteria to aid in deciding the *order* in which action should be taken, sounds attractive but will be misleading in practice. For example, *selection* can be based on criteria such as importance, rate of increase, irreversibility of damage or cost-benefit ratio, while *order* can be based on technological readiness, political acceptability, programmatic feasibility and overall economic capacity to carry out the activity. The failure of such a two-part device is illustrated in several examples which follow.

How much of the available funding or other resource such as staff and committee attention, should go to even the highest rated problem? A single problem might easily gobble up all the resources available for that class of problems or even for all classes of problems. An approach to this issue used in New Mexico was to describe three levels of award —minimal, intermediate and optimal—and to suggest that state budgeting for environmental activities be required to fund every accepted problem at the minimal level before any were budgeted at the intermediate level. Similarly, it recommended that all be funded at the intermediate level before any received maximal funding.[23] This approach makes me very apprehensive.

The nature of problems is such that minimal coverage for Problem Number One might require a million dollars per year, while maximal coverage for Problem Number Two might take only $50,000 once. Yet, any funding less than the maximal of full $50,000 for Problem Number Two might waste the entire expenditure, while starting Problem Number One with as little as $10,000 might be very useful (or vice versa). Minimal or intermediate or maximal can be described meaningfully only in terms of what can actually be accomplished, not by how much is invested. In a different situation minimal funding for large Problem One produces a huge net saving, but maximal funding for small Problem Two could never approach the size of these benefits. Should Number Two ever be funded?

In the initial study of problems, usually only the planning body's own resources are being allocated. Commitments from cooperating agencies may well determine how many, even which, problems are to be studied. If the Heart Association were willing to undertake the main support of a heart disease problem investigation and analysis, the planning body might be wise to let them proceed even if it is on a rather low priority problem, particularly if the Heart Association could not or would not work on a problem with a higher priority. By cooperating in this way with other organizations, the planning body may implement study of a greater proportion of significant problems than its own resources could allow. Our conclusion is, then, that extent of allocation of planning resources to problems with fair to high priority ratings would further depend on:

Ability to get others to carry the main load for the problem.

Level of resources needed by a given problem study to anticipate breakthrough or results.

Seriousness of a problem compared to other high ranking problems in the minds of significant sectors of the public.

Because some issues undoubtedly have a threshold financing level below which payoff is nil, because some take years to firm up, because others have such spectacular potential, and because a good many may be happily taken over by cooperating agencies, the planning body must correlate its priority ratings with specific constraints posed by each of the proposals that were rated highly, before making final selections for study.

Some issues cannot be reduced to numbers, at least not initially, and surely, the spread of planning resource awards and the proportion of planning resources allocated to each problem will remain among the major legitimate intellectual activities for the planning body after use of the decision-making tools previously described has brought them this far. Conceivably, a council may select a problem completely out of priority, but it would need justification for doing so. This justification would clearly have to counter such notions as:

The council used meaningless criteria.

Their criteria were weighted erroneously or not in accordance with beliefs.

They did a very casual job of rating.

They succumbed to illegitimate influences.

A List of Usable Criteria with Suggested Weights and a Rating Scale

The simplest way to present the nature and variety of the criteria available for problem rating is by means of one figure (which also includes the criteria for solutions since essentially the same list of criteria may be used for both). This list was formulated by guidance from innumerable lists of criteria. Figure 6.1 is followed by an elaboration of the meaning of each criterion, because the titles may be a bit cryptic. The explanations are also phrased in terms of application to solutions as well as to problems.

Two criteria are shown as absolute. The failure of a problem to pass either of these two criteria would presumably table it, and significant degrees of failure on goal conformance and plan conformance would do likewise.

FIGURE 6.1
CLASSES OF CRITERIA, THEIR WEIGHTS,
AND RATING SCALE

Criteria	Weighting	Rating Scale
Technological Aspects*		
Technology Possible	Absolute	Pass or Fail
Technological Feasibility	5	−10 to +10
Manpower Requirements	3	−10 to +10
Balanced Attack on All Phases of a Situation	3	−10 to +10
Balanced Attack on All Phases of the Environment	3	−10 to +10
Health Aspects		
Problem Likely to Go Away by Itself	5	−10 to +10
Probable Duration of Problem if Undisturbed	4	−10 to +10
Deaths	3	−10 to +10
Disability	3	−10 to +10
Disease	3	−10 to +10
Discomfort and Pain	3	−10 to +10
Condition Size or Numbers	3	−10 to +10
Condition Severity	3	−10 to +10
Condition Duration	3	−10 to +10
Distress or Danger to Others	2	−10 to +10
General Social Concerns		
Legal Conformance	Absolute	Pass or Fail
Ecology	5	−10 to +10
Environment	5	−10 to +10
Equity	5	−10 to +10
Resource Consumption	5	−10 to +10
Time to Consummation**	5	−10 to +10
Goal Conformance	5	−10 to +10
Public Concern	4	−10 to +10
Public Dissatisfaction	4	−10 to +10
Political Feasibility	4	−10 to +10
Flexibility**	4	−10 to +10
Speed of Change**	4	−10 to +10
Effectivity	4	−10 to +10
Productivity	3	−10 to +10
Overall Costs	3	−10 to +10
Net Benefits Level	3	−10 to +10
Community Involvement	3	−10 to +10
Avoidance of Other Significant Predicted Problems	3	−10 to +10
Protection of Next Generation	3	−10 to +10
Balance of Quality & Quantity	2	−10 to +10
Efficiency	2	−10 to +10
Cost-Benefit Ratio**	2	−10 to +10
Employment	2	−10 to +10
Esthetics	2	−10 to +10
Segregation	2	−10 to +10

Coordination between Levels of Government	2	−10 to +10
Coordination between Public & Private Interests	2	−10 to +10
Science Merit	1	−10 to +10
Can Others do the Necessary Planning?	1	−10 to +10
What Would People be Willing to Pay?	1	−10 to +10
No Other Way to Go	1	−10 to +10
Consideration to Special At-Risk Groups	?	−10 to +10
Planning Concerns		
Plan Conformance	5	−10 to +10
Leverage	4	−10 to +10
Public Education Re Planning	2	−10 to +10
Balanced Planning Body	2	− −10 to +10
Long-Term Planning Body Involvement	2	−10 to +10
Planning Body Image	2	−10 to +10
Planning Process Image	3	−10 to +10

*Technological issues are generally applicable to selection of intervention, and only by inference to selection of problems.
**Not applicable for Problems.

Descriptions of Criteria Applicable to Technological Aspects

Technology possible.   If there is no way to proceed technologically, there is no point in evaluating a proposal further (unless the effort is to be research designed to overcome a specific technology gap; and even then the research proposal must demonstrate the probable technological feasibility of breaking the current impasse).

Technological feasibility.   There are varying degrees of complexity involving issues of worker skills, delicacy of instrumentation, and so on. Problems and solutions which face significant technological difficulties rate low.

Manpower requirements.   These are always a potential bottleneck. Two factors are to be considered: (1) qualified manpower; (2) pool of adequately educated potential pre-manpower. Ratings for each of these might be averaged, or weighted and then averaged, to obtain the overall rating. Problems of shortages or solutions that alleviate manpower shortages would rate high.

Balanced attack on all phases of a situation.   This criterion emphasizes, for example, that perfection at the diagnostic end of a tuberculosis control effort, with failure to follow through on treatment, rehabilitation or evaluation, would not be valuable. Consideration of the whole picture for attainment of the most overall control would rate high. The rater must remember that many problems and solutions are specifically selected to patch up a deficient area or improve one area. They are not to be downgraded just because they do not do everything, but only if they are so out of line that the overall situation will not really be improved.

Balanced attack on all phases of the environment. This is a special case of the preceding criterion, and it emphasizes that all-out control of one element, such as avoidance of pollution of the air, without concern for water or soil, simply moves a problem blindly from one critical receiver to another. The more a problem or solution promotes this concept, the higher it rates; one running counter to it rates negatively.

Descriptions of Criteria Applicable to Health Aspects

Problem likely to go away by itself. A problem or a solution for a problem may on reasonable scrutiny be seen as predictably resolving itself over a period of time not much longer than planning proposals could offer. Where the probability of self-resolution is high, the proposal would get a low rating; where it is low, the problem would get a high rating.

Probable duration of problem if undisturbed. A problem likely to continue for a long time unless specific new effort is put into its control rates high.

Deaths. Also recognizable as life span, this concern includes at least three factors: (1) numbers involved; (2) probable duration over which the deaths-causing situation will continue to operate; (3) prematurity of the deaths to be prevented. (Do not assume that a life spared from one cause will then necessarily have a normal life span or one free of disability, disease, discomfort, or dissatisfaction.) Ratings for each of the three factors may be averaged, or weighted and then averaged, to obtain the overall rating. Problems involving loss of many man-years rate high. Solutions controlling large losses rate high.

Disability. At least six factors are of concern: (1) numbers involved; (2) degree of disability; (3) probable time over which disability will continue; (4) prematurity of the onset of condition; (5) irreversibility of damage; (6) probable duration of the threat to society; (7) irreversibility of the damage created. Ratings for each may be averaged, or weighted and then averaged, to obtain the overall rating. Problems dealing with much disease rate high. Solutions which avoid much disease rate high.

Discomfort and pain. At least five factors are of concern: (1) numbers involved; (2) severity of distress to the victim; (3) degree to which others are distressed by the victim's discomfort; (4) probable duration of discomfort or pain; (5) probable duration of underlying situation if uncontrolled. Ratings from each can be averaged, or weighted and then averaged, to obtain the overall rating. A problem involving much discomfort rates high; a solution effectively controlling much discomfort rates high.

Condition size or numbers.   These are included as part of many specific criteria already listed, and are applicable only where not already taken into account.

Condition severity.   The same considerations apply as for the preceding criterion.

Condition duration.   The same considerations apply as for the two preceding criteria.

Distress or danger to others.   Essentially the same considerations apply as for the three criteria preceding.

Descriptions of Criteria Applicable to General Social Concerns

Legal conformance.   This criterion involves compatibility with *requirements* of laws and with regulations of bodies by which the council is bound. True, the planning body could decide to fight for changes in such constraints.

Ecology.   This criterion involving risks of significant ecologic worsening, or disruption of an unpredictable kind might be divided into four parts: (1) time of onset to effects; (2) condition size; (3) severity; and (4) duration. Ratings for the four parts may be averaged, or weighted and then averaged, to obtain overall rating. A problem perceived as having significant ecological damage factors would get a positive rating and a solution a high rating if it overcame or avoided them.

Environment.   The same considerations apply as for ecology, but they are more limited in significance and more specific in concerns.

Equity.   Inequities in this discussion are limited to those situations in which groups of persons have less than their fair share of opportunities generally, or less than their fair or reasonable share of resources to cope with their adverse conditions. Considerations might extend into failure to have the additional resources appropriate for such conditions as infancy, motherhood, aging, disability, or dying. A problem perceived as having large inequity factors rates high, a solution creating them would be rated negatively.

Resource consumption.   This criterion has at least four subdivisions: (1) quantity; (2) duration; (3) level; and (4) time to onset. Ratings for each may be averaged, or weighted and then averaged, to obtain the overall rating. Problems which involve a large consumption of resources rate high. Solutions which eliminate high resource consumption also rate high.

Time to consummation.   This criterion partially overlaps the cost-benefit criterion if discounting is utilized; it should not be allowed therefore to exert influence in more than one place. Solutions which require longer periods to go into effect get a lower rating.

Goal conformance.   Problems and solutions are rated on conformance with major, general, long-range goals set by the planning body. Gross violation of such goals or reversal should be grounds for tabling a problem or solution altogether, no matter how good the other ratings.

Public concern.   Public interest may be widespread and palpably high for an issue that has no merit or possibility of success. The high rating of a problem on this criterion may be its only good rating. Notwithstanding, such interest may mean that the issue may not be abandoned and that if it cannot be defused more simply, it may have to be taken up just to get its true status clarified to the public. Interest may sometimes be high in one sector of the populace and nonexistent in another; that is, teenagers, the aged, legislators, property owners, and parents may have quite disparate interests on a given issue. Ratings for each of these groups may have to be shown separately, or might be averaged, or weighted and then averaged, to obtain the overall rating for problems or solutions.

Public dissatisfaction.   This negative aspect of public concern may be one of the most critical of all criteria. *Disease, discomfort,* and *disability* may be much better tolerated, but diffuse mounting *dissatisfaction* may really represent unfulfilled aspirations and rising value gaps that could presage revolt. Issues which contribute to this condition are of more consequence than popularity or concern for an issue. This criterion has three major aspects: (1) the numbers of dissatisfied people; (2) intensity of dissatisfaction; and (3) probability that dissatisfaction will remain unchanged over time under the circumstances forecasted, will rise, or will fall. Ratings for each of these three aspects might be averaged, or weighted and then averaged, to obtain the overall rating. Problems with significant dissatisfaction rate high, solutions which promise serious dissatisfaction rate negatively.

Political feasibility.   Although closely related to several preceding factors, this criterion is primarily an estimate of the possibility of gaining favorable action from the recognized policy makers in government or other institutions. A problem whose study will get support and a solution which will get support rate high.

Flexibility.   A solution which locks a community into a given direction, removes opportunity for changing forces set in motion, or prevents the harnessing of forces for other ends at a later day rates negatively; one which maintains openness to a maximum of options rates positively.

Speed of change.   Some solutions create such a rapid rate of change that they endanger political approval for next steps once it is realized how fast the change really is. Where unusual speed is not a prerequisite of strategy or goals, it rates negatively.

Effectivity.   This criterion refers to volume and nature of desired outputs which are really created. Problems involving low effectivity of operations and activities, and solutions offering improved effectivity rate high.

Productivity.   Issues involving the labor force age group usually have a major bearing on this criterion of human productivity which has at least three main factors: (1) duration of loss; (2) level of loss; and (3) speed at which the loss is overcome (or sets in). Ratings for each may be averaged, or weighted and then averaged, to obtain the overall rating. A problem perceived as having a high loss of human productivity rates high, as would a solution promoting productivity. It should not be measured twice as would happen if it were also included as part of the cost-benefit ratio calculations.

Overall costs.   This criterion refers to straight costs without consideration for cost-benefit ratios or net benefits. High dollar costs or high usage of special or hard-to-replace resources (currently, primary care physicians) can exceed the tolerable limits by depriving other needs or causing bottlenecks elsewhere. High costs may simply exceed what we can afford. Some problems whose cost is felt to be unbearable would get a high rating, no matter how much we would otherwise like to leave them alone. Some solutions may have prohibitive costs, no matter how much we would like to implement them, and thus get a negative rating.

Net benefits.   The greatest payoff for the greatest number of people has many versions. (This is not intended to be the converse of the overall costs of a problem that is to be controlled.) This criterion might be broken into three factors: effects on (1) upper class; (2) middle class; (3) lower class. The ratings from each might be averaged, or weighted to favor one class and then averaged to obtain the overall rating. Problems and solutions indicating increasing net benefits would rate high; decreasing benefits would rate negatively.

Community involvement.   Several factors are of concern: (1) extent of public acknowledgement; (2) extent of public participation; (3) extent of community control over the issue; (4) potential increase or decrease the issue suggests for the community's role of being responsible for the study, decision making, responsibility, authority, provision of services, and so on. Ratings for each of these factors might be averaged, or weighted and then averaged, to obtain the overall rating. Problems or solutions promising more involvement would rate higher, less involvement would rate lower. (There are unusual situations where less involvement is actually desirable, and the ratings would be the reverse. For example, in the case of regional air pollution control with a history of locally created impasses, it would be important not to fan the embers of local autonomy conflicts which have kept improvements at bay.)

Avoidance of other predicted problems.   This criterion includes consequences of secondary, spillover or externality effects. Problems tackled, or solutions designed which promise avoidance of significant other problems which seem impending, rate high.

Protection for next generation.   Several versions of this issue exist. This generation may undertake to foot the bill for benefits for the next generation. It can also set the machinery in motion now and postpone the bill so that it is paid by those who benefit. We can also borrow against our children for something to be enjoyed by us now and to be paid for by them. Decision regarding the desired option has to be made on each proposal where these concerns are relevant. Rating is then based on how well the problem or solution performs the desired protection for the interests of the next generation.

Balance of quality and quantity.   This criterion calls for confronting such issues as improvement of quality in the face of need for expenditures on behalf of those who do not even get services of present quality. Decisions will have to be made about the directions desired before problems or solutions can be rated.

Efficiency.   This criterion often merges into one with effectivity at the operational level, depending on definition of objectives. It may be at the heart of problems such as service overlap, duplication, and gaps. Beware not to measure twice, once here and once in the cost-benefit criterion. Problems involving large inefficiencies and solutions proposing large improvements rate high.

Cost-benefit ratio.   This criterion involves a ration of dollar costs spent to implement a solution over the dollar value of benefits produced, minus disbenefits (untoward consequences or further costs). It is most suitably used to compare alternative solutions which have essentially the same objectives or outputs. The higher the ratio, the less favorable the rating.

Employment.   Increasing the level of employment would undoubtedly earn a problem or a solution a high rating in these times, and lowering employment would earn a negative rating.

Esthetics.   Provision of a higher level of esthetic influences would undoubtedly justify a higher rating for a problem or solution; a lowering would earn a negative rating.

Segregation.   Although conceivably a part of equity, this criterion stands alone. A problem or a solution carrying a removal of segregated status would get a higher rating, and one increasing it would rate negatively.

Coordination between levels of government.   Committed as we are to the belief that this could only be a good thing, a problem or solution that encourages coordination rates high, and one diminishing it rates negatively.

Coordination between public and private interests.   The same considerations prevail as in the preceding criterion.

Science merit. The criterion suggests that a problem or solution producing new knowledge would receive a higher rating.

Can others do the necessary planning? If a given proposal requires the use of planning body resources—when others can equally or better do a comparable job—and thus decreases the planning body's resources for other jobs of problem analysis or solution design, the proposal rates negatively.

What would people be willing to pay? This criterion should not be used if it covers the same concerns as "Public concern" or "Public dissatisfaction." Adam Smith popularized this approach, and Vincent Taylor restored it to health planning as a substitute for cost-benefit thinking.[24] Something for which people would gladly pay would get a positive rating.

No other way to go. Although usually more useful for solutions or for projects embodying solutions, this criterion may also be significant for some problems. It signifies that there is no other source of funding or authority available to do what is badly wanted or highly justified. The fewer options open to the proposal elsewhere, the higher the rating.

Consideration to special or at-risk groups. Although not shown in the figure as weighted, such a concern might be established with a low or high weighting because a given planning body and its community had strong feelings about favoring some heretofore neglected group or one whose fate they believed critical to community survival. (For example, infants, children, women of child-bearing age, the labor force, small farmers, job-creating industrialists, the aging, or the dying). Having chosen one group to be favored and assigned a weight commensurate with concern, the more any problem or solution offers to improve that group's welfare, the higher the rating.

Descriptions of Criteria Applicable to Planning Concerns

Plan conformance. This criterion refers to compatibility with higher level or overall plans and their criteria by which the planning body must abide. It applies to commitments and relationships either to (1) the multisectorial, horizontally integrated planning at the same level, or (2) vertically integrated planning with planning bodies below and above. Again, if the issues are deemed to be sufficiently important, the body can fight to change the more inclusive plans that invalidate its own interests. Although modest straying from the planning body plan commitments would lower the rating, significant violation would, like violation of goal conformance, prohibit proceeding, no matter how good the other ratings.

Leverage. This criterion refers to gain in stature, power, or capacity to do other things because of undertaking a given issue, or occurring as a byproduct of undertaking it (gain of a new level of capability, or obtaining a multiple utility, not merely more of the gains envisioned in terms of the original specific objectives). This criterion might apply to a problem, but most particularly to a solution. The more leverage created, the higher the rating.

Public education about planning. This criterion refers to evidence that a great many people would be involved in a way that would enable them to learn about how planning works. A high rating would be earned by issues offering such education.

Balanced planning body activities. As the name of this criterion suggests, a planning body might give all its attentions to one area or one type of problem or solution. It is suggested that a problem or solution would earn a higher rating if it promotes balance, and a lower one if it distorts the workload of the planning body.

Long-term planning body involvement. If undertaking the analysis of a problem or designing a solution were seen as the beginning of an excessive commitment of planning body resources for the future, a negative rating would seem in order.

Planning body image. This criterion refers to making the planning body look good and it has many ramifications. However, taking for granted that improved image is always a desired side effect, and on occasion a major goal, a problem or solution which enhances image rates positively.

Planning process image. This criterion refers to evidence that if the planning body tackles a problem or designs a solution, most people and interests will see the wisdom of planning. This would no doubt occur where serious conflicts had been worked out so that all parties felt a gain. A positive rating would be earned by issues promising such a result, a negative one by those threatening to denigrate the image of the process.

It remains to be stressed that use of criteria, weights and ratings cannot substitute for judgment, even though their use helps inform those who do the judging. Rather than providing a simplistic guide to setting priorities, the main utility of creating and using a rating scheme is to guide planning body members to consideration of what may be, for them, novel value systems; such considerations would then lead to a full view of the complexities involved. Members are also led to the necessity for a reconciliation among themselves of their differing choices of criteria, weightings, and ratings. At the same time, this exercise provides the community with an educational experience in how decisions might better be made. Moreover, this effort may be the first time that minority position holders have been given a chance to express their concerns in a way that is seen as socially relevant, not just as self-serving.

LIMITATIONS OF ASSESSMENT

The ever present limitations of the assessment process must be kept in mind. Since there never will be the capacity to carry out a thorough assessment, that particular deficiency is not regarded as excluding the use of planning. All collected data can be said to have been picked out for collection because from someone's point of view they are important as symbols of goals, of problems, or of successful or failing solutions. Data now available is necessarily "full of history" and reflects former practices and habits, and their ensuing results. Even the unlabeled effects of lien laws or the presence (or absence) of outpatient care for the poor may have determined the nature of the data about use, and thus be interpreted as evidence of need for inpatient care. Both past and current data can serve only when accepted with reservations. Failure to keep in mind the consequences of common shortcomings leads to a false security, particularly when data shows up in well-bound and well-presented folios. The hazards of assessment tend to arise from several categories of inadequacies, many of which have already been indicated in one way or another.[25]

Before trying to conduct assessment, we must acknowledge that our value systems do get in the way. They determine how we set up the questions and the criteria to define well-being. Physicians have barely arrived at the level of measuring prevention. Few of us in health circles can tolerate levels of human productivity as a measure when it is expressed in dollars. Considerations of self-satisfaction and self-realization find many of us in disagreement over the relative satisfactions from exertion of physical strength, intellectual or artistic prowess, and self-gratification. Upward mobility (and its motivation) is currently a difficult set of forces to reconcile with diverging value systems.

To overcome the most exaggerated of the initial distortions resulting from discrepancies in our value systems, we will have to create a joint measuring venture among many skills and many backgrounds. Even then, the views of a large section of our populace may not be represented on the issue of the meaning of well-being. Perhaps the variety of people that I insist should be on our planning boards can help find useful ways to measure the qualities of life which diverse groups savor, and the degree to which these qualities are achieved.

In setting up the measuring machinery to do assessment, the labels "good" and "bad" must have been erased from the slate. Whether people do or do not seek care for their health is to be determined; never is this good or bad. The facts are to be examined in the light of what shaped the situation, why the particular phenomenon occurred as it did, and what might change the situation if change is desired, and what other things would occur given the proposed means of change.[26] Value judgments exercised in advance can block a rational analysis.

After the measurements are in, assessment can and will lead to applications of values and of judgments which will, of course, label situations good or bad, and thereby indicate what is to be planned for. In this process of assessment, we can make clear how specific value systems, rather than so-called needs, have often dictated the nature and form of interventions. The presentation to the public of data, showing how values have distorted certain interventions and prevented other more useful interventions, can help to change value and belief systems which hold us all subject.

Assessment, first as an information-gathering tool and then as a process of creating judgments, has been offered as the means whereby (1) normative goals are selected and (2) problems are chosen for amelioration. Both the selection of the problems and the development of solutions for them must be guided by the normative large goals selected. Otherwise, problem amelioration may lead to solutions which violate our long-term ends, or what is worse, inadvertently direct us toward other ends which we would not have tolerated if we had perceived what we were about to perpetrate in the innocent posture of planner-problem-solvers.

Thus, assessment helps us begin the two major planning activities envisioned by developmental planning, normative goal seeking and articulated and guided problem solving.

REFERENCES

1. Andre L. Delbecq and Andrew VandeVen, "A Group Process Model for Problem Identification and Program Planning," *Journal of Applied Behavioral Science* 7 (July/August 1971), 466-92.

2. R.F. Logan, "International Studies of Illness and Health Services," *Milbank Memorial Fund Quarterly* 46, Part 2 (April 1968) 126-39.

3. Allan Blackman, "The Meaning and Use of Standards," *Health Planning 1969*, by H. L. Blum and Associates (San Francisco: American Public Health Association, 1969), chapter 2.

4. C. West Churchman, *Prediction and Optimal Decision* (Englewood Cliffs, N.J.: Prentice-Hall, 1964), 93-136. Leo G. Reeder "Community Health Indicators: a critical analysis and conceptualization of Issues" Dept. of Health, Education and Welfare Health Services and Mental Health Administration, Community Health Service, Technical Paper Series No. 2 April 1973.

5. California Medical Association, Advertisement: "You're suffering from an ailment doctors cannot cure." *Newsweek*, California edition, April 19, 1971.

6. C.W. Churchman, Ibid. no. 4, 93-136.

7. A. Blackman, Ibid. no. 3, chapter 2.

8. National Commission on Community Health Services, *Health Is a Community Affair: Report of the National Commission on Community Health Services* (Cambridge: Harvard University Press, 1966).

9. American Public Health Association, *Guide to a Community Health Study* (New York: American Public Health Association, 1961).

10. A. Blackman, Ibid. no. 3, chapter 2.

11. American Public Health Association, Committee on the Hygiene of Housing, *Planning the Neighborhood* (New York: American Public Health Association, 1961).

12. American Public Health Association, Ibid. no. 9.

13. Ruth and Edward Brecher, "The Disgraceful Facts about Infant Deaths in the United States," *McCall's Magazine*, February 1966.

14. Roslyn Lindheim, *Uncoupling the Radiology System*, Health Services Monograph Series, Hospital Research and Education Trust, 840 North Lakeshore Drive, Chicago, Illinois, 1971.

15. Michael J. Teitz, "Toward a Theory of Urban Public Facility Location," Working Paper no. 67, Department of City and Regional Planning, University of California, Berkeley, 1967.

16. Gerald D. Rosenthal, *The Demand for General Hospital Facilities*, Hospital Monograph Series no. 14 (Chicago: American Hospital Association, 1964).

17. A. Blackman, Ibid. no. 3, chapter 2.

18. E. G. McGavran, "Research and Public Health Practice," *American Journal of Public Health* 48 (March 1958), 348-52.

19. David Braybrooke and Charles E. Lindblom, *A Strategy for Decision* (New York: Free Press, 1963), 29.

20. P. T. David, "Party Platforms as National Plans," Changing Styles of Planning, Special Issue, *Public Administration Review* 31 (May/June 1971), 303-15.

21. H. Hilleboe, A. Barkhuus, and W. C. Thomas Jr., *Approaches to National Health Planning*, Public Health Papers, no. 46 (Geneva: WHO, 1972), 69-86. H. E. Hilleboe and A. Barkhuus, "Health Planning in the United States: Some Categorical and General approaches," International Journal of Health Services 1 (1971) 134-48. Vicente Navarro, "National Health Insurance and the Strategy for Change," The Milbank Memorial Fund Quarterly, 51 (Spring 1973), 223-51. American Association for Comprehensive Health Planning "Position Outline for Reviewing Federal Legislative Proposals," mimeograph, Alexandria, Va., (Oct. 1973).

22. State of New Mexico, Comprehensive Health Planning Council, Environmental Task Force, "The Environmental Plan," first draft, January 1970.

23. State of New Mexico, Ibid.

24. Vincent Taylor, *How Much is Good Health Worth?* (Santa Monica, California: The Rand Corporation, P-3945, 1969).

25. Irwin D. Bross, *Design for Decision* (New York: Free Press, 1953), 33-38. Darrell Huff, *How to Lie with Statistics* (New York: Norton, 1954). U.S., Department of Commerce, Bureau of the Census, Vital Statistics Reports 19:21, "Effect of Changing Birth Rates upon Infant Mortality Rates," by I. Moriyama and T. Greville. Vital Statistics, Special Reports 21 (November 10, 1944) 399-42. F. D. Norris and P. W. Shipley, "A Closer Look at Race Differentials in California's Infant Mortality, 1965-67," *HSMHA Reports* 86 (September 1971), 810-14. Amitai Etzioni and Edward Lehman, "Some Dangers in 'Valid' Social Measurement," *Social Intelligence for America's Future*, ed. by Bertram M. Gross (Boston: Allyn & Bacon,

1969). Raymond A. Bauer, *Social Indicators* (Cambridge: Massachusetts Institute of Technology, 1966). Bertram M. Gross, special volume editor, "Social Goals and Indicators for American Society," *Annals of the American Academy of Political and Social Science* 371 (May 1967). Henrik L. Blum, et al., "The 1948 Epidemic of Poliomyelitis in San Diego County, California," *Stanford Medical Bulletin* 7 (November 1949), 169-79. C. W. Churchman, Ibid. no. 4, 93-136. Melvin M. Webber, "The Roles of Intelligence Systems in UrbanSystems Planning," *Journal of the American Institute of Planners* 31 (November 1965), 289-96.

26.   F. J. Curry, "District Clinics for Outpatient Treatment of Tuberculosis Problem Patients," *Diseases of the Chest* 46 (November 1964), 524-30.

7. A Systems Approach to Analysis of Goals and Problems to Determine Suitable Interventions

Although I will concentrate on analysis of problems to explain the systems approach used, the same analytic approach can be applied to achieving normatively set goals. To separate the various stages of the planning process from one another is extremely difficult; Figure 1.3 tries to show the reiterative nature of the effort. At no point is it more difficult to hold the steps apart than during the sequence beginning with the analysis of problems (or goals). This sequence clarifies the opportunities where interventions are most likely to succeed, and the subsequent design and analysis of possible interventions directed at these points. New insights about opportunities or constraints may lead to reformulations of the original definition of the problems and their objectives, thus calling for a renewed round of problem analysis.

Allen Schick makes the very pertinent observation that analysis is not unlike evaluation in the concepts used and in the purpose served —primarily guidance of policy makers. But the applications do differ in that analysis is used in a period of optimism—new funds and new programs—while evaluation is used more in periods of uncertainty— loss of confidence, short resources, lack of enthusiasm for innovation. Thus two elements of planning are tied together in yet another way.[1]

Those of us in public health are accustomed to focusing on problems revealed by measurement of incidence or prevalence of disease in a given geopolitical area. At the same time, the nature and quantity of services intended to control the problem have been built to standards essentially unrelated to the nature or frequency of the problems as they occurred locally. Often the standards were devised at the national level by experts-away-from-home and conventionally built around the notion of the single agent as the etiologic cause of each condition (the Arden House syndrome). The programs usually have been unrelated to the activities needed for effective intervention in each condition in any given community. Such an approach can at best be described as engineering for an improved status quo. Its dubious contributions to significant downward trends in disease and death statistics on both state and national levels, and its continued failure to bring downward trends in resistant problems, reveal an overall failure of comprehension of the factors involved.

251

Because of the difficulties associated with isolating systems, we utilize an ecologically—more than epidemiologically—oriented systems approach which avoids the programmatic pitfalls, and articulates the problem to be solved with the rest of the world. This approach requires analysis of information in terms of probable or potential relationships which explicates the multicausality of most conditions.

In attempting to analyze health problem systems in order to intervene more rationally, there are two obvious approaches. We can try to analyze all the significant disease or problem systems at one time, a total study. Or, we can study selected disease entities. At one extreme, a good example of the analysis of one-disease system is given for tuberculosis by Lynn and by several other health planners.[2] At the other extreme, given in a most readable and conceptually clear way, is the scheme for the survival outcomes for the world as developed by Forrester[3] and Meadows.[4] These two levels of systems analysis are musts for anyone interested in analysis, the design of systems, and the forecasted outcomes based on alterations of forces or alternative interventions on those systems.

Because the combination of techniques that we are about to describe is new (although not unlike what is being done in some developing countries), it would seem reasonable for a planning body to make a beginning by analyzing just a few major problems.[5] In order to pick out suitable problems, a quick overview of the community under study has been suggested (Chapter 5), followed by a decision as to which problems deserve major concern (Chapter 6).

GOALS AND PROBLEMS

In Chapter 2, we pointed out that what constitutes a health goal or a health problem is determined by the viewpoints of individuals, created in turn by the nature of the system that is the habitat of the viewpoint holder. There is no fixed or firm point of reference about what should be—no lodestar by which all persons concerned with health may be guided in the choice of goals to attain or problems to eliminate. In this regard, Anthony Downs emphasizes that rationality is a term applicable to means but not to ends, since ends are basically issues of desires and values.[6] This does not invalidate our belief that we are acting rationally when we plan normatively and let our desires become our guides. For these and other reasons to be advanced in this chapter, it is important that a wide range of diverse viewpoints be represented among those persons assembled to come up with decisions about the improvements to be planned or worked for.

High Level Goal Selection and Problem Choice Go Together

One of the first selection difficulties is in part real and in part semantic: Should we seek to attain old or new goals, or should we first attempt to eliminate vexing problems? In Chapter 2, problem solving
was seen as one major part of the developmental mode of planning for
improvements, and long-term goal setting was the other. Without
guidance from high-level, long-term goals, problem solving by its very
nature is disjointedly incremental. One of the devices recommended to
guide problem solving was the conversion of high-level values or their
derived goals into criteria by which problems would be assigned priority for action (Chapter 6). Essentially the same criteria could then be
applied to selection of interventions for solving problems, so that they
would do no long-term harm, advertently or inadvertently (Chapter 8).

Selection of Problems Is Followed by
Specifying Working Objectives

Unfortunately, the word "objectives" is used in many ways, and is
commonly used interchangeably with the term "goals." In this book
objectives is the term used for specific end points for given
situations—that is, ends at a much lower level than the general goals
which are derived from major values. I, therefore, emphasize that high-
level goals are not the same as working objectives.

After problems have been selected for attack, there is a distinct utility
to an initial statement from the planning group of the obvious objectives for each problem chosen. If an excess of maternal deaths has
been categorized by a planning group as a problem worth attacking,
the objective is essentially a simple analogue—minimize maternal
deaths. Hopefully it would be possible to make this objective more
tangible by prescribing a reasonable set figure such as "by 50%." Some
problems do not necessarily call forth a unanimity of objectives, and
agreement must be reached on both the statement of the problem and
the objectives held out for it. If not, the problem analysis may be directed to many points, and all parties may be disappointed by the outcomes. The safest approach may be to begin the total problem analysis, however superficially, before settling firmly on objectives. Starting with concern prematurely limited to only a few objectives often
leads to consideration of only the one or two working objectives that
were thought of initially.

By accepting the complex problem as the initial base of analysis,
many wise and attainable working objectives may come into view. For
example, if a planning body chooses automobile accidents as a problem for action, the obvious objective would seem to be reducing fre-

quency. However, it may soon develop that the objective is not just to reduce numbers, but to reduce the human damage resulting from the accidents. In other communities the hurt of the problem that is to be assuaged may really be property damage, a chronic court calendar jam caused by auto accident litigation, or the costs of long-term disabilities.

All the desirable objectives may not be discovered before the situation is analyzed. As new objectives come into view, decisions can be reached whether they are to replace the initial objective, or are to be added to, or reconciled with it. The planner may wish to set limits to the ramifications of the problem. In the example of automobile accidents, the statement of an objective could be "minimizing the number and severity of casualties associated with automobile accidents." Such a working objective limits the guiding concerns by giving the study system boundaries; that is, not everything about autos or transport is included in the study.[7] However, a full analysis of causes or consequences of auto accidents in not precluded, and this initial definition of the system need not inhibit the development of other working objectives and interventive means as the problem analysis brings them into view.

However, if after reasonable scrutiny, the planning group remains insistent that only one consequence of automobile accidents should be chosen as the problem—for example, court congestion—then at least all those who participate in the planning will understand the limited nature of the objectives selected. And presumably they will not complain when the interventions proposed ignore the precursors or the other consequences of auto accidents and focus on the factors in legal actions, such as insurance or juries.

THE SYSTEMS APPROACH

Each community is a net of interlacing games, such as banking, health care, or schooling. The rules are made up by the actors in each game, under pressure from the aggregate of systems around them. Systems analysis can cut up this community in many ways, depending on what we leave out in order to get a tidier picture of the game we wish to study. The most significant activity in the technical effort of planning occurs here. The concept of a social system and subsystem utilized in Chapter 2 remains the basis for our concern of introducing change into such a system by means of planning.

Edward S. Rogers presents the dual background of what we shall propose.

> One approach, the more common, deals with an environment that is identified, intuitively or otherwise, in somewhat limited terms.

> For example, epidemiology is ecological in this sense when it inquires into the causation of a specific disease by studying its associations with, let us say, a half dozen or so of the more evident environmental conditions that are considered as likely factors in the causative system. The other approach . . . is holistic and seeks to detect every environmental relationship of possible consequence through an attempt to identify the larger system of interactions within which the event of particular interest may be expected to have occurred.[8]

I propose to approach the second of Rogers' methods, remembering that analysis in depth of a disorder which creates consequential disability might ultimately bring into consideration almost every facet of the circumstances of living. Ramifications of each form of ill health will be reasonably traced out into related disability fields and, in fact, the entire scope of its effect on well-being will become visible. (This is not the same as trying to analyze the whole world first, hoping to disclose practical approaches for control of specific conditions that are killing or maiming us.) As we ferret out the relationships of consequence for those few disorders given priority, planning experience will be gained at the same time that new relationships are discovered. Every input will eventually be seen as an output of some other system, and every result will point to other causal factors in a totally interrelated world. As chains of cause and consequence are watched from numerous vantage points, we will discover their propensity to reverse, interlink, or extend in new directions. We will learn how and where to interrupt undesirable linkages.

Although we will ultimately concentrate on presenting one technique of analysis, the principles underlying the many techniques now in use are not totally different. The techniques discussed under forecasting by Erich Jantsch,[9] such as relevance trees or morphological research, are systems approaches applied to analysis of different levels of problems or goals. Depending on the currency of the outcomes under consideration, one goes from problem solving or goal attainment to forecasting; depending on the quantity and quality of data used in the analysis, one goes from fairly firm data analysis to anticipations or the best guesses of experts. However, analysis and forecasting are never very far apart in any kind of problem solving. A variant of what we describe as problem analysis has been developed by Frank Baker, Verne Gibbs and Frank Anderson under the title of "Issue Analysis."[10]

One arm of the U.S. Public Health Service has undertaken a simplified and fairly direct approach by their use of a Relevance Tree, which graphically relates all the associated or related factors, up through a logical structure, with the purpose of describing what makes a condition occur.[11] They also use knowledgeable "voters" to estimate the size of the effect of variables on the occurrence of the condition. This step is, of course, part of forecasting.

A very flexible or intuitive approach has been called Zigzag Thinking.[12] The U.S. Department of Health, Education and Welfare has undertaken a more mathematical, rigid, and less politically-aware approach, based on the 17 major classes of disease from the "International Classification of Diseases, Adapted."[13] This approach reflects the orientation of the Department, working as it does with nationally accumulated figures, and given its responsibility to provide funds in accordance with the calculated relative national significance of each set of problems, rather than with the origins of various conditions and their susceptibility to attack. At the state and local levels, the realities of the ecological influences cannot so easily be ignored, since it is here that the laying on of hands generally takes place. For example, programs for tuberculosis cannot be lumped with those for lung cancer and virus pneumonia, as they have been at the federal agency level.

Included in an excellent general discussion of planning, the Pan American Sanitary Bureau presents an alternative approach for determining which conditions are to be given priority. It is based on related, but in effect, very different formulae.[14] It has become too rigid and we suspect ineffectual.[15] The Lynn[16] and Forrester[17] schemes already referred to are other versions of systems analytic exercise.

The utilization of PPBS for health concerns is worth a brief review. PPBS has been the force most responsible, in the United States, for popularizing the concept of the systems approach to analyzing problems, shaping alternative objectives, and designing and evaluating alternative means or interventions to attain the objectives. PPBS had its baptism in defense concerns of the federal government, but the logic utilized by PPBS is quite as much at home with major decisions for a village or even for a family. It is of interest that PPBS, when used by the federal government for other than defense purposes, has not always been synonymous with national level concerns.[18] It is one thing to see what the national costs and gains will be as a result of federally budgeted programmatic interventions as carried out by one sub-department of H.E.W., and quite another to see what effects might result from all interventions made anywhere in the nation in behalf of certain desired outcomes.[19]

PPBS was badly oversold and, as a technique, is disappearing from governmental applications. Neither its requirements in personnel, comprehension, and costs, nor the implied restructuring of the decision-making processes were clearly understood. However, its general thrusts will not be lost.

Richard M. Bailey has summarized what systems-oriented planning logic in the form of PPBS is supposed to be doing for the federal government.

1. To force a careful examination and specification of the objectives of each governmental agency.

2. To raise the level of consideration of objectives beyond those of a vested interest nature and to widen the number of alternatives considered at all levels of government.

3. To analyze the *output* of specific programs and drop the practice of counting activities accomplished.

4. To measure total program costs (more than one year) and hence avoid the practice of incremental budgeting.

5. To formulate objectives and programs with a view to the long-run (five years or more) so that agency heads who often spend only a brief time in offices will know where the major thrust of their efforts is needed.

6. To analyze alternatives using economic criteria so that the most effective means of achieving objectives can be found (effective is usually defined as least-cost).

7. To establish analytic procedures as a systematic part of the budget making and review process; to link policy and program analysis through the budget.[20]

ANALYSIS APPLIED TO PROBLEMS

I have chosen a particular approach to analysis which can be used for either *goals* or *problems*. It is applied to *problems* first because it is easier to present. The analytic process is divided into exploratory and definitive stages.

Exploratory Review of a Problem

The idea of a schema by which all problems can be analyzed is very appealing but at the same time may suggest an approach so simplistic as to be useless. Nevertheless, the procedure to be described has been useful in beginning the study of problems as varied as those of disease, undesirable conditions, sick or failing communities, inequities in receiving services, or inefficiencies and ineffectivities in the machinery for delivery of services. As the following sections make clear, many critical purposes are served by following the suggested schema. It reveals the value origins of how the problem came to be recognized as such; the nature of the problem, the extent, the probable future, the consequences, the causes; at what points interventions might be mounted; and above all, it clarifies which parties have, or probably will have, an interest in the problem or its solutions.

However, before each and every problem receives a serious analysis (analysis is not without significant cost), it should be put through the kind of rating process described in Chapter 6 so that it can be determined whether it has sufficiently high priority potential to deserve serious consideration by the planning body, which never has enough resources to study all matters brought before it. Unfortunately, use of the rating criteria depends on knowing the political, health, economic and social impacts of the problem, as well as the technological possibilities and costs of doing something about it. Must every problem be studied fully before it can be rated for acceptance? If so, why bother trying to priority-rate problems? A problem whose significance is not clear should be put through a relatively inexpensive staff level analysis by skimming over all the steps of the technique which we have found so useful—a bird's eye view, so to speak. This approach will help in rating problems effectively. It is also undertaken because it gives a quick summary of the steps of the analytic schema that will later have to be carried out in greater depth if the problem is found to merit serious study. It also gives a preview of who will have to be involved in the more definitive exploratory study.

Beginning with a quick staff preview, the planner and one or two interested and knowledgeable persons can run through the schema (see Figure 7.1) and obtain in an hour or two an idea of the kinds of data, experts, and heavily involved interests to be assembled for the exploratory analysis. Figure 7.2 shows the results of such a preliminary activity by a small local group devoted to a community-selected problem of dental caries. As a result of this effort, which also produced a sizable list of feasible interventions, it became relatively easy to decide which experts, which data, and which interests should be brought together for a one- or two-day exploratory session to make a more explicit study of dental caries. The one- or two-day exploratory study will provide information on size, significance, cost, and modes of attack, and will advise the planning body both about rating the importance of the dental caries problem in comparison with other problems and about the likelihood for effective action. If caries were then to be accepted for serious consideration, the work of the exploratory session would already have opened up the problem so well that a significant portion of the analysis would already be completed. As the result of the exploratory session, the planning body will have a clear enough picture of the issues to be able to decide on the instructions, major sense of direction, membership, and scope of concern it wishes to include with assignment of the caries problem to an anti-caries planning task force.

Summarizing the Work of the Exploratory Analysis:
Redefining the Problem:
Determining the Merit of a Definitive Study:
Estimating the Size of System Which Should Be Studied

The problem can now be redefined on the basis of the exploratory study. The statement will include a definition of the nature of the problem; the data wanted; data resources; parties at interest to be in-

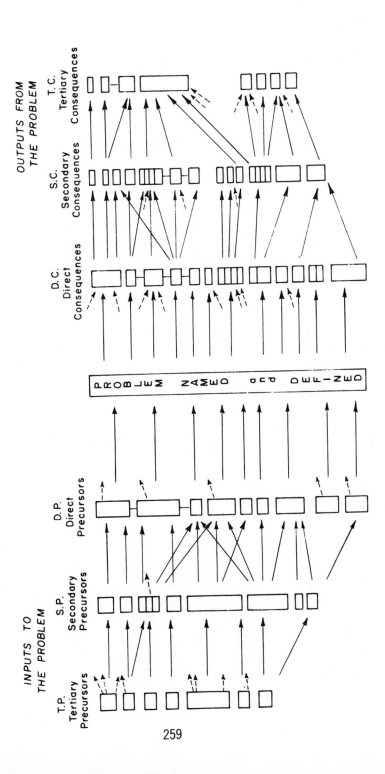

FIGURE 7.1

ANALYSIS APPLIED TO A PROBLEM

FIGURE 7.2.   DENTAL CARIES ANALYSIS

Input To The Problem			Problem	Output from the Problem			
Tertiary and More Remote Precursors	*Secondary Precursors*	*Direct Precursors*		*Direct Consequences*	*Secondary Consequences*	*Tertiary Consequences*	*More Remote Significant Consequences*
ignorance	malnutrition		D				
culture	calcium, phosphrous, vitamins, protein deficiencies		E	pain	distress and inattention at school	waste of schooling	dropouts
lack of money	soft diet	improper nutrients	N				
expensive housing	sweets		T			waste of time & money	poverty
bad housing	sticky food		A		pain		
poor markets	soft drinks		L	infection		psychologic effects	social isolation
poor transport	acid foods	deficient oral hygiene and other bad habits	C	loss of teeth	loss of more teeth	cosmetic effect	unemployment
advertising	fluoride deficiency		A		cosmetic effect		
vending machines	frequent food		R	other carious teeth	tooth displacement	speech changes	malnutrition
social mal-adjustment	suck bottle		I				
disrupted homes	inadequate brushing	inadequate dental care	E		further tooth loss	hearing changes	debility
neglect	no toothbrush		S			masticatory difficulties	
culture	manpower shortage	injury bacterial flora					
poverty	transport deficiency						
ignorance	no funds	genetics and race					
	fear						
	neglect						
	ignorance						
	no baby sitters						

vited; a listing of major causes, consequences, and possible interventions (which allow some quick judgments about the technical feasibility of doing anything at all); and the probable system limits. This summary should include a statement of the probability of successfully affecting the problem, as well as of the costs of assembling minimum information necessary to allow the planning body to make useful decisions. What expertise will be needed? Will surveys be necessary? Will pilot runs be needed to get data? Can any of these be obviated by studies of the literature or by good guesses? The statement on the size of the system and the related information on who needs to be involved also provides guidance as to long-or short-run possibilities, political acceptability, and the ultimate profitability of the analysis.

The relative current importance of this problem and its forecastable future importance can now be stated roughly, since the nature of the precursors and consequences has been visualized. By using the type of criteria referred to in Chapter 6 the problem can be rated and crudely compared with others placed before the planning body to assist it in reaching a decision regarding definitive study.

The planning council can also begin to explore how large a system they are willing to have the study team search, thereby delineating the scope of the problem analysis. For example, in the dental caries review, if it is decided to leave out the layer of remote precursors, then, interventions against ignorance, cultural beliefs, lack of money, and so on, need not be considered. If it is decided not to include malnutrition, even more elements can be ignored. Of course, all precursors can be ignored as being too difficult, that is, too broad in terms of the other issues that will be aroused if interventions are directed against them, and all efforts may be concentrated on caries and on their consequences. However, for many kinds of problems the latter approach is not wise; although it rocks a few boats initially, the best long-term community "buys" are likely to be built around interfering with one or more of the problem precursors.

Scrutiny For Underlying Social Factors:
An Opportunity to Attack
Many Problems (Or an Inducement to Procrastinate)

It is to be anticipated that analysis of a significant number of major health problems will disclose that several of the same major social precursors underlie many of the problems. Poverty, ignorance, and cultural outlooks will almost surely be among the major initiating, underlying, or predisposing factors to such problems as infant mortality, excessive disability, malnutrition, dental caries, and tuberculosis. This does not mean that each of these problems should be set aside to await the output of nonexistent social planners, at which time the problems at hand will melt away. Nor does it mean that the health planners must abandon any lesser interventions not directed at such social precursors. On the contrary, a careful analysis may reveal that specific, even if so-called suboptimal, interventions (such as specific therapy for tuberculosis) will control the problem. (Chemical therapy apparently controlled tuberculosis in Alaska without significant deliberate social interventions.) In other situations, the health planning body may, in fact, be in a position to mount social interventions that control the health problem at hand as well as help in other problems. In the Gibson-Geiger effort in Mt. Bayou, Mississippi, gainful employment was suspected of being more important to health than medical care, and action was taken accordingly.[21]

Because of their patently causative relationship, strong arguments can be advanced for mounting major offensives against such pervasive causative factors as illiteracy and poverty. However, certain cautions must be noted. A nationally declared war on poverty, the growing GNP, and a new era of affluence in America have not relieved us of the specific problem of poverty pockets such as Appalachia. Apparently, general measures without a study of specific areas of pathology may have only marginal impact on problem areas.

The national affluence of the 1950's and 1960's has not rooted out the hard core of tuberculosis which is so heavily associated with poverty areas. Nor has affluence done away with accidents associated with dangerous housing or inadequate vehicles. Affluence has helped remove jalopies from the road, thereby decreasing accidents, but it has also put more cars on the roads, more juvenile drivers in cars, and more liquor in juveniles.

The secondary effects of planning consequent to the broad reallocation of resources are obviously poorly anticipated at present. In the United States, formal social planning is currently limited to the health sector, and it would therefore seem prudent to expend the limited monies allocated for health planning where there are possibilities of successful breakthroughs and minimal dangers to our cherished way of life. Modest success with a few conditions that could confidently be observed and measured would be reassuring both to those involved in the planning and to those providing the means by which the planning is done—the citizenry and their delegated policy-makers. In other countries that are more goal oriented, it would clearly be exciting to press for big goals and, at the same time, to coordinate such planning with the solution of problems in the course of overall planning.

A final point of caution is that health planners as a group are not ideally equipped to evaluate conditions such as poverty and illiteracy in terms of their ecology. Some of these problems might be unraveled by carrying out studies conjointly with other interests, but initially it would seem more feasible for health interests to study the undesirable conditions which fall under the general understanding of health.

Orderly Utilization of the Concept of the Four Major Input Areas to Health

The problem analysis device depends heavily on the analysts' keeping firmly in mind the four major areas of inputs to health: heredity, medical care, behavior, and environment. (See Figure 1.1 and Chapter 3.) At each step of the analysis, a check should be made to see that these four areas have been considered. Consideration of the four areas of inputs to health is as relevant to the determination of the consequences as it is to that of the precursors, and is at its maximal utility when the study has come to the stage of designing interventions.

Definitive Problem Analysis

The major causes and consequences of the given problem were enumerated, and their size and nature estimated in the exploratory analysis. A more detailed analysis consists in large part of the same type of study done more accurately and in greater depth. This procedure, as shown in Figure 7.1, is set out schematically to gain an objectivity, conciseness, and clarity not always possible in writing. Furthermore, such plottings of problems can be kept and indexed for reference and comparison as the work of the planning body progresses.

How Did the Specified Problem Come to Be Identified and Given Priority?

1. How did the problem get defined? If it has not been defined, a definition must be obtained.
2. Now that the definition is clarified, can we be sure that the community still wants to attack this problem?
3. What was the nature of the assessment and the anticipations about this problem and its relative importance compared to other problems?
4. Further definitional changes can be expected as the analysis gets underway and the problem, its causes, and consequences are seen more clearly. In fact, the problem may be put aside as being of less concern than one of its causes or consequences, which will then be chosen as the problem for study.

What Are the Consequences of the Problem?

1. Multiple generations of consequences. Firmly identify direct, secondary, tertiary, and so on, major consequences both *bad* and *good* to which the problem gives rise. These are usually in part synonymous with the reasons which created awareness of the situation as the problem or as an unachieved goal. (See Figures 7.1 and 7.2.)

2. Contributing factors. In some consequences other identified factors besides the original problem may be either participating, initiating, or predisposing forces. In Figure 7.1 these contributing factors are indicated by broken-line arrows among the consequences. For example, malnutrition and emotional stress are claimed to make sizable contributions to the condition of that fraction of persons infected with tuberculosis (*Tbc*) who then go on to have active clinical diseases. All of which does not take away from the fact that the original infection with *Tbc* was the problem we started with. On the other hand, if we were working out the various consequences of the problem defined as malnutrition, activating the *Tbc* process could well be one. In that case, infection with *Tbc* would still be a necessary concomitant, and in our scheme would be the origin of a broken-line arrow. In other words, whether we were studying the mainstream of *Tbc* or malnutrition, in almost any part of the world, each would very likely enter as a contributory factor to a major consequence of the other.

3. Description of each direct consequence:

Name and suitably define each direct consequence for future reference.

Quantify by a numerical or other device each consequence in the community. (If there are significant consequences for other communities, these too should be recorded.) Figures may be known locally, may exist in the literature for presumably similar situations, may have to be estimated from various hypotheses existing in the field, or may have to be developed *de novo* by the study team. Upper and lower or outside limits should be given for guesstimates. With refinements, the probability can be developed that the event will fall within the outside limits of the guesstimate. Do not place full reliance on reports by experts.[22]

If there are different qualities or degrees of severity of a given direct consequence for victims or communities, the consequence should be subdivided and redefined, and quantities should be shown for each subdivision. In this way, secondary consequences relate to well described direct consequences rather than to diffuse or all-inclusive ones.

Indicate how long it takes the problem to cause each specific consequence and, if applicable, over what time span it continues to create the consequence.

Forecast size along a suitable time span for the consequence under study, to help determine whether the consequence is melting away, growing, or maintaining its status.

State some reasonably ideal or justifiable achievement over time for each direct consequence, with a brief justification for each.

4. Origin of secondary consequences. Direct consequences may not be the final or most important outputs of the selected problem.

For, in turn, direct consequences may give rise to another generation of events, which are called secondary consequences (S.C.'s). One direct consequence (D.C.) may give rise to none, one, or many S.C.'s. Several D.C.'s may be seen as creating the same S.C. One D.C. may join with other forces from outside the problem under analysis to create consequences that should be noted. One D.C. may also give rise to an S.C. which will in turn create a later consequence which is identical with another D.C. or S.C. That is, the same consequence may show up in two places or more.

5. *Description of each of the secondary, tertiary and later consequences.* Resulting S.C.'s need to be given much the same treatment indicated above for direct consequences. Some secondary consequences may in turn give rise to significant, perhaps even easily quantifiable, further or tertiary consequences (T.C.). These in turn should be analyzed as suggested for the S.C. and D.C. Further generations of fairly clear consequences may need defining and quantifying, particularly if a refined analysis is being undertaken.

6. *Consequences (outputs) may also turn out to be inputs or precursors.* Many T.C.'s and later consequences, even some S.C.'s and D.C.'s, will turn out also to be inputs to the creation of the very problem from which they arise. Where this is the case, these items must also be shown on the input or problem-causing side of the analysis. (Because I have used a simple linear graphic method in Figure 7.1 to describe the system, there is no way to diagram the complex feedback loops among its various elements.)

What Precursors (Inputs) Lead to the Problem?

1. *Multiple generations of precursors.* As a result of local observations, formal ecological, epidemiologic, or other cause-and-effect studies, a sizable number of known or hypothesized contributing factors can be identified. I call these factors precursors. It is easiest to begin by listing those factors which directly result in the problem. Then one can follow the causal chain back through one or more reasonably identifiable steps or generations and list those precursors.

2. *Precursor-produced effects of significance which are not related to the stream of events leading to the selected problem.* Any given precursor may also have a part in causing (or ameliorating) other problems. If such effects are of great significance, they are worth labeling. For example, an attack at an important precursor might clearly be a fine investment in terms of its total effect, although it might rate poorly as an investment in terms of its effect on the central or initial problem. The reverse might also be true. The precursor itself may be doing so much good elsewhere that we would not wish to attack it just to remove its undesired effect on the problem that was our initial con-

cern. Such effects are shown in Figure 7.1 by broken-line arrows, and serve as simple reminders of these other possible relationships.

3. Description of each direct precursor.   Those conditions, events, forces, or influences which seem to have a direct bearing on, creating, or magnifying the problem or are felt to be an immediate preceding step are classified and analyzed as direct precursors. The actual directness of the factor may be open to question. For example, sometimes the sub-clinical or carrier stage of a disease such as diabetes might better be shown among the generations of precursors or contributing factors to the clinical form of the disease, rather than lumped with the active stages of the disease or condition. However, the decision about how to lay out the study is made purely as a matter of choosing the easiest or most revealing way to present the problem in terms of understanding its origins and consequences. After identifying and classifying the direct precursors (D.P's), the following steps should be taken to describe each as accurately as possible.

—Identify, suitably name, and define.

—Assign a numerical or other rating in terms of size, frequency, consequence, and so on, for the community under consideration.

—Describe in qualitative terms the force this factor seems to exert in producing the problem. If the force acts much differently when weak than when strong, it may be divided into two or more parts and each quantified to give a more precise estimate of the contribution of this precursor to the problem.

—When feasible, describe the period of time for each precursor to create its effect in causing the problem, and if applicable, over what time span a unit of this factor continues to create more of the problem.

—Forecast its size along the time span assigned or selected as meaningful for attacking the original problem, so as to have a basis for deciding whether this precursor is weakening, continuing, or increasing in consequence, and thus determine how much we should be concerned with it.

—In a careful study, each identified precursor (of any generation) would be set up as a sub-problem for analysis. Thus, each precursor is seen as contributing not only to the original problem but perhaps to many others. Even when there is no intent to be so thorough, a list should probably be maintained of the other problems to which each precursor makes a major contribution. If these lists are indexed by the precursors which gave rise to them, they may have critical value at the stage of analysis when interventions are designed, for an effective intervention directed at a precursor factor should also have consequences on the other problems listed. In this case, the intervention would have values or benefits beyond those directed to the original problem, and thus would deserve a higher rating when priorities are set among interventions.

4. Secondary and tertiary precursors that give rise to direct precursors. The direct precursors may not encompass all of the major contributors to the problem. In some cases they may almost be more in the nature of identifiable way stations for a generation of preceding precursors which we call secondary precursors (S.P.'s). Many S.P.'s may lead to a single D.P., or one S.P. may lead to many D.P.'s. Any identified generation of precursors affecting the original problem may clearly lead to other significant problems as well. Similarly, the S.P. may be preceded by tertiary precursors (T.P.'s). Some T.P.'s may also give rise directly to precursors that are identified as primary as well as to secondary ones. (See Figure 7.1). These second and third generations of precursors need to be described as outlined, above, for direct precursors.

5. Other precursors. Usually, preceding generations of predisposing factors (precursors) will need defining and quantifying. Not a few of these may actually turn out to be, in part, outputs from the very problem under study (a reminder of the feedback relationships).

Existing Interventions As a Source of Information about a Problem or a Reminder of Other Precursors and Consequences

An analysis of the interventions currently applied is needed to determine their effects on the present status of the problem system under study. Much of the observable prevalence of a condition may reflect an effective (or ineffective) control or treatment program currently underway. The process of evaluation described in Chapter 12 can clue us in to the realities of how and to what extent current interventions do influence the situation. Upon examination, the effects may be seen as nonexistent or even adverse. An example of the latter is a disease that is driven underground because of the limitations placed on the freedom of its victims once they are identified. The level of effectivity of any one intervention also may throw light on the real nature of certain relevant relationships, and point to new or unexpected chains of cause and effect.

Another approach to the analysis of delivery systems, particularly those built around recipients of public programs, scrutinizes the relationships between the needs and wants of the client, recognition of these by others, eligibility and actual receipt of benefits. It begins by observing the forces from which laws arise, the programs and services which result, and postulates possible future developments.[23]

A recital of interventions—education, legislation, control, testing, and treatment—now being used or advocated to solve the central problem may also serve as a reminder of the postulated existence of precursors or consequences of the problem which were overlooked in the analysis up to this point.

*Analysis of Each Major Consequence or Precursor, Treating It
as though It were the Central Problem*

If one has occasion to be thorough about the significance of a certain
major consequence, that consequence in turn would be made into the
central focus for a problem analysis. This is simply a means of separating out the pieces of one problem analysis, so that each piece can be
individually examined in a less constricted way than might be induced
by constantly focusing on the original problem. The study of one significant consequence could reveal that it is more critical than the original problem which called attention to it. A shift of concern might
result from the discovery of the significance, acceptability, concern,
feasibility, or profitability of attacking the consequence as compared to
attacking the original problem. The same would be true for a precursor.

Opportunities for Interventions

The precursors, the problem, and the consequences must be studied
systematically to see whether they invite or suggest interventions
which could act to prevent their occurrence, neutralize their presence,
or intercept their consequences. From what has been said about the
examination of any particular problem system it becomes obvious that
a crude yet useful model of the system can be devised. For each relationship described in the model, there are potentially a number of
alternative methods of intervention.

The problem of the unsafe automobile, for example, can be attacked
from any one of several approaches: government payment to the automobile manufacturers to cover the cost of making a safer car; legislation to require safety features, the cost falling on the purchaser; a law
that the individual car owner must install and use safety devices. The
question of whether legislation or education is the better method to
deal with individual car owners suggests further options needing
study. The relationship of freeway construction and safety introduces a
secondary, but major, issue: Is the extended use of freeways an efficient
method of metropolitan transport? Not only accidents, but additional
factors of cost, deterioration of property values, air pollution, and slow
mobility must be considered. Rapid mass transit is a major alternative.
If freeways are not to be eliminated, appropriate interventions may
include safer design, or the introduction of electronic guidance devices. Better patrol is another possible approach to freeway safety, albeit there is little supporting evidence. Options still remain, dependent on whether the cost of interventions should be borne by the entire
community, those using the transportation system, or those using the
freeways. In the area of driver education, the search for alternatives

indicates that money might best be spent in finding out how effective education is, before any further investment is made in that sector.

Many intended interventions against most problems or their precursors are in effect now and these could have been shown as *good* precursors to a given problem. For ease of analysis, I have preferred to separate interventions from both the precursors and consequences. Interventions against consequences of most problems now exist in great numbers, and these can be included among the collection of interventions that will be designed and analyzed. Many naturally occurring phenomena also have favorable effects on problems and could therefore be considered as anti-precursors or anti-consequences, in the sense that they act like interventions. Again, for the sake of ease of analysis, they are best kept out of the precursor and consequence groupings, although their interventive potential must be kept in mind if they are currently or foreseeably available or manipulable. Examples of such natural interventions include the red cell sickling phenomena which spare certain groups from the effects of malarial infection, and the omnipresent antipolio immunity in most unhygienic, wet tropical populations. (Of course, each of these sometimes also has deleterious consequences, against which one would have to weigh the benefits of exploiting them as interventions.)

Linkages in the Problem Analysis at which Interventions can be Directed

A single intervention may actually be working in several places at one time. For example, chemotherapy for an active case of tuberculosis (*Tbc*) is preventing a potential T.C.—death from *Tbc;* it is preventing a potential long-term S.C.—a case of disabling *Tbc;* and it is also knocking out a D.P. by eliminating another source of the *Tbc* bacteria which potentially leads to new cases of *Tbc*.

It may be hard to decide whether an intervention is (1) acting just prior to and thereby preventing a consequence or precursor; or (2) acting directly on the consequence or precursor thereby eliminating it; or (3) enclosing the factor so that its effects cannot take place. Where this distinction is of importance it is more easily made. For example, therapy of an active case of *Tbc* knocks out the illness directly as well as controlling transmission; isolating the case simply stops one consequence—the transmission of disease—but allows another consequence to continue—the potential worsening of the disease which may further disable the victim or even cause his death. Similarly, the masking of a contact to *Tbc* is intended to intercept bacilli that might otherwise invade and make him a victim, but immunizing the contact is a direct attack to make him relatively invulnerable. It does not seem critical that interventions be labelled in terms of the pre, post or direct attack on a precursor or consequence, but each interventive possibility should be so defined as to clarify where and at how many places it is postulated as being effective, and in what ways.

Multiple Alternative Interventions at One Linkage Point

Any one possible point of intervention may offer an opportunity to apply many different kinds of interventions. Also, a single intervention may be applied in smaller or greater doses or in a more or less complete way. These variations must be named and defined but had best be grouped as qualitative or quantitative variants of a single intervention. Once major types of interventions are defined, minor variants of any one intervention can usually be compared and the most profitable of the variants kept as the prototype of that kind of intervention. This process reduces confusion in keeping track of potentially useful interventions and simplifies comparison.

Larger System Interventions

Some interventions may not be related to the linkage points commonly delineated in a given problem analysis. In fact, some of the most elegant interventions fall in this independent category. For example, a painstaking study of automobile accidents might easily have been carried out in such a way that no attention was paid to the fact that automobiles can be replaced almost entirely by mass transport. In other words, the problem or system under study (auto accidents) was only a part or a sub-system of a larger problem best defined as transportation. Analysis of that system might produce interventions which essentially eliminate or overwhelmingly modify the initial problem or system chosen for analysis.

Furthermore, auto accidents are not only a part of the transportation problem, but the transportation problem is a part of the galaxy of concerns in the supersystem of communications. Because much transport is for purposes of communication, new modes of message transmission might well substitute for transport of people. Interventions into supersystems may lead to analysis of that larger system immediately or only after completion of the original mission (study of the auto accident problem).

Because supersystem problems approach a more optimizing outlook (and the smaller systems a more suboptimizing outlook), much of the new knowledge required to analyze the supersystem will almost certainly reside in hands other than those assembled for the initial problem. Many more interests are involved, and decisions to act will probably involve many more sectors than those initially considered, or will call for other kinds of decision-making arenas and tactics. Thus the problem may be referred to higher (multisectoral, or, in many cases, national) levels of planning.

We clearly enter the realm of policy planning by raising our sights and attacking larger systems. Even though we began with problem solving, it is the more normative policy-setting aspects of the developmental approach which predominate as interventions are directed towards larger systems.

REQUIREMENTS FOR A SUCCESSFUL PROBLEM ANALYSIS

People with Requisite Knowledge and Outlook

Process Leader

The process leader need not have any particular background, but he must understand the analytic approach the study group is to follow, and have the feel, either from experience or from intuition, for the kind of give-and-take and flexibility that is required. He must sense when to prod and dig for further ideas or when to close off an area as unprofitable for the time being. He must have the capacity to lead, to influence people comfortably toward working with one another, trying new tacks and approaches. He must also have some mastery of the techniques of how to get groups involved in problem solving.[24]

Experts

Acknowledged expert(s) in whatever field(s) are almost certainly going to be studied, must be identified and invited to participate in the problem analysis. For example, if tuberculosis (Tbc) is the problem, those who are highly expert in testing, treating, and preventing Tbc should be on hand for the entire analysis. The exact mode of origin or creation of the problem and its consequences, and thus the possible points of intervention may not be known to others participating. Without this kind of epidemiologic or ecological understanding of the pathogenesis of the problem, an adequate analysis cannot be opened. Supplying size, numbers, or quantities for the various steps of the analysis also depends almost exclusively on these same experts. They either have knowledge of local conditions or can extrapolate from what is presented in the literature about experiments, and about levels in comparable or different neighboring communities or in other countries.

The unbelievable complexity of identifying the relationships of general factors such as education, nutrition, occupation, and habits to health has been well described.[25] The nature of the expertise required in problem analysis is a complicated issue accordingly.

Illchman and Uphoff indicate the costs and benefits of various levels of expertise and knowledge. They find that the more proximal the cause, the higher the probability of validity and utility; similarly, validity is lower and application is riskier for more remote precursors.[26] The price to be paid for knowledge has both time and money limits. If no real expertise is available, a more experimental or a very incrementalistic approach is justified.

Experts are also needed for counsel on the design of interventions that are known elsewhere or appear reasonable on the basis of hypotheses about the modes of occurrences of the various stages of the problem. They can provide probabilities within which interventions can be expected to work. And they usually can provide the best current cost estimates for application of suggested interventions. Many other kinds of resource experts may ultimately have to be brought in to verify the significance or nature of precursors, consequences, and interventions that turn up in the analysis but had not been foreseen when the problem was chosen.

Involved Parties and Interests

Care must be taken to include in the problem analysis *representatives* of individuals known to have personal or business responsibilities in the problem area, and representatives of agencies that have official, legal, or public responsibilities—health professionals, related voluntary organizations or agencies, and officially assigned agencies. Individuals highly identified with possible modes of intervention should also participate. All of these people have understanding which will contribute significantly to the analysis. And because they will be among the first interests to be hit by losses or gains from proposed interventions, it is better to have them observe how the problem is being intelligently and legitimately unraveled than to have them discover at a later time that their interests are somehow being threatened.

Victims and High-Risk Potential Victims of the Problem

Often victims or potential victims have insights into the origins of the problem, how one gets caught up in it, and how one can escape or fail to escape. They may see it as quite a different problem. This element of the so-called consumer viewpoint may be the most critical ingredient in creating fresh outlooks on old problems.

Experience will demonstrate how indispensable these varied viewpoints are to a thorough problem analysis and substantiate how planning truly is a brokerage of technology and politics, and that it is impossible for a planning technologist to bring an analysis of a problem to a successful conclusion without assistance.

Summing Up with a Cross-Check: Look at the Problem in a Totally Different Way

With the addition of a few socially knowledgeable and respected scientific heretics, it would be wise to review the entire process for fatal flaws of logic, limited or perverted perspectives, social or technical biases, and tunnel vision. A logical analysis might have been made that calls for interventions to make inroads on mental illness through attacks on poverty, because poverty was considered to be a precursor of mental illness. The data on which the logic rests might indeed appear formidable, and the expected interventions might appear to promise high payoff. However, someone of philosophical bent might feel justified in reviewing some of the critical data which gave rise to the working hypotheses and, to everyone's consternation, might make a much more convincing case from the identical data that in fact poverty arose from mental illness, and not vice versa. Even if data is trustworthy, many equally valid interpretations can often be placed on the same data, depending on the point of view brought to bear. One can cultivate a "perverse" point of view (witness columnist Art Hoppe) and learn that such a view often provides more evidences of sound thinking than the conventional wisdom. A very sophisticated and charmingly disarming statement of how to go about enlarging capacity to look at things differently is presented by C. West Churchman as counter planning.[27] This approach sets an analysis off on a new track. Interestingly, many of the same or altered interventions may reappear, in great part because many outputs from the problem are also among the inputs, and even reversing consequences and precursors may not create a totally new picture.

If the new approach to the analysis ends convincingly, a new, preferred batch of interventions will emerge which needs to be compared with the first batch. Where there is a justifiable doubt as to which approach is more legitimate, one of several decision-making paths may be chosen.

—Apparently good interventions that occur in both analyses may be given priority because they are seen to be safe whichever way the reality lies.

—A decision may be made to follow the interventions derived from the logic of one of the analyses and to forget the other.

—Accepted interventions may be further qualified, so that preference is given to any that avoid significant adverse social consequences as postulated by the contradictory analysis.

—Interventions that offer high payoff may be selected from both schemata, provided they do not promise to neutralize one another.

—Both analyses may be abandoned if there were no "good" interventions in common, since there is no security about the analysts' understanding of the problem.

—A research experiment may be undertaken, using one critical intervention capable of demonstrating which of the equally attractive hypotheses is in fact accurate. This experimental intervention will help decide which, if either, of the analytical approaches was right, or it may offer a key link in the chain of facts to the correct hypothesis—a link which was not perceived in either of the contrasting initial analytic attempts.

Evaluation as Another Kind of Check

It is important to note that, for a given problem, one set of causal factors may have been operative at one time or in one place, and a quite different set may be operative at another. Moreover, what appears to be an identical problem may really be something else. (Witness the confusion among several pulmonary infections for many years.) These are two reasons for the critical need for continuing evaluation of the actual success of problem analysis and design of interventions. Even if analyses are well done and interventions are correctly designed for the problem at one period or one place, they may be irrelevant, or become so, at another period or another place. Only evaluation will tell a planning body about the adequacy of its substantive knowledge and about its prowess at problem analysis and design of interventions.

ANALYSIS APPLIED TO GOALS

At times desired improvements can best be reached by looking directly at the major goals and analyzing them as the means by which to design interventions.

When to Select Goal Analysis

An example from the health care field offers the options of approaching design of an intervention either from the position of ameliorating problems or of working from goals to build a new system. The analytic steps to be taken would be determined by whether a planning body has decided (1) to set a goal of good care for all or (2) to study the present delivery system in terms of each of the problems that its community had pointed out as deserving priority. If the planning body chose the grand goal route, it would seek to analyze the goal and design a system capable of reaching such a goal. If instead it went after each problem in existing machinery, it would seek to analyze each problem to point out interventions that would attack either its causes or consequences.

I suggest emphasizing the goal route for the design of interventions in situations where the interventive system is built on well understood or predictable phenomena of natural science, or is reasonably open to further investigation and comprehension. Where less well understood or less predictable behavioral and social science elements enter into interventive design, there is increasing justification for a problem solving or incremental approach. In the case of health care services, notwithstanding the many behavioral elements, the normative or goal directed planning still offers many advantages over incrementalism. Using the problem-solving route, we can foresee a delivery system of even more extensively gerrymandered proportions than the present confusion and chaos brought about by limited target interventions.[28] By contrast, a reasonable way of providing "good" care for "all" is not beyond conceivability. At least a dozen countries have developed delivery schemes which do rather well in the eyes of their citizenry.

In the analysis of man-made (man-machine) interventions such as health care delivery, I agree with Nadler[29] in opting for normative or ideal planning approaches. I am not, however, suggesting that man-nature systems can always be attacked from the position of the ideal or goal outcomes. Starting from a goal statement and working backwards deductively is a suitable method of attack for a goal of health care delivery or a mode of transportation, but not for most diseases or conditions of ill health. For example, diabetes cannot be eliminated or controlled by working back from a goal statement to that effect. It can be controlled only by a problem-oriented design which shows how to intervene.

The sick community tends to fall midway between the two situations presented. There, goal statements can provide one base for analysis and design, while problem study must provide the other if there is to be community acceptance.

Steps in Goal Analysis

A Concise Goal Statement

The goal must be so stated that it is as comprehensive as desired. This usually involves a series of descriptive elements that stipulate precisely what is wanted and thus become subgoals. Ultimately each such subgoal would also receive a quantifying statement. If all people are to be covered, all must be defined as 100%, 98%, 90%, and so on, and the circumstances set out under which exceptions would be made. If the goal is acceptable services for all, the acceptable must be specified in comprehensive terms. If care is to be acceptable to consumers, that must be stated; if it is to be acceptable to minority groups, as well as to the majority, that too must be stated.

Determination of Desired Intervention Outputs

If the goal is good health care, one looks at the entire life span, or perhaps divides it into the seven ages of man. These are more concise segments which facilitate determining the basic needs that require service or the nature of ideal services at each age. Of course, conditions occurring at one age often represent consequences of unfilled needs at an earlier time. Two general approaches are open. (1) The problems at each age may be given the kind of problem analysis already described, to get an idea of the health care interventions that are possible and reasonable. The collected, selected interventions describe the nature and quantity of services which are required by each age. Since a thorough analysis of this sort is not likely to be undertaken by any given community, only some of the major conditions are carefully analyzed initially. These, in combination with information about what is currently provided and what remains unprovided, define the needed aggregate services. (2) So-called ideal care services are postulated for each age and are aggregated to define a total of needed good care. In either case we then must design systems which put together the necessary resources to generate services which satisfactorily serve either the problem needs or the ideal care prescriptions.

Determination of Major Intervention System Elements and Relationships

If the goal is good health care for all, it must be visualized that health care is composed of consumers plus services, and that services must be synthesized by a delivery scheme or system that appropriately interrelates manpower, technology, facilities, and finances in such a way as to meet with the consumer in the right times and ways. (See Figure 7.3.)

Examination for Major Attributes of Each System Element or Subsystem

If each subsystem is to contribute to the goal set up for the system as a whole, its major attributes must be delineated. Figure 7.3 presents the major subsystems of the health care system inside the dashed line. The three other contributors to health are shown outside this system, as are the various proposed environmental constraints on it. Figure 7.4 describes the goals for *health care received,* 7.5 for *consumers,* 7.6 for *care services delivery organization,* 7.7 for *manpower,* 7.8 for *technology,* 7.9 for *facilities,* and 7.10 for *financing* concerns of the system. Going into the system's immediate environment, Figure 7.11 presents elements of *surveillance and control,* and Figure 7.12 combines the *evaluation* and *planning* with *policy* setting concerns. The column headings on the figures 7.3-7.10 represent the major goal attributes of each aspect of the major subsystems of the health care system. The column headings of Figures 7.11 and 7.12 represent major attributes of the environmental forces desired to guide the system.

Nadler[30] uses a matrix which is a reminder of all the principal attributes for each major subsystem or piece of the overall system required to make the system work so as to deliver the desired goal. Other less rigorous schemes can be used, as we have done in Figures 7.4-7.12, because not every subsystem has comparable qualities. I make no particular brief for this set of goal attributes or their criteria. Many shown here, such as consumer participation or per capitation are purely personal preferences, although I believe they can be justified.

Creation of Criteria for Each Major Attribute of Each Set of Subsystem Goals

Each goal attribute must be further described, dimensioned, and constrained by necessary requirements or criteria. These descriptors or criteria are shown under the attribute or column head to which they belong in Figures 7.4-7.12. By way of example, refer to Figure 7.7 and see that under the subsystem of "Manpower" one attribute is "Recruit and Train." Under that attribute are listed further criteria or specifications of what it is and what it must do. As the analysis of the ultimate goal of "good care for all" progresses by working deductively away from the goal itself, it comes to the point where the output of the analysis becomes the design criteria. Here the planner enters the design phase. We are at this point switching from analysis to design, and because of the organization of this text, the design and analysis phase falls into the next chapter. So we will pick up and continue the design effort there.

BRINGING TOGETHER THE ANALYTIC TASKS OF THE PLANNING BODY

Several immediate issues face the planners as they set about their analytic tasks. These include:

The inevitability of systems overlap, which means that problems will also be found to be overlapping with one another and with goals.

FIGURE 7.3

A WORKING MODEL FOR THE HEALTH CARE SECTOR

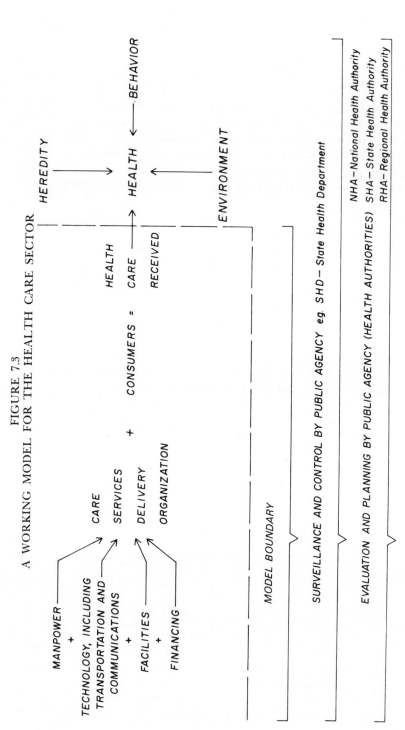

FIGURE 7.4

ATTRIBUTES AND CRITERIA OF "CARE RECEIVED" GOALS OF A HEALTH CARE DELIVERY SYSTEM (HCD)

Eligibility and Financial Coverage	Scope of Care	Access	Suitability	Quality
All persons, including those not signing up, given initial assignment by place of residency or work	All phases—preventive, maintenance therapeutic, and rehabilitative	Reasonable geographic distance or travel time, including provision of transport as needed	Acceptability of care to all ages, sexes, cultures, educational backgrounds to be served	Guaranteed HCD ascertainment of: patient results by category and practitioner
Freedom of choice among purveyors whenever reasonably possible	All conditions—physical, dental, emotional or socially disabling	Child care	Well-being and functional maintenance focus for all groups to be served, e.g., timely and function supporting in terms of job, family duties, etc.	Practitioner knowledge and competence as shown by his use of: tests services aides visits procedures drugs referrals autopsies
Freedom of choice and change among HCD's whenever reasonably possible	All services, drugs, prostheses	All hours indicated by community needs	Purveyors seek and respect patient participation in decisions about is health and the HCD system	Modern technology
All costs prepaid	All facilities, including home care, homemaking during illness	24-hour emergency care	Evidence of suitable utilization to be gathered as basis of how well each group is relating to health care	Modern equipment
Nominal co-payment is acceptable	For whatever period indicated	Working relations with all other relevant well-being support systems hospitals, education, library, ambulance services, etc.	Evidences of concern for societal well-being, as by wise use of resources, plans for replenishing key resources such as manpower	Provision of means to update all disciplines
	Connectedness of all aspects of care, including records and responsibility for costs and coverage			Utilization of updating
				All of the above determined by sample surveys conducted by committees of purveyors, outside super peers, and consumers

FIGURE 7.5
ATTRIBUTES AND CRITERIA OF "CONSUMER" GOALS IN A
HEALTH CARE DELIVERY SYSTEM (HCD)

Competency for Care	Competency for Participation in Planning and Governing
Evidence that consumers: seek and use health care "wisely" have good health habits (maintenance orientation) have adequate basic education so can participate in health activities and continue to absorb new health information have adequate health education as part of basic education so that they understand body functioning, importance of habits, environment, genetics, health care receive appropriate continuing health and health care education Incentives built in for wise habits and use of services Sanctions built in against poor health behavior, misuse (copayment no answer)	Opportunities, instructions, and incentives to participate as an equal partner in work of committees and boards doing: assessment of needs and demands evaluation of services planning design of care policy making and governance of delivery machinery Opportunities, instructions, support, and incentives to work on any level of health authority (planning boards)

The issue of which categories of problems should be tackled first and, similarly, which goals.

The use of the community as the base upon which studies are made.

Systems Overlap

For ease of presentation of the logic in the discussion of priority setting and analysis of problems, I have dealt largely with isolated problems. In practice, problems are apt not to be so discrete. They may represent the malfunctioning of small or large systems. It has been emphasized that the boundaries of the system (or the number of systems) to be dealt with are set arbitrarily by the planners on the basis of the evidence available to them and the breadth of their interests in tracking down the precursors and consequences of a problem. But even

FIGURE 7.6
ATTRIBUTES AND CRITERIA OF "ORGANIZATIONAL" GOALS OF A HEALTH CARE DELIVERY SYSTEM (HCD)

Integration	Machinery for Governing, Planning Operating, Controlling	Machinery for Evaluation	Constraints

Puts together four major resources: manpower, technology, facilities, financing, into a flexible, self-evaluating, redesigning, service-rendering operation; establishes outreaching linkages for all aspects of care it does not provide	Extensive internal participation (all levels of personnel)
	
	Extensive outside participation (all kinds of consumers in majority and control)
		Maintains internal evaluatory machinery in conjunction with RHA concerning:
		
		  coverage
		  relevancy
		  quality
			Cannot avoid competition or freedom of choice
			
			Operating under performance requirements set by SHA and NHA

Puts together the HCD organization and the consumer so that the care received is of high quality and relevant, i.e., appropriate, acceptable, etc.	Responsiveness, capacity to change; flexibility built into governance, planning, operations, roles, coverage, etc. Obtains contractual relationships to other agencies providing health or health related services	costs and investments efficiency utilization, under or over connectedness consumer participation training health status	Outside technical, financial delivery and general evaluation by RHA Outside general surveillance by SHD

Integrates all services, records, and financing required by clients with the clients, including costs, necessary referrals, transfers, transport, information transfer	Sets patterns for centralization and decentralization of services
	
	Sets quality and relevance measures
	
	Sets consumer support, education, and participation measures
		Publishes annual report showing above as well as expenditures made for such major categories as:
		
		  evaluation
		  administration
		  consumer education	

Maintains forceful relationships with environmental, social welfare, educational, health, etc., agencies with purpose of assuring that the community is a healthy place in which to live	Sets patterns for enrollment; switches, sanctions for misuse Sets patterns for financing Sets patterns for control, spending Sets patterns for manpower, technology, facility relationships Sets patterns for centralization and decentralization of planning and policy making, participation, inspection, controls, records, etc.	manpower or training investments services certain conditions or diseases of concern because of cost, possibility of control, etc.	

FIGURE 7.7

ATTRIBUTES AND CRITERIA OF "MANPOWER" GOALS OF A HEALTH CARE DELIVERY SYSTEM (HCD)

Define Uses of Manpower	Organize Working Structure, Provide, Distribute	Recruit, Train
Design and redesign modes of manpower distribution, teams, skill packages, or new disciplines, records, to suit community needs and to ensure connectedness	By location and in accordance with needs, including outreach	Participate in educational planning for general manpower pool from which health manpower is drawn
Guided by RHA,* SHA,* or NHA* for general standards, practices, licensure and provide feedback to health authorities on standards as well as all other functions	In relation to other skills, teams, transport, travel times, technology, and facilities of the HCD or contracted for	Share with education through recruitment to health skills,** taking into account issues of equity as to who gets to be a server by geography, sex, and race; and create incentives to get servers from underserved areas and groups, e.g., work with career counselors, provide materials, encounters, experience, encouragement
	Maintain control over practice under its auspices, e.g., newcomers must work in underserved area for so many years, or schemes of rotation	Participate in educational planning for current and newly proposed health skills
	Develop contractual, quality, quantity, reimbursement machinery	Participate in providing education for current and newly proposed health skills
		Participate in, or organize on and off the job training for horizontal and vertical skill changes
		Participate in or organize on and off the job continuing education for all skills
		Maintain connections with major teaching medical centers for educational purposes

*See Figure 7.12.
**Skills include related capacities, such as social, psychologic, or economic knowledge relevant to application of skills.

FIGURE 7.8

ATTRIBUTES AND CRITERIA OF "TECHNOLOGY" GOALS OF A HEALTH CARE DELIVERY SYSTEM (HCD)

Planning, Operating, Controlling	Provision and Distribution	Constraints
Plan for obtaining, maintaining, replacing	Provide what, where, and as needed, with reference to:	RHA finalizes decisions on issues of major capital outlay
Evaluation for utilization, cost, quality of results	necessary skills available for use	RHA evaluates utilization plans
Assist with R. and D. efforts as relevant	volume of use necessary to keep up skills, training, and research needs	RHA*(SHA,* NHA*) makes standards to be met
Correlate with manpower and training needs	volume to justify overhead, versus skill, travel, time, and cost tradeoffs vs. obtaining by contract elsewhere	(HCD's participate in such decisions)
Investigate need for new technology, possible areas of evaluation suitable in HCD	linkages with communications, transport, accounting, educational and other service system tie-ins as police, education, welfare, etc.	
Participate in standard setting with RHA*	Relation to use in or through linkages with adequate facilities	

*See Figure 7.12.

FIGURE 7.9

ATTRIBUTES AND CRITERIA OF "FACILITY" GOALS OF A HEALTH CARE DELIVERY SYSTEM (HCD)

Planning, Administrating, Controlling	Provision and Distribution	Constraints
Determine issues of competition between subunits	Provide suitable numbers, sizes, types, designs as needed for consumers and services	RHA* (SHA* NHA*) makes decisions on issues of major capital outlays services
Determine issues of economies of scale, convenience vs. special capacities, single vs. multiple dispersed centers, etc.	Connectedness internally and externally	RHA evaluates utilization, plans for, etc.
Determine issues of centralization vs. decentralization of operations	Correlate with technology, manpower, communications, transport, and education and research to be carried out, in terms of capacity desirability, cost, flexibility	RHA (SHA, NHA) makes basic standards decisions (HCD's participate in such decisions)
Determine local delegation vs. central policy making and operations	Provision of reasonable, optional, extra hotel-type services for consumers at their cost	
Set standards for maintenance, safety, hours		
Determine issues of capacity to enlarge vs. new units and specialized units, flexibility, durability, cost		
Participate in capacity and performance standard setting with RHA*		

*See Figure 7.12

FIGURE 7.10

ATTRIBUTES AND CRITERIA OF "FINANCING" GOALS OF A HEALTH CARE DELIVERY SYSTEM (HCD)

Planning, Administrating, Controlling, Constraints	Sources and Adequacy	Expenditure and Cost Control
Design income and outgo budgeting that avoids sudden changes in services or remuneration	Federal base required with diversity, stability, and reasonable means for growth	Use of devices such as per capitation to earmark funds
Design annual total care per capita budget for the population served (show facilities, major capital outlay, research, training, evaluation, administration, and planning separately)	"Progressive" type financing	Use of devices such as per capitation to pay key professionals used to fee-for-service to discourage their generation of more services and more take home pay
Present clear annual report showing major sources and expenditures of funds	Minimal expenditures to middleman such as insurance groups or sales promotions	Evaluation for needless work, extra procedures, meaningless experiments, lazy work habits
Guided by funds made available and policies and standards set by NHA,* SHA* and RHA* for:	Negotiable costs depending on level of community need for services	Comparisons with other HCD's to spot underuse, overuse, unusual costs, organizational and technologic advances or lags
levels and types of care	Standards for what care packages provide commensurate with financing	Rewards for better producing or more efficient subunits
research	Rewards built in for efficiency and high standards of operation	Studies of unusually good or bad production records
recruiting and training	Coverage provided in one package for all persons and for all aspects of health care as shown under quality and relevancy of care (Figure 7.4)	Rewards to customers who wisely hold down usage
external planning and evaluation (done through RHA, SHA, NHA)		Cost/effectiveness studies of various subunits, programs, projects that are expensive or whose costs seem excessive or which draw unfavorable consumer and/or personnel feedback
accrediting, licensing, surveillance, and controls		
administration, internal planning and evaluation		

*See Figure 7.12

285

FIGURE 7.11

ATTRIBUTES AND CRITERIA OF "SURVEILLANCE AND CONTROL"*
GOALS OVER A HEALTH CARE DELIVERY SYSTEM (HCD)

Facilities and Technology	Manpower and Services	Personnel Requirements and Administrative Practices	Enforcement
Inspection for basic standards of: safety cleanliness maintenance construction waste disposal etc.	Consumer acceptability Consumer access Consumer participation Consumer education Personnel education Personnel adequacy Personnel participation	Control, examine for and issue: licenses accreditation registration and, where above delegated to HCD, inspect for compliance Control, examine for: accounting procedures recordkeeping accuracy of reports	Carry out legally defined steps to obtain compliance Provide education as training institutes to enable HCD's to comply Carry out enforcement for failure to comply Close up or take over temporarily as required until failing HCD reorganized

*Surveillance and Control are envisioned as being done by a state health department (SHD) type of agency, or being a surveillance arm of a state health authority (SHA) which is seen as a successor to currently scattered agencies now doing licensing, accrediting, standard setting, facility approval, service control, etc.

286

FIGURE 7.12
ATTRIBUTES AND CRITERIA OF "EVALUATION, PLANNING AND POLICY SETTING" GOALS FOR ALL HEALTH AUTHORITIES

National Health Authority (NHA)	State Health Authority (SHA)	Regional Health Authority (RHA)	Constraints
Sets key national policies for SHA's, RHA's, re roles on HCD: organization manpower technology facilities financing health care standards utilization consumer participation	Sets key state policies for RHA's re roles in relation to HCD's organization and delivery	Carries out policies and roles re HCD's set by NHA and SHA HCD's set by NHA and SHA	All levels must have representation from: consumers victims vested interests politicians planners other sectors technologists such as M.D.'s economists, etc.
Sets key national policies on per capita costs, benefits, role of insurance, means of vendor payments, co-payments, etc.	Sets key state policies re costs, benefits under NHA policy and state legislation	Assures that all persons covered; no massive segregation by race, poverty, age; emphasis on highly available primary care; investigates all problems of delivery; assures input from all neighborhoods and consumer control of HCD's	Vested health interests must be in the minority
Allocates financing for care, training, manpower, facilities, evaluation, research, etc., as guided by federal legislation	Plans for and carries out policing, licensing, if so assigned, or works with state health department if it does control activities in accordance with NHA policies	Carries out policing, licensing etc., as designated by SHA	All plan designs must be based on serving the health of people, not on desires or needs of the purveyors or of the planners for bigger and better plants, HCD's, etc. To serve ultimate aim that all persons get health care in accordance with their needs, with no significant out

		of pocket expenditures (prepaid basis) and no possibility of bankruptcy from costs (absolute catastrophic coverage)
Advises congress on health and health care annually re: what has happened what will happen what is desirable what should be striven for means of so doing	Advises legislature on health and health care annually re: what has happened what will happen what is desirable what should be striven for means of so doing	Advises local planning bodies and local legislative bodies on health and health care annually on: what has happened what will happen what is desirable what should be striven for means of so doing
Guarantees that all states are covered by HCD's, SHA's, that all get a hearing, and settles all disputes between states or between states and their regions	Guarantees that all of state is covered by HCD's and RHA's and that all get a hearing, and settles all disputes between RHA's and between RHA's and HCD's	Guarantees that all of region is covered by HCD's and that each HCD gets a hearing, and settles all disputes between HCD's and between local and sublocal planning bodies, and between planning and HCD
Plans ahead for health care nationwide	Plans ahead for health care statewide	Plans ahead for health care region wide
Plans ahead for *health* nationwide and cuts unnecessary needs for health care, e.g. genetics, environment, behavior	Plans ahead for *health* statewide; cuts unnecessary needs tor health care, e.g. genetics, environment, behavior	Plans ahead for *health* region wide and cuts unnecessary needs for health care, e.g. genetics, environment, behavior
Carries out planning: do assessment overall establish major goals define key problems suggest changes and interventions	Carries out planning: do assessment overall establish major goals define key problems suggest changes and interventions	Carries out planning: do assessment overall establish major goals define key problems suggest changes and intervention

National	State	Regional/Local
evaluate prior year's capabilities and programs	evaluate prior year's capabilities and programs	evaluate prior year's capabilities and programs
Carries out duties of national level CHP* and RMP* which are incorporated into NHA	Carries out duties of state level CHP and RMP which are incorporated in SHA	Carries out duties of regional and local level CHP and RMP
Must be officially established at national level in accordance with federal law	Must be officially established at state level in accordance with NHA policy and state legislation	May be voluntarily established at regional, city, county, and neighborhood levels, even self-perpetuating if meets NHA and SHA policy; must have neighborhood units for those with serious health problems, representation from neighborhood units on RHA bodies

Note.—NHA and SHA and RHA each receive 0.1% of all health care funding to do tasks indicated, including expenditure of funds now allocated under 314(a-e) and RMP for reasonable operation.

Planning and policy setting for all of health care is seen as a major part of the duties of a national health authority (NHA), which relates to and provides guidance for state health authorities (SHA) which do similarly for regional health authorities (RHA). These are seen as successors to the plethora of one-purpose health agencies carrying on unrelated activities, of licensing, accrediting, standard setting, facility control, health planning (CHP), regional medical programs (RMP).

*CHP represents the current comprehensive health planning bodies set up by PL.89-949. RMP represents Regional Medical Programs set up under P.L. 89-239.

problems as discrete as tuberculosis also contain clusters of lesser problems—fear of being examined, diagnostic failures, therapeutic failures, and so on.

The "sick" community or ghetto neighborhood as the presenting problem appears to carry the obvious definition of the malfunctioning system, which is the ghetto itself. But we do not get off so easily, for the analysis of this problem reveals that it is typically a malfunctioning subunit of many larger systems. It may be the cross-whipped area of the economic, agricultural, educational and health systems. It usually is also a subsystem of the geopolitical city, metro, and state systems.

The two sets of systems described, and many others, cut across one another in innumerable ways. Both the ghetto and the posh neighborhoods are the resultant small area outcomes. How shall we proceed with the analysis of what ails the sick neighborhood? Shall we break it down into each of its clusters of debilities, tuberculosis, venereal disease, malnutrition, high infant death rate, crime, or unemployment and analyze each in turn?

This community—which may be only one part of a town or as much as half a dozen states—with a high work-accident rate, excessive pulmonary disease, widespread poverty, unemployment, delinquency, school dropouts, and generally depressed health indicators may, on careful study, reveal its secrets. It could, for example, be a one-industry town with worn-out marginal mines which are poorly timbered and poorly dust-controlled, operating irregularly in accordance with fluctuations in the market, contributing little to civic wealth or taxable resources, and in general discouraging, if not maiming, the residents. Such a state of affairs would not benefit greatly from the kind of health planning which might typically be applied to a high accident rate or to lung disease. What is needed is total economic redevelopment or relocation of the residents. Disease by disease approaches could squander available resources without creating meaningful change.

Neighborhoods are sometimes designedly the sole concern of planning efforts. The Model Cities concept originally utilized comprehensive planning insofar as possible within the constraints of a neighborhood.[31] Every aspect of well-being—health, employment, education, recreation, housing—is considered, for whatever man is thought to reasonably need is relevant to the planning of a model neighborhood. The logic of analyzing the ecology of a community is most importantly applied to those which are seen to be failing significantly according to many health and well-being indicators. It may even be said that failing neighborhoods spawn ill health.

When the systems analysis type of logic is applied to a so-called sick community, an analysis, conceptually similar to the analysis of a disease, is needed to discover in what ways community poor health arises.

(Analysts should not overlook the inputs shown in Figure 1.1, because any one or several of them may be important in determining the well-being status of the community.)

Where the maimed community represents a much more complex set of forces at work, as in the big city ghetto, somewhere among the precursors we can expect to see the consequences of the national policy of fighting inflation by unemployment and of abandoning central cities to blighted housing, dilapidated schools, and their aura of hopelessness. Perhaps behind these precursors also lies the uneconomic nature of small farming operations and national agricultural policies which essentially destroy small farms so that rural communities stagnate or die and force unskilled people by the millions to the cities to compound the grief of the ghettos. What magic can a city or community health planner find to counteract forces which have rendered the nation impotent in its internal affairs?

If we attempt to look at still larger collections of problems, we find ourselves even more pressed to categorize and relate problems systematically and systemically. One innovative attempt to put together a list of key problems as the basis for attempts to introduce planning into the myriad affairs of the State of California provides us with Figure

FIGURE 7.13
MAJOR DISRUPTIONS

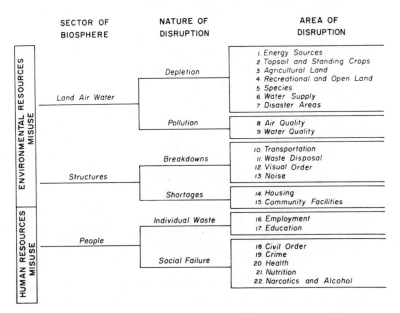

SECTOR OF BIOSPHERE	NATURE OF DISRUPTION	AREA OF DISRUPTION
ENVIRONMENTAL RESOURCES MISUSE — Land Air Water	Depletion	1. Energy Sources 2. Topsoil and Standing Crops 3. Agricultural Land 4. Recreational and Open Land 5. Species 6. Water Supply 7. Disaster Areas
	Pollution	8. Air Quality 9. Water Quality
Structures	Breakdowns	10. Transportation 11. Waste Disposal 12. Visual Order 13. Noise
	Shortages	14. Housing 15. Community Facilities
HUMAN RESOURCES MISUSE — People	Individual Waste	16. Employment 17. Education
	Social Failure	18. Civil Order 19. Crime 20. Health 21. Nutrition 22. Narcotics and Alcohol

7.13, which is taken from *The California Tomorrow Plan: A First Sketch.*[32]

The problems are not specifically defined, but are listed by the area of disruption in the right hand column. This is not a problem-by-problem approach but a comprehensive listing of all the threatening problems facing the State. Using this listing, more specific problem entities can be selected out of each area of disruption. By tying all the problems back to the sector of the biosphere most involved (the left column), the nature of the planning enterprises and how they must interrelate begins to stand out.

In comparison with such a comprehensive approach, the idea of health planning standing by itself, not surrounded by comparable ventures in the other areas of disruption and without means of dealing with interconnecting concerns, leaves one with a frightening sense of futility about isolated health planning, and with particular misgivings about proceeding with specific health problems in sick communities.

Which Type of Problem Should Be Analyzed First?

If particularly aggravated diseases, conditions, environmental problems, inequities, and sick communities with a superabundance of all kinds of problems were analyzed first, presumably the best interventions designed for each would then form the basis for plans to introduce changes into such delivery systems as health care. The planning body's analysis and reordering of health care would then start with the benefits of the solutions to various specific health problems.

Unfortunately, this sequence is neither logical nor ideal. Political pressures and the national purposes are obviously giving high priority to availability, accessibility, acceptability, freedom from worries of cost, and full equity of health care services. Therefore, it seems clear that planning for suitable health care machinery cannot wait for the "logical" analytic approach to be carried out for each major health problem or for the specific needs of sizeable "sick" communities before instituting any further delivery system changes. Granted, if planners follow the dictates of nationally accepted priorities, even the most expensive service machinery may not be designed optimally, for lack of a clear picture of who should be served for what purposes. But normal wear and tear and natural obsolescence will allow most of the "mistakes" to be retired after having rendered ample, if less than ideal, service.

The intervention or delivery systems in the health field are well established, and annually render many tens of billions of dollars of service. At the same time, the needs and opportunities to modify the means whereby they render care are commanding greater attention. In many cases, the advantages of creating new internal operating relationships or of utilizing new techniques are irresistible in spite of significant capital outlays and high continuing operating costs. The specific promises of more effective diagnosis and therapy with the saving of lives or the amelioration of disability provide ample justification for introducing changes. Sometimes these changes involve primarily the relationships between members of different classes of purveyors, as manifested by the growing ties between hospital, convalescent, and home care operations.

Strauss contends that even a limited approach to the analysis of delivery systems (acknowledging the mismatch between our methods of delivery and the population group with the heaviest load of ill health, the poor) would pay off handsomely.[33] He points out that almost every facet of the health care machinery is designed so that it cannot serve the poor, no matter how much money is put into their hands to buy services. Almost every aspect of their lives makes health care services as they are currently rendered essentially unavailable, inappropriate, and unintelligible.

We see no way technically or politically that a planning body can or should evade a combined or simultaneous analytic attack on problems (of disease, environment, sick community or current delivery scheme failures) while setting about its major chores, the normative planning for a healthier community and for an overall acceptable care distribution system. Where novel alternative breakthroughs in disease intervention are not easily visualized, we can justify provision of optimal modes of delivering the interventions now considered effective until planning studies point out new possibilities for intervention at more appropriate times or circumstances, and research clarifies the actual utility of such alternatives.

Use of the Relevant Communities as the Base for Planning

One of the better devices to ensure a drawing together of the study elements is the use of the aggregate of people represented by the "community" as the base upon which to make studies. The level of community at which the resolution of the problem or attainment of goals seems likely to take place provides such a base. (For a typology of communities see Chapter 11.)

Although this hardly seems like a revelation, I am continuously amazed to find service or facility planning done by comprehensive health planning bodies in terms of purveyors or facilities, without regard to full coverage for the major problems or goals of all members of the community. Planning is done service by service, program by pro-

gram, typically with each service group harking back to some historical norm or service cliche—or to the expected difficulties with financing—which justifies their carving out as much or as little (usually the
cream) of the needed service venture as they are predisposed to do.
This, of course, is the natural outcome of planning for solution of
problems by vested interests, without at the same time carrying on
planning for achievement of major community goals.

ANALYSES NEED TO BE CONDUCTED BY THE RELEVANT SECTORS AND LEVELS

Allocation of Analyses to Appropriate Sectors of Society When They Involve Issues that Embrace More than the Health Sector

Health planners doing analysis at any level will soon run into precursors and consequences which involve issues lying almost entirely
outside the health sector's expertise and influence.[34] Through its contacts with the general policy makers and higher levels of planning, the
planning body will have to make a strong case for reassignment of
such problems to the planning machinery in other sectors. (See Chapter 10.) This same concern also arises for allocations of potential
interventions.

Allocation of Analyses to Appropriate Levels of Planning Inside the Health Sector

In a comprehensive planning approach, literally thousands of potential assignments will be made by the health planners, which are to
be retained in the health sector. Added to these will be health-relevant
assignments coming from other sectors (such as education, welfare,
and natural resources) where the concept of comprehensive planning
is likely to be introduced also. From all of these, health planners must
abstract certain recurrent themes, as well as potential conflicts about
the needed interventions and the kinds and levels of skills and facilities
that are proposed for each of the services called for.

Because some issues can be resolved only at certain levels (licensure
of physicians cannot be done at the local level and is still unwisely
carried out relatively independently at 50 state levels), it is imperative
that problems be assigned to planning levels where something can be
done about them. Planning allocations to neighborhoods may also
have to go downward for some matters. (This subject is discussed in
Chapter 10.)

CONCLUDING COMMENTS

Concurrent attacks on major health goals and for major health problems in all categories, such as disease, environment, sick communities, equity, and delivery failures must be undertaken by health planning bodies. By the systems type of analysis the relationships between various problems and the systemic matrix in which health is embedded will begin to emerge. Simultaneous analyses done for large health goals will provide the knowledge and criteria to guide design and selection of interventions by means of which such really major ends as equitable distribution of health care for all can become a reality. At the same time, these same large goals will provide the needed guidance by which problems can be selected for priority attention, and interventions directed against them can also be preferentially rank ordered. By being engaged in analysis both for major goal attainment and for problem solving, health planners will also begin to find the necessary planning relationships as well as the intervention relationships that will lessen the hazards threatened by disjointed planning ventures, each of which is so likely to disrupt the others.

Perhaps the most critical task facing the health planners will not be to get their own game together, but rather to stimulate society's concern so that other sectors will begin planning as well. Just scanning Figure 7.13 makes us realize how hopeless the outlook is for meaningful health changes if simultaneous and correlated planning is not going on in transport, energy, agriculture, and so on. Health planners will not only have to use systems analysis of problems to assign developmental and programmatic tasks inside the health sector, but they will have to forcefully hand out planning assignments for other sectors via the overall policy makers, because health problems arise in those sectors and must be attacked there if worthwhile improvements are to be made. Health workers customarily treat the casualties made by others.

The educative aspects of planning for those now hurting and those interested in health problem alleviation can be the means of creating public awareness of the really major areas causing disruption and future failures. This awareness will not happen by itself, nor will it develop until health planning bodies commence to use systemic approaches to problem resolution, which will inform them of the necessary kinds of influences that they must help bring to bear.

Analysis of problems or goals leads not only to design of possible interventions but to the reconsideration of the preceding planning steps, such as goal setting and assessment. This final thought is added here to re-emphasize the circularity of the planning process shown in Figure 1.2. The analysis carries us forward from defining improvements to steps of designing, evaluating, and choosing the means of attaining them. But it may well carry planners back to the need for reconsidering goals or devising new means of assessment and problem selection if the planning steps already undertaken in the light of problem or goal analysis are now seen to be directed toward work that is unfeasible, irrelevant, or no longer desirable.

REFERENCES

1. Allen Schick, "From Analysis to Evaluation," *Annals of the American Academy of Political and Social Sciences* 394 (March 1971), 57-71.
2. Walter R. Lynn, "Systems Approach to Public Health," *Human Ecology and Public Health*, ed. by Edwin D. Kilbourne and Wilson G. Smillie, 4th ed. (New York: Macmillan, 1969), Chapter 9. E. Groth-Petersen, J. Knudsen and E. Wilbeck, "Epidemiological Basis of Tuberculosis Eradication in an Advanced Country," *World Health Organization Bulletin* 21 (1959), 5-49. M. Piot and T. K. Sundaresan, "A Linear Programme Decision Model for Tuberculosis Control," World Health Organization/TB/Technical Information/67.55, mimeographed. "A Planning Methodology for Tuberculosis Control Programmes," World Health Organization/Res/68.16, Geneva, December 2-10, 1968, Consultation of Experts on Research in Public Health, mimeographed. C. S. deVelle, W. R. Lynn, and F. Feldman, "Mathematical Models for the Economic Allocation of Tuberculosis Control Activities in Developing Nations," *American Review of Respiratory Diseases* 96 (November 1967), 893-909. Martin S. Feldstein, M. A. Piot, and T. K. Sundaresan, "Resource Allocation Model for Public Health Planning—A Case Study of Tuberculosis Control," Supplement to Vol. 48 of the Bulletin of the World Health Organization, WHO, General, 1973.
3. Jay W. Forrester, *World Dynamics* (Cambridge, Mass.: Wright Allen Press, 1971).
4. Donella H. Meadows, et al., *The Limits to Growth* (New York: Universe Books, 1972).
5. Albert Waterton, "Public Administration for What: A Pragmatic View," International Bank for Reconstruction and Development, January 11, 1967, mimeographed.
6. Anthony Downs, *An Economic Theory of Democracy* (New York: Harper & Row, 1957), Chapter 1.
7. H. Freeman, "Comments," *Milbank Memorial Fund Quarterly* 46 (April 1968), part 2.
8. Edward S. Rogers, "The Ecological Perspective," *Administering Health Systems: Issues and Perspectives*, ed. by Mary F. Arnold, L. Vaughn Blankenship, and John M. Hess (Chicago; New York: Aldine,; Atherton, 1971), Chapter 12.
9. Erich Jantsch, *Technological Forecasting in Perspective* (Paris: Organization for Economic Cooperation and Development, 1967), 109-239.

10. State of Washington, Office of Comprehensive Health Planning, "Issue Analysis," by Frank Baker, Verne Gibbs, and Frank Anderson, Olympia, Washington, 1970, mimeographed.

11. U. S., Department of Health, Education and Welfare, Office of Program Planning and Evaluation, Bureau of Health Services, *Management Summary of the PHS Social Forces "Project Navigate,"* Washington, D. C., April 1, 1968.

12. Edward deBono, "The Virtues of Zigzag Thinking," *Think* 35 (May/June 1969), 7-10.

13. U. S., Department of Health, Education and Welfare, Public Health Service, *The Principles of Program Packaging in the Division of Indian Health,* Washington, D. C., January 15, 1966.

14. Pan American Health Organization, Pan American Sanitary Bureau, *Health Planning: Problems of Concepts and Method* (Scientific Pub. No. 111), 1965.

15. Pan American Health Organization, *Report of the Technical Advisory Committee, Pan American Program for Health Planning,* Santiago, Chile, United Nations Building, February 12, 1971.

16. W. R. Lynn, "Systems Approach to Public Health" (see no. 2).

17. J. W. Forrester, Ibid. no. 3.

18. U. S., Department of Health, Education and Welfare, Office of the Assistant Secretary for Program Coordination, "Selected Disease Control Programs," 1966. U. S., Department of Health, Education and Welfare, Office of the Assistant Secretary for Program Coordination, "Maternal and Child Health Care Programs," 1966.

19. "Symposium: Planning-Programming-Budgeting System Reexamined: Development, Analysis and Criticism," *Public Administration Review* 29 (March/April 1969). S. T. Gabis, "Mental Health and Financial Management: Some Dilemmas of Program Budgeting," Department of Political Science, Michigan State University, East Lansing, 1960.

20. Richard M. Bailey, "Economics and Planning," *Health Planning 1969,* by H. L. Blum and Associates (San Francisco: Western Regional Office, American Public Health Association, 1969), Chapter 9.

21. Count Gibson and Jack Geiger, Report in the *Wall Street Journal,* Western edition, January 14, 1969.

22. Thomas Fulop, "Integrated Epidemiologic Surveys," *Milbank Memorial Fund Quarterly* 49 (January 1971), pp. 59-92.

23. J. S. Reiner, E. Reimer, and T. A. Reiner, "Client Analysis in the Planning of Public Programs," *Journal of the American Institute of Planners* 29 (November 1963), 270-82.

24. Andre L. Delbecq and Andrew VandeVen, "Nominal and Interacting Group Processes for Committee Decision-Making Effectiveness," *Journal of the Academy of Management,* 14 (June 1971), 203.

25. Bernard Benjamin, *Social and Economic Factors Affecting Mortality* (New York: Humanities Press, 1965). M. H. Brenner, "Fetal, Infant, and Maternal Mortality During Periods of Economic Instability," International Journal of Health Services, 3 (1973), 145-59. Robert J. Haggerty "The Boundaries of Health Care," The Pharos (July 1972), 106-11. Warren Winkelstein Jr. "Epidemiological Considerations Underlying the Al-

location of Health and Disease Care Resources," International Journal of Epidemiology 1 (1972), 69-74.

26. Warren L. Ilchman and Norman T. Uphoff, *The Political Economy of Change* (Berkeley & Los Angeles: The University of California Press, 1969), 260-73.

27. C. West Churchman, "The Role of Weltanschauung in Problem Solving and Inquiry," Internal Working Paper No. 94, Space Sciences Laboratory, University of California, Berkeley, November 1968. C. West Churchman, *The Systems Approach* (New York: Dell Publishing, 1968), 173.

28. E. A. Gardner and J. N. Snipe, "Toward the Coordination and Integration of Personal Health Services," *American Journal of Public Health* 60 (November 1970), 2068-79. Vicente Navarro, "National Health Insurance and the Strategy for Change," The Milbank Memorial Fund Quarterly, 51 (Spring 1973), 223-51. Victor Fuchs, "Health Care and the United States Economic System: An Essay in Abnormal Physiology," The Milbank Memorial Fund Quarterly, 1 (April 1972), 211-37.

29. Gerald Nadler, *Work Design: A Systems Concept*, rev. ed. (Homewood, Illinois: Richard D. Irwin, 1970), 507-11.

30. Ibid., 514 and Chapter 2.

31. U. S. Congress, House of Representatives, Committee on Banking and Currency, "Basic Laws and Authorities on Housing and Urban Development," 1967, 279.

32. California Tomorrow, *The California Tomorrow Plan: A First Sketch* (San Francisco: California Tomorrow, 681 Market Street, 1971), 3.

33. Anselm L. Strauss, "Medical Ghettos," *Trans-Action* 5 (May 1967). Taken from "Medical Organization, Medical Care and Lower Income Groups," a paper for the Institute of Policy Studies, Washington, D. C.

34. Stanislav U. Kasl, "Effects of Residential Environment on Health and Behavior—A Review," A Report written under Contract PE-R-69-30 to the Bureau of Community Environmental Management, HSMHA, PHS, DHEW, March 1972. Paul V. Lemkau, "Mental Health and Housing," A Report Written Under Contract PH-86-68-154 to the Bureau of Community Environment Management, HSMHA, PHS, DHEW, February 1970. Daniel M. Wilner, "Sociocultural Factors in Residential Space," A Report Written Under Contract PH-86-68-154 to the Bureau of Community Environmental Management, HSMHA, PHS, DHEW, March 1970. Kermit K. Schooler and Neal Bellos, "Environment and Aging: Some Implications for Policy and Planning," A Report Written Under Contract CPE-R-69-30 to the Bureau of Community Environmental Management, HSMHA, PHS, DHEW, April 1972. Albert Damon, "Residential Design, Health and Behavior," A Report Written Under Contract CPE-70-103 to the Bureau of Community Environmental Management, Consumer Protection and Environmental Health Service, November 15, 1969. John R. Goldsmith and Erland Jonsson, "Effects of Noise on Health in the Residential and Urban Environment," Prepared for the American Public Health Association, August 1969. Ido De Groot, et al., "Human Health and the Spatial Environment: An Epidemiological Assignment," A Report Written Under Contract PH-86-68-154 to the Bureau of Community Environmental Management HSMHA, PHS, DHEW, no date. Thomas

H. Holmes and Minoru Masuda, "Life Changes and Illness Susceptibility," Presented at a Symposium on "Separation and Depression: Clinical and Research Aspects," at the Annual Meeting of the AAAS, Chicago, Illinois, December 26-30 1970. John Cassel and Lynn Waller, "The Relation of Urban Environment to Health: Towards a Conceptual Frame and a Research Strategy," A Report Written Under Contract CPE-R-69-30 for the Bureau of Community Environmental Management, HSMHA, PHS, DHEW, July 1971. E. Laszlo, *The Systems View of the World* (New York: George Braziller 1972). Alan Sheldon, Frank Baker and Curtis P. McLaughlin, editors *Systems and Medical Care* (Cambridge Mass: The MIT Press 1970). Howard Brody, "Systems View of Man," *Perspectives in Biology and Medicine,* 17 (Autumn 1973), pp. 71-92.

8. The Systems Approach: Design, Analysis, and Comparison of Alternative Interventions

In Chapter 7, we examined the systems approach for analyzing community goals and problems and determining which factors led to a problem (or goal) and which resulted from it. Once a system is laid open, opportunities to interrupt its current functioning are disclosed. Fertile minds and divergent viewpoints see various means to affect the system so that certain goals are attained or certain problems are brought under control.

After the planning group has drawn up potentially useful interventions, a means is needed to assure that the interventions proposed will, in fact, do what is wanted without excessively adverse side effects, and at a price commensurate with the need and the outcomes. In addition, a means is needed for comparing proposed interventions to aid in making choices among them.

DESIGN OF INTERVENTIONS

Drawing up interventions is not a single step at any specific point in a problem or goal analysis, but rather occurs throughout the entire process. I have suggested certain steps during which a look at possible points of intervention may be particularly productive, but with no intention of limiting discussion of interventions to those times. The process may begin at the first session when a participant declares: "Something has to be done; I think we need more traffic lights," and will continue on through the study, hopefully widening as the scope of the study widens.

The details of the design process of interventions need not be extensively dealt with here, for we are devoting ourselves to planning at the community level. Thus, our concerns are with community desires, needs, goals, and problems, and our purpose is to help the community handle these in accordance with its purposes.

Community-Level Planned Interventions

The community-level planning body output for goals is not a series

300

of specific detailed interventive tools, methods or programs; it is rather a set of directing criteria drawn from three major sources.

Design Criteria Drawn from Normative Goals

To be more concrete, let us take a community's health care desires. The planning body has analyzed what its goals imply in the way of facilities, manpower, finances, consumer comprehension, and systemic wholeness. The general nature of the interventions (what is needed) have suggested themselves. This community level planning body now turns what is desired of the system into sets of stipulations about what the delivery system must offer, under what circumstances, and to what kinds of people. (A set of "ideal" stipulations for a health care system were presented as Figures 7.3-7.12, and will be dealt with further.)

Design Criteria Drawn from Significant Problems

At the same time, the community will undoubtedly have looked for its health care hurts, disease problems, and sick neighborhoods and will have analyzed each of these for consequences and precursors. Many sets of fairly specific interventions will suggest themselves: new cliches, special services, outreach, different hours, translators, consumers on policy boards, and so on.

Design Criteria Derived from a Forecast of the General Social Environment

An alert community planning body will have achieved a set of reconciled forecasts from all sectors, many of which will have a direct bearing on the two categories of concerns around health and health care—that is, desires and problems. The forecasts will include the likelihood of Federal financial support in behalf of the poor, and its nature, the toleration of new kinds of personnel, the likelihood of new relatedness between various now separate pieces of the health care machinery, and so on.

Setting Operating Policy (The Community-Level Planning Output)

A framework for planning (or action or operations) is set up for the community planning body from these three sources: (1) the sets of design criteria; (2) the intervention characteristics needed to overcome the major problems; and (3) the constraints anticipated from resources, traditions, higher levels of government, and so on. Using this information, the community health planning body begins to design and specify what service outputs are to be made available, and their timing; or it may go further and describe the system which is to create the outputs. Thus, it designs a current plan or set of guides. This design effort provides the criteria by which those responsible for output know what is required of them in the immediate as well as the more distant future.

The specifications made by the community-level planning body on the basis of its analysis of desires, hurts, and constraints then provide a planning framework for operating agencies. That is, the planning body does not usually (but sometimes it may) design hospitals or spell out how manpower is to be trained or how children are to be immunized. It points out what is needed, while those who create hospitals or train manpower or immunize children undertake the internal planning efforts of the operating agencies which must create the outputs to meet the social needs in the ways specified by the community planning body. The interventions stipulated by the community planning body are, therefore, not detailed designs but the specifications for the output of the systems whose efforts are involved. If the planning body's plans are implemented and the resources called for are available, presumably its design will allow the various systems and subsystems to perform and interrelate appropriately and on time, because the community's plan or specifications for output become the planning targets for the subsystem producers. With incentives and penalties—as well as resources—built into the community-level plan, its subsystem producers should get their planning as well as operations into the selected stream.

The design of the community-level interventions (plans) should enjoy the participation of those who will shortly have to do the agency or operative level planning and delivery. Therefore the community-level planning body should know well the technical, organizational, political and human resistances its design effort is going to encounter; and as part of its plan the group should have worked these through to a reasonable set of design expectations and participation. Thus, the design would presumably be realistic in terms of what the various elements of the system under consideration would have to organize and deliver.

Other Design Considerations

Individual Interventions

As the analysis of goals or problems is concluded, the work of the planning task force moves into the design phase. Possible points of interventions into a problem are catalogued. Objectives singled out as way points to goals are similarly listed. Opposite each are listed the major criteria for judging acceptability of an intervention, as well as any anticipated harmful consequences that would make an intervention unacceptable. These criteria specify that no less than $x\%$ improvement would be acceptable, that it must occur by a certain time, must spare infants first, and so on. Again, at each interventive point that seems feasible, the appropriate expertise and other involved interests must be on hand to explore the reality as well as the acceptability of the possible interventions. The interventions at each point are thoroughly checked out individually, if they look hopeful.

Packages of Interventions

The interventions that seem to fit the situation best are then put into a package for a given goal or problem. The use of time, materials, and methods networks schedule approaches, such as Program Evaluation and Review Technique (PERT) or Critical Path Method (CPM), enables the planners to see how well the individual interventive pieces can be fitted into a package which will move the issue along from objective to objective until a goal is achieved or a problem solved.

The interventions proposed for a given objective can be very diverse. Some interventions may carry the effort over or around many steps. A decision to medicate everyone in a population against tuberculosis generally obviates the also available interventions to skin test or X-ray for that disease. In other words, not every feasible attack need be mounted. Many interventions may be harmful or at least redundant and wasteful if others are used. The possibility of having prompt transportation for the sick, for example, has been known to cause some outlying health service units to go unused—they are bypassed because everyone prefers to get to a more elaborate center. Combining interventions into packages, then, involves study of the relationships among them. Some complement, some inhibit, some obviate others. Packages should represent the more useful and acceptable mixes.

Counter Planning

Goal definitions may be based on very distinctive outlooks of what is desirable. How a problem or goal is viewed may similarly have locked it into a given analytic framework which can yield only one set of answers. In the preceding chapter it was suggested that a cross check approach be applied to analysis. The designed package of interventions might likewise be considered in the light of some totally opposed set of notions of what is wanted and of what is going on in the system at hand. Because Churchman has made this kind of proposal so well, I quote his statement that "a counterplan needs to have certain characteristics. It must appear highly reasonable and attractive. Hence it must use all the data that were used to build the plan, but must give the data a different interpretation based on its plausible view of what the system is like."[1]

Although cross checking can be costly to planning resources if repeated excessively, it may prevent more costly errors to the community if carried to reasonable lengths.

Referral of Proposed Interventions to Appropriate Sectors or Levels for Study

The most significant choice decisions among interventions occur between those that represent changes to the environment or larger systems influences and those that affect only a small part, such as a subsystem of the system under study. To obtain the appropriate expertise and study for determining their real utility, a given health planning body may have to refer some potential interventions to other sectors, some to higher or more general levels of planning, and still others to more specific sub-units of the health sector. In many cases the implementation will also have to be pursued, at least in part, by the planning levels to which the interventions were referred for study.

Allocation to Other Sectors of the Economy

From a practical standpoint it may be wiser to joint-venture or to refer possible interventions to the sector or sectors of the economy which can best analyze the possibilities of potential interventions and their implementation. In making this determination, planners must consider the level of the planning and the policy-making machinery needs of a given issue. For example, some aspects for the care of certain diseases cannot be encompassed by a local community or even a state. Funds for intelligent medical training programs will have to be shared by several regions of the country—in fact, almost surely with other segments of the economy at the national level. The planning and policy-making bodies of each relevant jurisdiction have to be involved, or support will not be available. The example of automobile accidents can be used again to indicate how the assignment of possible interventions might be made, following analysis of the automobile accident system.

Safer cars. This problem, with accumulated data, would be assigned to planners in the economic sectors at the national level, so that both the federal government and the car manufacturing and transport industries could undertake the proper solution.

Safer roadways. The question of roads would be assigned, with accumulated data, to physical planning bodies and to economic planning groups at local, state, and national levels, so that approaches could be developed and estimates made on the cost of correcting or eliminating certain kinds of dangerous traffic.

Driver education. This problem would be assigned to local, state, or national educational planners to establish whether the current equivocal evidence that driver education improves driver performance represents a failure of the intervention, of its measurement, or of the teaching methods utilized.

Senility. The problem of the senile drivers, who are so heavily involved in accidents, would become a joint effort of the law enforcement agencies and health and general wellbeing planners at local and state levels.

Drug use. Accident related problems created by people using medications, habituating drugs, and alcohol (particularly its chronic use) might well be assigned to both health and law enforcement segments of local and state planning.

Better emergency care for victims. This problem would remain primarily a local concern, occasionally involving the state health planning body. Rapid transport of victims would be a joint effort with others such as law enforcement bodies.

Unfortunately, no one should assume at this time that planning interests in most sectors are ready, willing, or able to take on the intervention design tasks suggested. If health planning bodies were able to involve the appropriate sectors in problem and goal analyses, the joint ventures required would continue through the intervention design phase, with the technical load being transferred to groups with the required capabilities. Perhaps health planning bodies will have to organize massive, even Nader-like, pressures to evoke response from many sectors or their institutions for the design, or implementation, of anything new.

Allocations to Other Planning Levels or Subsectors of the Health Sector

Assignment of the study of the health service subsystems calls for decisions about the appropriate level of health planning and policy-making to be involved. Moreover, a particular intervention may have to be assigned, or reassigned to an existing subsystem or health unit to determine its actual utility. Some interventions need to be made which switch categories of outputs from one subsystem to another. For example, changes could be made in the insurance system, so that much surgery or diagnostic work for inpatients who are not bed sick could be done on an outpatient basis. This change would mean taking business out of the hospital and assigning work to other facilities, either outpatient departments of hospitals or freestanding nonhospital health services.

In talking about health interventions, we must guard against the erroneous assumption that the health system is unified—that a single system produces the various health outputs. Such a view does not square with reality. Also, police, welfare, public health and mental health agencies attack many identical problems from skill approaches based on varying points of view of etiology, categorical legislation, or local circumstances (see Figure 3.1).

Assignment of intervention studies should not be based on assumptions about the structure and function of any particular subsystem in the health system. Not all the subdivisions of the system are likely to be, or can be, functionally separable. Responsibilities may overlap or be incompletely specified. Considerations of stability, personality, and institutional inertia also influence the organization of the system. Consequently, systems analysts may look at a subsystem structure from a number of different viewpoints, depending on their orientation toward the administration, the processes of production, or the social and political behavior of the system.

A major difficulty is finding agency time and willingness to outline possible alternative patterns of production. One agency's analysis of implementation may lead to analysis of many other agencies, and choice among alternatives may point to the need for a coherent pattern of operation which may be quite novel in a given community. The possibility that the objectives can be achieved by customary means is then compared with the prospects unfolded by new programs.

A listing of the resources required for each intervention will point out whether the subsystem receiving the bulk of the assignment will have to turn over part of the chores to other subsystems, or will need help from other subsystems or even from major systems outside the health sector. For example, education must assist in developing new kinds of health skill outputs, and the financial quarters must participate in opening new funding sources so that educational services can be set up and made available. The complexities of joint planning between sectors and among levels are awesome, yet heartening examples are now emerging.

ON-PAPER COMPARATIVE EVALUATION OF ALTERNATIVE INTERVENTIONS

It is often possible to make exploratory forecasts. The proponent of a program or intervention proposal works out on paper and presents documentable evidence of the gains and the price presumably offered by alternative feasible interventions. By setting out this information in a methodical way, the planning body, the public, and the policy makers can see whether they might approve of what is to be obtained at the prices that must be paid. We say prices advisedly, because many kinds of costs besides dollars are involved in activating an intervention.

Nature of Benefits and Costs

Values as the Origins of Criteria to Be Used

Criteria used in judging goodness must be consistent with widely held value and goal hierarchies. The value and goal hierarchies pervading the work of a planning body cannot and need not be spelled out concisely. But the measures to be used as criteria to judge a benefit or a cost must be specified, and these are practical statements of values and goals. Criteria that are not representative of important social values, such as leverage or speed of change or a balanced attack (Figure 6.1), must be subservient to value-laden criteria, such as equity, ecology or avoidance of death and disability, and must not lead to decisions that run counter to highly value-laden criteria. (For an extensive discussion of the nature of useful criteria and how they can be used to weight and provide aggregate significance levels see, in Chapter 6, the discussion of how to give priority to problems.) In general, a cost means that some highly placed value has to suffer, and a benefit means that the value is satisfied.

Determination of Benefits Created by an Intervention

Benefits or gains are the tangible expression of what we intend to achieve. If the goal is minimizing deaths from cervical cancer, benefits are not going to be measured accurately by counting the number of women found with a positive cervical smear, or even those placed under treatment. What must be determined is the proportion of those women at risk who are actually brought to a disease-free state or a prolonged life by the specific intervention. The final estimate of benefits resulting from a particular intervention can be based only on the whole picture—the number of potential cases prevented, of lives saved, or of years of productivity saved. However, describing and quantifying the problem-solving effects of an intervention is only one aspect of the consequences. If interventions also result in other streams of desirable events, the time range and probability of the size and nature of these effects can also be considered. By somewhat arbitrary classification, the definitions, the desired consequences can be divided into several categories for purposes of measurement.[2]

Direct benefits include the prevented or saved costs of caring for or overcoming the problem. These may be in terms of services or dollars saved, or sparing of certain special or scarce technical or manpower resources.

Indirect benefits include the prevention of work losses, property damage, lawsuits, and so on. To calculate earnings, full (customary) employment is assumed and an estimate is made of the average length of working life of the persons, their working capacity, and so on. Indirect benefits also include intangibles such as happiness, spared families, and second generation and familial consequences, although we prefer to lump these in the next category.

Unintended benefits (externalities, spillovers, or secondary benefits) include any favorable consequences of the intervention on problems other than the one being analyzed.

The benefits concept can, therefore, be extended to three kinds of situations which are commonly hard to measure, although often not hard to identify. These are generally lumped under the rubrics of externalities or publicly felt effects, which may also be called secondary consequences or spillovers. At least three obviously related versions are of interest: (1) those which unavoidably shed consequences on bystanders, as when others are freed of risk when a case of contagious tuberculosis is treated successfully; (2) those which result from an unintended coverage of a second condition, as when penicillin is used to treat pneumonia and also cures syphilis present in the same victim; (3) those which result from a spread of awareness, as when a victim of tuberculosis is identified, his family also becomes an object of concern, and all are thereby put on a good diet removing the hazards of malnutrition and of succumbing to other conditions.

Determination of Costs Created by an Intervention

Costs also may be divided into several categories, the nature of which are more or less apparent from what has been said about benefits.

Direct costs include those incurred in studying the proposed interventions, the research and development called for, tooling up for the intervention, delivering it, keeping records about it, evaluation, and finally, the overhead necessary to keep the intervention going. Direct costs for a service may be *explicit* (what one pays) and *implicit* (what else goes into obtaining it). Implicit costs to the consumer have been shown to be as much as 90% of the total costs borne in getting care.[3]

Indirect costs include such things as subsidized care—costs paid by others over and above payments made by the individual or the program which may not show up in direct expenditures. Hidden costs for medical care may be those of building medical schools and training physicians—costs which come out of funding generally unrelated to payment of doctor or hospital bills.

Unintended costs (externalities, spillovers, or secondary costs) include the price of any disruptions and consequent changeovers in other activities as a result of implementing an intervention. Other unintended effects of interventions may also result—allergic or toxic reactions to drugs, breakup of families, overpopulation. The measured consequences of these adverse effects of the intervention need to be put on the costs side of the ledger or kept under a separate heading of *disbenefits.* Also not to be forgotten is the price of conflicts with other goals (see foregone opportunity costs). Costs include such disbenefits as alienation of political support (because of hostility aroused or fears the intervention raises which may provoke people into various undesirable activities). These can even be converted into dollar costs by determining the nature of tradeoffs needed to make interventions acceptable.[4] Other kinds of unintended costs are created when an intervention preempts some particularly scarce commodity or personnel from other uses, with consequent harm. Where scarce manpower is a problem, we compare secondary losses (disbenefits or costs) and gains (benefits) resulting from: (1) tradeoffs between different levels of skills, some of which are much easier to create or procure than others; (2) substitutions of new technologies or innovative use of facilities for manpower; (3) tradeoffs between skills, communications or transportation—phones or helicopters to bring in patients, rather than locating a physician in an isolated area; (4) tradeoffs between education for self-help and traditional care; and (5) tradeoffs with other methods of organization for delivery.

Foregone opportunity costs. Interventions always use resources which could be used elsewhere to produce other desired outcomes. However, in multiple comparisons, these general phenomena need not be calculated. That is, such foregone opportunity costs apply to each and all of the interventions. They are often hard to separate from the areas of unintended costs just discussed.

Costs and benefits which are commonly not counted must also be reckoned.[5] Failure to do so may seem innocuous at this point in our thinking, but shortly it will be demonstrated that they play a critical role in making traditional dollar-counting cost-benefit analysis untenable as the major or sole determinant of desirability among competing alternatives. Two collections of varied studies and proposals are available for identifying costs and benefits in the well-being field.[6] An excellent and well documented typology of the possible areas of benefits or costs from just one intervention, housing, is available as a prototype application.[7] A similar purpose is served for health by a paper from Wiseman,[8] of the contributions of health to the economy by Fuchs,[9] and for education and productivity by Leveson.[10]

Measuring Costs and Benefits

Quantifiable Units

Costs (at least most direct and indirect costs) can be stated in terms of dollars required more easily than can benefits. But clearly costs can often be stated more simply in terms of illness, lives lost due to reactions, political power shifted or withdrawn, and so on. Benefits are particularly likely to be expressed in terms of lives saved, days of disability or lost work saved, days of discomfort saved, homes spared, as well as dollars saved when hospitalization or damage is avoided. Many conventions are in use for converting all costs and benefits to dollar terms.[11] (Most will be seen as dangerous to such population groups as housewives, infants, the aged, and to many ecological balances, and are unnecessary for our purposes at this time.)

Taking Cognizance of Time Streams of Costs and Benefits: Discounting

The distribution of a cost or benefit over time can be critical because costs may be high initially, may continue to rise or they may drop, while benefits from the same intervention may do the same or behave quite dissimilarly. In other words, it is difficult to compare the costs against the benefits for an intervention, particularly when the comparison involves multiple streams of costs or benefits which may continue over a period of more than a few years. Even for a given disease (for example, an active tuberculosis eradication program) each of the following customary objectives can be seen to have its own time stream of benefits although the costs of the overall program begin at inception and costs of the different subprograms continue to varying levels over varying spans of years.

Decreasing illness—occurs promptly, reaching a peak decline in a few years.

Decreasing deaths—begins in a few years and reaches a peak decline in a decade.

Decreasing hospital construction—occurs immediately unless a serious deficit requires an initial expenditure.

Decreasing hospital and clinic service—rises initially but begins to decline in a few years.

Maintaining family stability—begins significantly in a few years and continues from then on.

Assuring society and families that children will not get this disease—begins significantly in a few years and continues from then on.

Among these objectives are several ranges of costs and benefits. Some of these, which will not occur as a major benefit for a decade or more, may, however, give us immediate satisfaction as we contemplate a future free of tuberculosis for our children.

The comparison is even more complicated when different interventions—each having multiple sets of different cost and benefit time spans—are to be compared to determine which seems to promise the highest payoff. The diverse nature of costs and benefits alternatives alone makes very critical Hill's admonition to avoid lumping together the costs and benefits for more than one objective of an intervention or set of interventions.[12] Attention must be directed to the potential cost and gains for each objective, and some hard-to-quantify items may stand out as a result.

An economic convention has been devised for returning all dollar costs or benefits, no matter how long enduring, to present-day value.[13] This is done by discounting each year between the present one and the year in question, not unlike the discounting forced upon long-term bonds to establish a present-day sale price or worth. Of special concern is the discount rate to be applied per year. If it is established at 10%, we automatically prejudice the chance that any venture which has immediate costs and delayed returns will be very competitive. If we utilize a 2% discount rate in the same situation, it can be said that we are willing to have interventions, the costs of which will be borne in this generation and the benefits reaped in the next. Thus, discount rates can be, and are in fact, an expression of value judgments about present-versus future-oriented payoffs or about desires for benefiting this generation versus the next. As a result, multiple rates are often used in analysis—a low, a medium, and a high (for example, 2%, 6%, and 10%)—to show policy makers the effect of each rate on the priority ranking of alternative interventions. (Since the significance of these different discount rates is rarely discussed, the use of multiple rates often does little more than add to the confusion surrounding alternative choices.)

How do we discount the delayed time stream of benefits for an intervention which gives us major satisfaction now, just in anticipation? Must we always discount what we claim to want most for our futures and those of our children? If we do, our grandest and inevitably long-range ambitions will always be the ones that look the worst in any comparison of interventions.

For purposes of comparing health and well-being interventions I suggest abandoning use of discounting procedures. I prefer to utilize diagrams of cost and benefit streams. (If aggregating must be done, use a single lumping of costs and another for benefits for a given intervention in several time frames—for example, years 1 through 5; years 6 through 14; and years 15 through 30.) In this way, policy makers can see the relative time streams, free from the landmark-erasing effects of discounting practices. Discounting appears to substitute for, or provide, finite figures to represent such unknowns as our feelings about specific problems, our current satisfactions over reordering the future, the probable nature of the future and its new problems, the effects of inflation, the possibility of substitutes and new technologies, and the desires and ability of future policy makers to disentangle themselves from commitments now being made for them. Furthermore, a planned intervention usually is built to satisfy more than one real objective and several ideational objectives. Thus, each objective will intrude its own time span into the picture and might, given its nature, justifiably call for a different rate of discount. Moreover, if we want something to happen, even years from now, why discount it? We *want* it *now* even though it will act *then*. The price we pay now is indicative of how much we want what we want now.

To add to the unwisdom of discounting, there is evidence that it is done with more than one purpose in mind. Downs points up three major grounds for discounting: (1) future events are less certain and so require higher stakes (liquidity preference theory); (2) present enjoyment is better than contemplation of future enjoyment (time preference role theory); (3) interest return, by economic logic, adds to capital (marginal productivity theory). Downs also points out the difficulty that government should or does have in applying discount rates.[14]

We conclude that discounting seems unnecessary and even risky at this stage in the maturation of goal achievement, and even in solution of current problems. A display of the different costs and benefits time streams is preferred because it will be more informative while avoiding the issue of high versus low discount rates and the value judgments they impose in terms of current versus future payoffs.

Applications of Economic Principles to Health Policy Decisions

I have been both excited and concerned about the concept of deliberately and knowingly being able to discriminate between alternative choices of health interventions on a basis that could easily be explained and widely accepted.

Cost-Utility Type Applications

Current concepts of health can be traced to a good many historical roots. Clearly, one accepted measure of a healthy populace is its ability to work and produce to capacity, that is, to be free from disability (see Chapter 3). Concern to quantify such phenomena can be justified. With the tentative acceptance of the logic of economics to help carry out this quantitation, we have begun to titrate the costs of caring for ill health as well as the costs of losses suffered from disability or premature death. Thus, we ostensibly pave the way for comparing the actual worth of alternative methods of improving the health of people by comparing the losses prevented. Dorothy Rice's landmark work brought scattered theory together into a working basis, and clarified the major requisite assumptions about the costs of death and disability.[15] The real or long-range consequences of applying those assumptions were not particularly well explored. However, the immediate new health applications of this tool were widely perceived and utilized under the prod of President Johnson's[16] mandate to improve all Federal level decision-making by utilizing PPBS, which has as one of its cornerstones the cost-benefit approach to quantitation.[17]

Although the terms *cost-benefit* and *cost-effectiveness* are sometimes used interchangeably with the more generic term *cost-utility*,[18] and even with one another, it is important to observe the differences between then.

Cost-benefit analysis. Where we accept the dollar or monetary value as the dominant or single criterion by which to be guided in our choice of interventions, we use the cost-benefit approach. In essence, we compare required spending to tell us where and what to buy, and the dollar sets the direction of our concerns. In the dollar-guidance situation where we include gains or losses to productivity for health reasons, productivity (essentially, its effects on the GNP) outweighs other factors and becomes the key decision-making criterion.[19]

GNP, of course, inadvertently includes both the cost of what can be called the bad or destructive things we accomplish, such as production of liquor or cigarettes, as well as the cost of the creative or useful ones.[20] Nor does it tell us of the backlog of damage that may be building, such as the 45 million dollars required to clean up Lake Champlain as a result of the contributions to GNP produced privately by one paper company. In fact, when the contract is awarded, the cleanup of Lake Champlain will be recorded as a 45 million dollar contribution to the GNP.[21]

Even worse, cost-benefit analysis which takes into account productivity or the GNP carries the assumptions of the free market, that government should not want things that are unprofitable, redistribute wealth, give veterans preference, maintain minimum wages, try for desegregation, and so on. Moreover, this kind of logic ignores the possibility that income may be eating up capital or that production may cause pollution and thus be destroying natural resources. GNP, productivity and cost-benefits, via traditional economic logic, seem restricted to very short-run concerns;[22] while those of us who are interested in health, equity, and ecology are interested in conservation and building resources, which are long-run concerns.

Cost-effectiveness analysis. Where, as stressed in this text, decision-making guidance is accepted from many values other than the dollar or productivity, the high-ranking values determine the direction taken and the objectives wanted. Thus, we use the cost-effectiveness approach to determine how we can get the best buy for the predetermined objectives.[23] The cost-benefit *(c-b)* technique is assumed to be much more comprehensive than cost-effectiveness *(c-e)* if it is utilized to convert every relevant consequence of a proposed event into dollars brought to present value. In reality, only with the aid of many and far-from-agreed-upon artifices and conventions, can *c-b* barely manage the simpler value conversion into dollars, and it cannot easily be used to measure alienation, stress, social disruption, inequity and so on. The *c-e*, which at first glance seems the simpler, is begun by rating competing interventions against many preselected and specified and weighted criteria including *c-b*, productivity, and so on (Figure 6.1). These, in the aggregate, are the sense of direction which *c-b* really lacks for any given issue, unless dollars and productivity can be accepted in lieu of all other specific desires.[24] (The common failure to clear proposed action with held values as expressed by policies, and the substitution of dollar measurement, have created a record of cost-benefit disasters which has been commented on.[25])

The specific dollar-counting step of *c-e* technique may then be applied to the interventions which have passed high on the criteria screen to determine which is the best dollar buy. If *c-e* is regarded as the entire criteria-rating and dollar-counting procedure, it is infinitely more searching and meaningful than *c-b*. If one regards *c-e* as only the dollar counting stage, then it is obviously simpler than *c-b*. The latter step has major efficiency uses and by itself might also be entitled "efficiency analysis."[26] Unfortunately, most users of *c-e* are unaware of the need for the criteria-rating process with which the technique must begin if it is to have long-term social significance other than dollar savings.

An internationally based report of the cost-benefit analysis of social projects undertaken by the United Nations Research Institute for Development gives examples of techniques and applications and concentrates on the deficiencies of the tools at hand.[27]

Limitations and Fallacies of Applications of Cost-Benefit Logic in Health Policy Decisions

Samuelson states that "Economics is the study of how men and society end up choosing, with or without the use of money, to employ scarce productive resources which could have alternative uses to produce various commodities and distribute them for consumption, now or in the future, among various people and groups in society."[28]

Heilbronner,[29] in a more focused definition, posits that economics exists for the purpose of enabling us to comprehend better the structures and tendencies of the economic order, that is, the situations and activities that affect the production and distribution of wealth. In particular, this definition clarifies the role that the principles of economics can play in a systems type approach to any analysis undertaken for the purpose of designing and selecting optimum interventions. According to this position, economics should assist with those aspects of the design of interventions which either shift, add to, or subtract from the tangible wealth of the community or its individuals. However, this expression of wealth does not include all of our concerns for well-being or our concerns for future generations which, of course, are very much a part of decision making by individuals and by communities when they vote on how their customary dollar-measured wealth is to be spent. We can rest for the moment with the assumption that the economics techniques or dollar-measuring wealth criteria make up only one piece—albeit an important one—of our choice or decision-making criteria for selection of better interventions.

In the course of applying the present generally accepted economics designed cost-benefit technique, many high-payoff, health-saving schemes have been visualized; but they are apparently not socially or politically acceptable, for few moves have been made to implement them.[30] Have we encountered an unexpected irrationality? What we have carefully counted, assigned dollar value, and can prove to be a best buy is somehow not explainable or acceptable to the policy makers or, presumably, to the populace, although the proposals can be clearly demonstrated to each and every citizen as a good investment, leaving society with more money to do more of what else is wanted. In many proposals, the overall payoff may be so high that the injuries of the few who would suffer a disbenefit can even be compensated in dollars as is done routinely in real estate condemnation procedures. What then can be wrong with our logic when the golden rule of converting all illness and health into dollars and only buying what pays off best for most of us is not acceptable?

In the light of the guidance from Samuelson and particularly from Heilbronner, let us examine what economists have been led to do in their hurry to convert health into a dollar-based measured currency which, by their implied definition, must result in creation of goods with a marketable value. Figure 8.1 shows the costs and benefits that Richard Bailey describes as usually measured in evaluating health interventions. In Figure 8.2 Bailey shows the customary results of these practices and thereby brings into full focus the discord between economic or wealth-producing efficiency and societal equity or fairness.[31]

Health policy decision making is concerned with the proposition that significantly different methods or plans to achieve certain health objectives or alleviate specified problems involve expenditures of different kinds of resources over different time spans. Each plan offers, of course, the promise of benefits, such as achieving certain health or life-

FIGURE 8.1
COSTS AND BENEFITS THAT ARE TYPICALLY MEASURED
FOR HEALTH CONCERNS
(Modified from Bailey)

A. A number of factors are counted as output that should better be counted as inputs:
   1. Expenditures for hospital care are considered to be representative of the dollar value of the output of hospital services even though they might also be thought of as an input to the patient, which, combined with other things, enables him to recover from his illness.
   2. Physician's services are represented by measures of gross expenditures (payments) to physicians—no pay, no value; high pay, high value.
B. Given the conceptual base of the national income accounts, the following measures are adopted:
   1. The value of housewives' services are counted as zero (no market transaction or as the equivalent of a domestic worker).
   2. Working women are valued less than working men (earnings are lower).
   3. The elderly (past 65) have no economic value (not working).
   4. Youngsters contracting serious illnesses have negative economic value (long-range consumption costs exceed potential value as producers).
   5. The poorly educated are valued less than others; so also are Negroes and other minority groups whose lifetime earnings are typically below average.

---

saving outcomes. These benefits save or restore productivity which would otherwise have been lost, and limit the resources which would have to be used up to treat conditions which would otherwise worsen or continue uncontrolled. Since health has values to an individual beyond avoidance of expenditures for medical care or maintaining earnings, many schemes have been devised to give those other values a quantifiable marker as well—for example, Klarman's assignment of dollar values to "stigma" and "consumer benefit" in syphilis.[32] This ostensibly can lead to our ability, with careful adjudication and public value voting, to put a dollar price on all things we hold dear. We could thereby encompass political rationality within economic rationality, or at least apply familiar economic or dollar markers to help us measure the political factors which are not traditionally encompassed in economic calculations. A dollar value might be given to every aspect of costs[33] (excluding the private cost of the votes lost by a politician who favors a particular health care goal or methodology), and to every aspect of benefits, such as the worth of a spared healthy mother to her children. The issue of unintended consequences or externalities might be handled similarly—the desirable ones added to the benefits side, and the undesirable ones, or disbenefits, added to the cost side of the ledger. The conventions used to measure these may be followed or altered as experience develops.[34]

Following the above logic, political decision making need only compare alternative proposals to see which offers the highest present dollar-value of benefits per dollar of costs. Such constraints as how many dollars we can afford to spend altogether may, of course, rule out some very high payoff schemes which are simply too large. Is this approach feasible? Can all desires and values be given a dollar price tag? Can all parties who expect to feel a gain or loss be identified and their gain and loss assigned a dollar value commensurate with the intensity and extent of their concern? Can planners prepare an overall cost-benefit dollar appraisal as they prepare packages of alternative interventions for action by policy makers? We doubt it for many reasons, some of which strongly violate widely held, health-related values. (Review Figure 8.2.)

Because, for economists, the dollar value of a life is best equated with its potential in terms of production, the loss of production due to

FIGURE 8.2
IMPLICATIONS OF USING COSTS AND BENEFITS
AS SHOWN IN FIGURE 8.1
(Modified from Bailey)

1. To direct even more health resources to the care of those who are best able to pay for the services.
2. To reduce the quantity of government health services made available to the elderly, minority groups, incapacitated youngsters, etc.
3. To shift further from the poor to the affluent the already recognized maldistribution of health resources and accept market forces as being permanent—those persons who value health highly and can pay for health services get them; those who either do not value health highly or cannot pay for health services are denied access.
4. Allocations of public funds altered to:
   a. favor the young over the old
   b. favor service (short-range) versus research (too much uncertainty about long-range value of research output)
   c. favor the educated over the uneducated
   d. favor the rich over the poor
   e. encourage treatment of acute illness and downgrade concern over chronic illness
   f. stress preventive care for some age groups; disregard it for others
   g. provide more funds for high income states and local areas; deny funds to the less affluent
   h. encourage more private health outlays; reduce the share of total health expenditures made by government.

premature death or disability is easily converted into a dollar loss. However, putting benefits into dollar terms is not always a happy maneuver in health planning. For example, because the aged have little potential for significant production, programs directed toward saving or prolonging the lives of the elderly would show low dollar-benefits. In fact, the total or per capita years of life saved for this group might also be small in comparison to other age groups. Moreover, the years of life saved might be spent in a hospital bed or in a nursing home at a high dollar cost compared to the limited costs for care that would have resulted had there been no intervention and a speedy death.

Measuring the dollar value of a program for the elderly is similar to measuring the dollar value of a birth control program which prevents potentially valuable lives from coming into existence.

If every life is to be given a value depending on age, sex, race, education, and earning capacity, a comparison of cost-benefit ratios would force us to accept a preponderance of programs which serve the young adult, white, college male because he has the highest and quickest expected earnings for the longest period of time.

From these examples it becomes apparent that the cost benefit formulations may easily be carried to *reductio ad absurdum* in the field of health, where humane values are still important and the retarded and infirm are not to be starved to death or "liberated" from this world.

Desirable as quantifying process is, it does depend on a cost-benefit logic which has further problems:

Opportunities abound to make situations appear as better measured or more measurable than they are.

Many unverifiable assumptions are made about what the inputs really had to do with the outputs.

Real gains are often guesses. As a matter of fact, not only do all "saved" victims not become well, but many remain high-cost nursing home or hospital casualties. As Sanders has shown, current prolongations of life are bound later to result in increasing general levels of chronic and costly disability.[35]

Attainments will never reasonably be measurable in dollars; the actual value of a mother to the needs of a child or the increased happiness of a family when an ailing child recovers must be described in vague and highly value-laden terms.

Externalities, spillovers, or secondary effects can never be adequately judged. For example, current analysis from the health field reports needs for 100% more radiologists, 200% more general practitioners, 50% more nurses, and so on. The solution to the problem of medical manpower shortages is presented as relatively simple—at least another 50 large medical schools are needed, or the output of present schools should be doubled.

Designers of interventions proposed on the basis of such projections will find it hard to consider the future implications of such an approach. Academia would be strained beyond sensible limits to support this number of schools, and would have to withdraw a disproportionate number of the better practitioners from practice to carry the teaching load. In fact, the scramble to produce new doctors would probably also divert attention from the evidence already mentioned, that expensive physician skills are poorly utilized now.

Secondary benefits accruing from the alternative approach of substituting health personnel at lower levels of skill for physicians are not insignificant either. The projected approximately million-man vacancies in health manpower cited at every manpower conference could probably be filled from the bottom of the ladder by the unskilled who need jobs, resulting in a real secondary economic and social good for the country. Obviously, costs and benefits of programs to society at large will not always be synonymous with the distribution of costs or benefits to various groups of individuals. In some instances, some pay and also gain; in others, those who pay may not be those who gain. Questions of equity and concerns for future generations must also enter into the choice between alternative courses of action.

Let us look at the major reasons that the cost-benefit has been so misleading and unusable. Because in this methodology all direct resources used and all easily measured economic changes induced by a proposal are converted into dollars, a serious slip in logic was allowed to operate in applications to the health field. It was carelessly assumed that because a handful of more prosaic satisfactions and values about resources had been converted into one common currency, *all values* were thereby included, and therefore, any number of proposals could be compared in terms of the amount they would cost and how much they would benefit. This process was mistakenly considered analogous with how an economically rational individual decides whether his next $25 should be spent for a trip, a medical checkup, or a bicycle for his child. In reality, not all of us have the same set of options (a confusing side issue, for some must clearly limit themselves to paying taxes and buying food and transportation to and from work). And, more fundamentally, none of us regularly does what traditional cost-benefit always tried to do, that is, decide which plan or procedure will produce the most *resources or wealth.* Neither the affluent man who seeks to spend $25 for an amenity nor the more restricted spender who must procure necessities is evidently thinking in terms of how his $25 will give him the most *wealth,* or of things equatable with wealth; each usually thinks in terms of which expenditures will provide him with the most *satisfaction* among his many values.

Clearly one should not be taken in by the non-sequitur that since traditional cost-benefit converts a handful of outcomes into dollars in a collective framework emphasizing marketable productivity, it should follow that this process is identical or even similar to how individuals behave as they compare the purposes served and the satisfactions produced by their expenditures. If society is to be asked to make decisions as individuals do, the basis for choice will not be what the next expenditure will do for *collective wealth* but rather what it will harvest in the way of *collective satisfactions*—what people would be willing to pay for something would be a better measure of worth than what that something produces.

Useful Lessons from Economics: What's "Right" about Cost-Utility Type Thinking

The logic of measuring and comparing the net gains in satisfactions to be derived from alternative proposals in terms of how much more or less they cost (losses or dissatisfactions) and how much more or less they benefit (gains or satisfactions) is good. But the counting and weighing implicit in cost-benefit analysis must be extended to the other pertinent values, and not restricted or converted to gains in wealth, as has been done in the past. Aggregating these countings and weighings for comparison purposes is, of course, not easy in a pluralistic, modern society with many operant value hierarchies.

Wildavsky's comment, "economic rationality, however laudable in its own sphere, ought not swallow up political rationality . . ."[36] deserves specific amplification, which can, perhaps, best be done by first pointing up what economic rationality has to offer. Because economics has a firmer, quantifying base of tangibility and practice than most other decision-making devices, I believe that using it as a prototype will help establish an orderly and quantifying way of thinking about measuring criteria other than wealth-creating or distributing types. Economics has learned how to relate both the input and output of a given intervention so that different interventions can be compared for cost (wealth-abstracting and redistributing) and benefit (wealth-creating and redistributing) factors. Economics has also offered a good concept, but a limited method, for dealing with the differing lengths of time over which a stream of costs or a stream of benefits is operant and how these can be expressed in present-day values (discounting), so that wealth-altering comparisons between interventions can be made more meaningful. It has further developed highly sophisticated means with which to determine the effects of further enlarging any existing or proposed activity in terms of changing the unit cost of production or the probable return from each new unit produced (marginal analysis).

Economics has even made us widely aware, although with much less rigorous methodology, of how wealth can be created unintentionally by new tangible byproducts known as technological spillovers, or by newly produced paper wealth (pecuniary spillovers) which involve not creation of any new products but just enhancement of the market values of old ones as a result of unleashing other forces, such as proximity. Economics has taught us how subtle and yet how gross can be the shifts of wealth from one group to another or from one community to another—unintentional but often overwhelming by-products of intended and desired changes induced by some monetary or fiscal policies, technological shifts, extension of certain markets, growth in the national product, and so on.

We know what these changes have done to the wealth of various sectors of our economy, such as the farmed-out farmers, the mined-out miners, and now the aired-out aerospacers. Moreover, economists are helping us understand that the non-economic or non-wealth-producing aspects of these same policies may be of even greater importance in the long-run. They are pointing out that the dream of a 5%-10% annual real or inflation-free growth in the national product of our country (and as is often stated, hopefully for every other country in the world) has further disadvantaged most of the countries exporting a handful of natural resources. If this maintained rate of growth were really achieved, we would, moreover, probably be shortly confronted by a total ecologic holocaust, which we are now beginning to accept as a future reality.[37]

Economics has given us the intellectual weapons as well as the precedent to understand the wealth-depriving, the wealth-creating, and the wealth-distributing effects of social, political, technologic, and economic moves. It has also been useful in examining democracy and political power (Downs[38] and Ilchman and Uphoff[39]). The writings of Lee and Dyckman,[40] Netzer[41] and Keyserling[42] exemplify the utility and significance of the economics approach to examining situations. We have also learned that using only criteria based on creating and distributing wealth will not be enough to guide us safely. The inequities of creating Appalachias, the follies of locally produced ecological imbalance and the threat of impending, large-scale ecologic disaster are all evidence of the danger and inadequacy of growth patterns based on analyses limited to concerns of traditional economics or production of wealth.

Nonetheless, we believe that the quantifying logic underlying the techniques developed for purposes of economic analysis is valid if applied to the other major areas of man's concerns as well as to wealth, for that logic brings measuring tools to value areas long neglected, such as ecology, future generations, equity, and esthetics.

Returning to Heilbronner,[43] we can say with him that economics finds its applications to social reality by constructing algebraic or geometric analogues of social situations that help to explain and thus forecast social actions. Because this is done by limiting concern to the aspects of the social process which can now be quantified, primarily two kinds of social behavior have been highlighted: the phenomenon of supply and demand, and maximizing subject to constraint (marginality). These are valuable predictors, but they are not by themselves sufficient in various important circumstances: times of stress, such as severe illness; new situations, such as ecological disasters; and violations of other major values, such as equity. In fact, economics notwithstanding, we still do not know why what is going on is going on at any one moment, nor can we be sure of predictions based solely on the postulations made by economics.

However, let me attempt to introduce the logic from economics to the wider world of reality so as to extend our ability to be rational, our capacity to analyze and to predict. I will therefore use economic type thinking to help define desired goals, and particularly in the weighting and rating of the many criteria to be applied to possible interventions, rather than using it solely as a tool for the measurement and prediction of the dollar-measurable wealth that alternative interventions promise. Other very specific wealth distribution uses to which economic rationality can be put to improve equity as well as efficiency are summed up in Figure 8.3, adapted from Bailey.[44]

FIGURE 8.3
NECESSARY DESCRIPTORS OF THE BENEFITS
AND COSTS OF HEALTH SERVICES
(After Bailey)

1. Benefits
   a. What are the *forms* of benefits?
   b. What are the *magnitudes* of these benefits?
   c. *Which groups* of people receive the benefits? How much is received by the person being treated? How much is returned to government through increased taxes?
   d. Over what *time periods* are the benefits received?
   e. Do the benefits vary by the type of service that is provided?
2. *Costs*
   a. What are the *forms* or types of costs? Magnitudes?
   b. How are the costs *shared*, as between: the individual or family and taxpayers? income-classes of taxpayers? taxpayers at various governmental levels?
3. *Balance Between Benefits and Costs*
   a. Are the groups that receive the benefits of health services the same as those that bear the costs?
   b. Are there substantial numbers of persons who receive benefits but do not bear costs?
   c. Are there others who share the costs but receive little, if any, of the benefits?

Bailey[45] has also suggested that applying economic tenets may offer insights into other distinctions of importance to the health sector.

Private effects or social effects?   Economists call the effects on people other than the patient, external, social, or public, in contrast with the internal or private effects on the individuals receiving the care. The existence of external or social effects from health services is important because it raises the question of what proportion of the cost of health services should be borne by the individual and what proportion by the government. Perhaps, if the returns in the form of increased income to the individual are large, all of the costs of certain health services should somehow be borne by the individual. In other cases, where health services benefit society at large, in addition to the individual, perhaps provision of services should be supported in part by public funds. Rehabilitation of an accident victim can have important public and private benefits, in fact, the argument of potential returns to the government in taxes was used for many years to sell the vocational rehabilitation program in the United States. Udry and Morris also make very clear that activities which may have great value for society may hardly be worthwhile for individuals to pursue, given the small probability of personal risk.[46] Government use of both incentives and sanctions may be justifiable in such cases, and it may be necessary to increase the cost of individual nonparticipation now, instead of merely flaunting the threat of an increased cost later.

Should benefits accrue to the government jurisdiction footing the bill?   The out-migration of an individual who has received state-provided services involves a geographical relocation of the increase in tax base represented by his increased income resulting from his increased well-being—a relocation that removes the tax base from the original providing state in favor of some other jurisdiction. The attempt to equate the cost with the gain would point to national investment over state, and state investment over local. A case in point is the training of health professionals. Perhaps this training should be supported by national investment, because there is no way to guarantee where in the country manpower will serve.

Explicit money costs versus implicit costs.   A cost should be interpreted as something given up. The price of the health service itself is the explicit money cost. To obtain the health service, an expenditure of considerable time and effort may also be necessary. Time away from work may result in loss of income, and travel costs may be involved. These implicit costs may often be greater than the explicit costs. Thus, a person at the shaky edge of solvency may not be able to afford "free" service and may be regarded as incompetent or indifferent when, in fact, he is using good economic judgment by staying away from care.

Who foots the bills and how big will they be?   All money and other costs must be met somehow. Some are borne directly by the individual, others by philanthropy, others through insurance or governmental budgets. The source from which the money is paid out can be expected to influence the demand, and thus the cost, for health services. The cost for health services will, in turn, affect the total money cost of the health care system. An example is hospital insurance and the consequent increasing use of hospital facilities for tests and conditions that might be treated on an ambulatory basis. Obviously the method of financing and the total amount to be financed are inseparable.

Are health services investments or consumer goods?   To consider the effects of health services as income-generating implies a view of these services as an investment from which monetary returns are expected to flow; to consider them as consumer goods implies that we buy goods because we like them, not just because they will help us to raise our incomes. Consumer-type benefits from health services, like increased enjoyment of life, are particularly difficult to measure, but their relevance should not be dismissed. In earlier health planning experience, under the prodding of George Keranen, we came to feel that selection among alternative interventions according to the higher dollar payoff ratio under current cost-benefit analyses was only one way to go, and that priorities might better be set by asking people what they would be willing to pay to reduce the risk from particular conditions.[47] We have since observed that Prest and Turvey ask the same question, but do not try to answer it.[48] Klarman attempts to answer part of it in his consideration of "consumer benefit."[49]

Could such a new process help us out of the dilemma in which some people want their tax dollars to go to the aged, while others want those dollars to go to the poor, to law and order, to the educational sector, or to the health sector? Apparently, until the needs of an individual's priority area appear reasonably satisfied, no amount of traditional cost-benefit demonstrations can sway his priority-setting machinery. If this is true, then the present system of voting and lobbying (the political market place) is more direct and relevant to the allocation of resources according to a majority expression of preferences (or values) than dollar measuring cost-benefit technology. C-b would seem safe and useful only for choosing among methods which produce identical objectives and, primarily, only after all major decisions have been made about whether our money is going for such diverse things as war, moon shots, education, or health. Even within the health sector, our general value system decides whether resources should be used to alleviate the miseries of the aged, lead poisoning of the young, and so on.

In 1969 an article by Vincent Taylor[50] made clarifying inroads into the nature of the dilemma posed by the unacceptability of applying *c-b* logic in collective, major health policy decision making. He came up with a firm proposal that we should collectively do what individuals actually do—decide what we want most and pay for it to the point that our wants for other things will tolerate.

In conclusion, I am willing—in fact, I encourage planners—to utilize the economics type thinking that lies behind cost-benefit analysis. However, this position is built on the premise that this thinking be applied, as a rough counting method, to the losses and gains predicted from the impingement of each alternative proposal on each of the values selected to be used as judging criteria (Figure 6-1). A much more complex, multiple set of comparisons or ratios will result, but the utility of cost-benefit thinking should thereby be greatly enhanced. The customarily ignored transfer payments, such as welfare support, may now have to be weighed, because taxes are not only in disfavor but can never be applied in a non-discriminatory way. Discounting for measures that will ultimately protect our children may have to be abandoned or balanced against our satisfactions at knowing that our children will be safeguarded. Productivity as a clue to investment of health dollars will be weighed against the satisfaction of aiding the helpless, or more importantly, the satisfactions of those who are aided.

SELECTION OF INTERVENTIONS (SOLUTIONS) TO OVERCOME CAUSES AND CONSEQUENCES OF PROBLEMS OR TO ENABLE GOAL ATTAINMENT

A reasonable level of analysis of a single problem or desired goal leads to the development of many possible interventions. Interventions or packages of interventions to be used against a problem or to produce a goal need to be rank ordered so that the best can be selected for implementation. A process of choosing priority criteria and assigning weighting to each seems to be one of the simplest means by which a planning council can decide which interventions are best. This process is discussed fully in Chapter 6.

Comparison and Selection of Interventions

In addition to use of the more specific type of criteria shown in Figure 6.1, several rather generalized considerations deserve elaboration in the attempt to compare and select interventions:

The best price in terms of social and political acceptance. Many technically superb interventions run afoul of the values or mores of religious, social, cultural, or other subgroups. These interests may block adoption of the intervention or become alienated from the larger society or from its elected policy makers if the intervention is adopted. Policy makers can be presumed to prefer second or lower rated interventions which arouse no storms and make more friends than enemies. The fact that all policy makers do not follow such practices is evident in the current political history at all legislative levels.

Feasibility and acceptability.   Although the intent or the principle of the intervention may be acceptable, one of the specific techniques called for may involve questions of feasibility or acceptability. If annual, free sigmoidoscopy for all adults were possible and was determined to be worth the cost, the procedure still might not be acceptable. Any intervention based on use of this technique might attract only 50% of the population-at-risk. Ninety percent of the same population might very well tolerate some other appropriate procedure even if sigmoidoscopy were 99% effective for the purpose intended, and the alternative technique only 80% effective.

The best price in terms of a particularly scarce commodity.   An intervention which overall may be only modestly effective may still be rated best because it is the only one which makes minimal demands on an especially scarce element, such as one kind of highly trained personnel. Obviously, the rating of the proposal would change if the bottleneck to the scarce resource were overcome.

The "biggest bang for the buck."   Estimates of the costs and benefits involved as a result of Federal expenditures are illustrated by examples of cost-benefit applications to health services available in a series of DHEW publications.[51] The costs and benefits anticipated from each intervention e given at least a ball-park figure by people experienced in the field. To determine the costs or inputs required for each benefit obtained, several factors need to be considered. The total direct cost of the proposed intervention can usually be adequately estimated. However, if a particular measure can be put into effect at a presumed cost of so many dollars per capita, the proportion of the clients who can be involved and the proportion who can be effectively aided must also be determined. The true cost figure for the results achieved may be quite different from the initial cost figures estimated for the program. For example, if skin testing is to be done in a tuberculosis control program, perhaps only 90% of a given population can be reached by the promotion campaign, but the remaining 10% may have as much disease as the 90% tested. The test is only 95% accurate. Probably about 90% of those tested will return for a reading, and only 50% of the identified positives will agree to go on drug therapy. Perhaps only half of those beginning treatment will finish it, and the treatment is only 90% effective for those completing therapy. A thoroughgoing example of how to examine costs is now available.[52]

Issues of equity.   Sometimes an otherwise excellent intervention may require a large sacrifice from a few so that all the rest of society can benefit. Sometimes all of society must contribute so that a few benefit. Every intervention must be studied in terms of which individuals pay what share of costs, and which individuals receive what share of benefits. At the same time, the costs and benefits of an intervention to specifiable individuals or classes of individuals must be compared to the costs or benefits which accrue to the society overall.

The personal and societal costs and gains need to be shown so that policy makers can choose wisely. Will they prefer individually equitable interventions, those with overall societal gains of a very substantial nature, or those that avoid significant losses to certain classes of individuals? Will they be concerned with reimbursing individuals who are hurt by an otherwise societally profitable intervention, for example, the taking of private land for rapid transit? Will they try to recapture incidental high individual gains when these occur—such as the increased private land value which results from a public investment in transportation?

Freedom from worry. The capacity of an intervention to reduce tensions or relieve great buildups of anxiety is important, irrespective of other values. Some actions may strike at nagging fears of indecisiveness in a way that frees everyone from such a burden even though the intervention may not be much of a remedy for the basic problem.

Selection among interventions directed at one problem or goal. The comparative net worth of various interventions against a specific problem has substantially been laid out by rating each intervention against four batteries of weighted criteria. Unfortunately mathematical manipulation of these ratings does not give four comparative numbers which in turn could give an overall priority standing of each intervention studied. What the priority-setting process will do is provide understanding and guidance to the planning board and, through them, to the public and policy makers about which criteria are really being met and at what levels, and the source of the overall balance in favor of or against each intervention. Numerical priority levels should provide sufficient guidance for choice among mechanical interventions which achieve identical objectives. Manifestly, priority numbers alone will not be the deciding force between two interventions which produce equally valuable results at comparable prices for a given condition if one intervention favors children and another favors the aged.

Allocations among already favored "good" interventions which are directed at different health problems or goals. Interventions selected as best for one problem or goal often may have to be compared with selected best interventions for other problems or goals when they compete for similar interests and scarce resources. Comparisons need to be made between the value of priority interventions applied to tuberculosis, for example, as against lung cancer, to see if intervention investments would do more good (provide more benefits per dollar) against one lung condition than another. Again, purely dollar-measured priorities will rarely suffice, for many programs are directed to the aged, the retarded, the chronically ill and are often "losers" in dollar terms when compared with those which save more prime or productive years of life (particularly if productivity is included among the benefits of an intervention). Yet, cancer and tuberculosis each attract extensive program support from different groups which policy makers cannot ignore.

Once a problem or intervention has aroused public concern, it is not easily neglected even if more benefits can be expected from tackling other interventions. The four batteries of priority-setting criteria which reveal the weak and strong points of each intervention should theoretically be a more suitable source of guidance than public pressure. The averaged significance levels may not turn the tides, but rating interventions against the various criteria should provide information which will assist public and policy maker alike to face decisions about how and where to invest. When the public remains adamant in favor of a low-rated proposal, the planning body must acknowledge the value priorities actually held, even if they are different from what the planning body's weighted criteria would suggest.

Allocations among various sectors.   Comparisons need to be made of societal benefits that might be accomplished in sectors other than health or well-being—economic production, national defense—by dipping into the pool of dollars now reserved for health interventions, or vice versa. Experience indicates, however, that comparisons among sectors based on costs or gains may be less than relevant. This is pointed up by the simultaneous wars on the Viet Cong and on domestic poverty.

Selection of allocations for different purposes.   Listing potential interventions can also spot where research is needed. Potentially desirable interventions may hinge on technologies which are only conjured up at the time of planning. If new technologies seem feasible, or if they are now at work in other areas, research is indicated even though the extent of applicability in the new situation is not certain. Research is also indicated when the proposed intervention suggests the desirability of a totally new approach, such as immunization against a parasitic disease for which immunization has never been tried, or an economic incentive to get something into production that is ordinarily not available. In other words, postulating new interventions usually suggests priorities for areas of research that offer hopes of a high payoff. Presently, applied health research is often undertaken solely for the researcher's "kicks," and may or may not be directed to areas with hope of payoff. It may be directed, for example, to areas where interventions are already effective and where the payoff cannot be significantly improved. On the other hand, at another point in the same disease system or in another disease system, organized research might be the key to a totally new effective approach. Thus, setting priorities for research, supposedly a very formidable task, is one of the benefits of careful consideration of interventions that might be applied to a systems model of a problem or a goal.

Political advantages of interventions directed at precursors in disease or disorder kinds of problems. Attempting to correct recognized defects or their consequences with anything less than 100% application entails withholding care from individuals or groups and, therefore, the making of intolerable "God-like" decisions of who will and who will not be spared suffering, expense, or death. On the other hand, efforts directed at prevention of defects which require a test, an injection, or a diet, for potential victims may avoid the selected-neglect issues. Where the condition to be prevented comes predominantly from a definable high-risk group, no great concern is likely to be aroused among those at lesser risk if they are not served in order to keep the cost reasonable. That is, the low-risk persons do not feel shortchanged; they may even be happy to avoid some procedure or habit change. But once the same condition has been allowed to develop to the point where someone is victimized, then individuals, families, lobbies or associations will come forward who are unwilling to let others decide who is "too hard to find," "too expensive to care for," "too far gone" to be helped or "too useless" to be worth the investment. Often the political hazards of choosing who is to be served can be reduced by intervening at the less manifest levels or at the precursors of problems.

Comparison and Selection of Projects for Approval or Funding

Closely related to the selection of interventions is the planning body's review of projects prepared elsewhere for approval or for actual award of monies. Such projects also need to be rank ordered so that the most useful ones can be approved, the less useful delayed or discouraged, and the undesirable ones disapproved. The priority criteria chosen are the means of deciding which project is most useful. Two initial or special criteria seem indicated for projects of any kind, and proposals which rate poorly on these criteria should be sent back to their sponsors for clarification.

One such criterion is the definition and scope of the goal or problem that the project is proposing to attack. If, as is not uncommon, no goal or problem is really elaborated, or many problems are muddled together or implied in the course of projecting a "happy" solution, the project should be sent back for clarification because it may be intuitively sound and merely need more explicit thinking. The reasons for this prime criterion are simple enough. Solutions for unstated problems are not likely to solve anything.

The second criterion which a project should pass initially requires that the proposed intervention must give some evidence that other solutions and other points of intervening were considered and that the proposed attack or solution is likely to be one of the better ones.

Projects are typically of three kinds: (1) goal or problem analysis; (2) interventions or solutions; and (3) combination proposals. For combination projects which propose both to investigate a goal or problem *and* to apply a solution, it is suggested that a ranking be made on the goal or problem first. Only if it holds merit as a goal or problem should a separate rating then be made on the solution. If either portion ranks poorly, a combination project would seem doomed.

A point made in Chapter 6 should be reiterated here. Use of criteria, weights, and ratings does not substitute for judgment. The choice of criteria and the weighting and rating processes helps inform those who do the judging, provides an opportunity to include minority values in a decision-making process, demonstrates to planners (and eventually to the community) the complexities of the value systems operating in a given community, and points out possible ways of reconciling differences. Comparison of priority setting results with what all planning body members "know," may also force reconsideration of previous choices of criteria, and weightings that are clearly out of touch with community reality.

DESIGN AND EVALUATION OF INTERVENTIONS PROPOSED FOR HEALTH CARE DELIVERY SYSTEMS: AN EXAMPLE OF GOAL-ORIENTED DESIGN

To illustrate the design of a goal directed intervention, I will again use the example of a health care delivery system. I will postulate an endpoint of "good care for all" and will use the goal-achievement approach rather than the patch-up or problem-solving posture.

Normative Design of Health Care Delivery Systems

In view of the relative importance of the major inputs to health as shown in Figure 1.1 inadequate health care resources and their maldistribution are more a matter of equity than of realizable major improvement in the community's health. Many apparently poorly medical care serviced communities permit a comparatively long and healthy life because of the salubrious nature of their environment and, in fact, may not require additional care services for medical reasons.

Nevertheless, medical care concerns are among the most pursued of our national goals and may not be relegated to a back seat. Present hurts cry out for immediate attention. Persistent, gross inequities in the quality and quantity of available care have galvanized the nation into massive efforts to right injustices, even though little can be promised in the way of improved levels of health and much in the way of higher costs. For the short run, planning equitable delivery deserves top priority; for the long run, efforts must be concentrated particularly on study and interventions in disease and social systems, if health status is to be improved and the unnecessary burden of ill health and consequent demands for health care and its costs are to be lifted from our people.

Conversion of the Goal Analysis into the Design Criteria

The approach to designing, evaluating, and comparing the interventions designed to improve health care delivery began by analyzing the goals and indicating the systems which can deliver them (Chapter 7). This portrayal is built on the conceptual framework of the present modes of delivery and ignores competing modes, such as a computerized or highly technologic one, the counter culture's use of diet, meditation, mysticism and the occult, and other do-it-yourself "anti-scientific" schemata. Analysis of the encompassing delivery system is followed by an analysis of the major elements or forces (subsystems) which make it function. The subsystems are broken down into major attributes, and the requirements of each of these are listed. The series of Figures 7.3-7.12, which show how these analytic steps are used for design purposes, are addressed in order. From this analytic beginning, an ideal-oriented system is projected, and the performance-type criteria developed permit freedom to design many suitable, community-specific service delivery systems.

The more indigenously and ingeniously such health care systems are designed to accommodate local needs and utilize local strengths or resources, the better and less expensive we would hope them to be. Success is not to be measured by uniformity and conformance to a given configuration, but by ability to provide health care that reaches or exceeds the performance criteria established. Safeguards are equally necessary in the organizational aspects, such as requirements for specific kinds of participation, evaluation, controls, and so on, for without these the desired delivery cannot be promised. Again, neither the details nor their specific nature is spelled out. The initial critical element is the intent and the direction of the forces acting in and on the delivery system. Those forces must create an organization capable of delivering a product which meets performance specifications.

Since the basic ingredients of a care delivery schema remain on the whole the same anywhere, it seemed wisest to begin with a portrayal of the system and its modest contribution to health (see Figure 7.3). The general criteria of what constitutes good care were then spelled out in relation to each aspect of the delivery system. Because good health care is made up of good consumers and good health services, attributes and descriptors were provided which describe how consumers and health services are to be made good. Similarly, attributes of goodness were spelled out for organization, manpower, technology, facilities, and financing in Figures 7.4-7.10. Every piece of the paradigm was fitted out with the major descriptors or minimum criteria that a good solution must meet. In this way the entire theoretic framework was fleshed out for the key parts of the delivery system, including its organization. Because we expect that goodness for any one community can only be attained and maintained by intelligently and diligently applied planning and control agencies, we also suggested the need for and provided examples of criteria to guide the outputs of control, planning, and overall health decision-making machinery that helps shape the delivery system and watches over it to guarantee to the community a suitable level of care (Figures 7.11 and 7.12).

It is obviously not our intent to describe the *definitive* list of criteria needed to create ideal delivery, control, or planning systems. What has been presented is a possible list. Each planning authority or body, at least those at the state level, would create such a list. If there were any national source of guidance, it would provide a basic list of design criteria.

Operational versus Idealized Designs

Whatever delivery machinery is set up to intervene and achieve our care objectives must begin its work now, but the full attainment of its objectives may be scheduled for many years away, given the difficulties of financing, training, building, organizing and consumer orientation. Because phasing is at the heart of planning, there must be milestones of measurable tangible objectives along the way to the ultimate goals.

However, before we resolve these practicalities, we have to decide not only on the time rate of achievement but the level of achievement we really are planning for. Nadler[53] uses a set of targets for interventions which suits our purposes:

A *theoretical ideal* system based on the assumption that everything that we design can be made to work perfectly.

An *ultimate ideal* system which reflects our belief about what we can ultimately best possibly attain.

A *feasible ideal* system which represents specifically what we are targeting for and can attain at a specific set of points along the road.

It is from this latter target then that we select our intermediary objective achievement points.

The actual design. In order to determine achievable as well as desirable goals, the planning body will have to convert its design criteria into operating policy with the assistance of those called upon to deliver, as well as those awaiting delivery. This is the current operating policy—the output or the plan of the planning body. This operating policy must call for a meshing of short-run problem-solving schedules and long-run goal-achievement deadlines. In essence it must:

—Coordinate alleviation of hurts with overall goal attainment by: (1) assuring that the interim steps taken to achieve goals will also alleviate the problems selected for remedy or at least not worsen them; (2) assuring that the steps taken to achieve immediate or lesser objectives will not interfere or delay the master goal strategy.

—Indicate what the Health Care Delivery (HCD) systems must put into their schemes *now* to assure that the desired output will come to pass.

—Indicate *how* the HCD systems must get started to ensure that the outputs desired will come about. This is the most crucial step after the major design criteria. What the HCD system starts doing will in great measure determine what it ends up doing.

An example of this step might be how to handle the problem of "care for all. "The envisioned national financing for care of the poor is not likely to emerge, let us say, until 1976. The attribute of "Eligibility and Financial Coverage" shown in Figure 7.4 demands coverage for "all" from any system being designed in the years prior to that. We know that the delivery system cannot serve the poor until money is made available in their behalf. Yet, if a system is allowed to set up to serve only those with coverage presently, will it ever direct itself to also serving the poor when that becomes feasible?

A set of design criteria that could be built into the planning body's current operational plan to handle that future situation might be as follows:

—The HCD for a community must now show how its current plans can be extended to serve at least the same proportion of the presently poor and underserved as exists in the community, for example, 30%.

—The HCD must now begin negotiations with representatives of the groups of poor that it plans to serve.

—The HCD must now put on its governing board among the consumers the same 30% of the representatives of those unable to pay or to be served now but who will be served by the system as soon as money is made available. That is, if the community has 30% poor unable to buy in, the HCD board must now include among its consumer members 30% representatives of groups of poor with which it is now negotiating and who will be served when the monies in their behalf become available.

These are samples of current policy or design criteria which tell *how* the machinery is to be organized *now* so that *later* desired eventualities are most likely to occur. In each area of design where there are to be more fully developed later outcomes, the final outcomes must be planned for now, and guiding channels must be built into the paths the delivery organizations are to take between now and then. This does not preclude the entry of changes in goals or functions as soon as planners discover the need for such.

Making Comparisons among Proposed Health Care Measures

Comparisons among proposed schemes can be made by applying the same criteria which have been proposed as guides for the design of ideal systems. The attributes and criteria of good health care systems presented in Figures 7.4-7.12 can be the basis for a critical list of essential features against which all proposals can be checked or rated. Other elements or criteria have been suggested by Burns[54] and Somers[55]. These include: (1) evidence of specific health outcomes; (2) the effects on such key concerns as cost control and quality control; (3) consequences beyond health care, as on the economy, or inflation, and on political practices and precedents; or (4) a combination of goals such as administrative simplicity, general acceptability to providers and consumers, and pluralistic and regulated competition. Burns, for example, points out what the significance of full coverage is likely to be under a voluntary scheme. She also discusses the effects of including capital outlay for facilities as part of the overall health care scheme. She regards its inclusion as probably an unfortunate and splintering attribute. While we appreciate her point, we tend to feel that its visibility and relatedness to the whole system of health care would be enhanced by its inclusion, and that this outweighs the disadvantages of its being included. Somers makes the point that forcing the inclusion of financing, as well as the system of distribution, makes a measure politically hard-to-pass, and thus blocks legislative action. Such a bill would be poorly rated in terms of political feasibility.

A second mode of comparing or evaluating health care proposals lists comparatively the various major specific methods, services, recipients and so on which each plan covers.[56]

Evaluative judgment requires the use of many elements of comparison. As a minimum, we need both methods, the comparative statement of the provisions of bills and a digest of their probable consequences. Because the predicted consequences are the critical long-range issues, it is unfortunate that they must represent personal judgment rather than a statement of fact. A technician might prepare the list of a bill's provisions, but a table of consequences should be the considered work of a large planning committee which has before it all the proposals to be compared and allows the points of view of the diverse membership to come up with conclusions about probable consequences.

Even the selection of the criteria by which we test the interventions represents viewpoints at work and, therefore, criteria also need to be selected rather painstakingly by a diverse planning group. The ones offered in Figures 7.4-7.12 are of interest to me, but may not be to others, and they do not deal adequately with political and long-term outcomes to our society. However, they are mainly presented as a basis of discussion.

AN ALTERNATIVE APPROACH TO DESIGN OF GOAL-DIRECTED DELIVERY SYSTEMS

The material presented so far assumes that long-range goals can be meaningfully translated into more specific objectives which, in turn, have attributes for which criteria can be established. The criteria then become the specifications by which the designers carefully and completely create the delivery systems. Many different delivery systems can be designed which meet what predominantly are performance-type criteria. The criteria thus allow competitive models as well as opportunities to design individualized systems which serve special needs as presented by different communities or different parts of a single community, or systems designed to utilize unique resources.

In spite of the design feasibilities provided by the deductive approach just described, in many systems the nature of the currently desired outcomes can be seen well enough, but even limited forecasting reveals great dissatisfactions and the strong likelihood of startlingly different goals or altered interpretations of old goals in the near future. This, of course, is a typical present-day situation for most serious social problems. How is a system to be designed to meet currently desired goals with concomitant needed outputs, when it is known or suspected that different—but as yet poorly defined and presently unacceptable— outputs and outcomes are almost certainly going to be required not too far down the road? Should a delivery system be set up temporarily to do the current job—such as training needed physicians—and then be abandoned? Can it be converted later to train some other needed skills? Can we afford to set up and then disband systems as expensive as those which now train physicians, or can we design them in such a way that they can be easily redirected, without a great loss of investment, to, let us say, train new kinds of health technicians or even to entirely different purposes?

Let us examine two widely divergent health care futures that seem extreme to us now but are being discussed more and more and are far from unbelievable.[57] Illich is reported as defending a health care system which would use and distribute self-appliable information and simple self-applicable tools as a first step. This would enable everyone to achieve some "best" minimum before a select few could have access to the kind of "miracles" which are so costly that to vast numbers (the majority of people in the world) they can have little or nothing to offer in the way of care The lid on new advances would be raised as fast as all could participate in them. Equity principles would really be applied.

In contrast, Ingrasci is reported, in the same document, as desiring to go further faster with technology to build up a worldwide system of intelligence. His approach would put our health concerns into an inquiring and adaptive system which would respond promptly to massive needs in an ecologically relevant manner, and thus would deploy from a central control center whatever interventions are needed anywhere in the world.

Regardless of the implications about the kind of world-wide society that could or would request and support such approaches, or of what would happen to a society that did, these proposals clearly represent quite different belief systems at work. Neither is beyond the possibility of occurrence; neither is likely to make happy or economical use of what are now the major health tools and investments. Each would make massive new demands for new kinds of outputs and require undoing much of what is now done under the egis of the health care sector. In referring to Figure 1.1, we can see that if our sights and goals were to be shifted from health care to health, most of the more meaningful, although politically and culturally hard to sell, health promoting interventions would probably be mounted outside the health sector altogether. That is one possible way of going. Ingrasci apparently is speaking strongly to such a logic.

If we continue to focus on health care as the goal, it is also conceivable that we will come to accept such approaches as the medicine man, the Christian Science practitioner, the curanderas, or the mystic, contemplative, diet, and herbal approaches of our own counter-culture. The latter, although depending on wise-man leadership, is the most accessible to individuals and partakes of Illich's desire for more accessible do-it-yourself approaches, including those for basic health care.[58] It also obviates dependence on ritualistic, highly skilled practitioners who make people feel less and less capable and self-assured and who are progressively available to relatively fewer and fewer persons other than elites.

Beginning Implementation Before Completion of Design

Let us introduce a second stream of considerations about uncertain futures, and interventions which require years to design and years to implement before the first useful output is created. The education of health professionals makes a good case in point. The question of their future utility and the length of lead time for planning and implementation plus training time are mutually aggravating considerations. If we take a specific currently desired output, the family practitioner, two to eight years of training after high school may elapse from aspirant entry to practitioner exit from the training system.

From the time the exact nature of the practitioner is clarified, the curriculum worked out, the faculty indicated, the general nature of the plant determined, approval and funding obtained, the site procured, the building plans drawn and approved, the construction, equipping, and staffing accomplished, at least five years have passed before the training center can enroll its first student. Planning and the implementation plus training will therefore require somewhere between eight and eighteen years before the first usable output is available to serve the need perceived now. This combination—the uncertainty of the future and the outputs called for, and the planning-construction-throughput time requirements—makes it unlikely that society can afford a style of planning that calls for completed plans, extensive and detailed on-paper evaluation of alternatives, and acceptance before implementing the first step of a plan.

If implementation can somehow follow along with planning, there may be hope of achieving outputs while they are still desired and desirable. This is the full flowering of developmental planning. In this way we could also get early feedback, rather than having to wait until the entire planning venture has been put into operation and turns out its first products. We can also get guidance from our continued future mapping, as it makes contact with the moving future, so that we learn early if an altered course is necessary to bring us to newly perceived futures. Such fast-track and contingent forms of planning are increasingly being used, even for hospital construction.[59]

Let us continue with the example of training family practitioners for the United States in the 1970's and beyond, and retain the notion that a university might still be asked to play a major role in the task of education for skills in relation to health. Until one gets the spirit of the developmental strategy, the planning strategy (first perceived by studying Figure 1.2 and reinforced by what has been said in the preceding chapter and most of this one) might suggest that we do a thorough job at each step before we move along to the next one, and that our design, with alternatives well worked out, be essentially complete before it is submitted to policy makers for adoption and implementation or alteration. General observations, fortified particularly by discussions with Robert Biller, Peter Marris, and Ivan Illich, have led to serious reservations about such a tidy mental set. In fact, they have led to convictions that such a procedure, if not out-and-out irrational, must be limiting if applied to significant and complex social issues.

In the example chosen, the planners are aware of the current need for more physicians, but cannot foresee whether this demand will continue for more than a decade. Must they set up a typical 50-100 million dollar medical school to meet current demands? Should they become Lindblomites and do so and expect to alter or scrap the plant when it is no longer wanted for training physicians? Should they do the best possible forecasting and plunge ahead on the basis of anticipated future needs? And, if so, who will pay for a future-oriented system that does not deliver what is wanted now?

A better answer should be to devise a low-cost system which will rapidly produce what is wanted now, yet one whose design will be heavily guided by knowledge gleaned from our forecasts that physicians will probably not be the only or even the major product desired from the system in ten years. In this way we anticipate the future, at least in general terms, and minimize future losses by a system design which takes on specifications heavily guided by the need for inexpensive flexibility—a design which has the ability to withhold irretrievable and expensive commitments or resources.

How does this work? Evidence is clear that the distribution of physicians is bad. There is disagreement as to whether there is a shortage, or whether there may indeed be a surplus of doctors who are so trained and socialized as to be incapable of serving people in just those areas where there are not enough doctors of any kind. In either case, at this moment we need either a greater output of physicians so trained as to be willing and able to serve the underserved, because existing physicians will not easily be relocated. There is also the very pressing possibility that a mixture of technology and lesser skills will soon extend the productivity of the physician by performing many of his time-consuming, routine tasks.

What kind of a school should be set up, how complete should its designs be, before the regents, legislature, and citizenry are asked to authorize the start-up or take the first implementing step? If we are justifiably worried about shifting goals, not only the customary 50 to 100 million dollar capital outlay, but also the collection of teachers, researchers, and students may need turning about shortly after they are assembled. And if they are well selected for currently envisioned tasks, the faculty may well not be redirectable. They may have to be dispersed, or blindly continue training unneeded medical scientists, neurosurgeons, ophthalmologists, or general surgeons. Perhaps family doctors, too, may be a glut on the market in 15 years, and a new system created to turn them out will also have to be abandoned shortly after its first outputs are released.

Attention is therefore called to the utility of pacing implementation right on the heels of the planning procedure so that the first exploratory implementing steps are undertaken as soon as the normative guidance is clarified. Proceeding with implementation and planning simultaneously means continuous and developmental planning which must direct systems to produce satisfactorily now, while altering their makeup and their output to keep meeting new requirements which are being foretold from the continuing future mapping. We must escape from the mental set or paradigm which suggests that every alternative and element, as well as their prices have to have been determined before implementation can begin. The plan-implement approach may involve a careful, but brief, six-to-twelve-month goal and problem scrutiny, which lays out the likelihood and nature of major changes in the goals or in the more specific objectives and provides a rough schedule of the probable appearance of such changed demands. This approach will also clarify the specific outputs which must be sought initially.

The next step is to undertake a design which guarantees a maximum of flexibility under the constraints of legal, moral, and philosophic obligations to trainees, faculty, tax payers, and the university. The participation and points of view of legislators, citizenry, health care professionals, students, university faculty, and others are used. And in another twelve months the basic long-range schema as well as the specifics of implementing and getting underway can be completed. Basic laboratories and classrooms already exist on the general campus and very modest additional inputs of equipment and faculty can be used to provide basic medical training, even if classes must be held and facilities used at unaccustomed hours and places.

At the same time, clinical training is arranged for in community facilities and private offices or in existing medical schools, as is deemed appropriate to create the desired skills and attitudes and successfully grant degrees. Thus, although wisely begun with a small class, a medical school comes into existence almost concurrently with, or only one or two steps behind, the planning for it. The societally desired outputs might conceivably be delivered in time still to be of use.

Continuing incorporation of the feedback from the first attempts at operation with future feedback from continued forecasting provides a planning process that is never ending. Hopefully, the future and the present can be brought closer in the sense that what we undertake now will also be able to serve what is wanted then, and long delayed change and changeover need not be the contested, traumatic waste of resources they now are. If we can start implementation at pilot or full steam levels as soon as we get our bearings from initial planning the two can go on together. This logic also suggests why isolated pilot operations may not always be sensible and why they are so rarely widely adopted even if highly successful. By the time their results are in and verified, the original concerns are changed or gone or newer ideas have come into view, and the pilot project is stranded because the stream is now taking another course.

Figure 8.4 provides a summary of examples proposed for guidance

FIGURE 8.4

CAPACITY TO REDESIGN IN THE FACE OF UNCERTAINTY*

(Based on work by Robert Biller, 1971)

ITEMS	Away From These Criteria of TRADITIONAL OUTLOOK	Toward These Criteria of DEVELOPMENTAL OUTLOOK
Program design criteria	Try to design a program that is *correct*; try to anticipate contingencies and design it so that it takes as many as possible into account	Try to design a suitable program that is also *correctible*; try to *anticipate procedures that will allow it* to respond to contingencies
Length of educational programs	*Traditional* ones (e.g., 4-year MDs) or Shorter (e.g., 3-year MDs) or Longer (e.g., 5-year MDs)	Adjusted to individual need, taking into account prior relevant training, use of performance testing for levels of skills required
Faculty	Appoint as *large a permanent* one as you can afford	Appoint as *small a permanent* one as you can't avoid
Courses and degree programs	*Accredit* courses and degree programs subject primarily to initial *pre-hoc design review*. Make them *hard to start* (therefore hard to stop)	*License* courses and degree programs—subject primarily to periodic *post-hoc consequences* review. Make them *easy to start* and hard to continue unless utility is reverified (easy to stop)
Physical plant	*Build new buildings* where your funds allow it; rent only when you can't avoid it	*Rent space* where its availability allows; build only if you can't avoid it
Stance toward planning and implementation	*Plan long and thoroughly* to try to increase the probability of developing a sensible, high-quality proposal that has a good chance of being implemented	*Start creating as sensible* and high quality a program as you know how to do in order *to learn from the consequences of these implementation acts* and benefit from the steering they make possible, so that what is implemented has a good chance of having been worth the effort
Commitment and change strategy	*Don't act* before you have commitment to a complete plan from all the significantly affected parties	*Begin action* with a commitment to a sense of direction but *don't generate* commitment to any plan before the significantly affected parties understand empirically the consequences-in-action of a commitment

* Biller's "contingent planning"

of those planning for the training of the medical practitioners we have been talking about. It was elaborated by the sixth month of a planning effort designed to accept the first medical students on a general university campus. The most significant single design element in this case was seen as the capacity to change product according to need over time, at minimum cost in dollars, human resources, and anguish. The procedural criteria, which are applied at every decision point where choices must be made between alternative ways of proceeding, were particularly selected to facilitate major low cost changes required by the inevitable shifts in goals. They should also help create a frame of mind which anticipates rather than obstructs implementation of new societally selected goals.

REFERENCES

1. C. West Churchman, *The Systems Approach* (New York: Dell, 1968), 173-76.
2. U. S., Department of Health, Education and Welfare, Public Health Service, Health Economics Series no. 6, "Estimating the Cost of Illness," by Dorothy P. Rice, 1966.
3. United Nations, Research Institute for Social Development, Report no. 7, "Cost-Benefit Analysis, Education and Health," by E. R. Rado, April 1966, 121-29.
4. Burton W. Deane and S. J. Mantel, Jr., "A Model for Evaluating Costs of Implementing Community Projects," *Analysis for Planning, Programming, Budgeting,* ed. by M. Alfandry-Alexander (Washington, D. C.: Operations Research Council, 1968), 27-47.
5. U. S., Department of Health, Education and Welfare, Public Health Service, Publication no. 1178, "Economic Benefits from Public Health Services," by C. C. Linnenberg, Jr., April 1964.
6. E. R. Rado, Ibid. no. 3, 121-29. Robert Dorfman, ed., *Measuring Benefits of Government Investments* (Washington, D. C.: The Brookings Institution, 1965).
7. United Nations, Research Institute for Social Development, Report no. 7. "Cost-Benefit Analysis of Improved Housing: A Case Study," by Leland S. Burns, April 1966, 88-120.
8. Jack Wiseman, "Cost-Benefit Analysis and Health Service Policy," *The Scottish Journal of Political Economy* 10 (February 1963) 128-45.
9. Victor R. Fuchs, "The Contribution of Health Services to the American Economy," *Milbank Memorial Fund Quarterly* 44, part 2 (October 1966), 65-101.
10. Irving Leveson, Doris Ullman, and Gregory Wassall, "Effects of Health on Education and Productivity," *Inquiry* 5 (December 1969) 3-11.
11. U. S. Public Health Service, Ibid. no. 2. U. S. Public Health Service, Ibid. no. 5.
12. M. Hill, J. Francis, and G. D. Rosenthal, "Cost-Effectiveness Analysis Applied to the Treatment of Chronic Renal Disease," *Medical Care* 6 (January/February 1968), 48-54.

13. U. S., Congress, Joint Economic Committee, "Economic Analysis of Public Investment Decision: Interest Rate Policy and Discounting Analysis," 1968. Samuel B. Chase, Jr., ed., *Problems in Public Expenditure Analysis* (Washington, D. C.: The Brookings Institution, 1968). U. S. Public Health Service, Ibid no. 2.

14. Anthony Downs, *An Economic Theory of Democracy* (New York: Harper & Row, 1957), 167.

15. U. S. Public Health Service, Ibid. no. 2.

16. David Novick, ed., *Program Budgeting: Program Analysis and the Federal Budget* (Cambridge: Harvard University Press, 1967).

17. W. L. Kissick, "Planning, Programming, and Budgeting in Health," *Medical Care* 5 (July/August 1967). Fremont J. Lyden and Ernest G. Matler, *Planning, Programming, Budgeting: A Systems Approach to Management* (Chicago: Markham Publishing Co., 1968). U. S., Congress, Senate, Committee on Government Operations, "Planning-Programming-Budgeting: Initial Memorandum, Selected Comment, Official Documents," July 1967. U. S., Congress, Joint Economic Committee, "The Analysis and Evaluation of Public Expenditures: The PPB System, I, II, III," 1969.

18. A. R. Prest and R. Turvey, "Cost-Benefit Analysis: A Survey," *The Economic Journal* 75 (December 1965).

19. U. S. Public Health Service, Ibid. no. 2.

20. A. A. Berle, Jr., "What GNP Doesn't Tell Us," *Saturday Review* (August 31, 1968), 10-12.

21. "Environmental Currents," *Environmental Science and Technology* 5 (February 1971), 102.

22. Kenneth Boulding, "Economics and Ecology," *Future Environments of North America*, ed. by E. F. Darling and J. P. Milton (Garden City, New York: Natural History Press, Doubleday,1966), 225-34.

23. "Cost Effectiveness versus Cost Benefits for Public Health Programs," *Public Health Reports* 83 (November 1968), 899-907. A. L. Levin, "Cost Effectiveness in Maternal and Child Health," *New England Journal of Medicine* 278 (May 9, 1968), 1041-47. M. Hill, J. Francis, and G. D. Rosenthal, Ibid. no. 12, 48-54. S. N. Dietz, "Cost Effectiveness Evaluation Methods for Identifying Hazardous Highway Locations," *Analysis for Planning, Programming, Budgeting*, ed. by M. Alfandry-Alexander (Washington, D. C.: Operations Research Council, 1968), 65-69.

24. L. Hansen and B. Weisbrod, "The Distribution of Costs and Direct Benefits of Public Higher Education: The Case of California," *Journal of Human Resources* 4 (Spring 1969), 176-91. Joseph Pechman, "The Distributional Effects of Public Higher Education in California," *Journal of Human Resources* 5, (Summer 1970), 361-70. Robert W. Hartman, "A Comment on the Pechman-Hansen-Weisbrod Controversy," *Journal of Human Resources* 5 (Fall 1970), 519-23.

25. United Nations, Ibid. no. 3, 121-29.

26. Phillip R. A. May, "Cost-Efficiency of Mental Health Care," *American Journal of Public Health* 61 (January 1971), 127-29.

27. United Nations, Ibid. no. 3, 121-29.

28. P. H. Samuelson, *Economics* (New York: McGraw-Hill, 1970 (1), 4.

29. Robert L. Heilbronner, "On the Limited Relevance of Economics," *The Public Interest* (Fall 1970), 80-93.

30. U. S., Department of Health, Education and Welfare, Office of the Assistant Secretary for Program Coordination, Disease Control Programs: "Arthritis," September 1966; "Selected Disease Control Program," September 1966; "Cancer, " October 1966; "Motor Vehicle Injury Prevention Program," August 1966;"Maternal and Child Health Care Programs," October 1966. U. S., Department of Health, Education and Welfare, "Report of the Committee on Chronic Kidney Disease" (Compiled at the Request of the Bureau of the Budget), September 1967. Robert N. Grosse, "Cost-Benefit Analysis and Social Planning" *Analysis for Planning, Programming, Budgeting,* ed. by M. Alfandry-Alexander (Washington, D.C.: Operations Research Council, 1968), 129-4.

31. Richard M. Bailey, "Economics and Planning," *Health Planning 1969,* by H. L. Blum and Associates (San Francisco: Western Regional Office, American Public Health Association, 1969), Chapter 9.

32. Herbert Klarman, "Syphilis Control Programs," *Measuring Benefits of Government Institution,* ed. by Robert Dorfman (Washington, D. C.: The Brookings Institutions, 1965), 367-415.

33. B. W. Deane and S. J. Mantel, Jr., Ibid. no. 4, 27-47.

34. A. R. Prest and R. Turvey, "Cost-Benefit Analysis: A Survey," *Surveys of Economic Theory, III, Resource Allocation,* The American Economic Association and Royal Economic Society (New York: St. Martin's Press, 1967), 155-207.

35. Barkev S. Sanders, "Measuring Community Health Levels," *American Journal of Public Health* 54 (July 1964), 1063-74.

36. A. Wildavsky, "The Political Economy of Efficiency: Cost-Benefit Analysis, Systems Analysis, and Program Budgeting," *Public Administration Review* 26 (December 1966), 292-311.

37. Jay W. Forrester, *World Dynamics* (Cambridge, Mass.: Wright Allen Press, 1971).

38. A. Downs, Ibid. no. 14, 167.

39. Warren L. Ilchman and Norman T. Uphoff, *The Political Economy of Change* (Berkeley & Los Angeles: The University of California Press, 1969), 260-73.

40. Douglass B. Lee and John W. Dyckman, "Economic Impacts of the Viet Nam War: A Primer," *Journal of the American Institute of Planners* 36 (September 1970), 298-309.

41. Richard Netzer, *Economics and Urban Problems* (New York: Basic Books, 1970).

42. Leon Keyserling, "The New Health Care Economy: Forces Reshaping General Policy, Structure, Financing and Quality of Care," *Bulletin of the New York Academy of Medicine* 42 (December 1966) 1157-77.

43. R. L. Heilbronner, Ibid. no. 29, 80-93.

44. R. M. Bailey, Ibid. no. 31, Chapter 9.

45. Ibid, Chapter 9.

46. J. Richard Udry, "A Spoonful of Sugar Helps the Medicine Go Down," *American Journal of Public Health* 61 (April 1971), 776-85.

47. Henrik L. Blum and Associates, *Health Planning 1969* (San Francisco:

Western Regional Office, American Public Health Association, 1969), 8.22.

48. A. R. Prest and R. Turvey, Ibid. no. 34, 155-207.

49. H. Klarman, Ibid. no. 32, 367-415.

50. Vincent Taylor, *How Much Is Good Health Worth?* (Santa Monica, California: The Rand Corporation, P-3945, 1969).

51. U. S., Department of Health, Education and Welfare, Ibid. no. 30.

52. Martin S. Feldstein, M. A. Piot, and T. K. Sundaresan, "Resource Allocation Model for Public Health Planning: A Case Study of Tuberculosis Control," Supplement to vol. 48 of the *Bulletin of the World Health Organization*, WHO, Geneva (1973).

53. Gerald Nadler, *Work Design: A Systems Concept*, rev. ed. (Homewood, Illinois: Richard D. Irwin, 1970), 510-11.

54. Eveline M. Burns, "Analysis of Selected Current Health Insurance Bills," background paper for Committee on Health, Department of Public Affairs, Community Service Society, 105 East 22nd Street, New York, N.Y., January 1972, mimeographed.

55. Herman M. Somers, "National Health Insurance and Strategy," *The Paros* (Journal of Alpha Omega Alpha) 35 (January 1972), 10-13. Herman M. Somers and Anne R. Somers, "Major Issues in National Health Insurance," *The Milbank Memorial Fund Quarterly* 1 (April 1972), 177-210.

56. U.S., Department of Health, Education and Welfare, Social Security Administration, Office of Research and Statistics, "National Health Insurance Proposals Introduced in the 92nd Congress," May 1971. Allen Ferguson Jr., "National Health Proposals, the Neighborhood and the Poor." NHC Seminar Monograph Series no. 2, University of California Extension, October 1971.

57. Centro Intercultural de Documentation, DOC I/V 72-6., APDO 479 Cuernavaca, Mexico [As recorded by Fred Purdy].

58. Ivan D. Illich, *Celebration of Awareness: A Call for Institutional Revolution* (Garden City, New York: Doubleday Anchor, 1971), Chapters 8 & 9.

59. Delbert L. Price, "Fast Track and New Methodology in Hospital Planning and Construction" Hospital Progress, 55 (June 1972), 50-57, 68.

Part IV

ACHIEVING THE IMPROVEMENTS DEFINED AS DESIRABLE BY PLANNING

9. Creation of the Means to Plan:
The Planning Body Selects Roles,
Functions, and Modes of Planning

Seven years after the adoption of Public Law 89-749, the Comprehensive Health Planning and Public Health Services Amendments of 1966, the most common question encountered among comprehensive health planners is still: "What should we be doing?" and the second most common is: "How should we get started?"

Although no categorically specific answers will hold equally well from one locality to the next nor apply to all levels of community or government, can any guidance be offered? The answer seems, unequivocally, yes. Health has been defined in a way that describes what we must be concerned with, and planning has been defined in a way that says what must be accomplished. The functions and the styles of operation which a planning body can then undertake lend themselves to reasonable understanding.

The three major societal purposes which planning bodies are expected to achieve—define, obtain, and measure improvements—suggest the need for an internalized guide or sense of purpose that will make each planning body capable of serving its society's requests. Thus, the planning body is seen as a part of, or included in, the general social system. The client of the planning body is the rest of the system. Because this system values participation, it may not be advisable for the public planning body to assume functions more forceful, formidable or partisan, other than providing a center of exchange, expertise, formulation, and implementation as well as leading the way in search of new directions and better means. Chapter 2 reviewed the place for planning in the democratic creation of intended social change and defined a style of developmental (multimode) planning as being desirable for health planning. Planning bodies can begin to select their roles and functions from this theoretic base; the local situation provides the pragmatic criteria for further guidance to role selection.

In the following section, many possible roles for planning bodies are described. Some surely go far beyond what we have just postulated as the central guiding expectation or internal purpose of planning bodies in our society. However, it is perfectly possible and compatible with our democratic beliefs for the system to call upon the planning body to assume some of the more partisan or forceful roles. (The foregoing discussion is not in any way directed as an ethical prescription to the independent individual planner—as opposed to the planning body—for he may seek to serve any kind of client or cause or segment of society in any role that he believes is just or wise, and which his society will allow.) The chapter concludes with a review of the major, or popularly discussed, modes of planning and illustrates how each typically represents an emphasis or denial of one or several of the roles or functions described.

POTENTIAL ROLES AND DESCRIPTION OF FUNCTIONS SUGGESTED BY EACH

A list of roles and the functions required to carry them out are presented, because the three major purposes of planning will not come about by themselves—the planning body must assume certain basic stances. The list is intended, however, only as an elaborate reminder of the possibilities, not as a blueprint.

One might suppose that a planning body could pluck off for itself any and all roles and functions. But to proceed with reasonable comfort and without arousing massive community hostility or loss of support in key quarters—such as general legislative bodies, consumer groups, or purveyor groups—is not simple. With this caution in mind, the most obvious reaction might be for a planning body to confine itself to those roles and functions already commonly practiced and happily received in the community. Because health planning—or any kind of social planning—is new, if not unknown, it is fair to say that the latter approach is not likely to produce much of value.

Another less restrictive but safe approach is to carry out only those roles and functions which, whether new or enduring, are directly called for by assignments made under P.L. 89-749, by state legislation, and by councils of governments which have authority spelled out by their constituents and by such instruments as Bureau of the Budget Circulars A-80, A-82, and A-95.[1]

The third approach to selecting roles and functions usually follows from the one above and results from the planning body's perception of what is called for as it defines first, the improvements wanted; second, how to get them; and third, how to measure their achievement. As the planning body accepts its first assignments, usually community problems and goals, its sincere attempts to measure, analyze, design, and obtain what is needed will call forth the assumption of role after role and function after function. Naturally, the broader the scope of assignments taken, the sooner the planning body will enlarge its scope of roles and functions. Just as the planning body's sincere involvement with significant issues leads it to assume particular roles and functions (inevitably it must take on the roles of inquirer, coper/problem-solver, educator, priority setter, assistor, and activator), it will also commence to run counter to the desires of various interests. At this point, the role of self-survival will loom large on the planning body's horizon. That need can lead to inactivity or it can lead to more systematic work, to more public education, and to more systems level approaches that take into account more interests and attempt to reconcile these interests over longer time spans.

Because no two communities have identical arrays of problems or interests, the actual choice of roles and functions will vary widely at least in the initial years. Moreover, local mores and cultural influences will affect the amount of tolerance with which the community will regard its planning body's assumption of particular roles and functions. Because a planning body is supposed to be reasonably representative of all significant groups in the community, it will probably be aware of what is considered intolerable. The main problem here is the reverse: a natural tendency to overlook or at least avoid some of the roles, functions, or activities most needed just because the planning body shares the blind spots and prejudices of the community.

The successful assumption of a limited number of new roles and functions will undoubtedly enlarge the capacity of the planning body to take on other new roles. Its life depends on innovation, and success allows the extension of innovative capacity. Success should not, however, blind the planning body to the fact that assumption of some roles and functions can negate its success in planning. The search for authority, for example, has brought many planning bodies new tasks, such as approving construction grants. Unfortunately such authority need not contribute to more planning, and typically decreases staff time available for planning, thereby threatening survival of the planning body. For different reasons, some kinds of advocacy roles might similarly remove the planning body from the center of the planning arena.

Planning bodies need not—in fact, should not—select masses of goals, functions, and activities in advance. A broad listing can be used from time to time as a reminder of what might be done, and it was for this purpose that the following material was prepared.

Selected Functions Enable Role Achievement

The list of functions shown under each role is meant to suggest possible or feasible ways to carry out each role that a planning body may wish to carve out for itself. Several functions appear under more than one role, because they so heavily serve more than one role, and a good many others could also be shown as relating to several roles. There is nothing preemptive about the list.

Choice of Roles and Functions Is Likely to
Vary With Level of Community

On what basis can the judgment be made that a particular function is appropriate to planning bodies at a given level (neighborhood, city, metro, state, region, or nation)? Each level might find justification to assume any or all of the roles, and I have postulated which levels of planning bodies would find a particular function necessary, and the degree of emphasis it should be given. (The allocation of functions and the degree of emphasis by level of planning was influenced by the typology of the community or communities of solution advanced in Chapter 11.) For example, I have suggested that the neighborhood level planning body not undertake the forecasting function shown under the "builder of futures" role. At the same time the metro, state, and national levels are encouraged to emphasize this function. The logic is that the national level planning body must do a good job of forecasting before states can do much of a projection for themselves. Similarly, metros are dependent on the state but must in turn do a good job for their area of responsibility which includes all the local areas. Multistate regions can be guided by federal and state projections, and where metro authorities exist, their projections can guide cities and/or counties within the authority. Neighborhoods will rarely have the capacity to do more than react to overall forecasts or to various projections which involve them.

By contrast, it is suggested that no national level planning body or multistate (regional) level planning body undertake the activities of community organization and community development shown under the role of advocate. The logic is that each of the four lower levels may undertake, legally and morally, defensibly and desirably, to help an area get on its feet, learn how to study itself, fend for itself, and fight for its own interests. But there can be little justification for a planning body at either the national or multistate level to try to reach down inside states and communities and carry out these activities, although they may find it important to encourage the middle levels to do so.[2]

Decisions by planning bodies to assume certain functions may be said to hinge on considerations such as the following:

Likelihood of having access to the requisite skills.

Degree of dependence on higher or lower levels to function first or at greater depth because of legal requirements, capacity or precedence.

Geographic and meteorologic basin boundaries of the issues at hand.

Relation to the area or the jurisdiction which is involved, is generating the issues, or providing the key to the causes or control for the issues at hand.

Political decision implications or requirements.

Capacity to generate interest and required political support.

Nature of the market, transport, communications, social, recreational, and educational implications for the issues at hand.

Resource capacity for the issues at hand.

Delivery base or capacity for the issues at hand.

Clearly not all these constraints apply to any one function, and different constraints may apply to the same function depending on the particular issue under consideration. For example, because of the historical precedent of reserving to the states all residual powers not specifically allocated to the Federal Government, and because of reinforcement by Public Law 89-749, it seems reasonable to expect that the state planning bodies will undertake leadership in dividing responsibilities between different planning levels and in determining the jurisdictions of lesser planning bodies within the state.

However, in some states the deciding voice on such issues has been given to the general law political entities and to chartered communities. In other areas, political concerns might dictate similar behavior even without legal requirements. The varying nature of issue may also be handled in different ways. One type of environmental control may be spelled out in law as the responsibility of a specific level of decision-making or planning. Bureau of the Budget (BOB)—now Office of Management and Budget (OMB)—Circular A-95 dictates that many types of federal funding must be reviewed by the federally approved Councils of Government (COGs), a metro level authority.[3] Other federal funds may pursue quite different paths in the same community. The COGs may also make different rules about where planning must take place for different subject areas, and no two COGs need follow the same rules—and undoubtedly they should not if they are guided by the nine considerations listed above.

Wisely, no general or a priori determination should be made of the degree of emphasis a planning body at any level must place on a given function. This decision is as indigenous as the choice of roles and functions by a planning body. However, the desirability of providing emphasis can be projected in a general way and is indicated in Figure 9.1.

Descriptions of Potential Roles and Functions

Figure 9.1 summarizes possible roles for planning bodies and the functions which appear feasible to carry out each role. Because of the need to discuss who does what (developed in Chapter 10), Figure 9.1 also shows whether the particular function is most likely to be carried out formally by the staff of the planning body (S); the board of the planning body (B); both (S and B); or the staff using the board as a means of presenting or formalizing a particular function (S via B). The

FIGURE 9.1
SUMMARY OF ROLES AND FUNCTIONS OPEN TO
A COMPREHENSIVE HEALTH PLANNING BODY

ROLE	by*	Planning** Level	FUNCTIONS
EDUCATOR	B	1 2 3 4 5 6	Hearing and exchange of views
	S via B	1 2 3 4 5 6	Issue clarification
	S via B	1 2 3 4 5 6	General public education and information
	S via B	1 2 3 4 5 6	Education of planning board members
	S via B	1 <u>2 3</u> 4 5 6	Extend community horizons
	S via B	1 <u>2 3 4</u> 5 6	Create value awareness
	S via B	1 <u>2 3</u> 4 5 6	Create goal awareness
	S via B	1 <u>2 3 4 5</u> 6	Create standards awareness
	S via B	1 2 <u>3 4 5</u> 6	Create systems awareness
DESIGNER OF PLANNING TECHNOLOGY	S and B	2 <u>3</u> 4 <u>5 6</u>	Adopt or create planning methodology
	S and B	1 2 3 4 5 6	Design and establish policies of operation
INQUIRER	S via B	2 3 <u>4</u> 5 <u>6</u>	Design and popularize desirability of the data collection on social and well-being indicators; institute means
	S	1 2 <u>3 4 5</u> 6	Measurement
	S and B	<u>1 2 3 4 5 6</u>	Assessment
	S and B	<u>1</u> 2 <u>3 4 5</u> 6	Forecast
	S	1 <u>2 3 4 5</u> 6	Feedback
	S and B	1 2 3 4 5 6	Evaluation
	S and B	1 2 3 4 5	Intelligence See "Early Warning" and "Forecasting"
	S and B	2 3 <u>4</u> 5 <u>6</u>	Place inquiry system responsibility
	S	2 3 <u>4</u> 5 <u>6</u>	Operate the inquiry system
PRIORITY SETTER	S and B	1 <u>2 3 4 5 6</u>	Design priority criteria
	S and B	1 <u>2 3 4 5 6</u>	Design priority weighting policy
	S and B	1 2 3 4 5 6	Apply priority criteria to choice of problems
	S and B	<u>1 2 3 4 5 6</u>	Apply priority criteria to choice of interventions in creating solutions
	S and B	<u>1 2 3 4 5 6</u>	Apply priority criteria to selection of projects for approval

*S—Staff; B—Board

**—neighborhood or small city or county; 2—larger city-county; 3—metro; 4—state; 5—multi-state region; 6—nation. (Underline indicates that the function is particularly relevant at the level underlined.)

ROLE	by*	Planning** Level	FUNCTIONS
COPER AND PROBLEM SOLVER	S	1 2 3 <u>4</u> 5 <u>6</u>	Early warning
	S and B	1 2 3 <u>4</u> 5 <u>6</u>	Quick reaction
	S and B	1 2 3 4 5 <u>6</u>	Adaptation
	S and B	1 2 <u>3</u> <u>4</u> 5 6	Identify health problems
	S and B	1 <u>2</u> <u>3</u> <u>4</u> 5 <u>6</u>	Measure size, severity, location of problems
	S and B	<u>1</u> <u>2</u> 3 4 5 6	Determine priority rank of the problem
	S and B	1 2 <u>3</u> 4 <u>5</u> 6	Clarify nature of issues within the problem
	S and B	1 2 3 <u>4</u> 5 <u>6</u>	Analyze chosen problems
	S and B	1 2 <u>3</u> <u>4</u> <u>5</u> <u>6</u>	Design and analyze alternative interventions
	S and B	1 2 <u>3</u> 4 5 <u>6</u>	Designate systems boundaries and necessary linkages
	S and B	1 2 <u>3</u> <u>4</u> 5 <u>6</u>	Establish priorities among solutions for each problem
	S and B	1 <u>2</u> <u>3</u> <u>4</u> 5	Design of plan package
	S and B	1 2 3 4 5 6	Design and promote implementation for chosen solutions
	S and B	1 <u>2</u> <u>3</u> <u>4</u> 5 <u>6</u>	Influence and promote the implementation for apparently useful solutions
	S and B	1 2 3 4 5 6	Conflict resolution
BUILDER OF FUTURES	S and B	2 <u>3</u> <u>4</u> 5 <u>6</u>	Forecasting
	S and B	2 <u>3</u> <u>4</u> 5 <u>6</u>	Exploration
	S and B	1 2 3 4 5 6	Exploitation
	S and B	1 2 3 4 5 6	Innovation
	S and B	1 2 3 4 5 6	Experimentation
	S and B	2 <u>3</u> 4 5 <u>6</u>	Research
	S and B	1 2 <u>3</u> <u>4</u> 5 <u>6</u>	Cope with forecasted futures
	S and B	1 2 <u>3</u> <u>4</u> <u>5</u> <u>6</u>	Normative goal design based on projections of current values
	S and B	1 2 <u>3</u> <u>4</u> 5 <u>6</u>	Normative goal design based on predicted values
	S and B	1 2 <u>3</u> <u>4</u> <u>5</u> <u>6</u>	Normative goal design based on creation of new values
	S and B	2 <u>3</u> 4 <u>5</u> <u>6</u>	Long-range design
	S and B	2 <u>3</u> 4 <u>5</u> <u>6</u>	Optimization
	S and B	<u>3</u> <u>4</u> <u>5</u> <u>6</u>	Ecological survival
ASSISTOR AND SYSTEMS FACILITATOR	S	1 2 3 4 5	Information and referral
	S	1 2 3 4 5	Advising and consulting
	S	2 3 4 5	Assistance with analysis or design
	S and B	1 2 3 4 5	Building cooperation
	S	2 3 4 5	Exchanging information
	S and B	2 3 4 5	Building coordination
	S and B	1 2 3 4 5	Linking levels
	S and B	1 <u>2</u> <u>3</u> <u>4</u> <u>5</u> <u>6</u>	Linking sectors

ROLE	by*	Planning** Level	FUNCTIONS
ADVOCATE	S and B	1	Negotiation or brokerage in behalf of a client
	S and B	1	Advocacy for a client
	S and B	1 2 3 4 5 6	Advocacy for a goal or belief-system
	S and B	1 2 3 4 5 6	Advocacy for a means
	S and B	1 2 3 4	Community organization
	S and B	1 2 3 4	Community development
	S and B	1 2 3 4 5	Lobbying
ACTIVATOR	B	1 2 3 4 5 6	For ends
	B	1 2 3 4 5 6	For means
	B	1 2 3 4 5 6	For resources, action, timing, scope
	B	1 2 3 4 5 6	For placement of responsibility
	S and B	1 2 3 4 5 6	Generate legislation
	S and B	1 2 3 4 5 6	Mobilize resources
POWER MODIFIER	S and B	1 2 3 4 5	Identify proximal and real clients
	S and B	1 2 3 4 5 6	Politicize
	S and B	1 2 3 4 5 6	Broaden participation
	S and B	1 2 3 4 5 6	Increase choice
	S and B	1 2 3 4 5 6	Extend community horizons
	S and B	1 2 3 4 5 6	Design strategy
	S and B	1 2 3 4 5 6	Bargain
	S and B	1 2 3 4 5	Scandal proofing
	S and B	1 2 3 4 5 6	Maintaining power
	S and B	1 2 3 4 5 6	Changing or shifting power
	S and B	1 2 3 4 5 6	Creating power
POLICY PLANNER	S and B	2 3 4 5 6	Design pathways for social change
	S and B	1 2 3 4 5 6	Assist in policy formulation
	S and B	1 2 3 4 5 6	Renew the planning cycle
CONTROLLER OF PLAN IMPLEMENTATION	B	1 2 3 4 5	Representativeness of planning board
	S	2 3 4 5	Advice and guidance
	S	2 3 4 5	Guidelines
	S	2 3 4 5	Blueprint
	S and B	1 2 3 4 5 6	Evaluation
	S and B	1 2 3 4 5 6	Overseeing
	S	1 2 3 4 5	Supervising
	S and B	1 2 3 4 5	Approving organizations and projects
	S and B	1 2 3 4 5 6	Approving financing
	S	1 2 3 4 5	Administration
	S and B	2 3 4 5	Enforcement

ROLE	by*	Planning** Level	FUNCTIONS
REGULATOR	B	2 <u>3</u> 4 5 <u>6</u>	Establish findings on needs
DECISION	S and B	2 <u>3</u> <u>4</u> 5	Establish criteria as law
MAKER	S and B	2 <u>3</u> 4 <u>5</u>	Determine eligibility and compliance
ADJUDICATOR	B	2 <u>3</u> 4 <u>5</u>	Adjudicate between competitors and alternatives
	S and B	2 <u>3</u> 4 <u>5</u>	Approve permits to fill needs
	B	2 <u>3</u> <u>4</u> 5	Adjudicate complaints; hear appeals
SELF SURVIVAL	S and B	1 2 3 4 5 6	"Looking good"
	S and B	1 2 3 4 5 6	"Something for everyone"
	S and B	1 2 3 4 5 6	Build a constituency
	S and B	1 2 3 4 5 6	Bridge schisms
	S and B	1 2 3 4 5 6	Popularize the "rules of the game"
	S and B	1 2 3 4 5	Broaden participation
	S and B	1 2 3 4 5 6	Become indispensable
EXPANDER OF	S and B	1 2 3 4 5 6	For society
CAPABILITIES	S and B	1 2 3 4 5 6	For individuals

planning level at which a function might be carried out is shown by coding from 1 to 6: 1—neighborhood or small city or county; 2—larger city-county; 3—metro; 4—state; 5—multistate region; 6—nation. Those levels of community or government where the function would seem especially important or particularly feasible are indicated by bold numbers.

The order of potential functions shown under each role resulted from an attempt to list the most obvious kind of role support first, as well as the functions most likely to be acceptable. Further down the list of functions suggested for each role come those which cut deeper—in the sense of requiring a stronger posture, a more active role, a more partisan stance, or a more controversial function under that particular role.

A brief account of the meaning of the role and function designations follows Figure 9.1.

Educator

Information Exchanger (analyzed further in this chapter, and certain aspects also discussed in Chapters 10 and 11).

Hearing and exchange of views. Provide the setting in which persons and interests can make known to the planning agency, to the community and to one another their positions on an issue or an activity of the planning agency, or state beliefs or opinions about needs, wants, points of view, information, attitudes, and challenges.

Issue clarification. Provide the setting in which the planning agency can make known to the community the nature of issues which have been brought to it, the reasons for real or apparent conflicts, and the points at which they occur. This information can be given by means of a description of the situation and an analysis, so that the situation can be better understood in terms of its precursors as well as its consequences.

General public education and information. By means of mass media, hearings, presentations, and so on, provide information to the general public about situations, conditions, events, activities, relationships, trends, interventions, costs, and so on.

Education of planning board members. By general consent of the planning board members, provide for special programs of education about planning processes, specific content areas, discipline areas such as economics theory, and so on.

Extend community horizons. By means of hearings and mass media, make known the diversity of community values, goals, and means, and the choices to be made among them; the possible positive achievements or hazards offered by new technology, alternative political processes, and planning. Create awareness of multiple options, interrelationships, causes and consequences, spillovers, and so on.

Create value awareness. By means of hearings and mass media, help make comprehensible the legitimate competing or contrasting value positions which underlie the differences in perceptions of issues, ends, means, specific interventions, or of priority-setting devices.

Create goal awareness. By means of hearings and public media, make meaningful the concepts of ecological relationships, interrelatedness, comprehensiveness, inputs, outputs, equilibria, vectors, and interventions.

Designer of Planning Technology

Adopt or create planning methodology. Select or design the means to perform such tasks as: inquiry or assessment; carrying out systems analysis of such problems as diseases, disorders, and sick communities; designation of system boundaries and critical linkages; establishment of priority-setting and weighting devices; design and analysis of alternative interventions; presentation of plans to public and policy makers; implementation as via scheduling, budgeting, and influencing.

Design and establish policies of operation. Adopt and keep current the rules by which the agency determines such matters as: representation on the board or its committees; nature of linkage to other planning entities; division of labor with and among coworkers and participant interests; and choice of roles and functions to be undertaken.

Inquirer

Designer and Operator of the Inquiry System

Design and popularize the desirability of data collection on social and well-being indicators. Define useful markers or indicators, explain their utility, and design the means to obtain data that will allow assessment of well-being.

Measurement. Carry out data gathering and analysis to determine changes and trends for the various aspects of well-being.

Assessment. Carry out interpretations of information to select problems and priorities.

Forecast. Extend the past through the present and into the future using both exploratory and normative approaches to gain an idea of where the community appears to be headed, as opposed to where it could, should, or does want to be headed.

Feedback. Design a means of obtaining data from operations that will indicate the success and relevance of planned operations.

Evaluation. Design a means of correlating feedback and assessment so that evaluation can be made of the validity of planning assumptions, planning processes, operational success, and new factors, thereby providing guidance for further planning.

Intelligence. (Also see "early warning.") Provide information of particular concern to the implementation phase such as: the key figures in the various relevant interest blocs; the thrust of these interest blocs; which interest blocs have key say-so or desired resources; nature of alignments among interest blocs with estimates of their strengths and durabilities; "noise level" among relevant interests and participants to gauge anxiety, antagonism, withdrawal, and so on; impending critical moves; and means of escalating decisions to other levels where desired kinds of consideration can be obtained.

See *"early warning"* and *"forecasting"* functions under "Coper" and "Builder of Futures" roles, respectively.

Place inquiry system responsibility. Take leadership in development of the joint inquiry system; allocation of duties, schedules; adoption of basic uniform criteria and indices among the planning bodies at various levels.

Operate the inquiry system. Undertake the operations of the inquiry system as well as planning for it, or assure satisfactory operation if it is in other hands.

Priority Setter

Design priority criteria. Examples of criteria which could be selected and carefully defined are: (1) compatibility with overall plans; (2) ecological disruption; (3) overcoming inequities; (4) increasing productivity; (5) technological implementability; (6) political or general implementability; (7) public concern. (See Figure 6.1 for a list of criteria.)

Design priority weighting policy. Criteria, based on avowed aims or goals, must be weighted so that they can be used in the selection of problems, interventions or projects.

Apply priority criteria to choice of problems. Decide which problems are to be attacked first.

Apply priority criteria to choice of interventions in creating solutions. Decide which solutions are to be recommended for implementation and provide a priority rating for guidance.

Apply priority criteria to selection of projects for approval. Select projects for approval by the planning body and provide a priority rating for each.

Coper and Problem Solver—Short-Range Planning

Early warning. By collection and analysis of meaningful data about events, services, attitudes, behavior, and so on, note early changes in direction or intensity of heretofore accepted trends and determine when and where such new knowledge might be relevant to well-being, to political support, and to future as well as current plans.

Quick reaction. Act promptly on new information by creating projections and suggesting their possible direct and indirect significance; rally support if the trend or events seems favorable, or create interference if it is unfavorable.

Adaptation. Respond to observable or projected new situations through planning that tries to make the best of the situation or to overcome any deleterious effects.

Identify health problems. Clarify the nature of the problem so that its significance will not be seen differently by different people.

Measure size and severity of problems. Ascertain their relative significance.

Determine priority rank of the problems. Inevitably, limited resources can not be extended to every problem. (See "priority setter" role.)

Clarify nature of issues within the problem. Aspects of this function are critical. I will describe in some detail a few of the common issues, because each tends to require a different analytical focus. Where objectives are not being met adequately but remain desirable, the issues may be to *improve efficiency or effectivity*. At other times issues of balance are the most significant:

Balancing equity. Determine who benefits and who pays in each intervention or proposed program, so that policy makers can see how to avoid making one group pay a disproportionately higher share for some basic services (for example, at present the poor spend a much higher percentage of their income for less medical care than higher income groups). Policy makers also need to avoid unintentionally penalizing or denying one group services for which they pay—this is a complex issue, for some taxes are institutionally designed as progressive (favoring the poor) and other are regressive (favoring the rich) in accordance with current beliefs and compromises about redistribution of wealth. Improving distribution is in part another aspect of equity; opportunities and services must be distributed so that needs and demands are reasonably fulfilled. Because need, demand, availability, and accessibility are all potentially different criteria for equity—and there are many others—equity must be defined in each given circumstance.

Balancing marginal gains. To get the most per dollar, policy makers must make their next dollar expenditure on each high priority intervention buy essentially equal amounts of well-being.

Balancing use and availability of resources. Focus on key resources that are being used up or those that are not being created rapidly enough. Compare interventions in terms of their demands on such existing scarce resources. A larger system version of this process is described as "ecological survival" under the "Builder of Futures" role.

Balancing time frames. Take into account the rate at which interventions pay off, and indicate how to balance those with an immediate return against those with a delayed return (to the next generation, for example).

Tradeoffs among the four balancing accounts. Take into account the four preceding balancing accounts. Each of the four balances tends to shift planning decisions along a different axis of concern, and no two necessarily point in the same direction or to the same order or priorities or allocations in solving any particular problem.

Short and middle range design. Focus on solutions which can be expected to produce desired results in fairly short order. These results are usually accomplished by acting on proximal or direct forces which will alter promptly in predictable ways, even though the changes may not control the long-term, latent, background or underlying forces which will continue to create the same problems.

Suboptimizing and satisficing. Focus on solutions seen from the narrow standpoint of fairly small systems that do not deal with underlying and typically less well understood forces (suboptimizing). The purpose of this focus is to achieve results in the small system which have benefits for enough involved parties that the operation will generally be found satisfying by elements of the small system.

Maximizing. Focus on maximal achievement of a highly desired objective without major regard for cost, side effects, or consequences of allocation of resources within specific limits of adverse effects.

Analyze chosen problems. Carry out analysis of specific disorders (diseases or conditions). Identify inputs and outputs. Design of disease models could be done at the national level for the major disorders, but it will also be done at state levels, frequently for lack of national leadership and competency. Carry out analysis of such situations as sick communities, inequities, and inefficiencies by identifying inputs and outputs and pathways they take, and indicate the size and forecasted trends and rates of change.

Design and analyze alternative interventions. Create interventions to act at various points, such as on the inputs or outputs of the problem system under analysis. Weigh costs and benefits, spillovers, externalities, or secondary effects. Determine priorities among interventions. The nature and source of each intervention provides further clarification of the boundaries of the system in terms of which actors and events must participate.

Designate systems boundaries and necessary linkages. Describe the relation of inputs to the issue at hand and describe the relevant agents whose inputs must be coordinated or altered to affect the issues of concern. The nature and origin of such agents and their inputs provides a general idea of the system or systems and their boundaries which must be taken into account.

Establish priorities among solutions for each problem. See "Priority Setter" role.

Design of plan package. Design the actual plans needed to achieve desired ends. The level of detail depends on which agency takes the responsibility for designing the delivery apparatus. This is usually not the community level planning body.

Design and promote implementation for chosen solutions. This function applies to those solutions that lie within the sector for which the health planning body is responsible.

Influence and promote the implementation for apparently useful solutions. This function applies to solutions that lie in sectors outside those for which the health planning body is responsible, such as in education and agriculture.

Conflict resolution. Provide the setting as well as the expertise by which conflicts can be overcome. Resolution can be brought about in some cases by demonstrating unperceived mutuality of concerns, irrelevance of differences, ultimate coincidence of interests, compensating benefits or offsets, and so on.

Builder of Futures—Long-Range Planning

Forecasting (predicting, anticipating). Foretell the future, assigning probabilities to the parameters of what is being forecast, for example, in terms of time of appearance, quantity, direction, quality, and results.

Exploration. In the sense of forecasting, project horizontally and vertically the shifts in technological and social progress and their probable results in one or many areas. In the sense of planning, try new, innovative, or untried mixtures of interventions that seem to be justified on the basis of careful situational analysis with the intent of achieving or simply looking for breakthroughs.

Exploitation. Use forecasts with high probability to guide planning for interventions which will mesh with forecasted states, and take advantage of them so that whether the forecasted events are desirable or undesirable, the planners can harness or utilize them to profit the interests for which they are planning.

Innovation. Plan in a way which is probably only slightly different from exploration. Innovation is perhaps more limited in that it tries to invent interventions, rather than using them to explore the situation. When applied to a style of planning, the term tends to take on other flavors—such as advocacy for an idea, a means, or a new goal which, in the minds of the planners, seems to have intrinsic high payoff possibilities for the general community.[4]

Experimentation. Plan in a way not unlike that described under innovation or exploration, but in a way which also suggests a high order of observation and evaluation, so that newly applied interventions are evaluated or rated according to such aspects as their utility and side effects in operation.

Research. Beyond the intention to search out information which is sometimes called research,[5] and even beyond experimentation, lie the efforts at empirical studies which provide the basis for hypotheses and theory building and field testing of hypotheses to verify their theoretic capacity.

Cope with forecasted futures. Utilize a limited type of planning that seeks to be ready to cope with undesired forecasted events as they occur, rather than trying to use planning to alter their occurrence.

Normative goal design based on projections of current values. Plan on the assumption that selected future points in time will find the community still holding the present value configurations. Goals for those points are chosen according to present values, and plans are designed which will work toward their achievement.

Normative goal design based on predicted values. Plan on the assumption that values held at future times will not be the same as current values. By utilizing current knowledge of value relationships, in combination with information about changes in activities, institutions, and behavior that have a bearing on values, planners predict the values, priorities, or interests likely to be held at a given future time. Goals for planning are then designed to meet those postulated future value sets. In this way, plans produce interventions that will be delivering outputs presumed to be desired at that future time.

Normative goal design based on creation of new values. Create and promote acceptance of values and beliefs which are not currently enjoying significant vogue. Once these ideals become current, they will call for new goals. New or previously subdued values can be promoted without totally reorganizing existing ideologies (for example, concern for nature only recently has been vividly reformulated as ecology). Planning will then set about to create outputs which will match the newly promoted set of desires.

Long-range design. Planning, designed to meet what is anticipated as a result of the forecasting activities, is focused on desires, needs or institutions as visualized ten and more years away. This design usually calls for interventions that stem from juxtaposition of trends, events, people, or institutions in complex ways that typically take many years to come about, yet still will create the outputs desired at that time.

Optimization. Planning is directed to the largest relevant or manipulable system revealed by analysis of the broad array of interrelated factors in any given issue. This goal of planning is not limited to any one aspect or to a sub-area of the issue, but is cognizant of all significant parts of the issue and attempts to achieve the best overall solutions or broadest objectives. Each of the sub-objectives may not be maximally achieved in the interests of overall achievement (optimization) of the major objective.

Ecological survival. Analyze existing and projected human needs, demands, and ideals in such a way that they are reconciled with the limits imposed by other ecosystems and natural resources. Interventions are designed to maintain a satisfactory ecological balance; they are built on the knowledge that no particular ecological balance is necessarily the right one. The emphasis is on awareness of what ecological changes are going to be introduced, and whether these are likely to be acceptable at the time they will occur.

Assistor and Systems Facilitator

For Agencies, Groups, Communities, Purveyors. (In the past this role has been carried out largely by purveyors and their associations.)

Information and referral. As called upon, provide information about conditions, trends, needs, alternative ideas, goals, standards, and so on. Make referrals to other sources about whose services the planning body attempts to maintain up-to-date coverage.

Advising and consulting. Provide advice about overall situations, specific problems, interventions, the planning process, campaign strategy, and tactics needed by a client (such as a hospital or neighborhood) which wishes to attack a given problem or to make a plan operational.

Assistance with analysis or design. Work out problems or design solutions for members of a given system.

Building cooperation. Use good offices of the planning body to bring together related systems or subsystems; facilitate mutual understanding; create environment of trust, respect, and support.

Exchanging information. Obtain operational information of use in planning, as well as plans and future goals, from the various related systems or subsystems, with the expressed intent of exchanging such information among contributors as a source of guidance for individual plans.

Building coordination. Build relationships between systems and subsystems to the point where service or function goals can be undertaken, with each system responsible for a specified part of an organized activity, so that a new overall output level or product is achieved.

Linking levels. Pursue and maintain connections with various higher and lower levels of planning and with the controlling and operating institutions that help shape the particular function or operation with which the planning is concerned.

Linking sectors. On the level at which the planning body is working, act to relate the planning efforts of other sectors, such as education, agriculture, industry, and religion.

Advocate

Advocacy is a more forceful and partisan stance toward a given viewpoint than advising, consulting or helping to work out a plan of attack. In the classic statement that justifies this role, Davidoff writes: "The right course of action is always a matter of choice, never of fact." In his concern for better planning, Davidoff sees the need for multiple partisan sources of planning in a pluralistic society.[6] Thus, competent advocates or planners are needed for each important position, so that the citizens are well informed and the final public product is based on decisions made with knowledge of all the alternatives. He does not suggest that the public planning body need be an advocate for positions but, rather, that advocates for positions be a means of keeping public planning honest and at a high level of competency. According to the position of the Davidoffs and Gold, in 1970, the exercise of planning functions is to be on behalf of specified individuals and groups, rather than on behalf of a broadly defined public interest.[7] The Advocate role, also discussed in Chapter 11, may include any of the following functions, which vary with the degree of aggressiveness and partisanship assumed.

Negotiation or brokerage in behalf of a client. The planning body represents the client in all matters and may speak for him in any decision-making processes involved in making compacts, changing, neutralizing or creating power, implementing plans, and so on.

Advocacy for a client. The planning body undertakes any and all activities in behalf of a client's desired ends, including not only planning but organizing, politicking, and harassing.

Advocacy for a goal or belief-system. The planning body undertakes strong representation to clients or to the community at large in favor of some goal or some set of goals which it feels must be given priority.

Advocacy for a means. The planning body undertakes strong representation to clients or to the community at large in favor of some approach or some set of approaches (to accomplish a stated goal) which it feels must be given priority.

Community organization. Bring together or organize the various groups or organizations already in the area, or create new organizations which would provide a spokesman for the community they serve, contribute to various planning activities, or support them (especially those undertaken by the planning body).

Community development. Undertake promotion of an interactional process through which individuals in their community of jurisdiction learn how to articulate, join forces, solve problems, and create pressures. Higher levels may assist neighborhoods to get underway.

Lobbying. Undertake active influencing of policy makers or of those who can and do influence them. The form chosen may vary from taking policy makers to lunch as a friendly gesture, a forceful siege with data, the use of influential go-between people, or an effort to increase out-and-out pressure on policy makers from voter groups or campaign contributors.

Activator

For ends. Focus attention and force decisions by policy makers on ends that plans indicate must be achieved.

For means. Focus attention and force decisions by policy makers on selected means to be utilized in achieving planned-for ends.

For resources, action, timing, scope. Focus attention and force decisions by policy makers, so that the decisions on ends and means are implemented in specified ways, times, manners, and extents.

For placement of responsibility. Focus attention and force decisions by policy makers which assign responsibility for carrying out parts of accepted plans so that there can be no question about who is to do what.

To generate legislation. Design needed legislation, and find groups willing to sponsor it and legislators who will introduce it.

To mobilize resources. Assist in gathering or organizing the customary and heretofore untapped resources which analysis indicates are invaluable to issues at hand—including dollars, manpower, power, and votes.

Power Modifier

Identify proximal and real clients. As issues are accepted and analyzed, identify true clients who are to receive benefits of the planning programs as well as proximal clients who are accepting or making plans operational.

Politicize. Bring planning issues to public awareness in such a way that they inescapably become a political issue for politicians, as well as among citizens generally, thereby creating a new level of concern.

Broaden participation. Extend the opportunity to participate in studies, planning, hearings, and reviews of the planning output. Because organizations and individuals who have been invited may not perceive their role, they also may have to be encouraged, induced, or prodded into such involvement. At the national or state level, execution of this function may well mean setting policy for other planning levels to follow.

Increase choice. Extend the range of types of problems that might be attacked, and by suitable analysis extend the possibilities of points and methods of attack. Provide or produce the information necessary to indicate how options might work, and their probable consequences.

Extend community horizons. (See "Educator" role.)

Design strategy. Select timing, approaches, participants, and so on, so that issues are seen in new ways or in new alignments.

Bargain. Give consideration to changing a position or accepting tradeoffs which allow some or more of the desired goals to be reached but which may change the time schedule, priorities, objectives, subobjectives, means, quantities, operational agents, and so on.

Scandal proofing. (Another way of describing how to help oneself or someone else to look good.) Take necessary steps to act appropriately on problems or to appear to act on problems; undertake studies or defuse issues by releases, hearings, rephrasing issues, or by making sure that any adverse fallout will occur to someone else. This strengthens the party protected, potentially weakens others who may absorb the blame.

Maintaining power. Assist those who possess recognized power (the ability to make others move) by involving them in a way that makes them look good; make friends for them; or actually reinforce or add to their power by placing them in decision-making positions.

Changing or shifting power. Act in such a way that, for example, power holders are placed in a position of taking stands which add to or diminish their control. Neutralize or fortify power holders with other or higher level interveners, or by surrounding them by persons in greater or lesser number who can activate or be activated by them, influence or be influenced by them.

Creating power. Bring together formerly powerless groups so that they are assisted in organizing; or place their representatives on a policy-designing (planning) board or committee to get visibility, or in such numbers or with such allies that they appear and, in fact, commence to have decision-making power. Provide veto power to certain persons, groups or bodies heretofore not having a say. Previously powerless groups, not given positive power but only a veto, may in fact extend their veto power to many issues of no direct concern to them, and thus use it as bargaining leverage for things they want.

Policy Planner

This role, which is elaborated upon in one aspect or another in almost every chapter is one of the most critical roles for planning bodies.

Design pathways for social change. To indicate ends is not enough; the means, to make appropriate ends desired and actively sought after, involves influencing value systems and behavior.

Assist in policy formulation. The inevitable function of the planning body is formulation of potential policy. A firm commitment to this idea bodes well for the creation of plans which can then be readily implemented.[8] This does not mean that the planning body should undertake such careful scrutiny of the physiognomy of fate that only plans with a high probability of being adopted are turned out, for such "plans" describe primarily what was about to happen anyway. Thinking in terms of policy formulation means that need, resources, demand, technological alternatives, and maximal public participation will be kept in focus all through the planning process in such a way as to accomplish the kind of public education that will encourage legislators to adopt the plans proposed.

Renew the planning cycle. Once planning is effectively established, there should be fewer surprises and fewer specific terminal points, because plans will receive continuous reworking and legislators will more often be modifying trends than setting frenzied new drives in gear. In addition to newly stated partisan demands and to opportunities unlocked by insight and technological advances, instructions from the legislators and advice (occasionally threats or cajolements) from the elected head of government will specify the limits for planners, or indicate directions that they should take during the coming year. Planning bodies which perceive their exclusive mission to be advising governing bodies or executive offices (particularly those which are creatures of such bodies) may find that the limits set for them preclude investment of further time or money in particular areas. The planning bodies which see the community as their major responsibility will receive a new round of data, prognoses, demands, and suggestions from an ever-widening range of "clients" for the succeeding rounds of planning.

Controller of Plan Implementation

Representativeness of planning board. Appropriate interests should be selected for service on the planning board, so that what is going on as well as what is planned receive well-directed scrutiny and guidance—the most basic form of control.

Advice and guidance. Give advice and assistance to relevant interests in the form of technical advice or information about the limits, direction, timing, and so on, of matters that fall under the jurisdiction of the planning body and comply with the planning objectives of the planning body, particularly those within the scope of adopted plans.

Guidelines. Provide relevant interests with formal directions, and limitations on the scope, timing, methodology, or priorities which are in accordance with planning objectives. (These are not seen as having the force of law unless they have also been formally adopted as regulations under authorizing laws, or have been adopted by relevant policy-setting bodies that have jurisdiction.)

Blueprint. Provide relevant interests with formalized, appropriate, and detailed directions and limitations on any or all aspects of matters which fall under the planning agency's jurisdiction and are in accordance with their planning objectives (perhaps foreclosing many options).

Evaluation. Scrutinize all operations which fall within the planning agency's jurisdiction and scope of concerns, so as to determine and publicize the degree to which operating agencies or social outputs correspond with those called for by the relevant plan.

Overseeing. Provide constant scrutiny of how the planning body's plans are being operationalized, note and report progress, deviations, and obstacles, thereby forcing public recognition of unplanned changes that the planners feel were unwisely introduced. Observe new events that need to be taken into account so that the objectives can be achieved through appropriate alteration. Avoid sabotage or blind pursuit of plans in the face of ignored or unforeseen consequences.[9]

Supervising. Undertake formal scrutiny of all operations which result from the planning body's plans or are affected by them, thus ensuring that the operations are in fact being carried out in a way consistent with what the plans call for.

Approving organization and projects. Make findings as to which organizations or projects are acceptable and which are not. Forward findings to funding or implementing agencies which have the final say, or approve directly if the planning body has the decision-making authority.

Approving financing. Decide which activities or projects are to be funded and to what extent. Forward decisions to funding or implementing agencies which have the final say, or approve directly if the planning body has the decision-making authority.

Administration. Carry out the actual operations of the units whose activities resulted from or were significantly affected by the planning body's plans, to ensure that operations are totally consistent with the plans.

Enforcement. Maintain the necessary controlling machinery through reports, inspections, and hearings, and take the legally defined steps in controlling conformance. Penalize, close, constrain, take over, or depose, in accordance with authorizing legislation. Issuing permits to operate with powers of revocation is a standard tool.

Regulator, Decision Maker, and Adjudicator

This role is relatively new, and is often unforeseen by planning bodies as they draw together the parties needed to plan. At this point, it may be requested as clout or power, presumably to obtain the authority to get their planning adopted.[10] Unfortunately, the power delegated is not likely to be specifically for control of planning implementation—but rather to control activities in the field being planned for—and has serious potential for decreasing planning capacity. In California, for example, some of the lawmaking, regulatory, or adjudicatory functions which were thrust on health planning bodies need not be regarded as an obvious part of the planning efforts required.[11] All of the functions to be described under this role assume that the legislature has delegated adjudicator, regulation-making, and decision-making authority to health planning bodies.

Establish findings on needs. Determine, from planning assessments and derived goals, the targets to be striven for, and what more is needed of specific services in specific areas. Establish those as the regulations to be met.

Establish criteria as law. This function, as much as any others under this law-making role, relates to ensuring that planning criteria are adhered to in any changes made in the health sector. However, the criteria here are not the broad, general kind called for under priority setting; rather they are composite, simplified, and fairly specific measuring sticks, such as full coverage, accessible within so many minutes, at maximal per capita annual cost, and so on.

Determine eligibility and compliance. Review those performing or desiring to perform services, to learn whether they meet capability, quality, quantity, promised coverage, and so on, in order to determine their fitness to continue, retrench, discontinue, enlarge, or enter other service arenas.

Adjudicate between competitors and alternatives. Consider which competitors seem most suitable to service a given need. This may amount to weighing which alternative will best cover a need; this decision may of itself then determine which competitor(s) still remain in the field.

Approve permits to fill needs. Review needs with those applying to fill them and issue approval accordingly.

Adjudicate complaints, hear appeals. Provide for public hearings between consumers and purveyors, purveyors and purveyors, planning body decisions versus consumers or purveyors. Act as an appeals body to revise plans or decisions within the legal scope of the planning body. Act as an airing point for concerns beyond immediate capacities as decision maker, and transmit any matter felt to be of concern to the appropriate planning and decision-making centers.

Self Survival

Looking Good. Take every opportunity to look interested, to be helpful, effective, friendly, and above all, to exert effort to make the public aware of this "fine agency."

Something for everyone. Look for problems and then for solutions in such a way that all significant interests apparently receive current, visible benefits. The long-term significance of this approach need not always be unfavorable.

Build a constituency. Undertake solution of major concerns for large public groups that carry votes, or power, or both, and be reconciled to be guided by them in return for their vigorous support.

Bridge schisms. Reconcile conflicting interests in a way that encourages all parties to seek out the planning body as an arbitrator as soon as they feel aggrieved. This position is difficult and Solomon-like, but need not interfere with long-range planning.

Popularize the "rules of the game." By involvement, commitment, publicity for successes, and exposure stressing the democratic, rational, and moral nature of the planning process, convince the public that the work of the health planning body is critical to the goals of improving health or of establishing equity in the receipt of care.

Broaden participation. Much as the doctor's office is often the locus of a patient's search for a concerned listener, so the planning body can—with proper exposure, use of committees, involvement of groups—become the place where all those concerned with health and health care issues get an intelligent, satisfying, and helpful hearing.

Become indispensable. If and when the body becomes effective it will—through its recorded deeds and the achieved results—have made itself indispensable.

Expander of Capabilities

This role could be the outcome of a composite of many, if not all, of the prior ones, but it deserves a place of its own because of the sense of direction it can impart. It may, in fact, be important enough to deserve being placed among the "Purposes of Planning."

Expand society's operational capabilities. The successful planning body should expand society's area of capability in the field of operations for which it is to provide leadership. This extension of societal maneuverability can best be illustrated by contrasting the social significance of the activities of the comprehensive planning body for health with those of the popular ad hoc official and voluntary committees set up—for lack of a planning body—to study and formulate recommendations in a given area of concern. Such synthetic planning groups are commonly known as blue ribbon committees, others as legislative study or interim committees. Usually, all of the special interests (and a few of the general ones) are represented on such bodies, or a point is made of seeing that they present testimony. Staff for the committee is limited in terms of career job opportunity; it is sometimes borrowed; often it is nonexistent. The committee is charged to come up with a proposal, but rarely is it requested to develop alternatives, amplified with the projected costs and consequences of each. In spite of the historic utility of blue ribbon committees, what often takes place in their work is the pitting of one special interest against another. This sort of a girdling set of forces may result if each special interest presents its own case with its own data which negates those of the other proposals, so that all forces tend to agree only on a minimal solution that is mutually the least disadvantageous. Too often, the works of such bodies result in monumental straining and striving, with much imput but little or no output. On occasion, it is a runaway for one or another interest that can achieve a coalition that overcomes opposition irrespective of social values, benefits, or losses. The special ad hoc committee is a device which often limits society's operational capabilities to patching the status quo, and it often constitutes a very dubious substitute for planning. It often sets the stage for majestic reversals of direction or for stalemating of progress at a later date.

Contrast the above situation with the work of a planning body dedicated to analyzing the systems of concern, proposing alternatives, and figuring out their direct and indirect costs and consequences—all this with the assistance of a widely representative board and an open forum for all interests. Certainly, the special interests must be present; but in such an environment, the presentation of their preferred options is likely to be worked out better than they could have done for themselves. At the same time, the costs and the consequences of these and other possible options are determined. The mixes that are being considered for priority take into account all important losses and gains; and, where overall gains are the guiding principle, losses can be recognized and means devised to overcome inequities. Special interests will have had ample opportunity to participate in the planning; given sufficient warning, they will be able to change direction if necessary. Plans will not be designed that casually destroy legitimate vested interests; every business has assets, employees and beneficiaries to be taken into account as part of the nation's wealth. As a result of impartiality, partisan drives for special positions will be minimized or blunted, open as they are to comparative scrutiny by planners and public who have before them all the significant alternatives created by the planning body. Modern comprehensive planning bodies create the expectation that they should be able to expand society's ability to achieve equitably what its members want, at less cost and with less trial and error.

Expand individual operational capabilities.   The planning process also offers each participating individual an opportunity to change his perception of himself, his needs, his organizational affiliations, and his spectrum of choices, both of wants and of ways to proceed. By involving a greater diversity of people in consequential community decisions, particularly at the local and sublocal levels, health planning can have an important impact on the quality of public participation by individuals. The following are some of the effects participation in community-level planning might have on citizens:

Make more individuals aware of their roles and of the possibility of altering them through planned change and, even more immediately, through taking part in planning (feelings of capability as a result of participation).

Make more individuals aware of what social and societal[12] planning can offer in the way of tangible program, citizenship obligations, and the legitimacy and the feasibility of redistributing power and creating new capabilities.

Make more individuals aware of new information about current achievements, trends, probable and conceivable achievements, and outcomes.

Make more individuals aware that choices are an exercise in integrating values, desires, and technology, thereby introducing them to ways of modifying currently held values.[13]

Make more individuals aware of how to utilize organizational, inducement, and incentive approaches as well as the customarily accepted conflict or coercive techniques to achieve change.

Help people perceive the possibility that they can formulate and modify personal goal choices that go beyond specific shortrange means-ends schemes, thereby bringing more directional consistency to their own endeavors.

Help people become aware of the continuity, the permanency and the genuine inseparability of the physiological, emotional, and functional unity common to all men, and at the same time increase their comprehension of the origins of different cultural and behavioral responses among men.[14]

ROLE-IMPLEMENTING ACTIVITIES OF A PLANNING BODY

Specific activities of a planning body—the daily visible chores—are the means whereby the functions are carried out and the roles effectuated. The distinction between a function and an activity is open to debate. As I use these terms, a function does not or need not specify the tool or method used to achieve it, whereas an activity tends to be either a name for or a description of the use of the tool or method which achieves a function. The use of some tools or methods practically specifies certain functions and so, activities and functions may be hard to keep separate in discussion. In practice, such distinctions may be pointless if the function is understood and is being achieved to the degree desired.

A given activity can often be seen as serving all three described purposes of planning, and any given activity may serve a great number of functions and many roles. Thus it is desirable to consider any or all of the extensions of an activity, for it may commit a planning body to other functions and roles which were not intended or desired.

The Forum

One activity or technique is so important to almost all the roles that it deserves independent treatment. Providing a forum may be considered the mainstay of the Educator Role. I see the forum as serving all health-related issues and all elements of the community, allowing for the exchange of information, beliefs, and viewpoints among politicians, government departments, technologists, elitists, special interests, and consumers. The most significant activity of the planning body could be providing a forum.

Utility for Politicians and Government Departments

Established units of government, elected executives, and governmentally operated agencies, facilities, and services are seen as depending heavily on planning bodies to provide a neutral forum. In such a setting they can exchange more freely the views, concerns, needs, early premonitions, and tentative positions that may be difficult or treacherous to express from their own offices without prejudicing future votes, positions or administrative prerogatives. Although a governor or legislator is expected to make informal policy presentations to the press, when an agency administrator does so, he is often perceived as attempting to take advantage of his position to prejudice or special-plead a situation.

An elected chief executive, such as a governor or a strong mayor, can exercise his leadership role to deliver messages (particularly tentative ones) to the planning body. These will not be offered in quite the same fashion as messages directed to the legislature or to the press, where anticipated interpretation about support or opposition can influence what is said. Legislators face the same problems of finding nonthreatening forums where they can try out their views and listen to differing viewpoints in a situation where their vote is not being counted.

Few agency people now have means of asking questions or trying out answers for public reactions, except indirectly through news releases or trial balloons released by others. When questions or answers are tentatively voiced in public, the agency spokesman runs the risk of being seen as a fool if later he finds reason to change his mind (although this may have been the very reason for putting forth a tentative gesture). But, can agency executives always be expected to put forth fullblown, wise proposals on the basis of an initial tussle with a problem, realizing as they do that many other unidentified persons might make significant contributions?

Government agencies would presumably be happy to have a planning body through which their data, questions, opinions, and recommendations could be channeled to the public. If the planning bodies are legitimate and carry the brunt of putting the pieces of the future together, it would be difficult for either the elected executive or the legislature to order operating agencies to keep silent. Perhaps planning bodies offer agency heads with professional competence and pride the long-awaited advantages of a public podium.

Another difficult situation could be served. The numerous legislative bodies in any locality overlap partially and segmentally both in territory and function. And so they need a common meeting ground where, in the presence of planners and other interests, meaningful resolutions can be worked out without putting legislators on the spot by forcing them to appear publicly before another legislative body in any kind of negotiating posture.

All of us have had the opportunity of participating in a forum built around one or another issue and have observed the often remarkably candid participation of policy-makers and agency heads. Politicians and public agency administrators may enjoy the implicit freedom from "being counted" while thinking out loud with their constituents, and the chance to explore their own feelings in a reality-testing situation. A planning forum can serve as a permanent arena for such discussions.

Utility for Technologists, Elitists and Special Interests

It is hardly necessary to dwell on the special attributes of each of these groups, for they have many characteristics in common. They are all accustomed to having the ear of the politician, but seldom do they either talk or listen to the people who elect the politicians. The viewpoints of elitists and technologists as well as those of the well-organized and financially lubricated special interests will, of course, be forcefully pressed upon the planning body—with or without the presence of a forum. The special interest, private, and voluntary agencies in particular will bring to the forum the opinions, positions, and desires of the organized segments of the community and those of the professional groups and societies. These groups are in the forefront of the causes, and they are often the possessors of the hands, brains and technologic as well as traditional political knowhow. However, without a forum, other groups (such as consumers) will have difficulty in asking questions about the data, prognoses, or advice received from elitists, special interests, and planners.

Utility for Consumers

Consumers are the vast majority of the population—people who have no clear voice in government or policy formulation, either directly as individuals or through organizations in which they have significant voice. Today there is no simple way for the ordinary person to have his views on public issues heard by the legislature or administrators. Moreover, a high proportion of individual or group presentations made directly to a chief executive, a legislative committee, or a department are interpreted (or misinterpreted) as being critical. If the attendance of the press has been requested, no doubt remains in the minds of those about to hear the consumer presentation that the parties making it mean to be prejudicial or intimidating. If the presenting consumer goes to the press as his first step, his hostile intentions are presumably even clearer and his future reception by those in policy-making or serving positions is tailored accordingly.

How does someone without status go about presenting to the community a view of problems or ideas, new or old, critical or commendatory, without being labeled as a friend or foe, prejudiced without hearing, usually on the basis of how or to whom he makes his presentation? If planning bodies serve as a forum for the public, a marked improvement should occur in our ability to communicate meaningful suggestions and queries to one another.

The benefits of receiving information or statements of minority positions or outlooks will probably come about only if the forum function is highly developed and publicized. In particular, individuals within the community who have not organized have nowhere to present information they possess. To provide them with an opportunity to be heard may be of considerable consequence when the attitudes and receptiveness of any particular grouping of such individuals are in question, because the possibility of their future participation may be at stake. Not only does the forum provide a meaningful audience of planners, it also allows minority views to be brought out where they can be scrutinized and discussed before plans are formulated. In addition, persons or groups presenting their views can usually be persuaded to listen to the problems of others as well as to participate in the implementation of plans, when they see their own contributions helping to shape the community.

Although blocked or bypassed communications are often blamed when community political processes break down, common experience shows that no real attempt to communicate or encourage communication with the politically less organized is made in public life. Sporadic attempts at times of crisis are of little value. The longwinded and longworded facade erected by the sophisticated and the technically trained is a familiar barrier which infuriates the less well-educated and the plain-spoken who cannot get a question across or elicit an answer that seems relevant. In turn, consumers may appear to be obtuse, abusive, and stubborn about an issue that the sophisticated are sure they themselves understand and have already explained away. Long practice and much goodwill are needed before the haves and have-nots can talk together meaningfully.

Utility for Community Communications

The planning forum engenders an awareness and an understanding of the origins and beliefs held by others out of which new values can develop. As pointed out in Chapter 2, value systems—with their dual origin in tradition and in current life environment—commonly conflict even within a single individual. Ideologies based on "tribal" value systems may quite literally call for the elimination of persons with different characteristics. Only by repeated exposure, and by quarreling over rights, values, and how each person or party arrived at the position he now holds, can each of us learn tolerance. Interaction at both the intellectual and the gut level may, of course, lead to polarization, but this is already happening and can hardly be an argument against bringing together people who hold different values. The forum setting, in which a search is begun for solutions to meaningful problems of community health, offers at least the possibility for resolution of conflicts. If confronting the issues that keep us from enjoying reasonable levels of health results in successful discussions, new common values will emerge and new ways will be developed to achieve them through joint effort.

The planning forum teaches the art of participation and renews the sense of community. Although socialization among groups goes on in all walks of life, people from different social groupings rarely meet and participate in satisfying activity across the boundaries that usually separate them. Participation in the broad concerns of a community at the city or neighborhood level, even at the regional, state, or national level, is usually seen as a tug-of-war. Whatever one group wins, another expects (often justifiably) to lose. The individual sense of concern for general well-being has been vitiated or divorced from effective action.[15] If complex, intertwined issues can be discussed in a situation freed from the threat of limited partisan action, the sense of community enjoyed by the citizens of an earlier American democracy may be reawakened.

Utility for Conflict Resolution

The planning forum creates a multiplatform stage for working out resolutions of traditional community conflicts, particularly those relevant to planning for health and well-being on a community level.

Conflicts over who should have the major say in making formal health policy go on continuously among the professionals (technologists in or out of government), politicians elected to help establish policy, lay groups, and special interest groups. Each group has its own view of what the problem really is and its own convictions about why the remedies do or do not work. Without a public forum, these four groups have no meeting place and no opportunity to try out their views, each with the other, to work toward applicable and acceptable solutions.

Conflicting interests between different levels of community are perennial sources of political campaign material. Conflicts occur between state and regional interests, between regional and local interests, between local and sub-local interests, and often all of these are in conflict with the federal government. There is little doubt that neighborhood interests have too often been ignored, that metro-level planning seems more necessary than ever, and that new opportunities are at hand for citizens to work together with federal support through Public Law 89-749 and Bureau of the Budget Circulars A-80, A-82, and A-95.[16] It becomes possible now by means of the planning forum to override current political boundaries and traditional state inertia in tackling urban problems and multijurisdictional questions, thus enabling self-fulfillment at various levels of community.

Ideological conflicts continue between proponents of the idea that government must take the lead in providing needed services and those who would rather do without such services than see government strengthened. The battle over private versus public control usually precludes the kind of joint endeavor between government and private interests that might bring about far-reaching changes in service patterns. The Hill-Burton Act of 1946 at least showed the way, but many communities, and physician groups in particular, fought off for over a decade this attempt to bring in partial public financing of health facilities. New trends in joint venturing between large industries and government, begun in World War II, are spreading to make new patterns of cooperative enterprise in the health field a very viable alternative. They probably need the opportunity and spotlight of the public forum to become a significant reality.

Ideological conflicts smoulder and occasionally flare over the concept of community planning. Planning itself has been suspect in some quarters as a symbol of the total government control associated with the communist countries and their five-year plans. Only recently has there been wide acceptance of the idea that all significant enterprise—public, private, or personal—calls for planning if goals are to be successfully chosen and attained. Nevertheless, conservatives still see planning as socialism and, realistically enough, realize that individual options for future enterprise will be limited by long-term community commitments created and supported by public interest. Extensive publicly authorized forums with dignified purposes may be a means of exchanging views and calming fears.

Conflict has not died out among the various segments of the tax-supported health system and between various health agencies or groups in the private subsector. The bitter infighting on both public and voluntary sides has blocked internal cooperative effort and has prevented the two from coming together in support of broad health issues. The county hospital is often the enemy of the county health department, while both ignore or fight off or try to absorb a mental health program or a rehabilitation program which may derive authority from the state or from a combination of voluntary and public efforts on the local level. In the private subsector, agencies or facilities compete with one another for funds, for community prestige, and often for a particular segment of the consumers. Organized medicine has done battle against group practice, and even with the principle of health insurance. The vicious fight between public and private health interests is only now beginning to subside, as both sides condemn segregated care for the poor and urge government as the producer of segregated care to give way to government as the consumer of privately produced health services in behalf of those who cannot pay for care. Only in the spotlight of a community forum can these issues be resolved.

Conflicts, of course, exist within the health professions. Typical of this internecine warfare are the battles between specialists and general practitioners, and the struggle to control hospital admission standards and practice privileges (which results in large numbers of doctors without hospital connections). The skill lines, drawn by professions, are further hardened by state professional examining boards. For example, in some states a dental hygienist may not look into a child's mouth without the express individual authorization of a dentist. These nonsensical boundaries in turn are frozen into civil service and union job descriptions. Only in recent years has there been professional admission of the shortage of primary care physicians or dentists, or any acknowledgment that lesser levels of skill, so superlatively used in Europe (midwives) or in our armed forces (corpsmen), might make a contribution. This compartmentalization is tied in with the apparently inevitable desire of most skills for professional status, a drive which is forever directed toward excluding those without a special brand of training, setting up new requirements, and building higher fences—a lengthy farce which is antithetical to planning. The planning forum will bring into the open the public's stake in resolving such matters.

Utility for Generation of New Solutions

Because the planning forum generates broad public interest and creates new channels for dissemination of information, many more people than those who actually attend planning meetings receive the information presented. Moreover, the broadly representative nature of the planning body sets up a potential network reaching into the community. Because of the extent and diversity of persons participating, the forum function may elicit and even stimulate ingenious and imaginative approaches to health problems, bringing into view heretofore unimagined possibilities for intervention and high payoff. The combination of nonprofessional and specialist participation tends to break down rigid thinking and encourages innovation. In addition, the systems analysis approach pictorializes the factors relevant to each problem and suggests the points at which interventions can be made to intercept movement toward an undesirable outcome. Bringing together people who do not know the traditional answers, the experts who do, and groups actually at risk who desperately need answers drives the discussion onto untraveled ground.

There is sufficient reason to believe that public debate over how to meet health needs, even creation of public awareness of the existence of those who are shorted in health care, will create an environment in which we can get past the initial stage of blame and accusation and can focus, not on facesaving panaceas, but on using our prized American ingenuity to cope with the problems at hand.

Hazards of the Forum

A number of hazards built into the forum approach have already been indicated. Some people have raised the issue that the kind of responsible public involvement described would make planning into a new base of power and would threaten current power centers—surely the legislative, the executive, the administrative, and the technologically oriented,[17] perhaps even those built on poverty or minority-group interests. If this is so, what has been envisioned for planning might soon be scotched by these traditional power centers, singly or in coalition. However, this fear seems farfetched, for P.L. 89-749 was adopted by the Congress and has been promulgated by bureaucrats and professionals alike, with full knowledge that the law is geared to massive consumer participation, increased rationality in decision-making, and to returning some power to local levels of government and generally, to more people.

VARIOUS PLANNING MODES OR OUTLOOKS EMPHASIZE DIFFERING COMBINATIONS OF PURPOSES, ROLES AND FUNCTIONS, AND EXCLUDE OTHERS

As was explained in Chapter 2, most modes or types of planning depend on a particular outlook or concept of the purposes or uses of planning, and build accordingly. A brief review of some of the more commonly discussed planning modes reveals that each is typified by an emphasis on particular collections of the roles and functions which we have outlined as being available to planning bodies. Sometimes a mode is concerned with scope—the breadth or narrowness of the work; other modes emphasize particular stages of overall planning operation, such as the program aspects of planning; another mode concentrates on time span participation, and so forth. Most modes or outlooks dictate the use of certain roles, functions, and even activities to carry out their emphasis on a purposive theme and thereby emphasize the overall planning thrust, such as allocative, participative, or advocacy planning.

The value system of the planner and his clients is the basis for the choice of outlook emphasis, which in turn leads to use of various measuring devices and to acceptance of the constraints built into that outlook. When certain tools, such as cost-benefit, are used, they preclude some planning options and open up to others.

A Sampling of Well-Known Planning Modes and Outlooks

Figure 9.2 shows over 80 of the terms in common usage to describe some 50 distinguishable, but often overlapping planning modes or outlooks. They are grouped into eight categories according to what seems to be the major orientation or most critical attribute of the mode, although many of the modes do not truly belong in just one category. The categories chosen do not fall along a continuum of any particular attribute. But taken together, they do point out some of the major role emphases that have activated the skills of planners.

Some of the categorizations may seem rather arbitrary. Nevertheless, perusal of the *adaptation* orientation produces, for example, a group of outlooks or modes that have as their dominant theme the idea of making do, coping with, or overcoming adverse situations. Moreover, this set of outlooks is generally expressed in terms of what the present offers or the past has brought. The span of the *boundaries* category may be even harder to manage intellectually. Concepts of integrating across or keeping issues separated behind intellectual, geographic, and sectoral boundaries are all included in that category.

Unfortunately, there is much confusion over terminology. Although the approaches attributed to *normative* and *function* modes in the *idealistic* category are all considered to be normative, the appellation may, in fact, be a bit far-fetched for many *mission, target-based* or *substantive* plans. In addition, many terms are used for totally diverse purposes—*strategic* being used in two widely different senses. My term *developmental* speaks to a particular broad comprehensive approach to planning, elaborated on in Chapter 2, that is quite different from development planning directed to growth and change of developing countries. The mode known as *comprehensive* in United States health circles (P.L. 89-749) is often indistinguishable from *national* as used in WHO circles.[18] Moreover, the term *national*, when used in the United States, speaks to planning either done by the federal government or for the entire nation. Hopefully we have not added any new confusion in our attempt to compare, relate, and categorize the various planning outlooks with which we all have to contend.

FIGURE 9.2
TERMS IN CURRENT USAGE TO DESCRIBE PLANNING MODES
(grouped by dominant theme)

I. *Adaptation, also a Heavy Present and Past Orientation*
   Laissez faire, non-planning
   Cooperative
   Coordinative
   Problem Solving (Disjointed Incrementalism), diagnostic-inductive
   Reactive (directed against events), counter
   Adaptive, accommodative, contingency, reactive (alerted by events)

II. *Future and Intellectually Interventive orientation*
   Ad hoc opportunism
   Allocative, comprehensive, balanced, projective
   Resource based
   Economic development
   Explorative, prognostic
   Experimental
   Heuristic
   Exploitive, opportunistic
   Stimulatory

II *Idealistic or Value Promoting, as Well as Future Orientation*
   Deductive, problem solving (articulated and guided)
   Innovative, unbalanced, strategic, creative, contingency
   Normative, anticipatory, directive-prescriptive
   Function, product, mission, target based, substantive
   Ecologic, ideational, utopian
   Total, totalitarian

IV. *Client or Participative Orientation*
   Participative
   Advocacy
   Nondirective, indicative
   Elitist
   Egalitarian
   Top Down
   Bottom Up

V. *Control Orientation*
   Inducement
   Command, prescriptive, coercive
   Regulatory
   Administrative, program, managerial, operational
   Centralized
   Decentralized
   Fiscal

VI. *Time Span Orientation*
   Short range
   Middle range
   Long range

VII. *Implementation Oriented*
   Action
   Strategic (in sense of achieving adoption)
   Evaluative

VIII. *Boundaries Orientation*
   Comprehensive
   Developmental
   Integrative
   Macro
   Micro
   Regional
   Sectoral
   Segmental
   Middle Bridge

Following, in alphabetical order, is a brief description of the various modes, in terms primarily of their dominant emphasis or general outlook.

Accommodative.[19] Focuses on coping with problems as they occur; not unlike *disjointed incrementalism, short range,* but most like *adaptive.*

Action.[20] Dedicated to implementation as the critical purpose of planning, but not necessarily focusing on the strategy aspects of how to obtain the implementation; assumes that planners will not plan in terms of turning their product over to decision makers or wash their hands of it at this point.

Ad hoc opportunism.[21] Moves towards present goals only when an inexpensive opening or opportunity presents itself.

Adaptive.[22] Alert to parameters, constraints, higher level control, opportunistic to present opportunities; a response to externally induced developments; similar to *accommodative* and *reactive* (responds to) and corresponds to a good many attributes of *problem solving;* sometimes is used quite differently to mean *innovative.*[23]

Administrative. Same as *managerial* or *operational.*

Advocacy.[24] Generally meant to be client oriented in that client needs or concerns create the priorities; may also be for a cause.

Allocative.[25] Focused on obtaining the most marginal gain from marginal increment of investment societally; also used in the sense of balance or equilibrium and interrelatedness and gradualism between various needs and sectors; same as *balanced.*

Anticipatory. Same as *normative.*

Balanced.[26] Concern with reasonable advancement of all sectors, bringing up the retarded ones and slowing up unnecessarily advancing ones; like *allocative.*

Bottom up.[27] Planning and goal setting for specific or local issues are used as the basis on which broader or higher level goals and plans are built.

Centralized. Done at one central seat, presumably the key political center of the given community—by the city council for the city, or by the national government for all sectors of endeavor and all regions of the nation functioning under it; at its apogee it is national planning for everything by the national government—not unlike *total.*

Coercive. Same as *command.*

Command.[28] Utilizes sanctions to create enforcement of what has been prescribed.

Comprehensive.[29] May be used in the sense of *allocative* or *balanced;*[30] also commonly used in health circles today to encompass all the forces which affect the health status of a given group or population; although it must reach well beyond health care and work with other sectors of endeavor, health remains the focus; this mode takes a broad view compositing long and short range, regional and sectoral, normative and incremental, bottom up and top down; I have called a variant of it *developmental;* sometimes used quite differently to mean *total.*

Contingency.[31] Similar to *adaptive,* but the focus is on creating conditions whereby effects of contingencies or unforeseen crises can be deflected or absorbed at minimum cost or inconvenience; borrows from ideas of safety factors and insurance. Also similar to *fast track.*

Cooperative.[32] Joint study and agreement for action between related parts of the sector for any kind of endeavor; generally a provider created and oriented effort related to improving the capacity of providers to do what they want.

Coordinative.[33] Joint study and agreement for action between related parts of a sector for any kind of endeavor, generally a provider created and oriented effort related to creating new capacities or products as the result of joint efforts by providers.

Counter.[34] Focus on countering other existing or emerging plans; also used as similar to *reactive* and *accommodative* in the sense of reacting against situations and events.

Creative. Same as *innovative.*

Decentralized. Done at many centers, such as by sectors of endeavor or by regions or by segments within a given community or society; the opposite of *centralized* or *total;* not necessarily coincident with so-called political ideology. (Communist Yugoslavia has national planning and decision making which, notwithstanding, calls for heavily decentralized planning and decision making.[35])

Deductive.[36] A goal or set of goals from which a plan is deduced and put down as a blueprint even before the first steps are taken toward its realization; to reach overall goals, it tends to concentrate on simple cause-and-effect relationships and highly directed programs to control them; focuses on the whole and derives the parts necessary for achievement. Partakes of normative.

Development.[37] A politically oriented, technological effort directed to develop, mature, mobilize, and utilize resources (achieve a high rate of cumulative investment); used particularly in terms of a developing country. "The concept of development is process rather than content oriented and is on that basis to be distinguished from the concept of modernization. . . . Modernization refers to those symbols, products and modes of life associated with modernity . . . which a unit or its members may acquire. . . . Development would refer to the rate at which symbolic content was being accredited."[38]

Developmental. As used in this text, refers to a composite or comprehensive approach to planning, based particularly on an interweaving of normative and articulated and guided problem solving; it is extensively described in Chapter 2, and utilized throughout the book to guide planning.[39]

Diagnostic.[40] Concerned with short-term planning to resolve existing situations and problems; not unlike *problem solving.*

Directive. Provides direction for operating or producing units; may be used interchangeably with *normative;* occasionally used in the sense of *command.*

Economic. Although focusing on increasing the production, consumption, and distribution of wealth, the term generally has become synonymous with *development* planning.

Egalitarian. Focuses on the wide involvement of all kinds of persons and interests to achieve goal participation and opportunity for participation in directing planning and selecting goals; similar to *participative.*

Elitist. Focus is on those persons who carry out the planning and who are thought to have some particular attribute such as knowledge, social status, freedom of vestedness, or heavy investment which qualifies them to direct the planning and select its goals.

Evaluative. Concentrates on evaluating the outcomes of various programs of policies so that results will be available to influence the future.

Experimental. Clearly explorative, but with additional intent to introduce experiments whose results, when evaluated, can be used for guidance in future planning.

Exploitive. Future-oriented and opportunistic, taking advantage of what probably will occur or can be aided to come about.

Explorative. Very future oriented, with its focus on determining what is possible; in that sense sharing some of the *exploitive* outlook; generally governed by a significant *normative* component or direction toward what is desirable.[41]

Fiscal.[42] Planning future budgets; how much money and how to spend it.

Function. Similar to *normative* but generally meant as having a limited area or function, such as good delivery of health care.

Heuristic. Not unlike *experimental,* but with a built-in air of optimism which suggests that evaluation or cultivated serendipity will play a part in providing new insights, and thus guidance for further planning.

Ideational. May be used in the sense of *normative* but also as *utopian, total,* or *totalitarian.*

Indicative.[43] Criteria used to guide outcomes come particularly from currently involved purveyors, and are then used to shape large public planning concerns; private and special interests thus influence the public planning process which comes up with what amounts to a joint planning venture, indicating to purveyors what would seem to be the suitable activities to implement; government plans with, rather than demanding or requiring compliance of private producers.

Inducement.[44] Emphasis is placed on incentives rather than on advice, structure, laws, or sanctions to obtain compliance.

Inductive.[45] Focus is scattered; rests on pragmatic, piecemeal attempts to correct problem situations; similar to *disjointed incrementalism*, but with emphasis on the parts of a system to be corrected.

Innovative.[46] Focuses on a selective resetting of criteria for goals by making values operational; is concerned with mobilization of resources to be guided by feedback from accomplishment; very close to *normative*.

Integrative.[47] Focus is on crossing boundaries of purposes, fields, sectors, or regions to make a more meaningful whole (optimizing).

Long-range.[48] Focus is on events and outcomes to occur ten and more years away; oriented to changing the system as well as to more humanistic goals, so that it partakes of the characteristics of *normative*.

Macro.[49] Concerns are focused on settling larger societal issues as between sectors, between modes of raising and disbursing resources (private versus national health insurance) or between efficiency versus equity issues; also used in the sense of *comprehensive.*[50]

Managerial.[51] Generally constricted to planning for the activity of an operating agency; may include planning for its future.

Micro. Concerns are focused on small, methodologic or procedural issues, but not necessarily restricted to one small operating entity, may include all of the small types of transactions in a large sector.

Middle bridge.[52] Focuses on articulating and guiding short range with long range; similar to *developmental*, as used in the text.

Middle range. Focuses on events and outcomes to occur within five to ten years; not to be confused with *middle bridge*.

Mission. Similar to *normative* and particularly to *target based* modes.

National.[53] Done from or at the national level; done for the entire nation; in terms of health planning, may not necessarily be comprehensive, as it may be limited to health services or just to their financing; at the other extreme, it may include all health concerns as part and parcel of overall national planning for all sectors.

Normative.[54] Focus is on future ideal outcomes, and works back from them to set up plans for today which will enable achievement of the long-range ideals; creation of a desired and desirable image of the future usually over a broad range of concerns, such as for health or all of social well-being, with the intent of changing the behavior and outcomes of the system.

Operational. Same as *managerial*.

Opportunistic. Same as *exploitive;* compare with *ad hoc opportunism.*

Participative. Extensive involvement of all interested or potentially interested parties in decision or various key stages and issues of planning; may extend to include heavy involvement in all aspects of the planning process.

Policy planning. Same as *normative.*

Prescriptive.[55] Criteria used are more societal and for long-term idealized "goodness" as seen by some general rather than exclusively involved group; planning is made to conform to larger plans so that it prescribes to all significant involved interests; close to *normative;* may occasionally be used in the sense of *command.*

Problem solving.[56] Exists in two versions; one, disjointed incrementalism, plans for each problem by itself (similar to *diagnostic*); another version is guided and articulated (see Chapter 2) and begins with problems, relating them to long-term societal goals and to all factors influencing the problem.

Product. Same as *mission* or *function;* shares a sense of being *normative,* but is restricted to a given product such as landing on the moon or delivering care to an underserved group.

Program. Same as *managerial* and *administrative.*

Prognostic.[57] Concerned with the long-term issues of reaching specific desirable states; similar to *explorative.*

Projective. Similar to *allocative;* assesses and determines where we go from here; may also have elements not unlike *exploratory.*

Reactive. Alerted by events or directed against events, similar to *accommodative;* also used in the sense of directed against other plans, and the same as *counter.*

Regional.[58] Concern with balanced growth between the regions of the country, continent or the terrestrial world; sometimes narrowly construed to give the opposite meaning of concern for the balanced growth of all the peoples and sectors inside a region; in either case the focus is on the concept of *balance* between groups.

Regulatory.[59] Restricted to design of key controls so that other planning or operations are guided into some activities and prevented from going into others.

Resource based.[60] Planning from what is, or can be made, available; occasionally used, however, as planning for resources needed, which obviously is very different; somewhat similar to *allocative,* but differs in that resources are the central factor in the *resource-based,* while in the *allocative* mode, balance among outputs is the central concern.

Responsive. Same as *accommodative.*

Sectoral.[61] Concern with balanced growth between the sectors of the economy; sometimes narrowly construed to mean concern within the affairs of a single sector; heavily influenced by the concept of *balance.*

Segmental. Concern for a subunit like a region or subregion or for a sector or subsector; done for each segment as a whole suboptimally, without concern for other segments.

Short range.[62] Focus on events and outcomes to occur within a few years, and generally limits its concerns within the system as it now is; has an efficiency perspective and is also related to *allocative* and *problem solving;* may be *bottom up* or *top down.*

Stimulatory. Concentrating on inquiring, evaluating, and educating functions, without intent to design or produce policy or direction.

Strategic.[63] Used for planning which focuses on those aspects which will ensure implementation; sometimes used in the sense of *innovation.*

Substantive.[64] The planning of objectives, ultimate and intermediate; may partake of much or little *normative*—see *product.*

Target based.[65] Planning towards present targets; same as *substantive* or *product;* has a strong *normative* component.

Top down.[66] Concern with broader societal or national level goal setting done at high levels, from which more locally carried out planning stems for smaller or more local issues.

Total. Concern with all aspects of all concerns, such as we think of when we use the term *totalitarian* planning; infrequently used to describe *comprehensive* or *national* planning.

Totalitarian.[67] Planning undertaken by a dominant or in-power elite who presumably have the interest of the entire country in mind and arrange the planning according to their perceptions of what the best interests are; may be contrasted with *participative* and is often assumed to mean *total* or very detailed *comprehensive* planning, but that assumption does not necessarily follow; also assumed to be highly *centralized,* but in fact may be significantly decentralized.

Utopian.[68] Emphasis on a lofty and broad purpose which can be seen as a magnet, perhaps an unreachable ideal, but nevertheless inspiring and worthy of aspiring; sometimes planning itself is placed in the context of being the good towards which we are to aspire; similar to *ideational.*

Another valid approach to understanding modes of planning is to contrast certain pairs; the contrast helps clarify the key ingredient of particular views or purposes of planning. This is a significant refinement over the categorization approach used in Figure 9.2. Contrasting pairs might include deductive versus inductive;[69] exploratory versus normative;[70] allocative versus innovative (Friedman);[71] command versus indicative;[72] top down versus bottom up (Chapter 10). This listing further strengthens our belief that there will indeed be resolutions rather than polarizations of these contrasting pairs of modes when planners become more deeply involved in the larger social issues raised by concerns for health.

Standards as a Substitute for Planning

Although not included among the planning modes, utilization of generally promulgated standards often represents a mode or an attitude which may be used as a substitute for carrying out much of the process described in the text as being encompassed by planning. However, if one begins in a normative mood and sets goals, drops to a deductive mood and creates criteria which would satisfy or clarify when the goals are reached, and continues on to design, and then to a strategic frame of mind to obtain implementation, the result might well be a day-to-day set of criteria or standards by which proposals and outcomes are to be judged. These indigenous planning-derived criteria must be distinguished from generally promulgated standards. They differ in that much planning was done to fashion these criteria to suit the specific community condition for which the planning body is responsible. The factors of special intent and local design are distinguishing and critical differences between plan-made standards and the standards usually acquired from typically national pronouncements by special groups—pronouncements which may well be irrelevant, if not dangerous, for any given area or group of people.

Length of life or freedom from disability levels prevalent in one community may become the goal and in a sense, therefore, the standard for achievement in another. This kind of standard is often the means by which planning is stimulated, to which it is directed, and by which its success is measured. Using widely accepted standards to describe large goals, therefore, seems much more useful than using standards to describe means of achieving goals. It is particularly this latter use which seems to defeat the purposes of planning, because nationally accepted standards—for numbers of facilities, services, workers, dollars, procedures—are all means which do not necessarily describe ends. To be useful they must vary with the nature of local needs as well as with local capacities and ability to use specified inputs. Therefore, following generally promulgated input or service standards will obviate the need for local planning and may well dispose of all available resources. (See Chapter 6.)

Generally promulgated standards are, therefore, probably most useful when describing a widely desired set of ends or goals, and are, with due concern for their treachery, conceivably of some value as guidance in checking whether local calculations have strayed irrationally in estimating the nature and extent of means needed to achieve accepted goals.

CONSEQUENCES OF FAILURE TO MAKE A CONSCIOUS
SELECTION OF MODES, ROLES AND FUNCTIONS

In my field experience, I have found that planning staffs and bodies rarely announce or identify their planning outlook, and more importantly, are unaware of their choice of roles and functions. Commonly, there is no understanding that alternative possibilities exist; sometimes silence seems to be the result of fear that a public statement would be an academic posture demeaning to men of the world. The easily observable direct consequences of this nonexplicit posture are interesting. In some cases, the state planning agency declares that its intent is to be the servant of the metro and local agencies. Observation often reveals, however, that it undertakes no function that is of use to the local agencies, and moreover, that the state agency often at the same time designs territories and requirements for local agencies which strongly suggest the master or control outlook rather than the avowed servant role. Nothing about any of this is seen as irrational by anyone, although the actual practices are obviously often felt to be objectionable. Roseman[73] points out the discrepancies that occur between what planning bodies claim to be doing, what they are doing, and what they are perceived to be doing.

Horizontal and vertical relationships are fouled up by failure of the planning body to clarify for itself and for everyone else what it means to do and how it is attempting to do it. And internal work often goes around in circles as a consequence. The combination of no output and no sense of utilization of any particular set of roles can, and easily does, discourage constituencies or willing coventurers in planning. Furthermore, a real credibility gap is created as to what purpose is being served, beyond prolonging and confusing the status quo. In the agencies where this situation occurs, improvement is often seen as depending on heavy grants of authority, usually to perform regulatory and control-type functions for which the planning body is even less well-prepared at the staff or board level than for many other roles and functions.[74]

SELECTION OF OUTLOOKS OR MODES OF PLANNING,
AND OF ROLES AND FUNCTIONS

At different times and for different situations, individual planners have found it necessary to concentrate on one or more aspects of the ingredients of planning. For the very reason that each of the planning outlooks has at one time or another been dignified as the centerpiece and name of a mode of planning, it is important to remember that each significant planning venture calls for its own outlooks and set of roles and functions. Granted, its users may be strongly influenced by one of the better publicized modes that have been described. The choices among planning modes are discussed extensively by Friedman,[75] Arnold,[76] Peterson,[77] Bolan,[78] Jantsch,[79] among others.

Mary Arnold[80] suggests that there are many kinds of rationality depending on the kind of problem involved, and I would hasten to add, depending on the situation in which the planning is going on. She utilizes Diesing's[81] five kinds of rationality: logical rationality (understanding of cause and effect); economic rationality (understanding of cost, benefit, allocation, and efficiency); social rationality (understanding of maintenance of social interaction and integration); legal rationality (understanding formally prescribed courses of action); and political rationality (understanding of the nature, place, and actors involved in making public policy decisions).

These additional guidelines to logic help us use our value machinery and our sense of purpose in picking out roles. We can then go another step by exploring when our choice of outlook and roles and functions would vary. Because modes represent an outlook-oriented selection of roles and functions, the discussion inevitably drifts from one element to the next. However, role selection is emphasized as the most significant choice issue.

Outlooks Change Over Time and With Stage of Development

In conversations with Peter Marris I was forced to agree that we commonly had neither the logic nor the rationality to adequately analyze significant health problems or to make intelligent statements of normative goals by which to guide our analytic efforts. To be normative under these circumstances would therefore call for a more heuristic planning mode. True, heuristic planning in this case is solution oriented, but in addition it consciously undertakes design and implementation of intuitively approvable interventions to learn how the system responds to clearly defined and mounted interventions. It thus offers opportunities to learn about the system while proceeding in a way that is approved both politically and socially. This apparently not too highly directed approach may even be necessary for community acceptance of the efforts of a planning body in its early stages. Foreseeably also, mature and sophisticated planning agencies might return to heuristic planning as they approach the limits of what they can accomplish by their goal-guided, problem-solving capacity and their cause-and-effect knowledge.

Modes and corresponding roles that are seriously considered early in the life of a planning body include the cooperative and coordinative, apparently in almost all cases. Constituencies and friends are sorely wanted and inexpensive progress—progress pretty much left in the hands of purveyors—may look good while skills and power still remain with the purveyor. At the same time the short-range and adaptive planning modes somehow also seem to fit the planning body's lack of capacity.

With increasing experience and more professional capacity, the logical move is toward allocative, innovative, middle and long-range outlooks, and particularly to various control-oriented roles to enforce compliance with planning body outputs. New demands and capacities are particularly likely to result in the accretion of an increasingly large array of roles, as the planning body approaches a more comprehending and comprehensive outlook on their very complex assignment of improving health.

A listing of likely requisite tasks for a health planning body as it becomes activated might well begin with such activities as compiling inventories, goal setting and establishment of priorities and timetables. Subsequent activities would include development of review procedures, policy, projections, design of projects, and finally establishment of a comprehensive set of health plans (criteria for system outputs).

Outlooks Change With Needs and Problems

A planning body changes its work as it matures—in great part in response to the needs and the problems of the community served. In addition, these community needs and problems will continue to change for reasons outside and beyond the influence of the planning body. The first problems coming before a planning body are likely to be those which are particularly aggravated. These vary so much from community to community that there is no point in attempting to indicate any probable progression of the needs that will emerge. Predictably, however, a major local shortage of health services, or a frightening level of locally produced air pollution will call for planning modes that emphasize action and problem solving roles, and they may set the stage for adaptive or reactive postures as well as for a controlling one. By contrast, different or shifting needs could easily lead to normative, exploratory, or exploitive emphases, particularly for a planning body with evident capacity which is faced with poorly served people in ill health arising concomitantly with long-term and widespread poverty, bad housing, and educational deficits. The new pressures that occur with change in needs and problems also affect assignment of authority for adjudication, appeals, permits, and so on. Curran[82] questions whether agencies which have adopted roles oriented to goal setting and cooperating will be equipped technically or suited psychologically to add a control set to their armamentarium.

Outlooks Vary With the Level of Community Doing the Planning

Major decision-making processes are formally lodged in state government, as are the state level health planning agencies. However, the majority of local health planning agencies are not based in local government nor are they closely related to it, in most cases. Its capacities, and ultimately the demands placed on the planning body, will vary in accordance with what is perceived as its role in influencing decision making. Of course, these are not the only influences at work in determining role choices at the different community levels. Particularly at the state level (and conceivably at the national level, if any health planning were going on there), pressing demands for allocative thinking will be made to guide budget makers. However, state and national levels also seem to have the freedom and inducement to indulge in normative thinking. Probably all time ranges and many control-type outlooks will be encouraged, demanded, or simply placed on bodies at the state level because of the historic role of states in regulation, licensing, or distributing resources.

At the metro level, where formal government exists minimally in the United States today, pressures towards cooperative, coordinative, and adaptive planning modes and corresponding role assumption may be surmised. At city and county levels, there may be many diverse pulls, but it can be expected that allocative, geographic boundary, short-term and adaptive outlooks will be tempting. At the same time, client-oriented and participative modes will present serious choice problems, particularly when P.L. 89-749 constantly reminds health planning bodies that consumers must constitute 51% of board membership. At the neighborhood level, every conceivable outlook may come into view—from the most normative to the most adaptive, from laissez-faire to stringent control. In other words, the historic outlooks of each level, modified by current needs and the maturity of the planning body, will indicate mode and role selection.

Outlooks Vary With the Planning Environment, Operant Forms, and Institutions

Of the four determinants of social change, two—structure and self-regulation—are particularly operant in determining the outlooks a planning body can or must take. As a planning body looks forward to having its planning made operational, it becomes very cognizant of the political entities to which it is obligated for its existence and for implementation of its plans. This dependence is almost total at the state level, but still very evident to the three local levels of planning agencies who—just because they usually do not have firm ties to formal government—are becoming keenly alert to the difficulties of getting a meaningful hearing from government. The formal public decision-making bodies operating at these three local levels are having no easy time of it, and in turn are beginning to put planning to work in serving the political processes. Uses to which local health planning bodies have been put include: (1) symbolic representation of progress, modernity; (2) mobilization of external resources; (3) redistribution of the relative influence of participants in a diffused power structure (strengthening a political leader or scientist or consumer); (4) helping build a consensus on fundamental values; (5) stimulating an acceptance of development; (6) encouraging counter planning.[83] These clearly call for specific planning outlooks and utilization of various roles and functions by the planning bodies, if they are to meet these expectations while they plan.

Political structure and relationships may well determine whether the implementation or action frame of mind will dominate the planning picture.[84] They will surely be among the major influences determining the control, time, adaptive and future stances of the planning body. Concern with consumer protection and with consumer representation on policy-making boards will also be reflected in the roles chosen by the community planning board.

Outlooks Vary With the Nature and Source of Energy

The remaining two of the four determinants of social change—impetus and mobilization—are most representative of the energy sources and, as a result, heavily influence the planning outlooks or modes to be selected by planning bodies. Elaine Walbroek, coordinator of the University of California Comprehensive Health Planning field studies, has interviewed many executives and board members of planning bodies and has impressed us with the impact made on the modes of planning adopted by planning bodies by the nature and source of energy which brought the body into existence. Although her field data has not demonstrated consequences consistent with the nature or intent of the initiating energy, she has noted several kinds of energy sources that seem to have a major impact on choice of roles and modes of planning. They represent a modification of the notion of entrepreneurship which Peter Marris left with us over several months of recurrent discussions.

Positive sources of energy that have been identified as related to the origins and the planning outlooks of comprehensive health planning bodies include the following:

Desire for money or profit.
Pressure of an apparent goal or opportunity.
Need for services to get something done.
Desire to save money, improve efficiency.

Availability of other related resources.

Presence of coalitions on issues, crises, or community progress.

New social institutional forms made available and attractive.

Desire for personal or group power or control.

Drive for personal or group ego satisfaction of accomplishment.

Strong beliefs about equality, well-being, opportunity, and democracy.

Negative sources of energy can be as effective as positive ones in establishing the style of a planning body. Some of the anti-planning types of energy or motivation observed at work originate in:

Desire to maintain life situation (fear of change).

Desire to maintain institutions (fear of change).

Desire to maintain power or control (fear of loss or of gain by others).

Concern for costs in money, leisure, and so on (fear of loss).

Concern for social standing or prestige whether actual or relative to gains foreseen for others (fear of loss or of others' gain).

Neutral or non-motivated, low-energy positions held by significantly involved interests, surprisingly, may have a bearing on how a planning body comes into being, and may determine its outlook on planning modes and, thus, which roles and functions are undertaken. The neutral or non-energy position tends to be identified with postures such as the following:

Apathy—no wants, no hopes.

No feeling of relevancy.

Never involved before.

Have other more pressing concerns.

Will take planning responsibility on because somebody has to do it.

Why not try it?

Will serve as a compromise choice.

On a case-by-case basis, the mixes of these forces or sources of energy seem to be one of the significant factors in the creation of an indigenous outlook that then determines at least the initial choice of roles and functions made by a planning body.

Outlooks Vary With the Nature of the Problem and the Resources Available to Planners

Cyril Roseman, in discussions of the influences which determine choice of outlooks and roles, has suggested that the very nature of an issue is a significant factor. He pointed out that planning for health, as part of social planning, might be forced currently to take more short-term and highly interventionist approaches. In contrast, health planning as part of planning to take care of demands upon the physical environment might be much more controlling. It is also very evident that when a planning body has almost no resources, it is likely to turn to adaptive or reactive approaches, because it never has the opportunity to map out guidelines such as might be built out of normative or problem solving activities.

DIFFERENTIATION, SYNTHESIS, AND CONVERGENCE OF OUTLOOKS AND ROLES

How can the varying planning outlooks be made to relate to one another as needed? How can they be made part of a coherent, rather than a competitive, fragmenting set of guides? Martin Meyerson advanced the concept of broadening the functions of planning, even at the price of some capacity to carry out, into truly long-range planning,[85] and Ira Robinson recorded ten years of progress along those lines.[86] One broadening purpose Meyerson saw in 1956 was implementation—not the customary project formulation and implementation, but rather a set of currently implementable projects to be guided by long-range comprehension of the wholism to which the projects were contributing. He called this the middle-range bridge. Melvin Webber brought this concept another step along the way. He asked for utilization of the sort of decision-aiding devices that support incremental, multi-centered processes of decision and action, thus expanding the probabilities that decisions would be undertaken more rationally.[87] Meyerson emphasized the following functions: (1) central intelligence and information and analysis (our Inquirer role); (2) pulse taking (also part of our Inquirer role); (3) policy clarification (overlapping our Priority Setting, Policy Planning and Builder of Futures roles); (4) detailed development plan (our Designer of Planning Technology and Coper/Problem Solver roles).[88] He clearly saw the need to bring together correction of urgent hurts on a short-time basis, with a more significant goal seeking or long-range direction of our affairs.

E. E. Schattschneider pointed out that democracy is a competitive political system which can only function well when competing leaders and organizations define public policy alternatives in such a way that the public can meaningfully participate in the decision-making process.[89] If planning is to assist with both the comprehension and the phraseology, so that meaningful and meaningfully different alternatives will be available to choose from, it must repeatedly select and synthesize some of the conflicting, competing, and supplementing planning modes and utilize the roles required by each. Unless it does so planning may simplify and perhaps skillfully eliminate meaningfully different alternative approaches. Without doubt, this attempt to utilize a spectrum of outlooks and roles is placing a Herculean task before planners, but there seems to be no alternative to explicit recognition of the major relevant roles and functions that are involved as a planning body does its homework preparatory to assisting with definition of public policies. It is of interest that changes in styles of planning are now frequently commented on as though they were more secular phenomena than perspicacious choice.[90]

The developmental approach to planning, described in this text, is built on the normative and on the articulated and guided problem-solving modes of planning, but is not restricted to those two modes. It requires understanding and use of many modes, and thus of many roles and functions.

REFERENCES

1. U.S., Executive Office of the President, Bureau of the Budget, Circular No. A-80, January 31, 1967; Circular No. A-82, Revised, January 10, 1969; Circular No. A-95, superseding A-82 after September 30, 1969.
2. Daniel P. Moynihan, *Maximum Feasible Misunderstanding* (New York: The Free Press, 1969). Peter Marris and Martin Rein, *Dilemmas of Social Reform, Poverty and Community Action in the United States* (New York: Atherton Press, 1967).
3. Circular No. A-95, Ibid. No. 1.
4. John Friedmann, "Planning as Innovation: The Chilean Case," *Journal of the American Institute of Planners* 32 (July 1966), 194-203.
5. Henry Fagin, "Organizing and Carrying Out Planning Activities Within Urban Government," *Journal of the American Institute of Planners* 25 (July 1959), 109-14.
6. Paul Davidoff, "Advocacy and Pluralism in Planning," *Journal of the American Institute of Planners* 31 (November 1965), 331-38.
7. Paul Davidoff, Linda Davidoff, and Neil N. Gold, "Suburban Action: Advocate Planning for an Open Society," *Journal of the American Institute of Planners* 36 (January 1970), 12-21.
8. Richard S. Bolan, "Emerging Views of Planning," *Journal of the American Institute of Planners* 33 (July 1967), 233-45.
9. Paul Davidoff and Thomas A. Reiner, "A Choice Theory of Planning," *Journal of the American Institute of Planners* 27 (May 1962), 103-15.
10. William J. Curran, "Are Planning Agencies Ready for Community Decision Making Role?" *Health Planning Perspectives* 6 (December 1970), 1. William J. Curran, "Health Planning with "clout": Certificate of Need Legislation," American Journal of Public Health 62 (1972), 1549.
11. Ibid., p. 1.
12. John W. Dyckman, "Social Planning, Social Planners, and Planned Societies," *Journal of the American Institute of Planners* 32 (March 1966), 66-67.
13. J. R. Seeley, "Central Planning: Prologue to a Critique," *Centrally Planned Change*, ed. by Robert Morris (New York: National Association of Social Workers, 1964).

14. Pan American Health Organization (WHO), "Man and His Environment: Biomedical Knowledge and Social Action," by Rene Dubos (*Scientific Publication*, no. 131), March 1966.
15. Sidney Verba, "Democratic Participation," *The Annals of the American Academy of Political and Social Science* 373 (September 1967), 53-78.
16. Bureau of the Budget, Ibid. no. 1.
17. Guy Benveniste, "Toward a Sociology of Planning," Department of Education, University of California, Berkeley, 1966, mimeographed.
18. World Health Organization, "National Health Planning in Developing Countries" *(WHO Technical Report Series*, no. 350), 1967.
19. John Friedmann, "Notes on Societal Action," *Journal of the American Institute of Planners* 35 (September 1969), 311-18.
20. Ibid., 311-18.
21. R. S. Bolan, Ibid. no. 8, 233-45.
22. Ibid., 233-45. John Friedmann, "A Conceptual Model for the Analysis of Planning Behavior," *Administrative Science Quarterly* 12 (September 1967), 225-52.
23. Russell L. Ackoff, *A Concept of Corporate Planning* (New York: Wiley Interscience, 1970), 6-21.
24. P. Davidoff, Ibid. no. 6, 331-38. R. S. Bolan, Ibid. no. 8, 233-45.
25. J. Friedmann, Ibid. no. 4, 194-203. J. Friedmann, Ibid. no. 22, 225-52.
26. World Health Organization, Meeting on National Health Planning, September 17-23, 1968, New Delhi; Reported SEA-PHA/64, November 18, 1968, 13-4.
27. Ibid., 13-40.
28. J. Friedmann, Ibid. no. 22, 225-52.
29. Naomi Caiden and Aaron Wildavsky, *Planning and Budgeting in Low Income Countries*, (New York: John Wiley & Sons, 1974), Chapter 4.
30. John Friedmann, "The Future of Comprehensive Urban Planning: A Critique," *Journal of the American Institute of Planners* 37 (May 1971), 315-26.
31. R. S. Bolan, Ibid. no. 8, 233-45.
32. Nancy N. Anderson, *Comprehensive Health Planning in the States* (Minneapolis, Minnesota: Institute for Interdisciplinary Studies, American Rehabilitation Foundation, December 1968).
33. Gerald Rosenthal, "Planning, Policy Tools and the Implementation of Health Care System Objectives," Department of Economics, Brandeis University, Waltham, Massachusetts, November 21, 1967, mimeographed draft.
34. Ray H. Elling, "Health Planning in International Perspective," *Medical Care* 9 (May/June 1971), 214-34.
35. Albert Waterston, *Planning in Jugoslavia: Organization and Implementation* (Baltimore: Johns Hopkins Press, 1962).
36. William Petersen, "On Some Meanings of Planning," *Journal of the American Institute of Planners* 32 (May 1966), 133-42.
37. R. S. Bolan, Ibid. no. 8, 233-45. J. Friedmann, Ibid. no. 22, 225-52.
38. Robert P. Biller, "Some Implications of Adaptation Capacity for Organizational and Political Development," Department of Political Science, University of California, Berkeley, 1968, 23.

39. Amitai Etzioni, *The Active Society* (New York: The Free Press; London: Collier Macmillan, 1968), Chapter 12.

40. World Health Organization, Ibid. no. 36, 13-40.

41. Erich Jantsch, *Technological Forecasting in Perspective* (Paris: Organization for Economic Cooperation and Development, 1967), 29-38.

42. U.S., Congress, Senate, Committee on Government Operations, Subcommittee on National Security and International Operations, "Decision-Making in Large Organizations: Planning—Programming—Budgeting, Selected Comments by Charles J. Hitch," 90th Congress, last session.

43. Stephen S. Cohen, *Modern Capitalist Planning: The French Experience* (Cambridge: Harvard University Press, 1970). Gerald Sirken, *The Visible Hand: The Fundamentals of Economic Planning* (New York: McGraw-Hill, 1968), paperback.

44. J. Friedmann, Ibid. no. 22, 225-52. G. Rosenthal, Ibid. no. 33.

45. W. Petersen, Ibid. no. 36, 133-42.

46. J. Friedmann, Ibid. no. 4, 194-203.

47. Erich Jantsch, "Integrative Planning for the Joint Systems of Society and Technology: The Emerging Role of the University," *EKISTICS* 28 (November 1967), 371-80.

48. John W. Dyckmann, "Of Time and the Plan," *Journal of the American Institute of Planners* 28 (May 1962), 141-43.

49. World Health Organization, Ibid. no. 26, 13-40.

50. N. Caiden and A. Wildavsky, Ibid. no. 29, Chapter 4.

51. N. N. Anderson, Ibid. no. 32.

52. Martin Meyerson, "Building the Middle-Range Bridge for Comprehensive Planning," *Journal of the American Institute of Planners* 22 (May 1956), 58-64.

53. World Health Organization, Ibid. no. 18.

54. E. Jantsch, Ibid. no. 41, 29-38. Hasan Ozbekhan, "Towards a General Theory of Planning," *Perspectives of Planning*, ed. by Erich Jantsch (Paris: Organisation for Economic Co-operation and Development, 1969), 47-155.

55. World Health Organization, Ibid. no. 26, 13-40. J. Friedmann, Ibid. no. 22, 225-52.

56. Mary F. Arnold, "Philosophical Dilemmas in Health Planning," *Administering Health Systems: Issues and Perspectives*, ed. by Mary F. Arnold, L. Vaughn Blankenship, and John M. Hess (Chicago; New York: Aldine; Atherton, 1971), 209.

57. World Health Organization, Ibid. no. 26, 13-40.

58. Miles M. Hansen, *French Regional Planning* (Bloomington: Indiana University Press, 1968).

59. N. N. Anderson, Ibid. no. 32.

60. World Health Organization, Ibid. no. 26, 13-40.

61. Ibid., 13-40.

62. J. W. Dyckmann, Ibid. no. 48, 141-43.

63. J. Friedmann, Ibid. no. 19, 311-18.

64. C. J. Hitch, Ibid. no. 42.

65. World Health Organization, Ibid. no. 26, 13-40.

66. Ibid., 13-40.

67. R. H. Elling, Ibid. no. 34, 214-34.
68. W. Petersen, Ibid. no. 36, 133-42.
69. Ibid., 133-42.
70. E. Jantsch, Ibid. no. 41, 29-38.
71. J. Friedmann, Ibid. no. 22, 225-52.
72. World Health Organization, Ibid. no. 26, 39.
73. Cyril Roseman, "Planning Structures, Functions, Roles and Relationships," paper presented at Advanced Comprehensive Health Planning Seminar sponsored by the American Public Health Association, Yakima, Washington, March 30, 1969.
74. W. J. Curran, Ibid. no. 10, 1.
75. J. Friedmann, Ibid. no. 4, 194-203. J. Friedmann, Ibid. no. 19, 311-18. J. Friedmann, Ibid. no. 22, 225-52.
76. M. F. Arnold, Ibid. no. 56, 209.
77. W. Petersen, Ibid. no. 36, 133-42.
78. R. S. Bolan, Ibid. no. 8, 233-45.
79. R. S. Bolan, Ibid. no. 8, 233-45.
79. E. Jantsch, Ibid. no. 41, 29-38.
80. Mary Arnold, "Tools for Planning," *Health Planning 1969*, by H. L. Blum and Associates (San Francisco: Western Regional Office, American Public Health Association, 1969), Chapter 12.
81. Paul Diesing, *Reason in Society* (Urbana: University of Illinois Press, 1962).
82. W. J. Curran, Ibid. no. 10, 1.
83. J. Friedmann, Ibid. no. 22, 225-52.
84. J. Friedmann, Ibid. no. 19, 311-18.
85. M. Meyerson, Ibid. no. 52, 58-64.
86. Ira M. Robinson, "Beyond the Middle Range Planning Bridge," *Journal of the American Institute of Planners* 31 (November 1965), 304-11.
87. Melvin M. Webber, "The Roles of Intelligence Systems in Urban Systems Planning," *Journal of the American Institute of Planners* 31 (November 1965), 289-96.
88. M. Meyerson, Ibid. no. 52, 58-64.
89. E. E. Schattschneider, *The Semi-Sovereign People* (New York: Holt, Rinehart, & Winston, 1960), 141.
90. "Symposium on Changing Styles of Planning in Post-Industrial America," *Public Administration Review* 31 (May/June 1971), 253-403.

10.   Creation of the Means to Plan: Planning Body Organization

Having outlined the many options open to a planning body in the choice, arrangement, and chronology of accepting roles and undertaking the functions and activities to satisfy these roles, we will now consider how the structure and organization of the planning body affect its success in fulfilling its purposes.

THE RELATIONSHIPS OF STRUCTURE AND ORGANIZATION TO PURPOSES, ROLES AND FUNCTIONS OF HEALTH PLANNING BODIES

Preoccupation with organization and structure typified the first three years of activity of the health planning bodies instituted by P.L. 89-749. I believe this emphasis has been a serious strategic mistake and will outline the reasons and the order of the steps I think should have been taken.

A better beginning for health planning would have been made if the purposes of planning had been more clearly identified initially. To repeat, these are: (1) defining improvements and goals desired; (2) securing improvements; (3) measuring improvements achieved. The next most useful step would have been for each planning body to decide on the planning modes it would start with, and then to select the roles it might best assume in order to carry out the purposes of planning for the community it serves.

Purposes determine roles and roles call for certain functions. Thus, logically significant decisions about structure and organization should be among the last made in establishing a planning council, because it must be able to organize itself so as to facilitate execution of the chosen functions. Chandler has made the point well, that structure in the nation's largest business concerns resulted from strategy decisions about their functions and growth.[1] If the choice of structure has fixed a prematurely designed organizational pattern, this pattern may preclude, or at least overlook, the possibility of assuming particular roles, thus retarding the achievement of the three primary purposes as well. If the council is structured before its functions are chosen, it may not be able to carry out many of those functions for which it will opt. Figure 10.1 makes these points diagrammatically.

The planning body obviously must participate at the heart of social interaction, and is not expected to stand apart from its society while it makes plans or develops potential bases for decisions. The planning body must be at the hub of social action, receiving an endless chain of social bits and pieces—demands, feelings, suggestions and informa-

FIGURE 10.1

SEQUENTIAL RELATIONSHIPS BETWEEN PURPOSES, ROLES,
FUNCTIONS AND STRUCTURE

PATTERN I

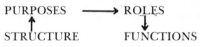

Structure has commonly been set up as the first step in creating a new institution such as comprehensive health planning. Structure tends to shape Purposes, which are then seen as calling for certain Roles. This pattern seems to be the result of "needing" the security of an edifice before defining its utility.

PATTERN II

PURPOSES   ROLES
↑   ↓
STRUCTURE ◄——— FUNCTIONS

Others see Roles and Functions as the starting point and proceed to Structure. Purposes tend to be rationalized from this set of structured and functional influences and are likely to remain unclear. As a result, the choice of Roles and Functions may be illogical or inconsistent and the Structure inadequate to do more than the initial comprehension called for.

PATTERN III

PURPOSES ——► ROLES
                           ↓
STRUCTURE ◄——— FUNCTIONS

Purposes visualized as the starting point are then seen as the determiners of Roles. Roles require that certain Functions be performed. Functions, then, place demands on the Structure of the planning body. This is the logic of setting up a planning body to which we subscribe. Once a Structure is conceived in this way, the probabilities are greater that the desired Functions will be performed. This in turn should contribute to Role success and lead to the fulfillment of the Purposes which gave rise to the planning body in the first place.

Note.—Source: modified from Cyril Roseman, "Planning Structures, Roles and Relationships," delivered at Advanced Comprehensive Health Planning Seminar, Yakima, Washington, March 30, 1970.

tion. From these, the planning body can choose what to analyze, and from its analyses it creates projections, understandable syntheses, and proposals for proceeding. These it delivers back to society for criticism, consideration, and utilization. The criticism or implementation, or both, of these syntheses, proposals, and analyses, and an awareness on the part of the community or special interest groups of new happenings, new perceptions and new desires, result in an enlarged stream of further inputs. The functions undertaken will in great part determine whether the planning body remains at the hub and what it becomes involved with. Involvements in turn require new organizational patterns, if the work and required contacts are to be coped with successfully.

This chain of logic begins with a statement of planning purposes, leads to a choice of roles, and subsequently to a choice of functions. The smorgasbord of functions provides the framework for the planning and implementation of activities. The functions and activities selected will, in large part, determine the most desirable organizational pattern, and thus the basic structural requirements for the planning body.

As satisfying as this logic might seem, several critical flaws would soon appear if it were followed as an absolute guide to structuring and organizing planning bodies. The general purposes remain legitimate. But the precise choice of roles with the attendant supporting functions and activities will probably not be apparent to the planning body as it begins its task. Even with access to a listing of potential roles and functions such as is described in Chapter 9, initially the planning body will have only vague notions as to which roles and functions it might assume. Only after the inquiring role is undertaken can the planning body begin to make decisions about how to select problems for study. As these problems are analyzed, the planning body will be able to separate the issues or forces which lie within its environment but outside of its sphere of direct influence from those which it can influence. From encounters with problems, forces, and relationships which are highly specific to its immediate scope of concern, the planning body will develop an idea of the degree of control desired, how much power it will wish to alter, and the extent of such functions as education or activation it will wish to undertake. Almost every role also indicates the planning body's necessary relationships to its environment.

Obviously, different community problems (as well as planning outlooks) call for different roles. Moreover, the choice of roles probably will vary over time as the planning body pursues goals and problems through the various phases of community alteration which result from the efforts of the planning body. In other words, the demands posed by newly accepted roles will continue to change the shape of the structure.

Of necessity, some enabling power must describe minimally at least basic structures and relationships (although not necessarily organization), before a group, funds, or authority can take form as the planning body which can begin consideration of the issues of roles, functions, or structure. How then does the planning body organize and structure itself within the freedom allotted it by enabling legislation? It should study the roles and functions it is likely to meet (the entire list presented in Chapter 9) and others that come up indigenously. It may see a few that it cannot conceive of ever undertaking, given legal exclusions and local traditions, culture, and beliefs. Therefore, focus should probably be on a minimal initial organization within the legally designated minimal structure, an organization which allows performance of the tasks designated as first order, as well as maximum flexibility so that as new roles and functions come into view, the organization, if not the structure, can be modified simply and rapidly. Needs for different representation, public stances, degrees of control, or education will vary endlessly. And so, organization and structure have to allow for making such changes reasonably expeditiously, unless obstacles are being intentionally inserted. Where enabling legislation has yet to be formulated, it should be framed in such a way as to give the planning body maximal leeway to change its organization and activities as needed, so as to easily include activities that come to be recognized as prerequisite to planning for different issues.

It is intriguing that the legislative rhetoric which set up comprehensive health planning suggests that it is to be the "top" organization, invited to "subordinate" all the existing organizations planning for health. Thus it will probably have to undertake nearly all the roles outlined in Chapter 9. Comprehensive health planning, therefore, presents a special case of fitting organizational structure to a very broad problem area and to particular desirable (purposeful) activities. Ritva Kaje has pointed out that in comprehensive health planning we still have some freedom in designing the formal organization, whereas in most other social problem-solving situations we have to find ways of getting new problems solved by existing old organizations set up for other purposes.

Each of the other issues discussed in this chapter has a bearing on structure and organization, and not all of the forces call for the same forms. Community constraints of a traditional, economic, or political nature may not permit the organizational form presumably best suited to serve all the needs of the planning body.

WHICH CAPABILITIES ARE REQUIRED?

Many capacities might be discussed; I will select only those that have particularly attracted my attention in contacts with health planning bodies. No excuse can justify denying planning bodies the specific means to do the job the community desires. Yet not every capacity will be agreed to, because some capacities are no more than the immediate means to carry out roles which are still highly controversial. The capacity to enforce sanctions is a good example of a far-from-settled role issue.

Contributions from Board and Staff

Health planning bodies in the United States are usually composed of a professional staff and a guiding board. To clarify the operations of health planning bodies it is necessary to indicate the difficulty of separating the functions of the relatively professional planning staff from those of the board or council. Board members may or may not be professional planners or health professionals, but boards have access—as well as claim—to the expertise of most major professional groups as well as to the wisdom that comes from living—whether it be a sophisticated life or one that is little more than a fight for survival. At the state level, a third element enters—a legislatively designated planning agency which employs and directs staff and carries out all the legally imposed instructions. This agency is guided by a policy board or advisory council but is very likely to receive its specific orders directly from the executive or legislative branch, from a joint venture formed by both, or from an operating unit in the state department of health or the state planning department. In each of these situations, direct authority comes from one source—the government—and much of the moral, spiritual or popular guidance comes from an advisory body, which usually has no other governmental functions, even though its membership typically includes a few key figures from the legislative and executive branches. Relationships between the staff, agency, and the board (council), the division of responsibilities, the allocation of power—whether implied, explicit or in doubt—are all of major import to the organization of a planning body.

The general purposes of society in setting up planning machinery are the source of guidance for this agglomerate of staff, board (council), and planning agency, which is called the planning body. The roles selected by the planning body are given tangibility by the functions that the body undertakes. Functions sometimes tend to separate out by whether they are carried out primarily by the staff or by the board (or by the agency, if it is a separate element). Because all local and most state agencies are heavily guided by their council, we will, for purposes of discussion, lump together agency and board as though they were one. However, where they are clearly separate entities, their relationships will vary significantly. Whether the agency, the board, or both jointly take on what can be described as board functions, will depend on their relationships. Figure 9.1 indicates the likelihood that each function will be assumed by staff or board or both, whichever seemed most suitable.

The allocations of functions in Figure 9.1 are only suppositions based on a limited and not totally consistent set of observations— modified, obviously, by the quality, caliber, and capacity of staff and board, as well as by circumstances. If left to chance, many critical functions indicated in Figure 9.1 as belonging to staff or board may fail to be activated because neither the board nor the staff has an explicit assignment or even an understanding that the function needs to be done.

Relationships of Staff to Board

There are two power groups in the planning body: the staff or technologists, who earn their status from their skills and possess the ethics and biases of planners determined to do good planning; and the board, which has no one skill but takes its status from the stature of the appointees who tend to develop the ethics for good health. For the sake of operations, can the titles which seek to separate staff from board be removed and staff and board be assigned to committees and task forces as equals? This seems a futile gesture, because staff usually is left with the basic work load. However, too many agencies preserve an antiquated etiquette that calls for staff anonymity in the presence of board members, and silence at all public or committee affairs, unless staff is specifically called upon.

The reverse situation, in which staff take over, is usually a matter of default where few board members have the capacity or willingness to chair a meeting or a committee. However, in innumerable situations, staff should be highly visible and should conduct meetings on request. Ideally, the partnership would be built on capacity and strengths, not based on formalities or imagined differences of rank between staff and board members. The intricate intertwining of the functioning of staff and board members is most easily brought out in the issues raised by the question: Who are the clients of planners and planning bodies? (The section of this chapter devoted to representation continues that discussion.)

Continuity of Operation

Continuity of operation, including the clear promise of continuity of responsibility and of funding, is essential to modern planning. Feedback can direct planning only if the capability for planning is assured an ongoing status. Notwithstanding its blue ribbon status, a remarkable product was created by the California Governor's Committee on Medical Aid and Health,[2] which tried on a one-shot basis to set up long-range plans for California's role in health services. Many of the conclusions were astute. And the committee's representativeness enabled it to get remarkable support and implementation. But the one outstanding piece of advice in the report went unheeded: Planning needs to be continuous and a planning body must be permanently established. Failure to keep the committee alive and staffed found the state in a tragically retrogressive planning position eight years after the committee expired, which meant that P.L. 89-749 had to start from scratch. A plan is meaningless unless reviewed and recast continuously, and each revision must profit from the knowledge gained from prior successes and failures. The element of continuity applies equally to the budget, a basic cadre of technicians, an ongoing but fluid council membership, and a stable legal vehicle which makes clear to whom the planners relate and report.

Sanctions

Exercise of sanctions, both positive and negative, remains a question in the operation of an effective planning body. This issue has been brought up repeatedly, while evidence has accumulated in support of both favorable and unfavorable views. Some see the authority generated by a planning body as commensurate with its success in representing the interests of the community and as arising from its recommendations which are translated into action. Others ask that the planning body have an initial grant of sanctioning powers so strong that it can exercise authority from the beginning without needing to develop further authority. Where the intent is to enable the planning body to insure that its plans are carried out, the planning body becomes a formal vehicle of government decision making. Even though this grant of sanctioning powers would have come about by legislative authorization, the planners in essence assume the policy-making role. The strongest antagonists to this point of view say that this grant of far-reaching sanctions to planning bodies is nothing less than government by technologists, and foretells the end of the democratic process.

Planning commentators with a stronger health care orientation see no alternative to health authorities which specify criteria of acceptability for health delivery organizations and the products they provide.[3] But in either case, the question must be faced as to how much of the planning output will be lost if another agency is to convert it into operating requirements; or if the planning body does perform the work of an authority, how much planning will it accomplish? This issue is approached from another set of considerations later in this section.

Some quasi-authority alternatives already in existence give planning bodies ready-made vestments of authority. How do these work?

The planning body is frequently given authority to approve or disapprove plans emanating from lesser or more specialized bodies. Similar authority may have been granted to the planning body with regard to proposals for specific projects or undertakings. This authority is not unlike the responsibility given to administrative agencies to license a hospital, license a doctor, or inspect and close a food plant.

In other words, if such powers are legislatively authorized, there is no reason why, under the terms of the authorization, certain areas of discretion cannot be delegated to the planning body. Physical planning bodies usually work this way in relation to physical plans. They also depend on official planning departments, which they advise or partially control, and which do the routine approval or disapproval of projects in accordance with the plans which have been legislatively adopted. Planning body authority and actions relevant to plans are usually subject to ratification by the responsible legislative body which may adopt, revise, or cancel any and all plans, and even revoke the authority of the planning body. At the same time, higher authority is available both to those enforcing the plans and to special interests— the courts may be asked to rule on the legitimacy of the legal basis on which planning or legislative bodies make their findings, or on the legitimacy of their findings. Obtaining access to these judicial processes, however requires a significant investment of cash and persistence.

Another alternative to granting sanction powers is the stipulation, by sponsoring or acknowledging government bodies, that all significant health proposals must be given a public hearing before the planning body. The planning body is then charged with the responsibility of rendering a public opinion on the merits of such proposals. Although without "teeth," the judgment of the planning body often has significance to the public as well as to banks and other loan agencies whose support is often critical in enabling major investments.

Still another alternative is to allow planning bodies to impose sanctions, with legislative review available only if the legislature wants to review their decisions. This option, created by law, is proper, and it is commonly used by legislative bodies as a supervisory tool over functions long since clearly spelled out and assigned to executive agencies or special boards.

Another fascinating alternative source of sanctioning powers came into prominence as a result of legislative and executive actions at the federal level. Federal executive agencies and their branches have, under administrative and congressional prodding, seen the wisdom of coordinating their efforts in any one metropolitan area. They have created their own coordinating center, and require that a broad range of federal well-being and support services—for which national funding is sought locally—be cleared with a locally created, comprehensively oriented metro planning body approved by the coalition of federal agency offices serving the area.[4]

Among the potential hazards of placing power with such groups are the often limited planning capacities and qualifications of metro planning bodies. Skilled health planners are typically not available to them. Their jurisdictional boundaries may be poorly chosen. The planning body may be made up of appointees and of persons elected to local offices not related to the functions of the planning groups. Notwithstanding evidences that the metro planning body may be unrepresentative of either citizenry or the multiplicity of local governments, and that its disapproval of plans and projects may not be binding, the responsibility for approval of plans is a tremendous power in the hands of such a body. No individual, organization, or governmental unit competing for funds will freely antagonize such a body or casually attempt to override it, or there is always the probability of having to come back to that same body with another proposal.

The most dubious features of this federally stimulated source of sanction power for a metropolitan level planning body are the remote origin of its power and, in all but a handful of metros, lack of a policy-making body at the metro level. Hence, control over the sanction power of the metro planning body rests in part with the Federal establishment, in part with the many local government units that make up or sponsor the metro planning unit. What is more, because the federal agencies do not retain the control over this freely dispensed sanctioning power, it is not clear how metro planning bodies, many of which have been haphazardly selected, will utilize their unexpected authority. The hazards that can be conjured up do not, however, leave us without hope of countering restraints. If sanctioning excesses are indulged in frequently enough, or if the planning competency of the sanctioning bodies is not rapidly escalated, we can expect mounting congressional concern as citizens reach their federal legislators with increasingly shrill complaints. Bad metro-level performances may move the citizens to change the composition of such a sanctioning body, even if they cannot get rid of its power to approve local plans and projects which are to be federally funded. Or, possibly, some entirely new alternative, such as the approval of grant applications by state or federal districts or agencies, may be proposed.

It is doubtful that health planning bodies will automatically receive extensive sanctioning powers from on high as have the metro level, all-purpose planning bodies. (See Chapter 11 for the generation of authority by a planning body.) What can be hoped for is the creation of health authorities with a major planning arm and an equal or lesser policy establishing and franchising arm. Responsibility for routine surveillance and control should probably go to the agency now set up to do it—the health department.

Technological capability

A full range of technological skills is required to devise and carry out assessment of health status, resources, services, and unmet and overmet needs. Technological capability is also needed to analyze systems and design models which indicate crucial relationships, thus permitting the invention of the alternative interventions which are the key to planning. Technology is also needed to devise the costs-and-benefits approach to be applied to criteria used in weighing alternatives. Not only is an economics approach required, but also an imaginative input-output psychology which can foresee and estimate secondary and spillover effects. Another kind of skill is needed to begin the implementation phase and the planning for client participation without which the plan may never be adopted, or, if adopted, may never be utilized. Still another set of skills is needed to design the information flows and feedbacks necessary for ongoing evaluation of major outputs.

Such a spectrum of skills is rarely available or purchasable on a full-time basis by any but very large communities. If such skills are to be obtained, it will be necessary to share them among the various planning entities. Because not all of these skills are needed continuously, technicians from operating agencies can be utilized part-time. Or they may be available on a consultant or job contract basis from private (profit or nonprofit), community, and government agencies. Figure 10.2 presents some of the potential strengths and weaknesses of the various ways of assembling staff.

Often, the only sensible way of doing a job is by contracts for special skills or tasks, but there are some dangers in this type of arrangement. Outputs may be heavily geared to the survival of those receiving the contract. Whatever their level of competence and whether they operate for profit or not, the concern of the contract consultants for future use of their services has a bearing on what is done and what is reported, and that concern is all too often apparent in the product.[5] Contracts are an ideal way to get technological supplementation, but a dubious way to carry on a basic operation. As a result of depending on contracts, the contracting agency often neglects to build its own staff capability, which may well impair its ability to judge the products produced under contracts. Outside technologists are probably best used as consultants for limited advice or for specific technical products, rather than for the design of a full plan.

A critical technological capacity of the staff (which should also be available on the board) is the ability to draw out information, attitudes, beliefs, analytic suppositions, and suggestions for handling problems and goal establishment. Although public hearings are highly touted and indeed necessary, they do permit abuse by highly vocal

FIGURE 10.2

EXPECTATIONS OF ATTRIBUTES ACCORDING TO THE SOURCE OF STAFF

SOURCE OF STAFF

ATTRIBUTES	Solely Independent* Agency Staff	Solely from Health Department	Solely from Planning Department	Work Done Solely by Contract with other Organizations	Solely from Private & Voluntary Agencies	Combined Sources
Loyalty	+++	+ −	+ − + − + −	+	+ −	++
Initiative	+++	+ − + −		++++	+ − + −	++++
Responsiveness to Planning Body	+++	−	−	+++	+ − + −	+++
Avoidance of Much Civil Service & Government Restrictions	++	−	−	++++	++++	+++
Freedom from Fear of Legislature	+++	+	+	++++	++++	+++
Health Knowledge	++	+++	−	+++	+	+++
Planning Knowledge	++	+ −	+++	+++	+	+++
Community Knowledge	+	+++	+++	+	+++	++++
General Public Acceptability	++	++	++	+++	+++	++++
Effectivity	+++	+	+	++	+	++++
Efficiency	++		+	+++	+	+++
Freedom from Service Agency Bias	++++	−	++	++++	++	+++

Ratings vary from very high ++++ to low—

* Independent refers to a planning agency which is not a subsidiary of an operating agency nor part of an overall government or quasipublic planning agency such as is developing in many councils of government (COGs).

and often quite vested, unrepresentative, or even irrational voices. The nominal and interacting group process, associated particularly with the name of Delbecq,[6] is a particularly useful technique for any group of up to 75 persons—and perhaps more—who have been gathered to help a planning body set its course of action or work on an issue. This technique—of eliciting participation from every attendee, of avoiding group control by dominating individuals, and of actually extending the quantity and quality of the contributions of group participants—has worked simply and effectively.

Many of the skills which are most valuable for inspiration, for balanced judgment, equity, and reasonableness may never be purchasable, yet be no farther away than board or committee membership. If those who appoint the board for a planning body realize the requirements, many planning bodies can have—at virtually no cost—the highest level of services from demonstrably wise and dedicated community members, at least for a few hours each week.

Freedom of Operation

Freedom of operation, a major capability requirement for the planning body, has many facets.

Freedom to receive, seek out, and consider points of view or expressions of concern from individuals, groups and public bodies.

Freedom to negotiate with organizations, enterprises, governmental bodies and agencies thereof.

Freedom to undertake studies, research, investigations and hearings. (Personal experiences with ill-defined constraints placed on a statewide health facilities planning body have made clear to me that this body was robbed of its ability to make critical decisions. Yet, its active existence led the state to assume that the planning body was doing the meaningful job which, in fact, its members felt they were not allowed to touch.)

Freedom to select non-council members to serve as participating consultants, committee members and witnesses.

Freedom to collaborate with, transmit to, or receive from the various levels of government and planning the tentative or final products of planning.

Freedom to structure itself internally as desired. (Perhaps the most important aspect of this ability to restructure comes into play at the local and metro levels, particularly when permanent or semipermanent subsidiary neighborhood structures for planning are necessary to attract needed information or to create participation.)

Freedom to hire and dismiss staff to maintain the scope and caliber of capacities required.

Freedom to hold public hearings and publicize various alternatives, their costs and consequences. This capability brings us full circle to the educational function described in the first point, and is closely related to the forum function discussed in the preceding chapter. The major problem in this kind of community exposure may be the necessity to make public every aspect of the planning body's records. Naturally, the planning body is not likely to receive certain kinds of data if everything in its possession is open to public and press scrutiny. There is no easy solution to this problem except trial and error. One aspect can get particularly sticky. In the past, implementation and citizen health behavior were not commonly the concern of planners. Therefore, data in this area were not gathered or, if gathered, not analyzed at the visible level. These kinds of data would surely make exciting reading and, when presented at public meetings, would not infrequently blow everything sky high as soon as it could be observed that strategies were being designed to coerce, neutralize, or otherwise remove opposition. (See Chapter 11.) Potential consensus will be pursued by a wise chairman; saliency will be promoted where it can build interest or neutralize potential opposition. Where clear-cut opposition is seen as unavoidable, a facilitating committee—tucked away in an inconspicuous spot, and including some staff along with key council members—will have to decide on the critical strategies to be included in the planning.

Many believe that conflict resolution will go on continuously if planning is done in a comprehensive manner with high visibility and high levels of public participation. As consensus is built by the formation of plans, particularly the middle and long range ones, an occasional dissident group may drop out of some portion of the planning. However, such groups will probably be so heavily involved in other parts of the planning that they will go along without doing more than expressing a minority position. They may, of course, withdraw and attempt to do what they can politically to stop the measure from moving. Because comprehensive planning does not usually hinge on any single, isolated crisis item, opposition to one small part should not be effective on overturning plans. Nevertheless, if every single portion of a comprehensive plan has one small but determined enemy, the aggregate of these enemies might represent a large portion of the citizenry and could halt the whole matter.

Freedom from the influences of operational and supervisory duties. The planning body that is only an arm of an operating agency may find that its planning is a target for interests opposed to the operations carried out by the agency's other arms. Or the operating budget of the parent agency may be threatened because of displeasure over the planning. This double vulnerability is such a major threat to legitimate planning that all the advantages claimed for placing the planning agency in an operating agency[7] are likely to be nullified. Moreover, relevant agency heads need not be excluded from the planning; through open invitation, or preferably through regular or ex-officio representation on the planning council, they can be party to the planning. (See the section on "Representation" in this chapter.) Even the release of a report needs to be done from a relatively secure and separate base, such as a government agency which is free of threat from hidden legislative reprisals that might be made against operational aspects of such an agency's budget. Daniel Bell[8] pointed out similar needs for a social report which, of course, is equatable in great part with the assessment function of planning presented in this text.

Other disadvantages of placing general planning duties in operating agencies include the inevitable inroads made on the think-time of all operational agency personnel to put out fires. Many of the planners would end up with operation duties occupying a large part of their time as well as narrowing the scope of their concern. At the same time, the staff of operating agencies would be hard put to overcome their customary limited field of vision and concern. Only with remarkable personnel can the operating agency be free of bias in scrutinizing its own affairs. An advisory planning council will also have difficulty facing problems that involve the service activities of the planning and operating agency to which it provides guidance. For example, planning placed in the health department may end up in conflict or competition with a board of health which has similar overall citizen advisory functions in relation to the operating aspects of such a dually functional service and planning agency.

The planning body that is itself the health authority—or to be exact, the health authority that has as its major function health planning—can, with proper precautions, keep its planning from becoming an occasional adjunct to its regulatory role. This effort will probably depend on the wisdom of the board and the sources of revenue.

Above all, it seems unwise to put one of the parties to the health delivery system in charge of planning, preparing the agenda, and controlling the direction, quality and quantity of staff planning work. Small wonder if organized medicine and others long hostile to governmental health agencies would find work difficult in such a planning partnership.

Responsibility for Evaluation and Supervision

In addition to the requisite capabilities already discussed, there are several others about which a good deal of disagreement may be expected for some time to come.

Evaluation

One capability on which a decision will probably be made sooner than others is the planning body's obligation—not just freedom—to evaluate the progress being made on the various interventions under way, and on those which arise as a result of partial or total implementation of the planning body's own efforts. Because assessment of the existing situation is a prerequisite for planning, evaluation of the outcomes of current interventions (services and programs) has to be made by the planning body. As a result, the planning body will be the most comprehensively oriented of the institutions capable of doing evaluation. Its major problem will be to get the necessary information. To do so, the planning body will have to include in its plans categorical definitions and descriptions of the kinds of data wanted from both public and private agencies and from individuals carrying out the operations. If its plans are adopted and resources allocated accordingly, information will, of course, start to flow in through the built-in feedback system directed to the planning body itself. (See Chapter 12.) The planning body, whether operating agencies do or not, must be able to see what has resulted from the implementation of the interventions planned. No doubt, many agencies will also study their inputs and outputs by means of these same data, as will special units of governments and grand juries.

Supervision

Another potential capability of planning bodies which may lead to violent disagreement is supervision, or at least the ability of the planning body to look over the shoulders of those who are carrying out plans. It is easy to imagine that an adopted plan could be rapidly vitiated by an obstinate or stupid operating agency board or executive. This kind of problem is particularly aggravated in a health services system because of the lack of a single source of overall control. If the agency which is to do part of a job—home visiting, for example—provides incompetent help, the problem is shifted to the hospitals which are then forced to receive some patients who would not ordinarily require hospitalization, and to keep other patients longer than necessary. If the training of a new category of worker is inadequate, some other operations will function with difficulty. The possibility of foul-ups is great; they may occur in timing, use of multiple levels of skills, production, available services, and facilities. How then, in this field served by innumerable private as well as public agents, can assurance by gained that at least key services and relationships envisioned by planners will not be jeopardized? Inevitably, the question arises of whether planning bodies need to be concerned with enforcement as well as planning.

Two alternatives are apparent. The first would give the planning body authority to review progress, and even additional authority to enforce plans with whatever sanctions were built in when the plans were adopted. These sanctions could include taking over the operation, capturing security bonds, cancelling licenses, and replacing or taking over management. The alternative approach, which I urge in preference, is that the planning body exercise the limited functions of receiving and analyzing data from operating agencies and of publicizing its evaluation of accomplishments. Inability to get stipulated data from program and service agencies, the receipt of inadequate or erroneous data, evidence that adopted plans are being poorly carried out—all these would become public knowledge as a result of routine planning body reporting. If public discussion of such failures or inadequacies does not suffice to put derailed agencies back on the track, the job of inforcement would fall to a customary enforcing agency which could guide the operators or, of need be, put them out of service. The agents or agencies designated to step in would be specified in the original plans adopted by the legislature, and the requirement for public hearings in case of any breakdown in implementation would also have been written into these plans.

In my opinion, such enforcement of take-over functions should never fall into the hands of the planning body itself. Accreditation boards might enforce some aspects of hospital plans; hospital inspection and licensing bodies could enforce other parts. Similar groups might ensure the continuation of planned professional education programs; licensure boards would carry out the licensure sanctions against professionals who fail to perform or elevate their skills. Obviously a single basic enforcement agency, such as the state health department, is a more logical agent to do surveillance and enforcement of all the types mentioned.

By separating the responsibilities of the planning agencies from the duties of operating or enforcement agencies, planning bodies will be able to do what they know best without getting bogged down in operational details, or being torn apart by demands on staff and board to operate or police innumerable (and they are truly innumerable) agencies with whose operations they cannot possibly be familiar. Moreover, health planning bodies will have initiated plans basic to health concerns which, in fact, would finally be developed by other sectors, such as the industrial or the educational, where they would be put into operation. If those sectors fall down on the job, the planning agencies set up primarily for health can hardly be expected to step in and effectively run such operations.

Will planning bodies ever be given the freedoms and the means to generate useful planning? Will planning bodies be given resources primarily to regulate, rather than to plan? If so, the present day planning boards are poorly structured and prepared for their work.[9] They have never been given the resources nor found staff capacity to match the planning roles which they must sooner or later assume if they are to be more than an obstruction to planning.

MANDATE, PLACEMENT AND RELATIONSHIPS

The issues of mandate and placement fall very close together, because assigned roles, or the liberty to seek out roles, are a part of the specifications surrounding the birth of a planning agency. A key attribute of structure, in assisting the agency to fulfill its purposes, is its placement in relation to public decision-making activities.

The Mandate to the Planning Body

Public Law 89-749 gave a very broad scope of duties to all the comprehensive health planning bodies, without specifying roles or functions. The legislation was shortly followed by explanations and amplifications from the U. S. Public Health Service which did not seem totally consistent. However, because legislative intent is often more important than the exact wording of laws, the combined impression given by P.L. 89-749 is that all aspects of health—not just health care—were the concern of CHP bodies, and that potentially their duties included at least parts of all the roles listed in Chapter 9.

However, it is useful to scrutinize P.L. 89-749 for any ambivalences which might make a CHP body have second thoughts about the range of its roles. Vicente Navarro succinctly points out how minimal is the actual power of CHP bodies, for they really have only veto power over minute sectors of the health care monies and activities.[10] Moreover, in reality, all kinds of health planning activities proceed independently, such as those for mental illness, mental retardation, rehabilitation, and Regional Medical Programs. More or less simultaneous changes—in the form of a new national agency for environmental control—have further weakened the likelihood that HEW will support CHPs in undertaking an environmental role, since HEW is essentially removed from the major thrust of environmental control. In more recent times the CHP mandate, as explained by HEW, has shrunk to health care rather than health, so that CHPs need have no guilt feelings about abandoning concern for the general social, as well as the physical environmental forces which probably are the major factors in the occurence of good or ill health.

What can CHP agencies do about health care planning? The national mandate, which provides only a small percentage of the dollars needed to plan, seems to be little more than an invitation to see what can be done with just the encouragement of a high-sounding federal law that at best can provide 50% financing for every fourth health planning agency for which it calls. However, sentiment and proposed legislation in 1973 suggest that much more tangible national support is in the offing.

The perforce slow progress of CHPs under heretofore flatulent federal stimulation has received minor support by state decisions to grant CHPs authority over Hill Harris funding for facilities construction. Particularly in California, CHPs have been given increasing veto power, as well as more health facilities regulatory work. Financial support for local CHPs at the same time was shifted to taxes on facilities. This responsibility has not been a total blessing. Reacting to various facility plans has kept CHPs off balance, as planning is pushed aside by the need to begin regulating, even though this means that regulation occurs without benefit of any particular sense of direction.

Placement of the Planning Body

Several aspects of the issue of placement can be approached by considering the auspices relevant to the various levels at which we expect health planning to take place. Because government is apparently moving into the critical areas of health care financing, and because all health purveyors exist under some kind of publicly granted license and many of their major means of operating are enforced by the terms of such licensure, comprehensive planning cannot very well be carried out without formal acknowledgment by government. Even when planning is done by voluntary agencies in behalf of government, the need for planning stability and assurance of serious public consideration of its proposals calls for governmental involvement.

There are several currently operative basic alternatives for the effective placement of a comprehensive health planning body below the state level. All involve a clearcut relationship to government, even if the body is not a part of any formal jurisdictions.

Placed independently (also typical of traditional planning councils). In health planning, there seems little doubt that the CHP must be designated as an official advisory and planning group by one or more of the following: chief executive of the government of the jurisdiction; the quasi-policy-making boards already in existence, such as the board of health; one or more governmental agencies, such as the health department; or the major multipurpose legislative body for the area.

Set up under legislation to operate independently (typical of many health and hospital planning bodies) but designated by law as official planner and advisor to the elected executive or legislature or both. A CHP which becomes part of an independent, legally established health authority may be designated by state law to do the planning, as well as franchising or otherwise establishing the qualifications of health care delivery systems.[11] This is the authority-laden version of the form.

Made into a strong advisory body, working in partnership with an agency of government (as most physical planning bodies do now). Usually such bodies have appointed citizen policy boards advisory to a government agency which is run by a civil service, appointed staff. The planning body acts as a formal part of government, with tasks assigned in accordance with provisions set up by law.

Set up as a section of a more general purpose planning body. Some councils of government have such a planning center—possibly as their major activity—of which health planning is a regular element. In other situations there is a possibility of a free-standing multi-purpose planning agency, and health planning may also be a part of economic development agencies and Model Cities multi-purpose planning units. In the few existing metropolitan governments and in all the state governments, good possibilities exist for making the health planning unit a part of the general planning department. Some general purpose planning bodies outside of government at the local and metro levels, such as health and welfare councils, maintain a strong health planning section. In such a case, they need to be designated as the official health planning bodies, as described in the independent placement described above.

Set up as part of a health center or health care delivery network. At the neighborhood level, such a planning body may undertake health planning for their area, not unlike Model Cities operations, but with a scope limited to health matters. Hopefully, this planning would be for the health of citizens of the area, not just for the services rendered by the health care organization. Where these bodies are recognized as part of Model Cities activities, they have official status, but they would have to develop ties to local or metro level CHPs to relate to the major stream of health planning being done about them.

Set up as a staff arm of an operating health department, with an advisory council attached. The undesirability and vulnerabilities of this situation have already been discussed under "Supervision" and "Freedom from the influences of operational and supervisory duties."

The merits of some of these forms are suggested in Figure 10.3.

The separation of the comprehensive planning machinery into two

FIGURE 10.3
PREDICTED STRENGTHS OF HEALTH PLANNING BODIES, AS AFFECTED BY THEIR AUSPICES

STRENGTHS	AUSPICES			
	Independent (voluntary), with own funding & staff	Set up under legislation with own budget and staff, reporting to executive & legislature	Advisory, reporting to one department of government	No council, a government staff agency or part of an operating agency
Offset bureaucratic centralization of power in government	++++	++	++	+
Freedom from coercion by prior estimates of government body's attitudes	++++	+++	++	–
Freedom from coercion by concerns for the political fate of the governing bodies and elected officials	++++	+++	+	–
Aware and concerned with government's role or stake in matters under consideration	+	++	+++	+++
Aware and concerned with great diversity of organized influences that need to be consulted	+++	++	+	+
Aware and concerned with great diversity of kinds of people with problems and needs whose plight needs consideration	+++	+++	++	+
Aware and informed about great variety of ways in which nongovernmental and governmental agencies exist and function	+	++	+	++
Able to get immediate hearing by top governmental and nongovernmental interests	++	+++	+/–	+/–
Able to develop power commensurate with successful production of high quality plans and with use as a forum for education	+++	++++	++	+

418

Able to avoid or overcome "derogating" status of being part of operating government	++++	+++	++	+
Able to avoid or overcome "derogating" status of being a "bunch of do-gooders"	+	++++	+++	++
Able to develop effective working relations with various operating government agencies in fields of concerns	++	+++	++	+
Able to avoid ambiguities of limits, purpose and functions of agency staffing them or to which attached	NR*	NR	++	–
Freedom from concerns of fund raising in the voluntary sector	–	+++	+++	+++
Able to face and tackle serious problems of all complexions whether full of potential controversy or not	+	+++	++	+
Able to order priorities fairly, irrespective of private, government, or voluntary agency nature of alternatives	++	+++	++	+
Board (or agency head) able to keep leadership role vis-à-vis the expertise on the staff	+	++	++	+
Expertise on the staff will not be overlooked by council or agency	++	+++	+	+
Create one more source of power in a pluralistic setting	++++	+++	++	+
Retain maximal feelings of independence and freedom from trivia and methods of government	++++	+++	++	–
Freedom from restrictions on quality of personnel posed by civil service procedures and government salaries and prerogatives	++++	+++	++	–
Freedom from limitations on function of staff in public appearances	+++	+++	++	+

Ratings vary from very high ++++ to low –

*NR – = not relevant

419

not necessarily related entities—an advisory council and a staff which is part of a state agency—is one of the great disabilities P.L. 89-749 encourages at the state level. The two parts should make up one whole, with the council directing the work of the staff and taking responsibility for the entire planning output.

The meaningfulness of an appointment to the appointees depends largely on its origin. An appointment made by the governor (mayor) or the state legislature (city council or county board) indicates significant public recognition, and also implies that the appointing body will subsequently listen to its appointee, who would obviously be affronted otherwise. Moreover, a council so appointed, receives due press notice. Its releases, which are automatically beamed at the appointing key policy executive or policy-making body, are public and receive wide publicity and consideration. Figure 10.4 provides my viewpoint of the relationship of source of appointment to general effectivity of planning board members.

Beyle, Seligson, and Wright drew some interesting conclusions about factors which determine success of planning at the state level: Performance is best when an agency is close to the governor, is regarded as relevant, and is run at a low or modest expenditure level. Partisan politics was not found to be an obstacle to effectivity. The current tendency in the United States is to move state planning agencies close to the governor. In 1960, five planning agencies were in that position, and in 1969, 27 were.[12] Whether this shift reflects clarity of mandate more than structural position is not revealed, but the key spot next to the governor should promote a better quality mandate, if only because of propinquity.

In contrast, committees appointed by lesser figures, such as health officers or independent planning bodies, do not have comparable official government recognition. Unless formally acknowledged as advisors to the top elected policy-making figures, these committees may have great difficulty getting key people to serve, awarding recognition to those serving, or gaining policy body hearing and publicity for their work.

Boards which are self-selected and self-perpetuated, like those of traditional health and welfare councils, may in some cases be designated by governing bodies as their planning units. This appointment enhances the so-called community aspects of the planning work by co-opting groups long interested in planning. However, the benefits of acknowledgment may be offset by the notorious unrepresentativeness often found on such boards and the status quo attitudes of many persons selected to serve. Such a council is not likely ever to be as close to the hearts and interests of the policy-making authority as one whose members it has itself chosen.

FIGURE 10.4
EXPECTATIONS OF THE EFFECTIVITY OF HEALTH PLANNING BODY BOARD MEMBERS ACCORDING TO THE SOURCE OF THEIR APPOINTMENT

EFFECTIVITY	SOURCE OF APPOINTMENT					
	By executive and legislature with agreement of special interest	By executive with agreement of special interest	By executive and/or legislature	By special interests themselves on invitation of executive or legislature	By health officer	By board self-selected and perpetuated
Obtain participation of major special interests	++++	++	++	+++	+	+
Obtain general community respect	++++	+++	+++	+	+	++
Be of superior professional caliber	++	++	++	+	+++	+
Be interested in comprehensive planning	++	++	++	±	++	+
Community oriented	++	++	++	+	++	++
Give adequate time	+++	+++	++	+	++	+++
Work well together	+++	+++	++	+	+++	++++
Relate to governmental agencies	++	++	+++	+	+++	+
Obtain interest of governor	+++	++++	++++	++	+	++
Obtain interest of legislature	+++	++	++++	++	+	+
Obtain interests of local governments	+++	+++	++++	++	+	++

Ratings vary from very high ++++ to low –

421

Needed Levels of Planning Bodies

Figure 10.5 indicates all of the commonly advocated levels of planning. From each level of community the view may be quite different on any given problem. The so-called rape of Boston's West End was designed by the city of Boston to improve its tax position by removing an old slum and, in general, improving the outlook of the whole city for the future. Agencies on the national level authorized to fund urban redevelopment acquiesced in this particular view. But, any genuine

FIGURE 10.5
RELATIONSHIPS OF PLANNING AND POLICY BODIES

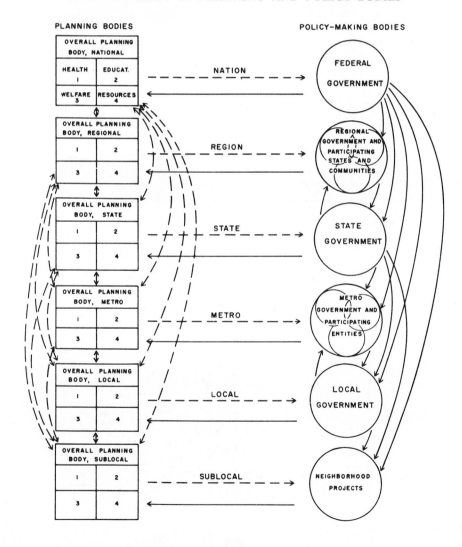

concern for planning for the people at the West End neighborhood level would soon have disclosed that this project was nothing more nor less than the destruction of a community and the liquidation of many families in a not-so-terrible ghetto.[13] Thousands of self-reliant people—who generally had a lower level of delinquency and dependency than people in most such communities—were to be dislocated, separated from their homes and from the small businesses by which they had been able to provide for their families and raise one or more generations. The displaced West Enders undoubtedly became an increased burden for Boston welfare agencies, because they could no longer sell their services to a long-standing group of neighbors and friends—all of whom were scattered as a result of the redevelopment. The welfare of the surrounding neighborhoods that had to pick up the homeless was certainly not given any consideration in these plans either. In all probability, the state of Massachusetts (and thus Boston and the outlying communities of Greater Boston) also suffered some significantly costly secondary effects.

The Neighborhood or Sublocal Level

Neighborhoods are defined by popular conception more than by technical standards. People identify with and recognize neighbors, boundaries, problems, and leaders. Neighbors are likely to have similar needs and come quite easily to internal agreements and priorities with only modest assistance. (See Chapter 11.) Neighborhood or sublocal planning efforts are necessary to attract key information, create participation, educate people to the existence of choice, and develop belief in the power of self-determination. The disappearance of the ward leader (or heeler) with the advent of federally-sponsored relief or service measures may well have left impoverished neighborhoods without any device except riots to bring the plight of some groups, even of whole neighborhoods, to the eyes of the public or to the decision-making centers.

However, I am not speaking to the need for an ombudsman[14] whose role is to create a shield against abuses by the helping institutions, but of a neighborhood (sublocal) planning council which, with technical assistance from its city or county level council, can be the means by which people and neighborhoods learn to formulate and support meaningful demands. Ways to accommodate to conflicting or competitive requirements raised by other equally important neighborhoods must be learned. In essence, the sublocal council becomes a crucible of energy for the development of a sense of community. This, in turn, promotes the growth of individual pride and a sense of power and worth, as more persons become involved, and each discovers that he has a hand in shaping destiny.

Although the sublocal planning body is not seen as necessarily using the technical staff that might be made available to it from the local city or county level as *advocate* planners, a degree of that spirit among the planners is both necessary and inevitable.[15] Technicians and citizens will jointly identify with worthwhile neighborhood (and general) goals. As the technicians assigned sublocally develop both technical and personal involvement in plans they help to engineer, they are going to have the greatest of all responsibilities—the creation and utilization of trust.

Neighborhood planning bodies, always a tenuous experiment until now, are at serious risk of premature dissolution if their efforts are overriden by higher local level planning bodies, unless this is done in a very perceptive way that points out how suboptimizing in behalf of neighborhoods may, in fact, bring no remedy to the ills for which they seek a cure. Unless the same general nature of the goals desired by the neighborhood is incorporated at the higher levels, the only interpretation that neglected neighborhoods can make is that planning is an idle exercise. In one city,[16] where local planning efforts had resulted in a master plan, a not atypical government failure to uphold the planners dealt a mortal blow to the sublocal voluntary planning entities which had been active in creation of the master plan. At such a moment, the sublocals may fade away, or they may coalesce into a militant community-wide entity and force city officials and planners to justify their actions. If the latter occurs, the voluntary sublocal planning councils which have coalesced may form a shadow council to patrol the doings of the official city council. The official body will presumably either learn to work with these newly polarized interests, so that insightful and legitimate planning efforts can go forward, or it will go on fighting them until the side with the most muscle wins—hardly the planning approach.

The sublocals which currently demand most of our attention are those neighborhoods which in most cases have a minimum of daily mobility and of health services and which usually also carry an excessive burden of ill health. When they start to plan, few producers of health services are situated in their midst. Unless the locals sponsor sublocal planning efforts, and make staff time available, and introduce producer and administrative types, sublocal efforts can rarely be more than wailing walls or muscle-building organizations. In all but those neighborhoods which are middle class or above, the chances of analyzing problems effectively and coming up with rational alternative interventions, which can be meshed with city and higher-level goals, would be effectively precluded by the denial of technical assistance to the neighborhood planners.

Moreover, if each sublocal were encouraged to sponsor a planning unit without importing needed skills, in all probability sublocals would then converge at the local or metro level and bring highly polarized, suboptimal proposals into a clashing confrontation—a situation which is hardly an improvement over the present polarization of interest groups. Carefully volunteered assistance to sublocals by local or metro planning bodies should serve as a point of exchange for knowledge and should open consideration of choices which look ahead to the time when all the sublocals will integrate their interests at the local or metro level.

Richard Bailey has pointed out that a spectacular yearly rise in GNP, or the passage of legislation providing negative income tax or old-age assistance on a nationwide basis need not, and in fact will not, obliterate tragic pockets of poverty and ill-health.[17] Similarly, city or metrowide programs may do no better, if they settle for areawide statistics which may show an improving composite picture. Only at the neighborhood level can resistant pockets of social failure be recognized and the lack of utilizable services documented. At this level, the needs of real people rather than statistical composites are held before the planners constantly; these same real people also participate in the planning.

Viable connections for the sublocal or neighborhood level health planning body are critical, for in all but truly large groups, health planning is unlikely to survive by itself unless it is: (1) a well-defined and supported arm of a local or metro health planning body; (2) the planning arm of a neighborhood based health care delivery system; (3) part of the planning unit of a Model Cities structure. The attempt to go further and provide true neighborhood autonomy is indeed controversial.[18]

The Local (City or County) Level

The local level is frequently given short shrift as a useful locus for planning. The suboptimization and fractionization that locals bring to the metro scene has earned the ill will of many planners. However, until recently there have been almost no metro-level planning activities to which locals could relate, and so their plight is not an indictment of local planning. Local level planners of either the city or county have a direct relationship with a relevant government which is traditionally accepted as being close to the people. However, in the past, neither the people nor the local level planners have had metro government or metro planners to relate to.

One historical point worth emphasizing is that planning at the local level has been manifest primarily in governmentally authorized physical planning and in health and welfare council activities. In my opinion, neither has a consistent history of concern for those matters that have a real bearing on man's well-being. Nevertheless, multipurpose

local government is one of the ideal nodal points for current comprehensive planning, because it is in a key position to correlate a high
proportion of well-being planning and services and to set priorities
and mediate differences among sublocalities. (Health and well-being
concerns must surely be at the heart of comprehensive planning.) Discussion of the many reasons for maintaining local multipurpose government and extending local level planning from the physical to the
health and well-being areas follows:

The multipurpose city or county government does render a high
proportion of all governmentally provided personal services to citizens, and even a higher proportion of day-to-day environmental services. It has the machinery, the tradition, and, in many neighborhoods, citizen cooperation.

Some governmental entity has to levy the local share of public
costs; cities and counties already do, and the nature of that role could
only be replaced or eliminated with the greatest difficulty. (True,
their ability to do what is financially necessary is badly limited by
citizen or political tolerance and by state statutes.)

A multipurpose government is needed to force the issue of priorities in poorly interrelated areas, such as public works, education,
health, and jobs. The local government level, in spite of its splintering by single purpose districts, is currently the only body below the
state level that has major experience with resolution of problems of
priority and appropriate mixes. The greatest weakness here lies in
the division of responsibility and authority between cities and counties. Cities have been created more nearly in line with what aggregates of people want for themselves; counties were created as creatures of the state to carry out state-required functions. This problem
has become more confused as many counties have, by popular demand, grown into partial and realizable, but not always geographically and politically useful, substitutes for metro government.

City and county governments and their physical planning arms
are familiar and traditionally accepted units. Health-focused planning bodies at the local level would not be setting a totally new
precedent and should be accepted readily.

Local level decisions have to be formulated, and sublocal decisions integrated into them. In turn, these have to be transmitted to
the metro level. Viable metro-planning units exist largely in name
only today, created primarily in response to requirements of various
federal funding programs and by Bureau of the Budget circulars
A-80, A-82 and A-95.

The current assessment of people, needs, resources, and distribution, which makes up the basis of planning, is now done primarily by city and county government, although metro centers could also

carry out these tasks. Availability and utilization of data are still largely a local affair.

There is every reason to believe that local planning will lead into metro planning as assessment, problem analysis, and definition of alternative interventions at more than one level of government (and suboptimization) become understood. This is, in fact, the current trend. Failure of locals to plan comprehensively until now is hardly proof that metro-level planning would have been any more successful. Comprehensive planning was not understood at any level, and it does not follow that it would have matured sooner in the presence of more extensive metro government. Rather, pressure for metro government is more likely to be the result of attempts at local and national comprehensive planning which point to the need for more than local, short-run, suboptimal plans.

At the local level, the health planning body is likely to be found in any of the following positions, with my preferences going to the second, third, or fifth: (1) an independent body, (2) a legislatively initiated and supported but independent body, (3) part of a health authority, (4) an advisory body relating to a government agency, (5) a section of a general planning body, or (6) a staff arm of an operating agency.

The Metro Level

Although somewhat different in concept from the problem-shed "community of solution" introduced by the National Commission on Community Health Services,[19] the metro level of planning should become increasingly important once a multitude of conditions have been investigated, each showing up with its own community of solution. The vast majority of important communities of solution will undoubtedly have essentially the same boundaries, which will also be those of the most logical metro community. The need for multipurpose rather than individual planning entities (as well as service entities) should hasten the demise of single purpose districts which are antithetical to the whole concept of comprehensive planning. The overwhelming interrelationships between personal health and well-being services and social and economic institutions generally, the daily as well as generational mobility within the metropolitan area, the need for uniform availability of taxable resources over a metro area, the need to reintegrate the suburbs with the central city, transport with people, people with jobs, and so on, will force most of the major, so-called local decisions to the metro level and even across state boundaries into multistate, metro areas. One cannot help but agree with the persuasive arguments of Altshuler that the two levels least well represented currently by governmental or planning units—the sublocals and the metros—will be the dominant centers for planning in the future.[20]

The discussion of communities in Chapter 11 points out that planning body boundaries need not be coterminous with those of bodies rendering services (literally, an impossibility in the health industry anyway). At the regional or metro level, planning may not always have the same boundaries for all purposes. By using existing local government boundaries as building blocks, viable regional planning areas may be defined; each would serve several purposes but each need not have identical boundaries. For example, Regional Medical Programs will rarely match service or market areas, because they are based on medical centers, several of which may exist in the same area. Nor are they likely to match water or air pollution boundaries.

Placements of health planning bodies useful at the metro level have included all those described for the local level. However, the present disabilities of free standing types only seem to accentuate the nonexistence of metro government and point out that the absence of metro government is a particularly forceful argument for the combination of all metro-level planning bodies. Such a combination is desirable whether the planning bodies would be part of, or advisory to, the planning arm of metro government where it exists, or to councils of government and economic development districts, or would be part of an overall, free standing, metro-level planning enterprise. Unfortunately, the truly independent or legislated independent metro forms are likely to continue; but many will develop into metro-level health authorities to fill the needs of guiding and franchising health care delivery systems.

Unless locals and states do correctly identify and make planning use of the metro (as well as neighborhood) configurations, we can expect a continuation of the flow of decision-making to the federal level which has given more attention to neighborhood and regional problems than have our cities and states.

The State Level

The logic for planning at the state level seems clear, although as metros or multistate regions become the center of resolution for the multiple communities of solution, state-level planning may not retain the same roles it now has.

States are repositories of the vast untapped (as well as the authorized) powers which were not handed over to the federal government in our constitution. The tragic disinterest of states in urban centers and their people led to the one-man, one-vote Supreme Court decision, which broke one of the major 20th century political stalemates at the state level. However, the resulting transfer of state-level voting power to the suburbs from the central cities does not give much assurance that in the future states will plan or operate more intelligently, that local government can plan or act more effectively, or that metro formation will be sought. To dim the prospect of metro-level planning even further, minority groups begin to see themselves coming into power in the financially troubled central cities, while WASP groups see themselves reconstituting their forces in a privileged ring around the central city, with a permanent and increasingly violent energy contained within. Conflicting central city and suburban interests thus further threaten any hope of extending metro government, and thereby transfer the resolution of metro-level problems to the state where the same embattled metro and suburban forces tend to replay the same issues under the auspices of rural arbitration. Notwithstanding revenue sharing, the historical and now large and rapidly enlarging role of the federal government in local affairs[21] does not seem to be headed for a plateau, because the predictable impasse between these conflicting local interests are the same ones that can also paralyze state-level action.

Given the reality of mounting violence if not revolt in the central city, general national welfare will find the federal government either carrying the burden of forming creative relationships at the metro level, or pushing the states to clamber aboard the metro problem bandwagon through various federally provided incentives. Perhaps the states will take suitable action for fear of losing a vital place in our multi-tier form of government.

The necessary resolution of problems in health services finds most states proceeding at a reasonable pace to get health planning machinery set up, but very few indeed have as yet produced outputs that inspire confidence. As long as states confine their interests to health care matters, they will not encounter too many critical problems initially; but, at the same time, they cannot be very successful in resolving health deficits and thus health care burdens, which result largely from socioeconomic limitations rather than lack of health care. The states are presently in a position to begin resolving health service delivery problems, even if they are hampered by the ideological splits on socioeconomic issues carried over from the metropolitan areas. Various factors—the residual authority of states over local government, their general access to rather large pools of dollars, their authority over vendors of care, and their reasonable freedom to negotiate with one another—put state-level health planning bodies in an excellent position. The state is obviously one of the critical multipurpose nodal levels of planning and government, and can pursue statewide goals at the regional and national levels. Above all, it can create and utilize powerful boards that can move relatively freely to meld public and private interests in behalf of the general welfare.

The state level planning agency is commonly a unit (1) in an operating agency such as a health department; (2) in a specially created staff agency, such as a human services agency; or (3) part of an overall planning or economic development agency. Its governmental nature is a requirement of P.L. 89-749, designed to insure that at this level it be a bona fide part of formal government. The planning body, of course, could also be made into an independent agency or health authority because of the pressing demands upon government to take over control and supervision of health care delivery.

The Regional or Multistate Level

The multistate level of planning may be required by the many problems which do not originate or cannot be resolved within the boundaries of one state. The opportunities for joint action between states, or for states to allow contiguous local areas to join in planning and operation, already exist. The exact relationships feasible are presently not clear[22] because of the role of the federal government, although this is evidently much less of an obstacle than the divergence of interests among states.[23] When situations have grown desperate enough, the federal government has even created its own regional operations, as with the Tennessee Valley Authority (TVA). TVA did work closely with states and localities. Although it need not have done so legally, its political longterm survival no doubt required such multilevel cooperation. Placement of multistate agencies does not seem to be a pressing matter for discussion here, but it is worth noting that multistate economic development authorities, which are heavily planning oriented, might make a suitable home for another key planning concern—health.[24] Some already have made this marriage.

The National Level

Although the national level is the most critical level from the standpoint of creating wealth and protecting general interests at home and abroad, the national level of health planning is strangely neglected.[25] With the probable continued failures of states to resolve their own crisis-level problems—whether purely internal or shared with other states—national survival may force increased federal involvement in rural, urban, metropolitan, and megalopolitan well-being problems, of which health is a prime example.

There is a distinctive national agenda that has a direct and vital bearing on health. As a minimum it includes a neverending concern for such obvious health issues as:

Migration of people and problems.

Need for redistribution of health care resources which are national resources, such as manpower.

Coping with rare diseases and scarce experts.

Large investments.

Scarcity of planning, assessment, and related skills.

Facing realities that some issues can only be handled politically or financially at the national level.

These do not take into account comparable issues in other sectors which have a vital determining effect on the health of our people as well as on the resources available to cope with health matters.

Can or should the nation move to further such federal involvement without creating national planning machinery which is truly representative of the public? If planning is so critical at all the other levels, can the master level of federal enablement be left without comprehensive planning? Every major health problem to be analyzed by planners has critical social as well as technical and legal aspects, many of which can be resolved only by national level agreements or enablement. Local success in alleviating unemployment, illiteracy or discrimination —all sources or correlates of ill health—depends primarily on national undertakings. Overcoming shortages of professional personnel, achieving uniformity in the identification of skills, obtaining needed dollars to train personnel or purchase services are matters that cannot be planned individually by states, particularly not by those that create few of their own skills, nor by those that create a surplus. Moynihan clarified the hierarchical relationships well when he said that "in a national society more policies must be national while programming remains local,"[26] and this also means that national planning is a must.

To prevent the popular panaceas put forth by election-minded legislators and executives from becoming national policy, we need to plan, and national planning must not be the traditional "share a scheme" approach that federal administrative agencies and congressional committees use to design legislation. The outputs of community planning at all the levels described previously also need to be delivered topside, so that something more rational than the continued unplanned outpouring of dollars for health services will occur. Can the federal government be serious and give money, encouragement, and praise for comprehensive planning at lower levels and not provide for it at the national level? Or is the federal government going to pawn off the work of administrative and legislative committees as a substitute for planning by formally recognized and adequately staffed and guided planning bodies?

Placement of a national body anywhere but in juxtaposition—as a formally legislated advisory body—to the President, and perhaps to Congress, would seem anomalous. True, various arms of the U.S. Department of Health, Education and Welfare have been heard asking for this responsibility, but the output of such a group would be so tainted—because it would be one, two, or three echelons down in the hierarchy of that vast health-vested agency—that it could hardly be suspected of doing truly national, rather than agency-level, planning. Nor could HEW necessarily correlate its efforts with those of the larger socioeconomic issues confronting the nation.

The International Level

The United States has made extensive private and governmental investments worldwide for health purposes. With awareness increasing that general well-being concerns truly and immediately tie the world together, the multiple rationalities for these investments could be the topic for an exciting analysis. For our purposes, it suffices to point out that such unilateral efforts provoke serious reservations. The Jackson report[27] lists the reasons very well and points out that the United Nations' and other extra-national ventures in a given country (and also for any continental region) must be thought through and coordinated in order to contribute to a meaningful longrange set of goals. Even a very limited sum of outside dollars for a special purpose dear to the donor's heart, business, or self-preservation, may create temptations that substantially divert the recipient's own dollars into special channels. These may not only represent more important foregone opportunities for the recipient's use of his own dollars, but may be setting up new institutions and attitudes which preclude important and imperative ways of proceeding in the recipient country.

The center of world efforts at health planning are being seriously concentrated at the World Health Organization, but WHO's present real separation from such entities as the World Bank and the United Nations coterie of nations means that true cooperation on health planning for a given nation or international region still proceeds more by chance than by design. Nevertheless, WHO has taken the leadership in disseminating information, education, consultation, and investments in health planning throughout the globe.[28] Its American regional office, serving the Americas and the Caribbean (Pan American Health Organization) has the distinction of participating in development of the first thought-through western schema for health planning, now known as the CENDES (Centro de Estudios del Desarrollo) method, widely used in Caribbean and Latin American countries.[29]

Structural and Policy Relationships Among Planning Bodies

The issues discussed here concern the formal and control ties between the various kinds of planning bodies (horizontal), and then between the various tiers of health planning bodies inside the United States (vertical).

Horizontal Relationships

Study of concerns that are partially or predominantly health oriented is not confined to health planning bodies. All concerned may act in intelligent unison through joint committees composed of members from each of the several planning bodies involved (see Figure 10.5). It is possible to appoint a joint committee and assign staff task forces so that all the planning entities are essentially joined as one. Alternatively, each of the major planning sectors can function as a clearly differentiated section of one overall community planning entity. If separate sector planning bodies are joined in such a way as to make up one overall planning body, that body can make assignments to the sector bodies and ask for or appoint joint committees or strengthen representation in sector planning bodies as needed. This is essentially the scheme shown in Figure 10.5 as an overall design for interrelating planning and policy making bodies and their functions at each level and between levels.

Because the special field planning units at any one level are not necessarily sections or committees of the overall planning body, these subunits might ideally share a 5% or 10% membership with one another and another 5% or 10% with the overall body. They may each be heavily augmented by outside members who fulfill the requirements for representation and technical expertise called for by the subjects of concern and applicable laws.

One subplanning unit might be organized under auspices different from the others. For example, the health unit may be a voluntary entity, while the educational planning body may be a creation of government. A third planning body might be essentially an independent body with governmental support and recognized authority. All must, however, have equal status and be formally acknowledged by governments for the territory in which they are expected to plan.

Overall planning at any level might likewise exist as any one of these variants. Particularly at the state and national levels, the government-sponsored, appointed, supported, but highly independent overall planning body seems preferable to one which is voluntary or freestanding. (See Figure 10.3.) Moreover, as more control or rule making tasks are imposed on the planning body, the more likely it is that it will have to be a part of formal government.

Roland Warren has given us an example of how the various sectoral planning bodies could be expected to work at what we call the horizontal level.[30] Although his postulated pattern of interaction utilizes the community decision-making organizations (CDOs) rather than the planning ones, the probable roles of each seem so heavily intertwined that the same logic would seem applicable to both. (Warren uses the term value not in the normative sense but rather in the sense of an object having the capacity to satisfy a given desire.) Warren has written:

> It is "as if" the people of the community, concerned with a num-
> ber of different kinds of "values"—such as adequate housing, a
> viable economic base, the rejuvenation of the city's core, adequate
> transit, an appropriate array of social services, good schools, and
> so on—had parcelled these values out among a number of CDOs
> giving to each the responsibility for maximizing its particular val-
> ue—not absolutely, but in interaction with other CDOs. The
> CDOs have different, partially overlapping value configurations,
> with different types and amounts of resources at their disposal.
> Not all the values can be maximized simultaneously, either be-
> cause of inadequate resources or because some—like adequate
> low-cost housing, may conflict with others—like eliminating seg-
> regation, when they are pressed beyond certain limits. Further-
> more, the people of the community have acknowledged the right
> of these CDOs to speak for the community in their respective fields
> (i.e., given them legitimation) and have allocated to them money,
> personnel, and other resources with which to do it.
>
> Although the joint decision usually satisfies no one completely,
> it produces a resolution well within the bounds of acceptability
> for most important parties to the community dialogue. Such
> changes as are needed occur incrementally through the waxing
> and waning of the various CDOs (resource reallocation) and
> through changes in legitimation (shifting domain). Where the at-
> tempts of the CDOs to press incompatible values result in a crisis,
> the mayor or some other *deus ex machina* is called in to resolve the
> immediate dispute and perhaps to reallocate resources.

This presentation makes a significant plea that each sectoral policy (or planning) body keep its reasonable autonomy, but be related and guided by that of the other sectors.

Vertical Relationships

The relationships of one tier of health planning agencies with an-other seem to be simply indicated in Figure 10.5 in terms of output, which is reviewed below. However, Figure 10.5 utilizes broken lines between the planning tiers to indicate that no one planning level need be the home or base of support of others, but that outputs from any planning level should freely go to any other, as well as to policy-mak-ing bodies. In other discussions it has been pointed out that locals or sublocals may be the formal arms of metros, or sublocals of locals. In a few cases, the state level planning agencies have more nearly a parent-child relationship with lower level agencies. It is my position that for-mal hierarchial or governing relationships between the levels of planning bodies are probably unnecessary (if not unwise) except where a higher level body—such as the metro—must organize and direct or support local or sublocal units if they are to be viable. But even here, the supportive relationship which exists between many state health departments and their local counterparts might be used as a model; there is guidance, major rule setting, some or even heavy financial assistance, and general but not day-to-day supervision. In this case, local governmental bodies really see themselves as the policymaking center for their local health agency. Local levels thereby gain a maximum of autonomy and sense of strength and are recognized as the direct health planning arm for the local political jurisdiction, rather than being seen as the district planning operation of a higher level of government (which is likely to be suspect by local government). Local CHPs tied into other entities—such as those economic development agencies that have a strong state dependency—may likewise inherit any local government enmity for state-directed agencies.

Each local planning council is seen as having its counterpart in neighborhoods that have significant problems. Sublocals would relate primarily to the local level units. They have, of course, no comparable level government structures to relate to, and sublocals would no doubt deal with local level planning bodies—or with local government, if the local planning bodies could not or would not assist them—in attempting implementation of their goals or solution of their problems. Any staffing would probably have to be a contribution from the local level or metro-level planning body. Some states are considering making planning resources available to neighborhoods because of the poverty at local and metro-levels.

Working Relationships of Planning Bodies

For Planning Output

Exchange of plans and problems between lower, higher, or parallel planning levels or bodies is another major function which is meagerly served at present.[31] In analyzing goals or problems (Chapter 7), the need is frequently found to allocate the design of health improving interventions to other local or parallel planning sectors, such as education or natural resources. And some matters need to be sent up the line for national or state solution (for example, alterations in standards or licensure).

The ultimate in participative planning would be the development of plans at the local level and even the sublocal or neighborhood level. These in turn would, for much of their fulfillment in the health field, have to be coordinated at the metro level. (In no way are aggregates of local plans a substitute for metro level planning.) Metro planning, concerned with the placement of critical facilities and dispersion of services and dollars in accordance with what was planned for locally, would only modify or discard local plans which were needlessly wasteful or harmful to others in or out of the local jurisdiction, or not in keeping with metro level plans. In turn, state plans would facilitate implementation of metro or regional plans, ensuring that they, too, were wise and congruous with the state or national plans and standards agreed to in the various areas of endeavor. National planning bodies would make sure that state plans were in line with national ones and facilitate the realization of state plans. Public Law 89-749 sets up such a scheme, in part at least, by its requirement for state level planning and by its economic inducements to metro or regional planning, although it all but ignores truly local planning and completely ignores national level planning—a very serious threat to the overall future success of health planning.[32]

Public Law 89-749, the culmination of several streams of interest, is realistic in that it recognizes that state level planning is imperative under any circumstances, and that there may be no talent available to work locally except in a few metropolitan areas. (Presently, even the talent needed at the state level is largely underdeveloped.) But by failing to spell out the prerogatives of local involvement, P.L. 89-749 takes the risk that the states—which have been notorious for their unconcern over even monstrous local problems—will preempt the planning field and work at general solutions which only dubiously will come near to solving local and deprivation or "people-type" problems. Of course, in the health realm problems of standards of availability, accessibility, quantity, and quality call for solutions primarily at the state and national level, and these could be attacked without awaiting local level planning. However, we must reiterate that state and national planning could be designed more wisely if locally devised and desired options were available for their study.

Nevertheless, state planning can and must begin without further delay. Results can be modified as local plans start coming in and contributing the knowledge of specific areas and the imaginative proposals that planning on the local level may generate. The option of making local planning one of the major planning bases for the nation must be kept open. Increased participation in planning could also assist the spread of participation in our society and in the redemocratization so sorely needed.

The dissemination of planning output is indicated by dotted lines in Figure 10.5. The overall planning bodies are shown on the left side by the upper compartments. The subsidiary or related specialized elements which may well be autonomous are shown by the dependent boxes: (1) health, (2) education, (3) welfare, (4) resources and physical. These would seem to constitute a minimum of comprehensive planning units at any one level of planning. Above the sublocal (neighborhood) level, I cannot at this time conceive of a single planning body encompassing all the concerns of health, general well-being, and education without at least the four-way segmentation by area of concern as shown. Nor can I see a purely health planning body dealing knowledgeably with all the problems of the utilization of natural resources which have, as secondary or unintentional outputs, adverse effects on our physical and social environments.

The overall policymaking bodies (government) are shown by the outer circles on the right. The enclosed circles at the regional government level indicate the states and any cities and counties that might be joined together in a compact. The enclosed circles at the metropolitan level of government indicate the cities and/or counties joined in a metro-compact.

Horizontal flow in the form of data, alternatives and analysis, and suggested plans for action (shown in Figure 10.5 by dotted lines) is from the planning council to the community or participating government units which sponsor or relate to the planning council. (Output from policymaking bodies, elected government, is shown by solid lines.)

Vertical flow up or down is from planning councils to those of higher (more encompassing political jurisdiction) or to those of lower level communities and jurisdictions. These exchanges are of information, plans, and so on. Flow may be from one level of health planning to another, from health to the planning entity in another field, or to the overall planning entity. There will be heavy flow at each level from any one to any other planning unit, to the overall planning body, or from the overall to each of its planning subunits.

For Policy Output

Solid lines in Figure 10.5 indicate flow of policy and requests from policymaking government bodies or from the people in the communities to the planning bodies.

Horizontal flow is to the planning body from the community, generally via the governing body or bodies concerned, and is in the form of the planning body's charter, charges, resources and constraints. Constraints may also take form as the resources made available are specifically allocated for consideration of one area or problem or for the total planning output. Governmentally specified minimal or maximal tolerable limits for a given service or function or provision of funds for the planning effort itself may be the constraints. Guides may also come in the form of specific resolutions, or may be embodied in contracts, budgets, and compacts with and between various units of government, or between levels of government.

Downward flow is from higher jurisdictions, as from states to their included entities, and from the federal government to any level of government below. Regional (multistate) and metro (areawide) bodies may make policies for entities included in their jurisdiction in accordance with preagreements made by their constituent bodies. Metros are also bound by state-imposed limitations that specify what they can legislate or provide for constituent bodies. At the regional multistate level, the government entity may exist as a creature of contracting member states or as a creature of the Congress. In the latter case, the regional government legislates for its constituents in accordance with federal limitations. It may exist with approval of Congress and with duties and functions as approved by Congress. There are many variants and loopholes in the legislative framework for such compacts.[33]

Upward flow of policy between governmental bodies occurs primarily in two locations. A multistate body may derive all of its authority from its constituent states and may be dependent upon directives from them regarding the limits of its scope, jurisdiction, and expenditures. A metro entity might also be much like a federation and receive its direction, scope, and authority from constituent subunits.

REPRESENTATION

The representativeness of a health planning board is a critical ingredient for comprehensive planning for health. Careful thinking about what is needed in the way of skills and interests to achieve the functions already described, guides the composition of the board.

Need for Diversity

In all but small communities, there will be great difficulty in achieving suitable citizen diversity. Persons chosen to represent consumers at all but sublocal levels have tended to be technical or leadership types. Some are "professional consumers" who may have organizational connections but few real ties to the masses of lay consumers they are chosen to represent. Conversely, at the sublocal or neighborhood level, a good bit of importation has to go on to overcome a paucity of technical expertise, for it is grossly unfair to deprive the poorer neighborhoods of technical and administrative skills. True, at this time in history, outsiders to a neighborhood—particularly when ethnically distinguishable or identified as part of the establishment—may be welcome only under very special terms.

Representativeness and representation should not be confused. Planning boards need both. A Black Caucus representative may have quite a different set of rules to fulfill than one of the people he represents (the black citizenry). For example, the black community really is in need of at least three representative types to make its position clear: the apathetics, the militants, and those who want to join the middle class world.[34]

Similarly, a physician in the role of medical society spokesman may feel constrained to give a rigid organizational viewpoint (the party line designed to satisfy right, left and moderates). But if he is relieved of this special mantle, he may have quite different and personal views that may or may not be typical of other physicians in similar practices. One of the tests of the legitimacy of the formal representative for a group is whether he has a group to report back to and does so, and whether the group has the opportunity to keep him informed of their wishes and does so.

The following is a summary of the diversity of interests that would ideally be involved in comprehensive health planning, varying, of course, with the planning level.

Political interests.   Representatives of structured political groups, whether part of the national major parties or not, are needed: from the related political jurisdiction (citizens or elected officials); from levels of government, above and below, that have related interests; from the same general level of government or community but with parallel, overlapping, or related interests; and from associations of mayors, supervisors, governors, and so on, where they are available.

Specific public policymaking persons from the geopolitical area being served.   A planning body needs representation from the office of the chief elected executive (if there is one) to bring the problems of that office to the planners, and vice versa. Similarly, members from the legislative body (both houses if there are two) should be appointed. Where there is significant partisan activity, members might be appointed from both the majority and minority parties, if the planning body is large enough. In this way not only are the problems of decision making made known, but the intricacies of policies, elections, and implementation of plans are made comprehensible to the planning body—which must make planning for implementation part of its work.

Technical interests.   Participants are required from significantly involved skills, like doctors; significant special interests, like facilities; and significant minority positions (if any) among these.

Government and voluntary control or standards-setting associations or agencies in the subject area.   Participants are required from the same level of government with related interests (for example, special districts) and from authorities; from similar levels of government in adjacent areas; from agencies in government levels below and above the community level of the planning body; and from joint accreditation boards.

Voluntary health agencies. Those serving relevant areas are welcome coventurers.

Other government and voluntary agencies in other sectors of the same geopolitical area. Participants from agencies that ultimately or indirectly bear on health (for example, education, welfare, law enforcement, and religion) are important for many aspects of planning.

Planners. Participants are required from planning bodies in health work at the same level, at higher or lower levels, and in areas generally affecting health; from planning bodies related to or controlling health matters such as those in councils of governments, economic development districts or model cities.

Other sectors. Other key sectors such as agriculture, labor, finance, industry and commerce (often inaccurately called consumers) can be the key interests in shaping policy as well as in securing implementation.

Consumers. General community interests—particularly organizations with a cross-section of consumers, such as the Parent-Teacher Associations and Neighborhood Councils—are groups from which general legitimation is likely to come.

Victims or special need groups. This group particularly will shed light on what is wrong and what is needed. Included are persons who have suffered from the specific problem under consideration—for example, those who have been deprived of good health care; the various significant segments of the population who are known, or suspected, to have special needs or concerns; persons with insufficient means (potentially or actually), such as the retired, unemployed, relief recipients, low-income families, migrants, and parents of handicapped children; persons with unique needs, such as the aged, parents, commuters, and persons in redevelopment areas; persons with other kinds of special burdens, such as the ethnic minority groups, other significant sociocultural minority groups, and handicapped persons.

Specifically vested groups. Those interests perceived to be vested in issues under consideration will generate support as well as major obstacles in the form of highly financed and organized pressures. Examples include the Health Insurance Council Program for Community Health Action Planning (Insurance), the American Medical Association, the American Nurses Association, the American Public Health Association, and the American Hospital Association. Whenever an issue arises that seems significantly to involve interests of a specific nature that are not represented on committees or the board, representatives of those interests must be introduced before planning goes very far. Vestedness is one of the higher priorities in seeking representativeness. Special interest should be visible, or it will sneak into the deliberations by a devious route and confound the issues without being understood. Or it will wait in ambush for public presentation, seeking sympathy by pointing out that it was not informed or not invited to participate.

Experts. Specialists on particular problems are needed in accordance with the agency's agenda. Experts also represent a strong source of vertical integration because of their professional affiliations, their command of the related literature, and their own professional peer presence on advisory and technical bodies at all levels, within the nation and internationally. In this way health agencies and associations —both the voluntary which have strong national ties, and the governmental with well established relationships—help planners to look at all levels of a problem or distribution system.

Operatives.   Persons from the administrative level of the concerned service-providing agencies are necessary as vested interests and as experts. A planning body must have the key relevant opinions about what the operating agency knows and is doing or ought to be doing in the areas of concern. Government executives can be included as non-voting members if they are feared, or as technical consultants if only their information is desired. They are often present by law as chairmen or secretaries, probably an unwise gesture of confidence, unless the planning body itself selects the specific person for such responsibilities. Through such council memberships, data and staff work can be more easily obtained. At any given community level, these persons may well be the key means of establishing the needed horizontal integration of the service, control, and resource-producing operational entities.

Thompson makes a very good case for the involvement of operatives in planning.[35] They are a means of getting critical information and technical assistance. They can bring reality to the discussion, both in terms of what present interventions can and cannot be expected to do and in terms of what capabilities will be needed to mount new interventions and to estimate their effectiveness and public reception. The involvement of operatives helps to stop agency footdragging which is otherwise so common. It can diminish the inevitable paranoia of the person who is not in on the discussion of his particular agency and its work. The operator's bias for action and expediency-oriented moves is also modified by his participation in the planning environment, and, hopefully, his staff will assist in the preparation of data he needs in order to get his agency's viewpoint on the planning floor. With more concern and more foresightedness, the operative will be ready to lend his own staff members as their skills are needed on task forces set up by the planning board. Without jeopardizing planning by turning it over to operating agencies, their capabilities can be utilized, and at the same time, their own planning skills can be developed and used to advantage in their own agencies.

Other health sector workers.   Whether professional, paraprofessional, skilled artisans, or unskilled labor, these workers must be represented. They make up over 90% of the health cadre and have too often been forgotten, in spite of their major and increasing importance in the work of the health sector.

Selection Process for Members of the Board

A 1969 report stated that the bulk of consumers was still coming from the traditional or well established agencies, services, and community organizations, and that committees and task forces were the principal means by which consumer-citizens and providers get together.[36] My observations from 1970 through 1973 confirm that only a slow trend is developing toward the kind of broad participative representation that is necessary for successful health planning.

The largest problem will be in allocating the slots designated for "at least 51 percent consumers" required by P.L. 89-749. Which of the 13 groups listed shall qualify as consumers? The decision is not simple, for each interest represents a facet of concern relevant to planning. By growing consensus, more bonafide consumers and victims are coming on the board in the 51% category. Many boards now have up to 65% and 75% members who are not health vested.

For all but the two critical categories, consumers and victims, a board is able to select representatives fairly easily, because each of the other categories limits the people eligible to a relative few who are qualified. The choice among these is often by personality, status, seniority, capacity, congeniality, or to achieve a better balance among board members for other reasons, such as numbers of people from a given race, region, or profession.

Selection of "consumers" and "victims" is more complicated. Perusal of the literature on how to get representative representation has provided no better counsel than that the board must seek diversity and must remember that formal representatives of major groups and persons typical of such groups are often quite different—and both may be of real value to a board.

Generally, the middle-class community will accept middle-class people who have had experience and who are visibly "good" people because of their work with the PTA, League of Women Voters, Grange, Heart Association, and so on. Victim groups not only do not trust traditional middle-class participatory assemblages, but have few well- practiced, go-to-meeting participators of their own, and the persons who do qualify may not always be acceptable to a very wide segment of the victim communities. Some techniques that have been advocated to select victim (or consumer) representatives include:

Selection of "good" victim-type people by the overall planning body or its organizing committee. In this case the middle-class aggregate from the larger community is doing the selection of the so-called victim representatives on the basis that the selectees are: (1) well known generally for their ability to work in the larger community; (2) indicated by the results of a victim community survey or by word of mouth which reveal certain victim people as ideal, popular, trusted, with reputed power, or with evident power in the victim community; or (3) already selected or elected by the victim community to do other public tasks in their behalf.

Invitation to well-known victim action groups to select from their own people those whom they would like to have sit on a planning board.

Invitation to the victim community to produce a list of their selectees on whatever basis they wish—political, power, campaigns, by blocks, by races, and so on—from which the planning body will make its selections.

Invitation to the victim community to set up a nominating committee with members to be chosen by geography, race, need, education, preexisting organizations, and so on, and to select an array of candidates, which will either provide the planning body a list to choose from or allow a public election of representatives by the victim population.

Self selection of victim candidates by such means as attendance at advertised public meetings held by the planning body; participation in health and related issues opened up by the planning body; or calling existing organizations to a meeting and then asking them to select their representatives for the planning body.

Selection of representatives by the victim community at an open meeting called by the planning body, by means of general acclaim; various procedural devices such as nominating; or allowing each existing victim organization one vote for a representative.

Each of these methods has its virtues and its deficiencies. Some are better for getting one type of representative, some for another. All affect the power situation in neighborhoods in trouble. At present, the choice of method seems not to be a problem in most victim communities, because few there see the CHPs as having enough power to be worth their time; the probable result is that a planning body attracts fairly atypical people. However, as ghettos grow more power oriented, and as CHPs are seen as potentially more useful, the issues around selection for service on a planning board will become aggravated, and methods will be manipulated and invented.

For groups other than victims, there are some useful rules of thumb for selecting board members.

Formal Representation

Asking each group to select a representative, who is to be accepted by the appointing authority for the planning body, is probably hazardous. Comparable organizations will then have an excuse to demand equal representation, and there may, for example, be as many as a dozen parent-teacher or labor type organizations in a given community. Not all organizations choose representatives who are interested or capable of participating in planning. Many organizations perfunctorily appoint the person who has the particular officership or committee duty that appears to be related to this matter; a few will appoint their most antagonistic or disruptive member, or, as punishment, their most derelict, nonattending member. Self-selection by interest groups holds many risks.

More wisely, the elected executive or legislature can form a committee which will ask for the assistance of knowledgeable people in and out of government who are known to be interested in the fate of planning. These people in turn can suggest names from the health industry and other needed groups and for the general consumer segments. These names can be cleared where clearance in terms of acceptability is necessary. By choosing people primarily for their concern, intelligence, ability to work, and potential or demonstrated interest in planning, and only secondly as representatives, the appointing authority may offer a single name for approval (or several names for a choice) to each of the special groups concerned. Not every special interest group need be cleared in this way, however, and no appointee should be allowed to feel that his role is solely as a spokesman for a given group. Real effort should be made to indoctrinate each appointee with the nature of his responsibility to the entire community. In this way the council membership is more than a collection of instruments, each of which has a limited and prescribed range of concern. Members must play many parts and see themselves as part of an orchestra.

Representative People

The other type of representation needed at the planning table will present not the consensus or organized attitude but a personal point of view as a member of a given group, whether chosen to represent occupational, racial, or other interests. These selections can be made freely by the appointing authority once the larger and better organized groups are assured that someone who sincerely appreciates their views will be active on the board. This dual approach to representation assures that more than party-line vision will be operative, and that an expanding and open—rather than a contracting—set of forces will be operative. A Minnesota study[37] describes alternative council structures, styles, support, and so on, in terms of what can be expected from the council membership.

The choices at a state or metro level tend to focus on better known persons who are generally acceptable, and the victim-type selection problems become much more acute, as could be expected from the difficulties of selecting such persons at even local levels. As participation by victims improves at local levels, representatives can easily move to higher level bodies, although present experience indicates that they almost inevitably lose some touch and trust with their own people as a result of their prowess.

Who Are the Clients?: The Planner's Dilemma

Davidoff and Reiner[38] say that there are two kinds of clients: the proximal ones with whom the planner negotiates; and those who ultimately use the product and finally foot the bill. The two groups are rarely the same, even though the proximal clients do always claim to share the two attributes of the ultimate. However, they are also likely to have a lot more personally at stake than use of the product and payment for it.

Client Identity

The issue of the client's identity sounds academic but rapidly takes on dramatic qualities when planners begin to finalize their mode of studying a situation.[39] They suddenly face the fact that if they study the community's problem or goal design in behalf of the broadest interests (the larger system), some of the findings and viewpoints to be presented might be obnoxious to members of the community planning body who see the system differently or see the issue only in relation to a subsystem. This is most likely to occur where the community planning body is supposed to represent the community but is obviously overbalanced with persons of a particular background who see issues only as members of a subsystem would—for example, much as traditional medical and hospital interests see the health care delivery problem. A different but equally limited view of the issues can occur if only poor consumers are on the board, a situation often commented on in the context of governance of neighborhood health centers.

From the position of the professional individual planner, a moral dilemma can be set up (not to mention the practical consideration of surviving as a planner). Such a dilemma is not easy to resolve if the planner is intelligent enough to understand that the limited views of an unrepresentative or an ignorant and conventionally "wise" board may so prejudice his opportunities to work intelligently that he must slight major considerations. If he does so, he hurts many interests, and he may well be hurting the entire community, because plans based on the outlook of one subsystem may be so suboptimal as to harm all parts of the system, including the subsystem which has captured the planner.

From these considerations have emerged many dicta. One is that the planner must seek a diversity of views and examine the situation from each of these positions (potential clients,) so that it can be said that he is really doing pluralistic planning.[40] In this way, of course, the planner's final resolution or optimization of situations may not be similar to what his advocacy posture had worked out for any one of his potential clients, for he has taken into account all of their interests as well as he can. In a somewhat less elite role, he makes a point of helping all the major identifiable interests or subsystems viewholders to work with one another, so that the final planning analysis is as cognizant and responsive as possible to the pluralism of interests inevitable in any situation of sufficient consequence to demand planning assistance.

Naturally, there will often be interests of major importance for which no legitimate or even visible spokesman can be found. As a result, another dictum has it that those who are not heard from—often a great majority of the populace—must become the planner's particular client, since no one else is about to look after their interests. Sometimes the planner (or planning body) may be able to arouse spokesmen for silent groups with much at stake. In that way he rounds out the pluralistic approach to planning without having to continue as a specific advocate for the unrepresented.[41] Given the American credo (see Chapter 2), it will be hard for many liberally inclined planners not to assume advocacy in behalf of those who do not come to the planning table. If a planner is astute and comfortable in this role, he may carve out a respected niche for himself, provided that he does not so strongly identify himself with his silent constituency that he can no longer do —or be trusted to do—the overall planning required if all constituencies are to be kept under one plan.

Where the planning body, created in the name of the community, is either set up to serve or is taken over by a determined subsystem which will only look at things in its own light, the planner may have few options: he stays and tries to educate his board by gently putting other views in front of them; he stays and subversively organizes their natural opponents so that they take over, or at least join and modify; he stays and becomes the advocate of the subsystem; he leaves.

So far, we have considered only the situations that arise when a planner is employed by a so-called community body which has the ostensible obligation to plan for its entire community. In other situations, the planner is hired by or is a regular employee of one subsystem and is contributed to the cause of community health planning with ample fanfare. We see such planners recruited and donated by, among others, the largesse of hospitals, medical societies, health departments, universities, health care systems, voluntary health agencies, and occasionally, by large industry and labor. Again, the planner is unquestionably morally obligated to serve the entire community, but his pay, promotions, and even survival or recommendations to other jobs are controlled by a single vested subsystem interest. The conflicts for the planner are identical with those already discussed, except that when he takes this kind of job he can hardly avoid recognizing that he has a very specific boss with an explicitly constrained point of view.

Where the planner is absolutely assured that he is only to consider the larger community's interests, he would be wise to draw a few pictures for his salary-providing employer, illustrating how it might come to pass that planning based on community-wide improvement would be something less than promising for his employer in the short run, and occasionally even over the long run. True, he may have that one-in-a-million employer who wants the planner to do what the community calls for; more often he may simply come to an understanding of how far his employer will go in putting up with the concept of community primacy. Where the employer clearly advances his own position as the one by which the planner must be constrained, even while operating under the guise of planning for the community, the planner has only his conscience to deal with—for he is to be the tool that knowingly brings about the hoodwinking of his community.

Other and more complicated situations may confront individual planners in identifying their clients. Employees or representatives of a United Nations or WHO type of organization may be lent to national governments or local agencies. The planner may be the regular employee of a national or state agency loaned to state or local communities. He may be a university employee co-venturing with semipublic, private, or governmental agencies. One of the more complex situations may be illustrated by the university professor temporarily employed by an international health agency to assist another nation in planning at the national, state, and local government levels by means of a planning study team based at a university in the host country.

Such a planner may have the following systems uppermost in his mind as the client to be served: First, his own university which will reward him if he earns recognition, does good research, publishes his experiences, and creates good images of his university abroad; second, his own government which will perhaps even honor him if he promotes the image or interests of his country; third, the international agency which sought him out as the suitable person to carry out their contractual obligations, and which will honor him by future appointment if he generally enhances their image and fulfills their specified obligations to the country he was selected to serve; fourth, the host country whose citizenry is to be served and which will have many interests. These will include:

The members of the governmental health agency which worked out the contract, and who want to look good as a result of the planner's efforts.

The members of the national political hierarchy who countenanced the venture, who do not want their political holds to be jeopardized, and who want to come out looking very good, some because they want changes recommended and some because they want, not change, but time to maneuver.

The members of the state and local health and political hierarchies who have similar but more limited concerns as their national counterparts.

The host university that wishes to be seen as the source of desirable and accepted change by educators, the health professions, the health agencies, the political hierarchies and the citizenry at large.

The university study team that the planner joins.

The citizenry themselves in whose behalf the entire planning venture is presumably being undertaken.

It is not uncommon for planners to make a prompt identification with the citizenry and proceed happily until they have inadvertently placed their team or their host university in one or more binds, often with the citizenry itself. They may shortly find that if their efforts are to be taken seriously, major issues must be settled with and between each and every one of the clients lest the citizenry, their health agencies, the political hierarchies, and the university be soon pitted one against the other. When these issues are not settled or are settled poorly, the contracting international agency may subsequently be perceived as a subversive influence because it provided the planners whose work indicates need for changes that one or more host interests are not prepared to face. Because of the planner's nationality, he may make his own country *persona non grata* with one or more clients. He may even besmirch the reputation of his alma mater.

There probably are not many recipes for successfully identifying one's true client. In the example given, the planner's own country and university may be dismissed as key determining influences, for they simply imply a neverending source of constraint in terms of not tarnishing the image of country and university. The international health agency must be explicitly dealt with in terms of the constraints it imposes because it is the planner's hiring agent which has contracted to do a specific job for a specific client in certain ways within certain limits, and the international health agency's perception of whom it has contracted to serve as a client must be given precedence. If the agency has not thought this through, it must be aided to do so.

Unfortunately, the national, regional, and local agencies that may be contracting for planning in behalf of a community, often do not perceive the ambiguities of the client issue and, as a result, decisions about this complex matter may exist only as platitudes in the contractual instruments. Nevertheless, a little direct exploration with the agencies will soon determine what constraints they place on the operation, to whom they defer, and of whose ultimate interests they are most conscious.

If the preceding sets of potential constraints are not considered, the planner who joins the team at the host university, in the example given, may soon find that the client issue has never been faced—unless warfare has already broken out. It is not rare to find that each team member thinks he has a different client or clients. Identification of clients is best drawn out by discussions in which the team members attempt to agree on whom they must involve, to whom they must report, and whose interests and decisions must be respected. Such issues are not impossible to resolve once they are faced, for someone in the host country has signed the contracts under certain presumptions, and inside of that set of implicit or explicit constraints the actual role of the university and the planning team can be clarified. Whether any freedom is left to the independent planner's work in behalf of the well-being of the citizenry depends on the sincerity of the university, and the health and political hierarchies of the host country. The time to find this out is while the negotiations are being made, not after planning is under way and fears have been aroused by clumsiness caused by lack of awareness of client issues. While an agency or a country's leaders are bargaining for a planning venture, they will almost certainly make much firmer and more liberal commitments about what the planners are to do than they will later on.

Unfortunately, if the planners are already at work and disagreeable issues arise before clarification of clients has taken place, the planners almost always find themselves in the position of supplicants asking for permission to work. And by that time they often have too large an investment at every level of client to fight too hard for the recognition of the citizenry as the major clientele.

The same types of problems have arisen for planners as they have been borrowed, hired, or loaned from one environment to another within the United States to help out in Model Cities, in neighborhood health centers, or in general health planning ventures.

How Does the Planner Relate to His Clients?

In all probability, the more clearcut the client group is—particularly if it is clearly represented by those authorized to negotiate with the planner—the more he will be expected to do exactly as the client group dictates. He will be very much their well directed and supervised technician until he proves unfailingly and unflinchingly that he is one of them. He may be allowed to work as he sees fit, if he has the kind of capacity that earns him a a leadership role. He may become their submerged source of inspiration or their leader, with or without the visible spokesman role.

The more confused the client issue, the more roles are open to the planner. Some planners in this situation very easily submerge themselves in the pure technician role, carrying out every written word of contractual instruction. Others prefer to create outputs suggested by those who determine the planner's promotion or continuation of employment. In poorly defined client situations, more self-assertive planners may become very powerful figures, making personal constituencies out of major client groups. When that is well done, threats from those who have the so-called formal authority to chastise or fire the planner can be obviated. Other planners in these circumstances try to play a very elitist role in behalf of the silent majority of their clients or for the entire community. They do what is "good" for their clients without having too much occasion to consult with them, and usually build a strong base among the active philanthropic elite (not unlike the Lasker circle in public health).[42]

Some planners have a more assertive and advocative bent and formally put themselves at the service of a poorly represented group or community, with the intent of providing them with as much technical assistance as can be mustered on a slim budget or foundation grant. These operations are often short lived for several reasons: the advocate planner, who is usually a stranger, may be maligned, lose all of his client support, and be starved out of business; usually his clients are concerned only with limited difficulties and do not stay with him or the planning effort for significant long-term issues; unless he has unusual intellectual and financial resources, he finds the going hard under strong adverse pressures from established sources—pressures compounded by insecure support from the very persons he is serving. There are some happy exceptions, of the Nader type, who have captured the public imagination and whose work has even resulted in popular writings.[43]

As often as not, the advocate planner comes equipped with a cause or soon finds one, and he is more realistically described as an advocate in search of a client. He stays to work with whichever clients appreciate his cause as theirs and are willing to work with him if he can find or bring his own resources; occasionally they may be able to support him if he does not.

A kind of hit-and-run technical advocacy has been utilized by Burco and Henderson.[44] On limited sums of money, a skillful planner comes in to represent a losing faction and is able to create both a strong

enough political alliance willing to consider alternatives and competing plans that are sound enough so that the establishment planning
steamroller is rebutted or dumped. This mode, of course, is based on
planning better or more pleasing solutions on a stage already littered
by poor solutions. But it is doubtful that this kind of hit-and-run advocacy can arouse enough interest or have enough staying power to
find and analyze the problems and then develop relevant alternative
solutions needed by a community. Its utility is built on the ability to
rapidly overpower existing poor planning, at low cost. When goals are
vague and plans have aroused significant pockets of apprehension,
doubt or resistance, the intent of hit-and-run advocacy is to shed light
and arouse interest that will find a way of undertaking good planning.

The majority of comprehensive health planning agencies with
which I am familar fall in the 314(b) or local CHP category, with self-
selected boards who hire the planner as one of their first acts. To date
those boards either were initially, or have come to be, typically domi-
nated by medical and hospital interests which intend to serve the community by the means they deem best. Many depend heavily on their
planner to provide or get them guidance, and—except for clearly
voiced apprehensions about consumers "piloting the plane"—they
really expect the professional planner to do his best for the community
as they see its needs. In this typically ambivalent situation, the planner
gets to know the elites and the health interests very well, and infrequently has much comprehension about or inputs from the poorly
served or even the general public who his board assures him are its
clients. Because preoccupation with the ultimate clients may earn him
no Brownie points, the planner typically serves his board as though it
were his client, and he often tries—even if ever so gently—to get his
board to produce some good rhetoric about the mass of people who are
its clients. More aggressive, people-oriented planners then use this
rhetoric as a base from which to involve more people and bring these,
the board's clients, into the limelight, so that consumer concerns,
rather than those of the vendor, come to the center of the health planning stage.

The planner (or planning firm) who comes to work for a CHP or
any other group on a specific contract for a period of time, or for a
specific project or plan, may seem to have an easier time finding and
relating to his clients. He generally deals with a specific body, whether public or private, and is asked to negotiate with an officer, their
planner, a committee, or the board. He writes up his proposal with the
designated party, signs a contract, and goes to work. The nature of his
work, however, may expose him to all the ambiguities faced by the resident planner, whenever the rhetoric tells him to make the best plan for
the community. His terms of work may even have to guarantee working with or surveying the community, but his final output will still

usually be cleared with the persons who signed his contract, even if they do say that his plan must be designed to achieve community concurrence. Only if he acts as the planning body's executive, however, is he in quite the same confusing position as the resident planner over the issue of the board versus the community as client.

In general the professional health planner is asked to play a very normative role. He is often asked (1) how the planning agency should plan; (2) for what they should plan; or (3) to produce what he considers a good plan. These are all heavy orders, for when he is asked to describe the goals toward which the community should be aiming, he must usurp the community's role of goal setting. Planning morality would call for the planner to study the community, its needs and desires, and to submit possible goal sets for selection by the planning body and by the community. If the planner really feels capable of determining community goals, without presenting alternatives and reasons for and against each, and if the planning body accepts those goals as a matter of course, the planner has become the decision maker for the planning body. Fortunately, his output is unlikely to go unchallenged when it reaches policy or legislative levels, for the very reason that so little community input went into his planning efforts. And, for just this reason, very prestigious planning firms are sought, in spite of often inflated prices, to carry out planning, with the hope that political and technologic opposition to the plans will be smothered by the firm's reputation.

Participation and Consumerism

As Alberta Parker[45] and Sidney Verba[46] point out, the concept of participation has new connotations, actors, and issues. Traditional organizational behavior in the United States is currently changing. People who never before seemed to want to play in the health game now want a policy-making say about issues that were never previously brought to their attention.

New Actors

These new lay participants can be placed in at least six major categories:

The first group of new participants—whom we may call *victims,* because they get to consume so little or so poorly—are in total contrast to the traditional community participants. They do not care about looking good in the eyes of the professionals. They often feel that professionals were never professional in any but a trade union sense and that they are not to be trusted with important decisions involving the consumption of services. Moreover, those who were most victimized by professional neglect—the failure of professionals either to fight for or to provide adequate health care services within bearable cost limits—currently want most to participate. Anselm Strauss[47] has shown how unconcerned health professional have been even with the forms of addressing and dealing with the poor—one source of the animosity between the victims and the professionals.

A second group of new participants are the ancillary health personnel. They believe that most professionals regard their own take-home pay as sacred but think that ancillaries should welcome the opportunity to work at any wage, just to associate with the professional, who will make all the decisions, even about such matters as organization and finances, without considering the interest, competence, needs, or concern of others.

A third group of new participants is composed of have-nots and is much like the first, except that its interests are not in health or health care per se, but in jobs. Along with industry they have discovered the veins of wealth that can be tapped in the field of health care. The job opportunities there for persons with minimal skills are particularly important for minorities who have more job needs and less skill. Furthermore, Office of Economic Opportunity projects and rapid training programs such as New Careers paid for on-the-job training for openings available at health care centers. In this way, new participants have entered the health arena. They know from experience that little will come their way in the form of jobs, training, or services, unless they fight for all three in the form of service centers to be brought into their typically underserved neighborhoods.

A fourth new group of consequence in some areas is the counter culture. They, too, have demands for care but want them satisfied in different, less formal, less professional and less established or less "scientific" ways. Their language, dress, food and drug intake, personal styles and attitudes are obviously permeating society. Even if only in superficial ways, they have introduced new perceptions and new approaches to formerly procedurally oriented physicians and institutions.

A fifth group of new participators are the Libs. Because initiative and orginality are required of their leaders, this group is likely to deliver representatives who find it incumbent to place unusual demands on the decision-making machinery in health care, as they do elsewhere.

The sixth group of new participators is being drawn from poorly paid and modestly skilled blue-and white-collar workers and from the better paid trades and skills, because they are seen as the average consumer. They presumably are the typical Americans of modest education, means, aspirations, and politics. They are anything but homogeneous.

Issues of Participation

Domination by health professions has been accepted in most health care environments; perhaps the most striking example is hospital governance. Although health professionals still sit infrequently on boards of trustees, the typical attitude is: "We, the trustees, exist to make the hospital a good place for our doctors to bring their patients." Generally, health professionals hold that unplanned disposition of resources on the free market is the only rational way to proceed. Thus, they are also saying that the consumer is an adequate judge to pick and choose wisely in the medical market and, that by exercising choice he can influence the way medicine is to be practiced. The people who make this claim for consumer wisdom in nonplanning situations are often the first to declare that the consumer has no business at the planning table. Even though it is his money they spend, they say he is too ignorant to contribute anything meaningful to the discussion of planning. How is it that the same consumer has so much wisdom when he is on his own in the market place yet becomes so stupid when he is at the planning table?

Before any attempt is made to predict how professionals may react to a challenge of their historic domination, the term consumer needs to be put in perspective. Only a very small fraction of the consumers who now occupy the required 51% of board seats on CHP boards come from any of the six categories of new actors described above. The current consumer board members are predominantly of two types. The first is the middle-class, traditional joiner, volunteer-agency type who is sometimes involved socially with or married to persons employed in some aspect of the health care machinery. The second consumer type is the upper-class business and community leader, who is at least the social peer of the professional. Increasingly, however, consumer appointments to boards are being made from the six categories of new actors just discussed. Clean lines of separation cannot be drawn between these types. Some of the ancillary health group will share or lean toward the middle-class values despised by certain of the counter culture and victim groups. Some of the Lib group have the professional and social status of the providers, but share the anger of the victim group on issues of discrimination, inequity, and hardship. They may also share, along with the counter culture, a belief in militant and disruptive tactics.

In Figure 10.6, I have drawn on some ideas of Meisner's et al.[48] to indicate the remarkable potential for conflict between the traditional board member, the victims and the lower-middle class or working-class consumers, who are also being drawn into many boards. Naturally, the stereotypes presented are far from adequate. For example, the grossest discrepancies may occur among the victim types, who may indeed be the best of the conceptualizers, even though other aspects of the stereotyping shown in Figure 10.6 may still be valid for such a consumer.

Occasional studies are available to indicate what knowledge or attitudinal differences truly separate professional decision makers from the lay public. Utilizing the water pollution situation, Mitchell[49] observed that the more-or-less traditional laity has what we might call a "touching" faith that professionals know the answers. More interesting is that the lay viewpoints were found to be on a continuum rather than polarized. This finding supports the belief that joint lay and professional involvement and reciprocal education should be a major effort of planning bodies, and that successful community planning outputs should not be written off as an impossibility.

Experience indicates that nearly all parties get upset, that nearly all can learn, and that nearly all can grow in the sense of learning what makes the others tick (values, fighting symbols, and so on). New ways of working together, comprehension of the basics of health care and of health promotion, ability to define what is mutually wanted and how to set about obtaining what has been defined as wanted—these are accomplishments we have learned to expect of board members. Obviously, some terrific battles and periods of total frustration will ensue and will occasionally dismantle planning bodies.

Since the term *participation* now connotes largely the participation of victim-type consumers, what kind of contribution is expected from persons fitting the consumer, and particularly the victim, categories? Various authors have identified what may be expected of consumers at large, and these ideas are worth summarizing.[50] Expected planning functions of the consumer include:

Identifying and articulating health needs as seen from outside the viewpoint of medicine.

Providing clearer pictures of the inadequacies of the health care delivery systems.

Providing perspectives on use of resources for living in general, versus those earmarked for health services.

Shortening reaction time between patients and doctors.

Improving the realism of expectations on both sides.

Bringing diverse brands of expertise to bear.

Forcing improved communication between subsectors of the biomedical sector.

Reorganizing centralized decision making in the health industry by injection of political, social, and economic know-how.

Offseting both narrow-minded and self-centered professionalism and many racist attitudes.

Providing a meaningful feedback to consumers about inappropriate usage of health care.

FIGURE 10.6
ATTRIBUTES OF CONSUMER PARTICIPANTS ON A PLANNING BOARD

Traditional	New Average Type	New Victim Type
Have important roles that are perceived community wide	Have few significant roles except at neighborhood level	Are "nobody" or are active only in neighborhood or ethnic politics
Financially well-off; able to get and afford amenities and good health care	Modestly well-off; not always able to get and often unable to afford suitable medical care	Poor; little access to other amenities or commodities or health care
Well educated formally	Modestly educated formally	Poorly educated formally
Sought after as patients	Acceptable as patients	Disdained as patients
Catered to by professionals	Treated patronizingly by professionals	Ignored by professionals
Socially equal to the professionals	Socially lower than the professionals	Bottom of the social ladder
At home with the social graces and believe in them	Not handy with the social graces; may or may not believe in them	Direct, abrupt, crude, despise social graces
Accustomed to working through power plays	Expect power plays and to be victimized by them	Accustomed to confrontation and force; also expect to be victimized by power plays
Usually paranoid about poor and minorities as participants, but some exceptions	Paranoid about minorities and victims as participants	Paranoid about rich and professionals as participants
Defer to professionals	Defer, often bow and scrape to professionals	Less and less respectful of professionals

456

Casual appearing and acting at meetings	Casual appearing but easily aroused at meetings	Apathetic or intensely involved
No great personal investment in any given board or committee appointment	Significant personal investment in any given board or committee appointment	None or great personal investment in board or committee appointment
Socialize with provider members on board	Socialize with own kind of consumers	Socialize only with their own kind of consumers
Involved in other professions or business enterprises	Involved in jobs, small business, service, lesser professions, labor	Often unemployed, rarely have run more than marginal businesses; few in professions
Have come on to boards over the years, one at a time; well socialized to the board	Have come on to boards in recent years; not socialized to the board	Have come on to board in recent years; poorly socialized to the board
Involved in many similar ventures	Involved in few other similar ventures	Involved in few other ventures, with some remarkable exceptions
Share middle class values, but often tolerant of others	Share middle class values, and generally less tolerant of others	Oblivious to, antagonistic to or envious of middle class values
Middle age and older	Middle age	Young, middle and older
Few children	Average number of children	Many children
Adept at generalizing, conceptualizing, specifying	Slow to conceptualize; prefer tangibles	Avoid conceptualizations; more comfortable with specifics
Use written materials as well as oral	Use written, but prefer oral	Prefer oral; dislikes written
Keep issues impersonal	Try to keep issues impersonal	Personalize issues

Improving the scope of support and capacity, and thereby, help growth and change in the health industry.

Providing reassurance to consumers about the integrity of the system.

Providing access to a community power base for social action which no trade or profession can mobilize.

The specific utilities that consumers are expected to bring to the board speak to the several general roles that consumers of all kinds might fill. The simplest definition of a health consumer is "anyone potentially consuming the products who does not make his living directly from the health services industry and who is not involved in working in the industry or with it in any obvious way." This definition excludes from the category of consumer the professionals, ancillary staff, and the executives and nonpaid board members of voluntary and governmental health agencies other than health planning.

Preparing consumers for service on planning bodies and determining the proportion of victims among them are key issues, but no more so than the uses to which consumers are put. Arnstein created a ladder of user inputs[51] which went from the essence of nonparticipation (manipulation), through the steps of treating, to informing, consulting with, placating, partnership, delegated power, and finally citizen control. We are all aware of examples of health care ventures that operate with consumer inputs at each of these levels. The levels of consumer involvement which are shown in Figure 10.7 represent possibilities to achieve the basic planning functions. Whether the consumers are in an absolute majority does not matter, provided that victims make up a goodly minority. Experience has indicated that appointing a tiny contingent of minorities or of victims to a board does not suffice to encourage them to come to meetings or to keep them in activities. Token representation has too frequently soon meant no representation of these groups. Often, minorities or victims have been appointed to the board but not to major committees. Thus they are removed from all serious work and learning experiences, and they know or assume that they are being used and either behave accordingly or give up.

What does count is that the consumer and victim types be allowed to participate at every level of decision making. If they dominate the board but are kept off of planning and study committees, they may have the option of voting for or against matters, but they will learn very slowly about the cause-and-effect aspects of issues and the realities of how these are in fact interpreted by different view holders. The traditional type of board member will learn little in return. We must impart to one another the viewpoint that has been called relativistic, the viewpoint that takes into account multiple values and moves away from the dualistic, right-and-wrong, or single-goal frameworks which plague our organizational and decision-making activities.[52] (This position is similar to Warren's suggestions for new decision-making structures.[53]

Some committees are said to be purely technical—meaning that only biomedical types are eligible to participate; others are said to be purely economic—meaning that only business types may participate. Such gimmicks are used to avoid consumer inputs where they are most needed. As long as victims and consumers cannot affect the system by buying competitive products, they must swing their weight at the committee and decision making levels of planning.

The suggestion that consumers serve on all committees leads to remarkable confrontations with some technological or medical types who object to a "committee doing surgery." In reality, consumers rarely want even to be concerned with medical procedures except for such issues as cost, safety, or manpower, which are more consumer and societal than medical in significance. (See Chapter 4 for discussion of what is medical and what is not.) By agreeing in advance that consumers will not involve themselves in individual patient treatment, few problems need be anticipated. However, the presence of consumers on quality-of-care review committees is one of the few ways to keep such activities relevant and honest. As good a way—perhaps better in a political sense, because it alleviates initial anxieties—is use of outside,

FIGURE 10.7
LEVELS OF CONSUMER INVOLVEMENT IN DECISION MAKING

Meaningfulness (Level of input)	Nature of Involvement	
Very high	Participant in system 1) individuals as prototype consumers, or 2) as representatives of consumer groups	—majority voice overall —minority voice overall —participant in policy making —participant in policy design —participant in planning —veto —advisory
High	Independently organized to influence	—set up competition —adversary —advisory —supplicatory
Low	Reactive to services used	—make suggestions —make complaint —do not like —like
Very low	Utilization of care	—do not —do

highly professional, quality-of-care survey teams from institutions known for their integrity and quality; men whose territory is far enough away so that referral business and dangers of reprisal are unlikely. Good reviews of what is involved in consumer participation are now available.[54]

Not only the professionals who work in the system, but also the volunteers and nonmedical and nonskilled employees who make up two-thirds of the workers in the health sector, need representation. Often demands for consumer and victim participation include concern for worker participation. Perhaps this concern grows out of the fact that the unskilled workers often come from the ranks of the victims. Moreover, members of the victim group perceive that more meaningful participation may be the beginning of a job situation ranging from volunteer, trainee, unskilled worker, skilled worker, up to and including management and even top managerial posts.

We are indebted to Richard Bailey for pointing out that, as a minimum, we should look at the major viewpoints likely to be found on the planning board, if it is constituted according to our advice. Figure 10.8 is a chart of a few key attitudes about planning or outlooks that must be reconciled and worked through by a planning board before it can really do much of a job. Again, the stereotypes apply to no specific situations and are simply illustrative of the diversity that can be expected.

Adding the widely differing participant viewpoints toward planning shown in Figure 10.8 to the gross differences toward life in general shown in Figure 10.6 provides some real ammunition for a doom-and-gloom attitude toward consumer participation. New types of participants who are appointed to boards to fulfill the requirements for representativeness may have little familiarity or respect for *Robert's Rules of Order,* or for the traditional types of board members who are now coming under pressure to share their historic control. There may be little initial harmony because no suitable means of operating is generally accepted. Fortunately, if our surmises about the differences are correct, some interesting convergences will occur from time to time. For example, victims and planners both often see the need for comprehensiveness and believe that more than health care services must be worried about under the rubric of health planning. Therefore, they surprise one another by coming to agreements—a happening which has been verified innumerable times in our field encounters.

The mixture among consumer board members is likely to become heavier with both kinds of new consumers. What types of accomplishments are we hoping for from them, and what are the prognoses for accomplishment? Irrespective of specific health and consumer participatory goals, there is a basic set of goals toward which a board must work if it is to do a creditable job. An effective board must have what

FIGURE 10.8
DIVERGENT ATTITUDES AROUND THE PLANNING TABLE

ISSUES AND APPROACHES	TYPE OF BOARD MEMBER				
	CONSUMERS			PROVIDERS	TRAINED PLANNERS
	New "Victims"	*New Average*	*Traditional*		
Participation of All Kinds of Persons	strongly in favor	somewhat in favor	dubious	opposed (exceptions)	opposed (exceptions)
Time Range of Concerns	mostly short	mostly short	short to middle	short to middle	middle to long
Control over Planning Outcomes	tight, use sanctions	tight, use sanctions	moderate, use sanctions and incentives	moderate, use incentives more than sanctions	loose, use plans, criteria, incentives, sanctions, evaluation
Coping and Problem-Solving	heavy emphasis	heavy emphasis	heavy emphasis	heavy emphasis	moderate emphasis
Future Building and Idealistic	sometimes	rarely	sometimes	rarely	variable emphasis
Action and Implementation	heavy emphasis	heavy emphasis	moderate emphasis	moderate emphasis	variable emphasis
Comprehensive and Boundary Crossing	broad outlook, emphasis on health and health care	narrow outlook, emphasis on health care	narrow outlook, emphasis on health care	narrow outlook, emphasis on health care	variable concerned with health and health care

Alberta Parker[55] has described for the neighborhood health center as "good basic relationships" among:

The members of the board itself.

The board and the organization and staff which the board serves, either in an advisory or policy-making capacity.

The board and the community represented.

The board and the outside health system, as well as the larger social political system.

The board and the funding agency.

The very subtle, variable and complex internal commitments board members may have with regards to themselves, the board, the institution and the community.

Requirements for the board members of a planning body would seem to differ little, if at all, from the requirements described above for the neighborhood health-center board. In participant training attempts, these relationship objectives had to be kept in mind, and were at least as important as showing consumers how to participate in planning. The consumers' own well prepared, even if poorly verbalized, agenda generally revealed their needs for process as well as substantive information. As health planning bodies now commence to feel the same participatory pressures, they too need to develop perception of their relationships as well as comprehension of planning—the latter still being at an unbelievably low level among all the types of participants on boards.

The contribution of Parker just referred to and that of Geiselman and Nowlen[56] are particularly valuable as an outline by which to introduce training. They point out the need for a forum "away from home," at which board members can look at the roles and goals of members as well as those of the planning body. Parker is not sure that training for policy making is likely to be immediately transferable to the purposes of planning. However, I consider the effective policy-making health center board as a means for many board members to develop the kind of background that would make them ideal board members for health planning bodies, and also as a means to expand community and individual capacities.

An exciting and profitable outcome can be expected from the participatory approach to planning. What can be done to speed up useful interchanges? I subscribe to the belief that it is important for a board to accept the role of educating its own members. This education is most needed and apt to be most profitable (even if slow) where the participatory nature of the board is the highest. The process should also be only modestly costly of time and ingenuity. Many sources of information are available in this area which offer specific techniques, approaches, and materials.[57]

Other problems that affect participation by victim or poor consumers include the need for transport and child care. Boards must learn how to assist their board members who have few resources so that they can participate.

Community Versus Participatory Control

Going well past the participative stance is the proposed full consumer governance over health care matters, with all others involved in health care serving in either an advisory or an employee capacity. Of course, nonprofessionals have always controlled most health care facilities and a good many voluntary health agencies; in addition, there are elements of control by insurance carriers. However, community control has now come to mean real control by victim types over the services rendered them, including planning, policy, and administrative matters—that is, possession of the ultimate power.

Steven Jonas[58] has reviewed governance of delivery of services. He points out that, because facilities and services which now serve the ghetto are largely government owned and funded (and until there really is universally funded health care, this will continue to be the case), a victim-controlled service system can do little more than administer what it is given to work with. Even worse problems will befall the victims who capture the planning machinery and exclude all others, because the nonvictim types include not only the bulk of consumers but also those who operate all the machinery and personally render all the medical services.

Community control, of course, carries a strong inadvertent anti-integration intent with it. To capture and keep power it is necessary to gain control. Minority groups, usually tightly segregated, capture power most easily when services are decentralized, or when a community control pattern gives them control where they are in the majority. So where ethnic or similar issues are real, decentralization enforced by community control may well mean segregation as opposed to integration. Such was the case in Detroit's schools.[59]

With Jonas, I conclude that community control by victims is not all that meaningful an ultimate goal for them to fight for. Rather, for all of us who want an equitable stake in health care and health care accomplishments, participation in health planning, policy, or operations seems to be the wiser, less divisive approach. In thinking that somewhat parallels mine, James D. Carroll[60] stresses the growth and utility of participation in all the technological affairs of our country, not just in those of health care. He points up the need for participation to counter the alienation which seems to be growing as a result of the belief that technology and thus technologists are really our masters and that their efforts are uncontrollable. Carroll contrasts the litigation and ad hoc resistance approaches to control over technology with the approach of technology assessment or joint study of the directions in which technological proposals might be taking us. He argues that those who will feel the impacts must have a say, and he points up many difficulties to be faced in the process—difficulties not unlike those anticipated in the health sector.

Devices for General Consumer Involvement

Care must be taken to ensure that the representative and typical consumers who have been appointed do not become gate keepers[61] who may, intentionally or unintentionally, exclude contact with the groups they are supposed to represent and from whom they supposedly draw guidance. Community groups need to communicate directly with the planning body or its committees, to express what is on their minds and to hear what concerns them. Ways to facilitate such exchanges include:

Small neighborhood meetings to bring testimony before the board or board committees (circuit riding).

Conferences which bring in one neighborhood at a time to meet with the board or a committee.

Conferences to bring in mixtures of neighborhoods to meet with one another or with the board.

Newspaper review of board activities; this device is one-way unless the board contrives to put material in the form of requests to be answered and returned by mail.

Testimony presented before the board by experts who are paid by the board and who present the positions of neighborhoods as given to them by the neighborhoods (this might include indigenous neighborhood persons).

Circularizing materials and seeking responses from selected respondents.

Surveys for attitudes.

Surveys which leave information and request the return of opinions.

Feedback systems about participation with agency activity.

Feedback systems about health care received.[62]

Constituencies

By traditional definition, a legal constituency is the geopolitical group which has the right to select or elect a representative. In more colloquial parlance, a constituency is that segment of a geopolitical grouping which consciously and favorably regards some publicly appointed person (or group) as the representative whom they will support and nurture in return for his (its) actions on their behalf.

In these terms, the entire community is the legal constituency for CHP, but only a small fraction of the community is probably ever aware and mildly in favor of its existence. Client and representative participants on the board and its committees do not guarantee a positive constituency concerned with support or significant outputs. One of the reasons for this situation is that CHP bodies are—even at 51% consumer membership—not designed or intended to be the watchdog for the public over an industry or sector, as many local, state and national commissions and authorities are charged to be. Interestingly enough, most people have the feeling that watchdog boards typically become protectors of their charges anyway, rather than of the public. The CHPs are intended to be resolvers of differences and designers of ways around differences to new objectives. They are not likely to be seen as entirely pleasing to the health care industry—whose voice, it is to be hoped, they do not become—nor to the consumers, nor to other participants whose immediate interest they cannot always accept without reservations and compromises.

The credit for any good work done by the planning body is most likely to go, first, to the legislators who politically implement it and, second, to the operating entities which programmatically implement and deliver the product called for by the planners. Because planning is a complex phenomenon that is difficult to describe, it is not likely to be perceived by the public at large as critical or productive, except for those events which fall under its adjudicatory roles where decisions may earn as many enemies as friends. Clearly CHPs could profit from numerous and powerful supporters.

What then is the likelihood that the planning body will develop a positive constituency? One source of a firm constituency may be victim types, if they are treated fairly in terms of representation, personal consideration and shared authority. But they are not the most powerful constituency, except in some large cities where they have captured the vote. Furthermore, they have yet to be won over to what they generally regard as a powerless game. However, some victims are beginning to discover that—as weak a legislative base as P.L. 89-749 provides—when buttressed by their participation and increasingly significant state laws, CHP may be a means to generate power for disadvantaged communities, or at least for individuals on the board.

More obvious sources of support are the two groups who have been pointed out as likely to reap the rewards from good planning—the policy makers and the health care industry. The policy makers are so accustomed to poor solutions at ever mounting costs that some are hungrily looking for more rational advice about health expenditures, services and controls. True, the present advice they now get from planning bodies is not very good, but they get no better advice elsewhere. And the planning body, to which they can now refer as their source of advice, does get them off the hook of appearing to favor one or another of the competing forces in the two hottest areas, health care and environmental control. If the caliber of planning improves and if planning comes to include awareness of what implementation involves politically, legislators may come to be the strongest constituency CHPs will get. They are important constituents and clients who can award money and power directly.

The health care industry would like very much to come out of the current fray looking good. Because it is so bitterly embattled externally and because its leaders now get vocal internal support most often when they refuse to acknowledge the necessity for change, they are in desperate need of an impartial forum where they can be heard, and from which can flow generally acceptable change proposals for which the health sector leaders need not take too much blame from their own constituencies. Those who earn their living in the health care sector are not likely to suffer outrageously under any forthcoming health care planning proposals. Furthermore, the violent reactionaries in their ranks are usually aged and being replaced by more aware young people. And so it may come to pass that CHPs will be regarded as a godsend by the health care industry. In fact, much support for CHPs and P.L. 89-749 was generated by the private care sector, possibly for just these kinds of reasons.

If victims, legislators, and purveyors all find CHPs useful, the positive constituency needed is guaranteed. If these interests then succeed in getting a socially valid product out of the CHPs, the entire polity or legal constituency should surely become a positive constituency. Perhaps this is a roundabout and tedious way of countering the critics and pessimists in CHP, by reminding them that real planning effort— which keeps in mind health, social relationships, and implementation—will hasten the day when CHPs have a powerful constituency.

A nagging fear about the future of planning remains. At the national level, where there is no CHP and where the major health and environmental decisions are made without more than highly partisan advice, the national legislators might prematurely withdraw their support of CHP because they have no planning counterpart of their own under this law from which to benefit. For lack of a CHP contribution nationally, they may continue to seek simple panaceas without appreciating the potential utility of creating a national level counterpart of the comprehensive health planning machinery that they have given to the states and localities. Fortunately, there is a countering force. National legislators all come from localities and states; success of CHPs at those levels could bring such legislators plenty of support to continue the CHP mandate. A similar phenomenon happened to RMP in 1970. As tremendous cuts, on the initiative of the Executive and without much objections in Congress, became evident, the mail started to come in from back home. What looked like a dim future for an equally young—and in our opinion, less socially significant—venture was reversed rather effectively, at least for a time.

ORGANIZATION

Issues of how to structure the planning body, how to use committees, how the board relates to staff, where functions are to be assigned, and so on, would seem to parallel those of other agencies in health for which there is a sizable relevant literature.[63] Therefore, only a few isolated issues will be discussed here.

Committees and Task Forces

Because there often is confusion over the terms *task force* and *committee*, a few descriptors are provided which suggest why the two are not synonymous and indicate when each is more relevant, irrespective of what it is called. The term *ad hoc* applied to a committee in many organizations is the counterpart of the term "task force" as used here. (Figure 10.9.)

In establishing a planning body, the first structures would be task forces. One would be for goal setting. Because we believe that planning must start by detecting and then analyzing major problems in at least three areas—human disorders, sick communities, and distribution problems—a second major task force is needed for assessment. One is needed on structures and relationships and another on membership and functions. And a task force on setting up subarea planning units at neighborhood levels is a must for a city planning body; at

FIGURE 10.9
COMPARISON OF TASK FORCE AND COMMITTEE

Task Force	*Committee*
Defined task or end points	A general sphere, sector, or territory of concern
Time limited	Long-term
Task-relevant individuals	Organizationally trustworthy individuals
Analytic and synthesizing	Watch dog, evaluative, controlling
Activities may be quite innovative, sporadic	Activities are usually clear, endless or repetitive

city/county levels for a regional body; or at regional levels for the state planning body. At about the time that these first task forces are generating a picture of what needs doing and how the planning body might go about getting it done, a committee on technical skills and another on financing should be formed to produce the means required to meet long-term and recurring needs.

The original task forces can be expected to have completed their work by the time goals and special health problems emerge for study. Then they can be disbanded, and new goal- or problem-centered task forces created to study, for example, an equitable delivery system, problems such as alcoholism, accidents, certain sick communities, or maldistribution of certain services.

I question the wisdom of an initial structural division solely into committees for manpower and facilities, plus one or two others. Such committee assignments suggest to me that neither human disorders nor sick communities will receive an intelligent evaluation or analysis. And problems and solutions will tend to be approached in terms of normative standards or national averages for two factors only, manpower and facilities—both quite unrelated to the major causes of ill health.

A planning body whose board has a task force organization designed to facilitate planning logic is more likely to be operationally meaningful and to contribute a growing citizen expertise to government. Without such a working board, the operation of the planning body may be perceived as the work of professional planners nakedly competing with the legislative body for the decision-making status which the latter must retain.[64] The question of staffing has been discussed under Technological Capability.

Size of Board

The size of the body can limit diversity and representation. A statewide health planning board of 15 members holds little promise of capturing much credibility for representativeness, particularly if one or more of the majority consumer members are the wives or relatives of physicians or trustees of hospitals. Figure 10.10 presents views on the strengths and weaknesses of a board in relationship to its size. With the requirement of 51% consumer board members, the needed diversity of technical and consumer interests on a state or metro level board cannot be attained with fewer than 150 members. How useful are large boards? State legislatures may have hundreds of members and few of us would care to say that they do less meritorious work than the small local governing bodies in the same states. More often, local ineptitudes, petti-fogging, and the obvious capture of local bodies by special interests make the state legislatures look quite statesmanlike by comparison. Be that as it may, few persons in the United States can get up enough courage to urge that boards have more than 75 members, without simultaneously creating executive committees that usually take over and turn the general board into a rubber stamp.

Standing and ad hoc committees, heavily composed of nonmembers but built on a base of the council's membership, allow the equivalent of an enlargement of the planning body through appointment of persons who represent the necessary interests and factions in any given subject area. At the same time, surveys, polls and public hearings will

FIGURE 10.10
PROBABLE EFFECTIVITY OF PLANNING COUNCILS AS
RELATED TO SIZE OF MEMBERSHIP

	10-20 members	20-40 members	40-over members
Work efficiency (because of numbers)	+++	++	+
Avoidance of unduly prolonged nature of deliberations	++	+	−
Adequate representation to have all major interests and needs represented formally	−	+	++
Adequate representation to have effective subcommittees (composed of members) working on key issues	−	+	++
Representation too large to be "reached" by special interests	+	++	+++
Every part of community has the opportunity of feeling represented	+	++	+++
Avoidance of domination by individuals or small cliques	+	++	+++
Avoidance of an unforseen value orientation of board not typical of community	+	++	+++
Avoidance of opportunity for opponents of a plan to label it as the product of a few selfish interests	+	++	+++
Chances for avoiding extreme approaches	+	++	+++
Appropriate concern for secondary and side effects	+	++	+++
Probability of including representation of major conflicting viewpoints from major sectors of concern	−	+	++
Adequate breadth of concerns	−	+	++
Adequate familiarity and competency for scope of undertaking	−	+	++
Adequate familiarity with all aspects of community	−	+	+++

Ratings vary from very high +++ to low −

have to contribute or even become the backbone of representativeness for a planning body. It is impossible to get all shades of opinion and all concerns represented on committees or the board, particularly because not all interests will contribute participants who can or will be involved continuously. Guidelines for the composition of a subcommittee that must address a particular issue have been stated by Raffel:[65]

What is the nature and scope of the problem for which you are developing a plan?

What information do you need for developing a plan?

Who has the information, experience, and judgment required as an input in the development of the plan?

What groups and agencies do you expect to act on your plan?

One analysis of the responsibilities and the structure of a comprehensive health planning body goes into the potentialities of committees in terms of composition, organization, and duties.[66]

Financing

The opportunities for financing planning bodies include a multitude of possibilities. The voluntary body may be served by one or several of the following mechanisms, and in any proportion; government grant allocation from the same or a higher or lower level of government; governmental project or contract from the same or a higher or lower level of government; voluntary or private agency contract or allocation for specified tasks. The government sponsored but essentially independent model may use the same types of financing. Direct funding by the governmental unit that set it up, and grant and project funds from the national level would be the major sources. Occasionally, lower levels of government, private enterprises and voluntary agencies might assist with funding. A government planning agency, or planning done by a department of government, might be financed in much the same ways, but it is more likely to receive regular funding as an arm of government.

The refrain of "he who pays the piper" is a reminder of an ever-present and often subtle hazard. There is every reason to minimize problems on this score by preplanning. Obtaining monies from multiple sources is obviously a safeguard against pressures from one source of funds. Funding entirely from voluntary and private sources is unlikely to be adequate. Moreover, major financial dependence can create unwillingness on the part of the council financed from the nongovernmental side to rock the boat of the private sector supplying the funds. Where voluntary or private funds are accepted for specific tasks, it must be clearly ascertained that those tasks (whether intentionally or unintentionally) will not pull the planning body in one direction at the expense of others; act as a bribe to persuade the planning body to go easy on contributing sectors; or consume a disproportionate amount of the total available planning funds and energy to finance a specific undertaking which was inadequately funded at the outset. Restraint, intimidation, inducement, and rule-and-regulation excesses are all hazards attributable to one or another sources of funding. Diversity among board members should spare planning bodies from the most flagrant victimization by special interest or government funding. It is of interest that one study of planning effectiveness at the state level indicated that only a low or modest level of financing was needed for success.[67]

An Ideal Form

I have attempted to clarify the capabilities, relationships, representation, and organization of planning bodies at various levels of community. The logic, the strengths, weaknesses, or predispositions for each of the possible choices was indicated. This does not mean that a board designed to meet all of the outlined functional criteria is necessarily ideal for a given community. This ideal might lead to a hopeless schism in the face of tradition or strong minority or majority beliefs. By means of logic alone no one would dare presume to dictate planning body function or structure to a given community whose special circumstances may call for unusual affiliations or representation if its planning body is to be effective. However, when options under consideration include theoretically undesirable traits, those persons setting up the planning machinery should be alert to the possible consequences and sure of the need for their choice. A lively review of how a major neighborhood planning body was brought into being and what organizational decisions were made is now available.[68]

REFERENCES

1. Alfred D. Chandler, Jr., *Strategy and Structure* (Cambridge: Massachusetts Institute of Technology Press, 1962), Introduction.
2. State of California, Office of the Governor, Committee on Medical Aid and Health, "Report: Health Care for California," State Department of Public Health, Berkeley, December 1960.
3. State of California, Assembly, Science and Technology Advisory Council, "State Legislative Action for Promoting Systematic Change in Health Care Delivery," *Health Care Policy for California*, report of the panel on Health Care, May 15, 1971, 34-121.
4. U. S., Executive Office of the President, Bureau of the Budget, "Circular No. A-80," January 31, 1967. U. S., Executive Office of the President, Bureau of the Budget, "Circular No. A-82," April 11, 1967; Revised, January 10, 1969. U. S., Executive Office of the President, Bureau of the Budget, "Circular No. A-95," superseding A-82 after September 30, 1969, July 24, 1969; and OMB Revision of Circular A-95 Spring 1971.

5. Ida R. Hoos, "Systems Analysis, Information, Handling, and the Research Function: Implications of the California Experience," Internal Working Paper no. 68, Space Sciences Laboratory, University of California, Berkeley, November 1967.

6. Andre L. Delbecq and Andrew VandeVen, "Nominal and Interacting Group Processes for Committee Decision-Making Effectiveness," *Journal of the Academy of Management*, 14 (June 1971), 203. Andrew L. Delbecq and Andrew VandeVen, "A Group Process Model for Problem Identification and Program Planning," *Journal of Applied Behavioral Science* 7 (July/August 1971), 466-92.

7. U. Thompson, "Administrative Objective for Developing Administration," *Administrative Science Quarterly* 9 (June 1964), 91-109.

8. Daniel Bell, "The Idea of a Social Report," *The Public Interest* (Spring 1969), 22-84.

9. William J. Curran, "Are Planning Agencies Ready for Community Decision-Making Role," *Health Planning Perspectives* 6 (December 1970), 1.

10. Vicente Navarro, "The City and the Region—A Critical Relationship in the Distribution of Health Resources," *American Behavioral Scientist* 14 (July/August 1971), 865-93.

11. State of California, Ibid. no. 3.

12. Thad L. Beyle, Surenor Seligson, and Deil S. Wright, "New Directions in State Planning," *Journal of the American Institute of Planners* 35 (September 1965), 334-39.

13. Herbert J. Gans, *The Urban Villagers* (New York: The Free Press, 1962), 281-35.

14. "The Ombudsman or Citizens' Defender: A Modern Institution," *The Annals of the American Academy of Political and Social Science* 377 (May 1968). Walter Gellhorn, *Ombudsmen and Others* (Cambridge: Harvard University Press, 1966).

15. Lisa A. Peattie, "Reflections on Advocacy Planning," *Journal of the American Institute of Planners* 34 (March 1968), 80-88.

16. H. Keen, "San Diego Revisited," *Cry California* 3 (Summer 1968), 35-39.

17. Richard M. Bailey, "Economics and Planning," *Health Planning 1969*, by H. L. Blum and Associates (San Francisco: Western Regional Office, American Public Health Association, 1969), Chapter 9.

18. I. Kristol, "Decentralization for What?" *The Public Interest* (Spring 1968), 17-25.

19. National Commission on Community Health Services, *Health Administration and Organization in the Decade Ahead* (Washington, D.C.: Public Affairs Press, 1967).

20. Alan A. Altshuler, "New Institutions to Serve the Individual," presented at the American Institute of Planners Conference, "The Next Fifty Years," 1968, mimeographed.

21. R. H. Connery and R. H. Leach, *The Federal Government and Metropolitan Areas* (Cambridge: Harvard University Press, 1960).

22. J. M. Winters, *Interstate Metropolitan Areas* (Ann Arbor: University of Michigan, Michigan Legal Publications, 1962).

23. Lake Tahoe Area Council, "Compact Hope Now Rests on Teale Bill in Senate," *Lake Tahoe* 10 (April 1968), South Lake Tahoe, California.

24. Melvin A. Levin, "The Big Regions," *Journal of the American Institute of Planners* 34 (March 1968), 66-79.

25. Allan Blackman, "Local Health Planning Requires National Health Planning," School of Public Health, University of California, Berkeley, 1969, mimeographed. Joseph L. Falkson and Demetrius J. Plessas, "Towards Rationalization and Integration of Urban Health Bureaucracies," *HSMHA Health Reports* 86 (June 1971), 495-500.

26. Daniel Moynihan, "The Relationship of Federal to Local Authorities," *Daedalus* 96 (Summer 1967), 801-02.

27. United Nations, "A Study of the Capacity of the United Nations Development System," I and II, by R. G. A. Jackson (Geneva, 1969).

28. World Health Organization, "National Health Planning in Developing Countries" (WHO Technical Report Series, no. 350), 1967. World Health Organization, "Training in National Health Planning" (WHO Technical Report Series, no. 456), 1970.

29. Pan American Health Organization, Pan American Sanitary Bureau, "Health Planning: Problems of Concepts and Method" (Scientific Publication, no. 111), 1965. Pan American Health Organization, "Report of the Technical Advisory Committee, Pan American Program for Health Planning," Santiago, Chile, February 12, 1971.

30. Roland L. Warren, "The Interorganizational Field as a Focus for Integration," *Administrative Science Quarterly* 12 (December 1967), 396-416.

31. Roland L. Warren, "Toward a Reformulation of Community Theory," *Human Organization* 15 (Summer 1956), 8-12.

32. Kerr L. White, "Organization and Delivery of Personal Health Services," *Milbank Memorial Fund Quarterly* 46 (January 1968), 225-58.

33. J. M. Winters, Ibid. no. 22.

34. N. E. Cohen, "Summary Report on the Watts Riot: Two-year Study" (Institute of Government and Public Affairs, University of California at Los Angeles), *University Bulletin* 16 (August 14, 1967).

35. U. Thompson, Ibid. no. 7, 91-109.

36. Donna M. Anderson, "The Citizen as Planner (The Citizen and Comprehensive Health Planning)," *Researching a Growing Force for Social Change: Citizen Involvement in the 70's* (Minneapolis, Minnesota: Health Services Research Center, American Rehabilitation Foundation, 1969).

37. Minnesota, State Planning Agency, Comprehensive Health Planning Program, "Deliberations on Comprehensive Statewide Planning for the Delivery of Health Services," September 30, 1967.

38. Paul Davidoff and Thomas A. Reiner, "A Choice Theory of Planning," *Journal of the American Institute of Planners* 27 (May 1962), 103-15.

39. C. West Churchman, *The Systems Approach* (New York: Dell Publishing, 1968), Chapter 4.

40. Paul Davidoff, "Advocacy and Pluralism in Planning," *Journal of the American Institute of Planners* 31 (March 1965), 331.

41. L. A. Peattie, Ibid. no. 15, 80-88.

42. Elizabeth B. Drew, "The Health Syndicate: Washington's Noble Conspirators," *The Atlantic* (December 1967), 75-82.

43. Ralph Nader, *Unsafe At Any Speed* (New York: Grossman, 1965).

44. Robert A. Burco and Clark R. Henderson, "Transportation Planning Alternatives in the Tahoe Basin," Stanford Research Institute, Menlo Park, California, Project MSH-8854, February 24, 1971.

45. Alberta W. Parker, "The Consumer as Policy Maker—Issues of Training," *American Journal of Public Health* 60 (November 1970), 2139-53.

46. Sidney Verba, "Democratic Participation," *Annals of the American Academy of Political and Social Science* 373 (September 1967) 53-78.

47. Anselm L. Strauss, "Medical Organization, Medical Care, and Lower Income Groups," *Social Science and Medicine* 3 (August 1969) 143-77.

48. Lisbeth Meisner, et al., *A Training Program for Consumers in Policy Making Roles in Health Care Projects,* Continuing Education in Health Services and School of Public Health, University of California, Berkeley, May 1970.

49. Bruce Mitchell, "Behavioral Aspects of Water Management," *Environment and Behavior* 3 (June 1971).

50. Benjamin B. Wells, "Role of the Consumer in Regional Medical Programs," *American Journal of Public Health* 60 (November 1970), 2133-38. Claudia B. Galiher, Jack Needleman, and Anne J. Rolfe, "Consumer Participation," *HSMHA Health Reports* 86 (February 1971), 99-106. Rudolph V. Sellers, "The Black Health Worker and the Black Health Consumer—New Roles for Both," *American Journal of Public Health* 60 (November 1970), 2144-70.

51. S. R. Arnstein, "A Ladder of Citizen Participation," *Journal of the American Institute of Planners* 35 (July 1969), 216-24.

52. George F. Lombard, "Relativism in Organization," *Harvard Business Review* 71 (March/April 1971), 55-65.

53. R. L. Warren, Ibid. no. 30, 396-416.

54. C. B. Galiher, J. Needleman, and A. Rolfe, Ibid. no. 50, 99-106. Joseph L. Falkson, "Consumer Participation in Health: Control or Cooperation," paper read at the Conference on Health Planning, University of Hawaii, April 29-3, 1971. Society for Public Health Education, Inc. Health Education Monographs, *Consumer Participation in Health Planning,* Marvin Strauss, guest editor, (San Francisco, November 1972). *Public Administration Review* 32 (May/June 1972), 189-222.

55. A. W. Parker, Ibid. no. 45, 2139-53.

56. Lucy Ann Geiselman and Philip M. Nowlen, "Training for Consumer Participation," Center for Continuing Education, University of Chicago, 1971.

57. Paul Henry, "Pimps, Prostitutes and Policemen: Education of Consumers for Participating in Planning," *American Journal of Public Health* 60 (November 1970), 2171-74. A. Delbecq and A. VandeVen, "Nominal and Interacting Group Processes" (see no. 6). A. Delbecq and A. VandeVen, "A Group Process Model" (see no. 6). L. Meisner, et al., Ibid no. 48.

58. Steven Jonas, "A Theoretical Approach to the Question of 'Community Control' of Health Services Facilities," *American Journal of Public Health* 61 (May 1971), 916-21.

59. William R. Grant, "Community Control vs. School Integration—the Case of Detroit," *The Public Interest,* Summer 1971, 62-79.

60. James D. Carroll, "Participatory Technology," *Science* 171 (February 19, 1971), 647-53.
61. L. Meisner, et al., Ibid. no. 48.
62. D. M. Anderson, Ibid no. 36.
63. State of Minnesota, Ibid no. 37. Henrik L. Blum and Alvin R. Leonard, *Public Administration: A Public Health Viewpoint* (New York: Macmillan, 1963). Henrik L. Blum, "Research Into the Organization of Community Health Services Agencies," *Milbank Memorial Fund Quarterly* 44 (July 1966), part 2, 52-93.
64. P. Clavel, "Planners and Citizen Boards: Some Applications of School Theory to the Problem of Plan Implementation," *Journal of the American Institute of Planners* 34 (May 1968), 130-40.
65. M. M. Raffel, "Working Together to Achieve the Goals of P.L. 89-749," address to the American Public Health Association, 95th Annual Meeting, Miami, Florida, October 22, 1967.
66. State of Minnesota, Ibid. no. 37.
67. T. L. Beyle, Ibid. no. 12, 334-39.
68. Robert J. Daniels, James W. Wagner, and Morton Creditor, "An Example of Sub-Regional Health Planning," *Inquiry* 7 (October 1970), 25-33.

11. Implementation: Conversion of Plans Into Policy and Operations

ACTION OR IMPLEMENTATION AS THE MAJOR REASON FOR PLANNING

Implementation is discussed again not because it promises to be so fruitful, but because, to quote John Friedmann: "The idea that planning and implementation are two distinct and separable activities dies hard."[1]

Planning well performed, it would seem, clears the way for the adoption of its outputs, by public policy makers where indicated and by private policy makers where they are the concerned interests. Not only attention and intelligent consideration for all public and private interests, but also involvement of acceptable representatives during the planning, has been advocated.

Is Voluntarism Enough?

Looking at the issue of voluntary planning and private acceptance brings us to a rude halt. The path is strewn with obstacles. There is always an operator who can turn the situation heavily to his own advantage if, as others follow the plan, he simply goes on cutting corners—for example, by disbursing health care services only to the well-to-do or to easy cases. With the knowledge of this possibility before all, few competing operators will wish to proceed the planned way or to be taken advantage of. An even more difficult situation occurs where each operator might well be better off with a new practice, but each is afraid to change without a guarantee that all others will start in the same way on the same day, lest he bear the brunt of loss of business because he is the only one making the change. Such desire for action in concept is particularly applicable to situations such as leasing apartments to minorities or admitting alcoholics to a general hospital, and it could apply equally to a proposal to encourage health care delivery workers to participate in policy setting or to charge extra for any of the hotel or nonmedical activities which often are charged on health care bills.

From these and similar situations, we have learned that—although apparent industry-wide agreement has been obtained—the individual operators or institutions affected by an agreement may feel called upon to hold out for a public (rather than a private or voluntarily planned)

476

guarantee in the form of enforceable law or regulation which will assure their boards and clients that everyone in the like situation must also go ahead as per schedule.

The issue of whether there should be public declaration in the form of law or enforceable regulation is heavily influenced by the nature and tradition of the private decisions that need to be made to occur in an industry, such as health, where production is predominantly private. The health sector, in addition, has many needs—such as resources for training, building, covering catastrophic costs for anyone, and paying in behalf of all those who cannot afford care. The desperate need for cost controls and efficiency as well as effectivity has prodded the mass of the populace into support for major changes in the modes of collecting dollars, distributing dollars to producers, or organizing distribution systems so that everyone is covered and all reasonable economies are achieved. Moreover, even issues of manpower training have become public, for the present system trains people to be able to work comfortably only where there are already surplusages of skills, and does not properly train those who could and then would work in underserved areas. Obviously, vast reorganizations are coming. They will not suit all the vested interests and, therefore, will not come to pass unless they are publicly made with enforceable decisions, whether compliance is secured by positive or negative sanctions or both.

Meaningful health care decisions must change the present system drastically; minor adjustments inside the system are not enough. What is called for is a change of the system itself as it relates to the larger societal system. This is why participative planning is a major requirement at this time of shifting and uneven mixtures of official and voluntary planning.

If we raise our sights further and begin to plan for health, rather than for health care, we find that the health care sector is only of modest importance to health. Obviously, the drawing together of the kinds of interests and systems which bear upon health improvement would be even less likely to evolve through a private sector set of agreements. (Actually, present laws and taxation already provide significant direction to much of the so-called private activity.) In addition, new planning approaches and structures must be created so that if changes are demanded of the various multisectoral interests, they and the jobs and products they control will not be casually destroyed in the name of guarding one or another item of social and economic well-being. To improve health by one act and allow by-product, uncushioned, socioeconomic dislocations to destroy it elsewhere is senseless. Planning for promotion of health has nothing to do with a totality of planning or government in business. Our government has long been intervening in business by guiding the market place or increasing nonmarket islands. What is proposed is that from now on the required government actions in the market place in behalf of health or any other public good should be guided by sponsoring and then utilizing the outputs from widely participative planning.

Is Design Enough?

Is planning finished when it has set the stage by its designs for an excellent product? Because public and private interests may prefer different options, or may not really desire to go ahead with any, no formal actions of any kind may be the outcome. Most public planning efforts have met this fate. Are planning bodies justified in stopping when they have deposited their outputs in the laps of those who can and will make whatever decisions they are inclined to, or do planners go further? If so, how much further?

Some of the roles for planning bodies described in Chapter 9 suggest going a long way towards securing implementation. Here is a point of bifurcation. Are planning bodies to be given authority by the customary public decision makers to put into law all their plans (enabling legislation can easily do this), or are they to be given the opportunity to set a very well lighted stage, so that policy makers must either address themselves to the major decision choices, or, if they choose not to, display their inaction under circumstances of great visibility?

We tend to favor the second alternative for most planning outputs. However, the health planning body will also foreseeably be given certain health authority functions. The elected decision makers will define these functions. For such activities as standard setting or enforcement, the health authority will act in the same manner as any customary government administrative agency which is given the power to make rules and regulations. Further administrative duties, such as inspection or licensure, may also be wished off on planning bodies. These duties could, in fact, be carried out by other agencies, such as health departments and licensing boards which are now in such roles. Beyond the desire to have standards enforcement closely match the planning output, there is no remarkable justification for these inspectional and enforcement roles to be taken on by the planning body, as long as the implementation phase is moved forward by a suitably empowered agency.

The real problem remains: How far is the planning body to go beyond design? Are they to undertake a highly influencing role short only of being given power to adopt their own output as law? The sections to follow try to explicate the major issues that a planning body must learn to deal with once it agrees that the only reason for defining improvements as the first step in planning is to follow through with the attempt to achieve the improvements defined.

If any serious doubt remains about the necessary relationships of politics to the achievement of planned improvements, or about the correctness of our introductory remarks that planning is a wedding of politics and technology, let us look at the effects of political activity on health. We will see not only why politics must be utilized to effectuate planning, but that politics too must utilize extensive planning if improvement is to be achieved in our nation's health or in the health activities aided, encouraged, or induced by our government.

Figure 11.1, modified from Roseman,[2] points out how day-by-day political actions directly affect health and health care, and it makes obvious what it means for these actions to go on without planning. Figure 11.2, a composite of two figures presented by Falkson and Plessas,[3] points out very specifically just how extensively generally unrelated (unplanned) interventions from the federal level in a 10-year period have impinged on the area of local health programs. Wildavsky pursues this question of the use of planning without government implementation and the meaninglessness of planning if government takes actions that undo what it has helped to plan and bring into being.[4]

GENERATION AND UTILIZATION OF AUTHORITY BY THE PLANNING BODY

To make clear how important it is for the planning body to have authority to affect the decision-making process, we must clarify the terminology used, and discuss how authority can be attained and utilized.

Nature of Authority

Power can be defined as the ability or capacity to get others to take steps they would not otherwise take—for example, secure compliance.[5] Power is also described as the personal or structural possibility of affecting decisions and desires, whether operating from an *informal* or a *formal* position.[6] Power, the ability to secure *compliance,* generally derives from the net resource advantage of a regime, sector, group, or individual.[7] Clark has created a convertibility matrix of 14 resources upon which power draws.[8] Power is also seen as "the capacity to mobilize resources for the accomplishment of intended effects with recourse to some type of sanction(s) to encourage compliance."[9] *Capacity* speaks to *potential* power, and *application* of sanctions connotes *actualized* power.[10]

In a sense in which I do not wish to use the term, power is also commonly defined as the absence of dependency,[11] and therefore independence.[12] There are also in common usage quite different relative meanings of power and authority which we do not accept. In these, power refers to illegitimate, and authority refers to legitimate ability to influence.[13]

In an important summarization of power as the term is used here, Lehman begins his description of power with the statement that it is *relational, intentional, impositional,* and *potential* and that it has *inter-member* and *systemic* capacities.[14] He defines the resources available to the operation of power as:

Utilitarian, such as material goods and services which are useful in *inducement.*

Coercive, such as the ability to do harm to another's body or psyche, which is useful as a *constraint.*

Normative, such as symbols related to shared beliefs, values, and sentiments that indicate prestige, esteem, love, and acceptance, which are most useful to effect *persuasion.*

Lehman also feels that at the macro or societal system level, with which we are concerned in planning, power is likely to be:

A general capacity applicable to many causes, rather than a unipolar phenomenon (this is related to the spillover of power derived in one field, and often is accompanied by access to diverse important resources).

FIGURE 11.1

POLITICS AND HEALTH—EXAMPLES OF HOW POLITICAL ACTION AFFECTS HEALTH AND HEALTH CARE TODAY
(Adapted from Roseman)

Form of Activity	Example
GOVERNMENTAL	
Direct action	Veterans Administration, county hospitals
Assistance—largely financial	Medicare, Medicaid
Regulation	Licensing facilities, personnel
Action in fields affecting health but not identified as such	Antipoverty programs; highways
Inaction	Indifference to tobacco production and distribution
Research	Cancer
Legislation for planning requirements	Comprehensive health planning
Citizen participation requirements	Neighborhood health centers
POLITICAL PARTIES	
Platforms	Environmental pollution
Proposed legislation	Universal health insurance plans

FIGURE 11.2
GENERALLY UNRELATED OR UNPLANNED FEDERAL
INTERVENTIONS AFFECTING LOCAL HEALTH PROGRAMS
(Adapted from Falkson and Plessas)

Federal Administration Affecting Local Health Programs			*Competing Local and Federal "Coordinating Agencies"*	
Program	*Year established*	*Federal administrative agency*	*Local coordinating agency*	*Federal coordinating agency*
Medical assistance for the aged	1960	HEW	Community action agencies	OEO
Community health services	1961	HEW	City demonstration agencies (model neighborhoods)	HUD
Radiological health and institutional training	1962	HEW	Economic development districts	Commerce
Air pollution control and prevention	1963	HEW	Overall economic development program	Commerce
Communicable disease activities	1964	HEW	Cooperative area manpower planning system	Labor
Community action programs	1964	OEO	Concentrated employment program	CEP
Administration on aging	1965	HEW	Comprehensive health planning agencies	HEW
Medical assistance	1965	HEW	Neighborhood service centers	OEO
Dental services and resources	1965	HEW		HUD
Health manpower	—	HEW		Labor
Disease prevention and environmental control	—	HEW		HEW
Health services	—	HEW		
Mental health	—	HEW		
Comprehensive health planning and services	1966	HEW		
Comprehensive neighborhood health centers	1966	HEW / OEO		
Regional medical programs	1966	HEW		
Model neighborhood health programs	1967	HEW / HUD		

481

Based on multiple resources of the three kinds described above, and stemming from the need to influence different interests in different ways.

A crystallization of the symbolic capacity that represents the ability of a power wielder to trade on his reputation and wheel and deal under a kind of threat without using much or any of his power account (power plays).

Differentiated into systemic and intermember power, the systemic involving power as a capacity to set, pursue, and implement goals in behalf of the entire system, the intermember being the exercise of power in the competition for the individual's or unit's share of the resources in the system.

A few additional definitions will make the discussion more concise.

Coercion, of which force may be one manifestation, is exemplified when A is in a position to give B no favorable and only depriving alternatives.[15]

Force can be defined as the ability to move someone physically, to restrain or imprison him, or to take his life. *Sanctions* are not dissimilar, but they can be either positive rewards, affirmative acknowledgment, or encouragement, or they can be limitations or negative strictures to the point, and including the use, of force and punishment, such as fines, loss of liberty, or death.

Compliance with the desires of power holders derives from the net resources advantage of the holder.[16]

Influence is defined as actualized power[17] or the production of an effect on another person, group, or organization through the exercise of a personal or organization capacity.[18] Influence is also seen as social causation of any kind, while power is intended social causation. Neither influence nor power is the attribute of a single actor in isolation, they represent a relationship between people. Sources of power or influence may be dominant over one another to any degree, or may reciprocate and may vary for different issues among the same power holders.[19]

Illegitimate means A had no right to ask B to move.[20]

Clearly, these definitions are not totally tidy with respect to one another, but in general they allow a discussion of authority and power to continue without going in meaningless circles.

For our purposes, *authority* is defined as the investiture in a position, person, or institution (for example, the planning body) of the means to influence the behavior of others—that is, to exercise power. These capacities derive from occupancy of authority roles, and those who really have authority possess resources as a means to power. Although legitimacy (which may be regarded as a resource) clearly adds to authority in wielding power, it is not equatable with authority.[21]

Authority may achieve its impact by as little as an intimation of what is wanted, by request or proclamation, by demand, or by access to and use of force and sanctions.

The combination of known or anticipated force and sanctions is often the hidden but not forgotten threat which obtains acceptance of authority. Signs tell us of penalties; our education is largely concerned with laws and policemen, both visible and invisible. Private societies can wield the threat of expulsion or of social, political, and economic boycott whether announced or unannounced. As Form says: "Absence of observed conflict does not prove that sanctions are not being applied and that the phenomenon of power is absent."[22]

Pluralism of the seat of power may spuriously appear real even though a truly powerful elite may work effectively to keep the value scheme (the rules we play by) intact. As a result, the visible, so-called pluralistic power holders in fact regulate themselves and maintain the formal, structural controls, thereby ensuring the quiet, invisible, and unannounced supremacy of a very elite group who operate by ensuring allegiance to their value base.[23]

Authority is most valuable when scarce. A person in authority can grant another a spot in which he can exert influence, yet not share or hand out much authority (witness some CHPs that have only been granted the right to plan but which are making their influence felt as a result).

Chapter 9 indicated that the planning body may not be invested with any means of enforcement or with significant sanctioning powers. How then will planning bodies come to have real influence? What form will their authority take and how will it be guided, assuming that authority is necessary to the planning body's role of effective change agent with public and policy makers?

Figure 11.3 is an attempt to illustrate the relationship of what is meant by the terms *power, authority, force, sanctions* and *compliance.* Authority may have been legitimately created (columns 1, 2 and 3). In the first instance, it has been formally bestowed by the power (acceptance as well as expected threat of force) generated in legitimate government. In the second and third columns, it has been informally generated. In column 2, traditional acceptance of values, doctrines, and beliefs which have been institutionalized results in the tremendous respect and acquiescence commanded by ecclesiastical figures, university and corporation presidents, and so on.[24] In column 3 the personal qualities of leadership, great charm, heroism, intellectual prowess, wealth, or family status available to individuals (such as Nehru, Churchill, Edison, or J. F. Kennedy), are the source of respect and acquiescence.

On the other hand, authority may have been illegitimately seized as shown in columns 4 and 5. In column 4, we find that money, physical

FIGURE 11.3   POWER, AUTHORITY, FORCE AND SANCTIONS, COMPLIANCE
(Developed from ideas of Lucy Johns)

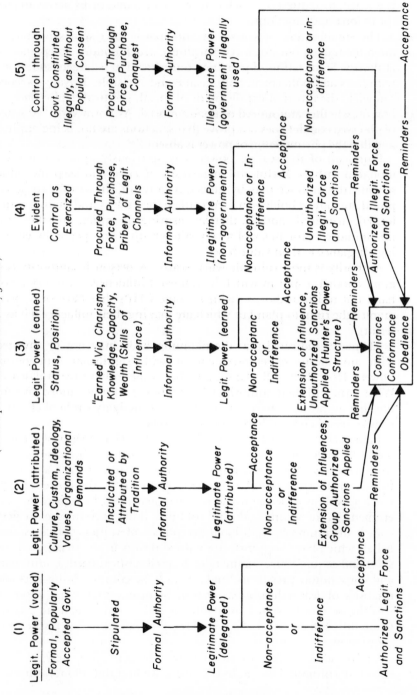

484

force, and political threat, can force individuals and communities to acquiesce (as in the operations of the Ku Klux Klan or the Mafia). In the fifth column the same pattern of influence either takes over government and actually runs it using force at the bidding of a few persons (Hitler) or operates government as a front through a so-called boss (Prendergast in Kansas City, Ruef in San Francisco).

Acquiescence to authority ranges along a spectrum, from those who will accept it with no more than a reminder that it exists, to those who will not accept it at any penalty. Authority and its acceptance vary, both for the issue at hand and for the nature of the constituency. Looking again at column 1, it can be pointed out that most people accept most government positions on the simplest of reminders (signs, printed ordinances, or visible policemen). The recent excitement over student revolt attests to how uncommon is nonacceptance of the rules of behavior established by so-called duly constituted government.

As an example of the power described in column 2, many people, even those who are not members of the Roman Catholic Church, accept or are influenced by the pronouncements which the Pope makes on peace, while only the most devout accept his position on birth control. Also, the standing of the institution itself varies from one decade to another, acts of individual popes can earn them authority which can be transmitted to the Church (Pope John XXIII, for example). Anyone who fails to accept guidance from this traditional informal authority can be coerced only if he values the support of the accepting members or fears their social, political, or economic boycott.

Column 3 indicates an authority of prominence. Air heroes, athletes, movie stars, scientists, and business tycoons may all be asked to support various issues because the opinions of so-called great people are influential. The degree of public acceptance will vary with issues, and with the nature of the audience and how it relates or identifies with the particular area of success of the authority figure. Professors are eggheads to some, oracles to others; movie stars are great common-sense leaders to some and tap dancers to others. The nonacceptance of authority stemming from such power figures is only punishable if and when the holder of the authority can so sell himself that those who hold with him are able to force nonbelievers out of a job, unseat them politically, boycott their business, withhold credit, and so on.

Column 4 describes what is often a surreptitious wielding of power against one or a few victims at a time. The very smallness of the number of victims may force them to succumb to threat; nonacceptance may presage a violent death.

Column 5 portrays a capture of the key public decision points through corruption or force. Public machinery is run for limited private gain or there may be an all-out bid to take over government and operate it as though it were duly constituted and legitimately accepted.

To label a government as legitimately constituted may be difficult, given the diversity of political and economic credos possible. We in the United States claim that the dominant criterion of legitimacy is popular consent, yet historians looking back upon the American Revolution may have reservations as to whether the new government was the result of an illegitimate, forceful seizure of control or the result of a formally constituted and legitimate popular demand. In any case, nonacceptance of this type of authority is subject to the same force and sanction power available to legitimate government, although force may be much more sternly and arbitrarily applied because of the shadow under which the authority was born.

An element of circularity is involved. Power is defined as the ability to move others. The various origins of that power lend authority to those in whose hands power is held. In turn, those holding the authority (for example, those making up a CHP body) now have power available to them by their position as the authority force.

Generating Authority

For some years to come, the duties and authority of most health planning bodies in the United States are likely to be heavily in the area of making plans and encouraging their utilization. How much authority can be generated under circumstances which fall short of granting planning bodies public decision policy making authority? Can such planning bodies generate enough authority to achieve implementation of their plans by influencing the legislators directly, or will their influence be acquired as they effectively reach the public so that legislators respond? The planning body can seek out and tap many potential sources of authority.[25] Those listed here have been arranged in a pragmatic way which cuts across Lehman's utilitarian, normative, and coercive types.

One potential source of authority is *client-based* and *extrinsic*, reflecting the authority already in the hands of the client. In the case of comprehensive health planning, government is the major client. Through P.L. 89-749 and the state and local planning entities created by this legislation, both federal and state governments are lending their traditional formal authority to the planning bodies.

A duly constituted government can confer authority on a planning body in various ways. For example, when it:

Fosters or requires and, in many cases, funds the planning body.

Acknowledges the presence and proclaims the importance of the planning body, even if voluntarily constituted. Government can, of course, go further and add formal authority by law and designate it as the relevant planning body for the particular unit of government.

Creates the planning body and appoints its members, making clear that government is directly investing formal authority. Government can go further and give highly visible ceremonial roles to the planning body.

Insists that its own members be on the planning body, to further ensure identification with government and to guarantee a hearing of the legislative body's concerns, while simultaneously implying legislative hearing for planning body proposals.

Asks the planning body to review and make recommendations on the work or proposals of others.

(When government goes beyond the planning-type grants of authority and lodges rule or regulation-making authority with the planning body—with or without enforcement, supervision, adjudication, project approval or control activities—the planning body is clearly in possession of formal governmental authority and the power that goes with it.)

A second source of authority is *participant-based* and *extrinsic;* that is, it resides in the person of each appointee to the planning body board or in the capacities and reputations brought into the agency through the personnel hired or the consultants contracted for. Individuals who represent major institutions bring informal authority from their attributed power. Similarly, individuals who are themselves of consequence to the larger community or to smaller groups—who have earned power as the people who "count" or who "have made it"— bring informal authority. Evidence is available that reputation is a major source of power in community politics, and that when reputed power holders unite, they do tangibly affect decisions in the direction they support.[26]

A third broad potential source of authority is *intrinsic;* that is, it is *earned* by the planning body. By a record over time of wise recommendations which have been followed, a planning body begins to take on institutional status and earns the traditional power that widely-accepted institutions come to wield.

Evidence that earns informal authority for the planning body accumulates when:

Plans have been wise and successful.

The planning body has sought out and taken into account all the significant community positions, satisfying most interests reasonably well most of the time.

Members attained prominence as a result of their participation, even if they had not been prominent previously.

The planning body showed the ability to harness the knowledge and energy of government agencies and to team them up with the voluntary and private sector.

It has been able to clarify values and relate goals to them, helping to redefine values, and thus serving as a center for democratic education.

New insights have been accepted and plans changed appropriately.

Distribution has been made of new and valid information which in the light of subsequent actions is evaluated as wise; errors and miscalculations have been acknowledged and proceedings updated accordingly.

The planning body has not sought to usurp authority to secure its own future at the expense of the community.

Outputs have been so engineered that they find ready channels and acceptance that either do no violence to those with power or do it so thoroughly that new sources of power take over.

The planning body has pulled politicians out of bad holes or made them look good.

Anthony Downs [27] suggests three other means of earning authority;

Offer leadership in the presence of uncertainty—the one place where leadership is most valued whether or not it is rational and inspired.

Provide evidence of reliability—an organization does what it says it will.

Demonstrate responsibility—hold to the organization's tenets, acknowledged roles, and behaviors, not maneuvering opportunistically or changing ideology or practices with each shift in climate as might be evidenced by results of elections.

Whether intrinsic authority is earned will depend heavily on the skills of influence that the planning body can muster. These skills can be made available on the staff and board or kept on call among dedicated friends of the planning body. Each situation will call for a different mixture of skills, and some situations may require the assistance of outside persons or organizations known to be able to carry out a particular skill role. The possibility must be kept in mind that not all the skills of influence are utilizable before authority has, in fact, been gained. The skills of influence have been outlined by Arnold and Welsh,[28] Miller,[29] Rein,[30] and Bolan,[31] and have been adapted into Figure 11.4.

Starting from another base, Martin Rein[32] suggests that the principal sources of authority for planners are really fewer than the skills of influence suggested in Figure 11.4. He opts for those of expertise, bureaucratic position, consumer preferences, and professional values. He analyzes where each takes the planner in relation to consumers, validation, source of guidance, and so on. This analysis leads Rein to consideration of strategies for acquiring authority, of which he discusses three in some depth.

Consensus of elites depends on forming a coalition of many old and new centers of power in both government and private agencies, with their powerful economic, political and socially important friends, and frequent friends in higher levels of government. But the effort of focusing on this coalition may cause the planning agency to expend more energy on creating and maintaining the coalition than on getting

FIGURE 11.4
SKILLS OF INFLUENCE

Intelligence

Interpersonal competence

Attributes of professionalism, expertise, or knowledge

For special problems the knowledgeable advice of a professional and an expert can be an influencer of behavior. For example, an attorney can influence actions based on his advice about the legality of the action.

Ability to weld together the various kinds of expertise needed in planning

Ability to manipulate symbols and to communicate

Influencing another to carry out an action is difficult unless he understands the action desired.

A wide network of socio-professional contacts

Ability to provide access to special and needed resources

More than having power and authority toward resources, this ability includes a knowledge of where resources can be obtained and how they can be tapped.

Ability to organize and arrange people and resources

in such a way that the desired action occurs.

Ability to engender enthusiasm and trust

or, conversely, to reduce fears of possible detrimental consequences of the action.

Ability to bargain and achieve conflict resolutions

Often action cannot proceed until conflicts of values are resolved or competing groups are mollified.

Capacity to obtain evidence of attitudes from the laity, special interests, and politicians

This may be a keener tool for sensing political feasibility than any other.

Ability to predict the effects of action or of non-action

The skills of prediction can also be skills of influence in that they aid in defining the parameters of action and expectations.

Ability to obtain bureaucratic and governmental support or position work done. Rein points out that national support for such coalitions was based on hopes that they would provide inducement to join forces, settle differences, and look for the real issues and solutions. They did provide ample involvement (which helped legitimation), but the involvement impeded innovation or meaningful planning. Since the latter is the reason for which legitimation was undertaken, this outcome is disturbing. Of course, these coalitions might have been very effective in getting implementation if they had produced something worth the effort.

The preceding discussion puts us in the middle of a long-standing controversy over whether power is in reality a unified or a dispersed attribute. Most people other than students of society (and many of the latter still do) probably accept the Mills,[33] Hunter,[34] and Lehman[35] position that holders of significant power are able to exercise it in behalf of innumerable purposes. Others suggest that power not only has multiple origins but is individually exercised by its holders only over limited areas.[36] By coalescence, a pluralistic—but none the less real—centrum of power may emerge from the individual centers. However, such individual centers may see no advantage to coalescing. For example, we have been witness to the significant and relatively growing divisiveness between the once inseparable companions of insurance, hospital, and medical interests. Curtis and Petras in their comparison of the evidence relevant to the power elite or stratification theory of power versus the pluralistic theories, showed very good correlation between the conclusions drawn and the methods of study used in all the major studies to date of distribution of power.[37] This finding suggests, among other things, that both theories may have validity.

Another of Rein's strategies of legitimacy or acquisition of authority is *rational analysis and the power of knowledge.* Good information persuasively packaged should indeed legitimate an operation like planning. Rein found these hopes far out of line with reality. Research-like or experimental approaches may, quite legitimately, intrude into capacity to deliver, and the constant need for operational changes secondary to political exigencies may result in the inability to keep knowledge-creating studies controlled or legitimate. Thus, Rein concludes that the process of obtaining first-class knowledge while doing planning under operational circumstances does not lead to a happy outcome, and that authority is not likely to be secured in this way.

I am not sure that Rein's concern, which is geared to eliciting new knowledge, involves the same considerations as the application of good available knowledge and logic to the planning situation. Therefore, I do not agree with his pessimism about the application of rational analysis to the creation of legitimacy. In fact, one of my major hopes for the generation of authority is that well-performed planning, in itself a kind of creation of new configurations of knowledge, will the most significant source of new authority.

The third of Rein's strategies is based on the concepts of an active constituency—*participation as a source of authority or the power of the people*. The white middle class has generally accepted the principles of participation through representation. However, at this time, participation of the poor and the counter culture portions of the new generation must often take place directly at the grass roots level rather than vicariously through representatives. Perhaps these groups have observed that most attempts to obtain participation of the disadvantaged or nonparticipating have come out of bureaucratic agencies which try to organize the poor to do something the agency wants done. Notwithstanding the low staying power or the tendency of these groups to personalize issues or obfuscate causes by forsaking them for the protests or organizations that are involved, Rein finds that the "process of involving the poor as a form of therapy and self-help on the one hand and legitimation of the activities of the planner on the other hand does not take adequate account of the potential role that citizen participation may have in politicizing the poor."

Generation of power from this source might include creation of power for a section of the community that had none previously. This could be done for purely normative reasons or could be combined with a strategy for creating a powerful group which would support the planning body. Simple techniques are available, such as providing a powerless block with veto power, or a key committee placement from which their representative could bargain in behalf of issues of more consequence to his own constituency.

Direct advocacy by a planning body can also be the role under which a powerless section of the populace is aided to become a participatory force. A discussion of the utility of advocacy planning as a means of gaining power for the poor (and thus for the planning body as its agent) resulted in views that advocacy planning may be manipulation of the poor, that it may waste their energy and delay their gains.[38] It may be nothing more than an arena to advance the concerns of the advocate planner who uses his particular tools expensively and, perhaps, erroneously in a situation where other approaches would help people much more effectively. I have no doubt that advocacy in the health field may also be the means of organizing the poor, educating them—often to grasp and use power, raising their sights, providing alternatives which suit their needs better, being a symbol to others and, finally, being a catalyst for desired gathering of power and reaching new ends.

Rosenthal and Crain cast doubt on any general proposition that wide or general public participation is helpful in passing legislation on issues of rancorous conflict, such as fluoridation.[39] Gamson also noted that participation did not particularly lessen rancorous conflicts.[40] However, these observations were made in situations without formal participative community planning, and where participation in such planning was not a possibility. Alternative interventions were never presented, their costs and benefits were obviously never publicly compared, and little was offered in the way of choice other than the opportunity to vote yes or no.

A distinct glimmer of hopefulness radiates from each of the strategies reviewed, and for different reasons in each case. Each appeals to an aspect of the democratic credo—the skills of influence carefully acquired should in their application appeal to all segments of the polity. The desire for consensus is particularly appealing to the elite. Reverence for science, fact, problem solving, and good plans is likely to be effective among the middle classes. Creation of power for the powerless should be appealing to that group. Validation of pluralism, diversity and conflict on which democracy presumably depends for its vitality should be appealing to all sectors, except perhaps to those who feel that they already have it made.

Rein's conclusions are that we need many strategies to acquire authority but that no one organization can hope to keep them all going under one roof simultaneously for long. The likelihood is that planning bodies must, and will, use all the strategies, but in varying doses at varying times for different issues.

Full reconciliation of the many polarizing issues that will be exposed as part of good planning is not possible, but as Rein says,[41] that is no excuse for not tackling what has to be faced. Even civil wars end. This phenomenon as it occurs in academia has been reviewed by Spiegel.[42] I am not recommending an all-out attempt to garner authority based solely on one of the strategies, but instead a situational analysis to see which amalgamations of authority are required for each. I do not see the planning body as committed to any one strategy exclusively or for all time. This posture does not imply that the planning body might not have a more prolonged effect if it were to create a strong and steadfast or positive constituency. After all, a powerful constituency is the critical source of authority in any kind of society. However, the planning body may attain a relatively positive and even broader constituency by approaching situations for what is in them, rather than with the specialized purpose of exercising a strategy to achieve authority. The latter approach could bind the planning body to one or another set of clients to the point of losing others, or to the point of rupture with its cultivated and strongest constituency, if planning issues are ever undertaken which annoy that constituency.

Various questions come to mind. Is broad-scope, formal authority always an unmixed blessing? Are there responsibilities that may dissipate earned authority which the planning body has established? Are there powers that the planning body might do well to avoid?

Many planning bodies constantly seek new power to augment their generally meager initial grant. They look hopefully at each new piece of legislation that gives them authority over one or another subject area as the means to strengthen their overall position, and presumably, therefore, their planning position. Grants of significant formal authority are now going to publicly constituted state-level (a) CHP agencies and to the more commonly quasipublic or privately constituted local (b) CHP agencies. Observations and speculations have been made about currently evident and potential outcomes.[43]

Grants of authority to regulate construction of facilities or to act as a hearing board on construction appeals may require skills not available on either the staff or the board of a planning body. The work may divert the little manpower and time available to planning bodies. As a consequence, the credibility of the planning body may be sharply diminished. Not only is planning not done, but the adjudicatory decisions made by the planning body are no better—in fact for shortage of skills and manpower they may be worse—than decisions made by other public and semipublic control authorities or by the market place.

Authority for nonplanning responsibilities, even for stern enforcement matters, may earn the planning body little in the way of authority for planning: if it takes away capacity to plan, the consequence may be erosion of planning authority. Because planning is an item of desperate shortage now in the health sector, it is of interest to witness that HEW (from another desk, to be sure) has awarded grants for health care planning to community health aggregates which have no relation to the formal CHP body in the area.[44] Could this be in part because the CHP is bogged down in seeking authority for nonplanning purposes? This designation of competing planning bodies promises a rapid loss of what planning authority the CHP has acquired.

How would the award of public policy-making roles affect implementation of planning outputs? If the planning body becomes a health authority with the duty of specifying performance, conduct, relationships, coverage, costs, or controls, it will doubtless be well on the way to achieving implementation for any of its planning outputs which fall under its policy-making duties. Whether such a situation will improve the quality of its planning is another matter. As it scurries to make policy decisions, the amount of planning may fall. However, what planning is done is likely to be implemented, and because implementation is a major purpose of planning, the search for direct grants of implementing powers seems timely in these hours of irreconcilable private answers to major health issues. It still, however, remains my suggestion that the planning body keep planning, politics, and implementation in mind, issue by issue and situation by situation, and that it not focus solely on pursuing the strategy of obtaining authority per se. It may well earn its legitimacy and authority, including significant grants of formal authority, even while satisfactorily fulfilling its vital purposes and legally required roles. Our reader is therefore referred to the preceding chapter with its discussion of representation and participation and to Chapter 9 for a discussion of roles open to a planning body.

Is it likely that a health planning body will get policy making authority beyond the control of health care delivery, for let us say, environmental issues? Presently, agencies like water quality control boards which have modest policy setting authority and which usually do very little planning, could easily be transferred to a health planning body as an integrating move. Frank Stead, the eminent environmentalist, makes a very strong appeal for placing real power in whichever planning body ultimately inherits a serious responsibility for the environment.[45]

In summary, a gift of authority—the opportunity to exercise power—can be made to a planning body by judicious selection of board members and employees, by the duties formally assigned, and by relation to governmental structure. We also recognize the legitimacy of CHP bodies seeking and being given, by law, significant policy (rule and regulation making) authority that is relevant to implementing the planning that has been adopted by the formal policy makers. But if such grants are extensive, it may be that the planning bodies will have to be more directly responsible to the citizenry. Perhaps their boards will have to be elected. There need be no pressure to award power for inspectional, surveillance, or adjudicatory roles, which can probably better be carried out by such agencies as state health departments.

In the United States, the act known as P.L. 89-749, 89th Congress, approved November 3, 1966, has for its first paragraph under "Findings and Declaration of Purpose" the following (emphasis is mine):

> The Congress declares that fulfillment of our national purpose depends on promoting and assuring the highest level of health attainable for every person, in an environment which contributes positively to healthful individual and family living; that attainment of this goal depends on an effective partnership, involving close intergovernmental collaboration, official and voluntary efforts, and participation of individuals and organizations; that federal financial assistance must be directed to support the marshaling of all health resources—national, state, and local—to assure comprehensive health services of high quality for every person, but *without interference with existing patterns of private professional practice of medicine, dentistry, and related healing arts.*

Whether CHPs have already been excessively handicapped, even by the founding legislation, is indeed the subject of argument.[46] If changes in the delivery system are prohibited, hope dims for the concept of comprehensive health planning. Fortunately, not even organized medicine has paid much attention to the limited intent of Congress, for which it so effectively lobbied.

Application of Authority and Power

Chapter 2 developed the idea of introducing deliberate social change by affecting one or more of the four determinants—impetus, mobilization, structural control, and self-regulation. Successfully operating planning bodies probably have assumed those roles which raise issues so as to provide *impetus* to large numbers of people, and thus each situation for which they are planning becomes a point around which to *mobilize*. Legislatively enacted planning proposals alter the *structural controls,* such as laws, formally established institutions, and service agencies by constraining or encouraging them to create the resources and means to achieve the desired ends. Even significant alterations in *self-regulation* are expected to occur as a consequence of planning outputs which change public awareness through promotional efforts provided by various health agencies and by obtaining normative legislation. (It is rare today in medical meetings to see any cigarettes or more than an occasional pipe and cigar smoker as a result of such influences.)

The work of planning concentrates on creating opportunities, incentives, penalties, constraints, new entities, new legalisms, or new resources. Thus, the major thrust of planning bodies in obtaining social change will obviously be in the political arena. As a change agent, a planning body might direct its outputs specifically to the legislative bodies at the level of community of solution appropriate for the problems or goals at hand. Outputs might be directed to the public in the expectation that the public will accept and respond by forcing the relevant legislators to comply. If the planning body follow our reasoning, it will analyze any planning situation to see what interests are likely to be concerned and will set about involving such interests, including relevant legislators, other associated power holders, consumers, and victims. In this way the planning body has a firm grasp on how to mobilize the impetus and where to involve the decision-making machinery. The usual means of introducing desired major improvements is to change the pertinent structural controls and, where necessary, the legislation. Constraints and saliency, well handled, also favorably arouse the self-regulatory concerns of the concerned segment of the public.

Clearly, planners have to be able to determine which decisions must be made in formal political arenas, and which will be made in other policy-setting environments, and then they have to act accordingly. In general, we concur that public policy actions will involve far more complex chains of decision making than private ones.[47] This is almost an axiomatic conclusion, because private policy actions remain private only as long as they are accepted sets of negotiations which adequately satisfy the parties involved. The minute such private agreements become unattainable or unenforceable, one or another of the interested parties will attempt to make a public matter out of them. Health care is moving into the public sector because the parties to what once was purely a private transaction could find no way to deal happily with one another. Health care for the military and for veterans was inevitably a public matter long ago. The need for public funding for care of the poor (once care became worth having) forced that issue into the political arena. The magnitude of that cost, the uneven distribution of resources among the states, and the changing character of the needs, as well as growing costs for education of the health skills are further examples of why decision making as a private matter is now further giving way to the public arena. This movement toward the public realm is in many ways a powerful force for putting power and authority into the hands of planners, as political stalemates develop or are foreseen.

AN IMPLEMENTATION TYPOLOGY OF COMMUNITIES FOR USE BY PLANNERS

One of the first considerations for planners interested in the implementation of their outputs is that implementation be possible. This determination requires taking into account the extensive network of communities, which not only multiply and embrace all of our activities, but in many cases have the law-making and taxing authority necessary for full or partial public choice and implementation.

Concepts of community are relevant to the implementation of health planning because issues do not all have the same reference points. Some are coterminous with geographic boundaries, some with kinds of people no matter where they are located. Often the means to attack a major problem will exist apart from the planning base or from the operational base capable of delivering the desired interventions. Constraints and resources of organization, financing, and enforcement may also have other bases which must be included in a planned approach to solving specific problems or attaining stipulated goals.

Implementation, and the design aspects of planning for health as well, raise the issue of defining the boundaries for which a planning effort is to take place. The usual way of handling this issue is to avoid it by speaking of planning for the "community." Little guidance is offered as to whether community refers to scattered persons with like interests or characteristics, or to the residents of an area bounded by geographic markers. In the latter case, there is often little clarification as to whether the community is a block, neighborhood, city, region, state, or the nation itself. The attempt to shed light on the problem of choosing the appropriate community for given special or general planning efforts has led us to replace vagueness with complexity. Nevertheless, suitable definitions may give an indication of how planning boundaries are to be determined.

Community is generally perceived as "a set of people living in a spatially bounded area that may or may not coincide with a legally bounded jurisdiction of government."[48] However, the study of community attitudes of activities requires more discrimination in defining the concept of community. Webber suggests two types of urban communities:[49] The *place* community in which interactions occur in a particular geographically definiable area; and the *non-place* community, in which the interactions may extend to widely scattered geographic areas when temporary or long-term interests create a focus of concern among people who may otherwise be similar or dissimilar and live nearby or far away. Several of the communities discussed will be seen as belonging to the first and several to the second of Webber's groups. He ties together the concerns of sophisticated societies that transcend urban places by defining an "urban realm" which includes both place and non-place communities sharing a common interest. The point to be made is that any examination of a given locale which does not explore the non-place exchanges that have become part of the scene cannot result in adequate comprehension. Various segments of the urban population have ties to one or more non-place urban communities, some of which may interrelate at other places in quite unexpected ways.

Some of the connotations of the word *community* are not clearly included in Webber's classification, yet would also seem necessary for an effective planning approach. To label specific meanings conveyed by the word *community* is desirable for planning purposes. The collection of labels in this text contains no startling novelties and covers only a fraction of the definitions in the literature;[50] but it tries to show the relationships between certain types of community which have a critical bearing on comprehensive planning in its various phases of community planning, organization and development, and community relationships to government.

Others agree that a single definition of community can no longer serve, and some have come to see community in such diverse ways as regulatory, integrative, structural-functional, ecological, monographical, and political-stratification.[51] Clark utilizes definitions which are based on political and economic autonomy, not unlike two of the distinctions to be offered here.[52] The typology I use has grown out of the needs which surface when the developmental approach to planning is applied.

The Face-to-Face Community (FFC)

The FFC was characteristic of the medieval way of life, in which a primary group shared for a lifetime a limited circle of contacts at work, at home, and at play.[53] The surviving FFCs in the United States indicate the continuing existence of strong forces, some of which are internal that give the inhabitants a consistent and relatively homogeneous outlook, some of which are external forces or social isolation. In all but sparsely populated rural areas, an FFC is less and less likely to be a political entity or coterminous with one; rather, it is most often only a part of a political jurisdiction—that is, a neighborhood.

The Neighborhood

The face-to-face community, with its person to person level of interaction and geographic compactness, is only one of many kinds of neighborhoods. The neighborhood is defined as a geographically-related and definable enclave of people who share a significant number of dominant characteristics. Whether the neighborhood is a distinct subculture,[54] such as a self-reinforcing, poverty-ridden ghetto and an FFC,[55] or a self-energizing, upwardly mobile executive community with a minimum of FFC characteristics[56] is not the issue in this definition. Rather the essence of a neighborhood is the presence of significant homogeneity in key sociocultural attributes of concern to planners because of their predictable effects on public decision making.

Donald Klein points out that this neighborhood type of community is, for many of us, the base of life and aspirations, where we are fed, housed, seek work, and educate children.[57] It is through this community that man discovers problems and their solutions, finds security and support during stress, and achieves self-realization. What is currently missing in many neighborhoods is the very quality of neighboring, or an easy and free relationship among neighbors. Klein also calls attention to the fact that many technologists and experts have personally escaped these kinds of ties and, as we see it, live more in Webber's non-place community than in the physical community or neighborhood which contains their home.

For practical purposes, neighborhoods can be demarcated geographically, environmentally, or by socially-defined traits. For example, a neighborhood is "on the city hall side of the railroad yards," is "old-line," or is "Bohemian." Unfortunately, some neighborhoods may be even further subdivided according to the many kinds of widely different interest-subcommunities whose individual members are interspersed in the area. Seeley describes well the different types of inhabitants of the slum.[58]

Obviously, not every member of any contemporary neighborhood shares all its dominant values. Even in a so-called socioculturally homogeneous neighborhood, such as the Negro ghetto, any supposed evidence of solidarity is shattered by the schisms which may be observed between traditionalists, militants, and those who are seeking to escape.[59] Nevertheless, a majority of the members of any homogeneous neighborhood can be expected to agree on most local, state, national, religious, or educational issues. A contemporary review of the significance of the neighborhood and whether it is declining or rising is presented by Felin and Litwack in terms of: (1) its viability; (2) the effects on its cohesion of mobility, heterogeneity, impersonality; and (3) effects of formal organizations.[60]

Although in health we are concerned with a great variety of communities, it is with the neighborhood community of living that we are probably the most concerned, the least effective, and the most needed. Lazarsfeld and Katz,[61] among others, have produced evidence that only in a small face-to-face community can ideas be transmitted in such a way that they are incorporated and come to represent individual learning or experience, opening the way to planned action.

The Community of Identifiable Need

Identifiable needs are those based on factually substantiated lacks which the overall organized society—such as the United States—feels can be rectified and deserve being rectified. The community of identifiable need is the needy group itself. In the case of the migrant farm workers in the United States, members of the community are scattered throughout the country.[62] Fortunately, other communities of need are more often bounded by a limited, geographically definable area. They might consist of several states that are short of water, or blocks of a large city where the population is inadequately housed, or subsections of a town occupied predominantly by minority groups which suffer (among other privations) extensive underemployment. In each of the latter examples, the small communities of need also become part of a larger community of like needs interspersed among cities, states, or the nations. The slum dweller has his counterpart in almost every city and every state, as does the underemployed minority person.

A community of need that might be seen as local in a specific setting might be seen as national in the aggregate; and the communities of ecology, concern, special interest, viability, action capability, resources, and political jurisdiction, shortly to be discussed, are only rarely the same as the one of need (unless and until we regard the nation as the all-encompassing community of communities). A need perceived at one level may obscure or prevent servicing the same need at another level. As an example, our stated desire that the people of Vietnam have freedom of opportunity is obscuring the need for augmented opportunities for our ghetto citizens.

The Community of Problem Ecology

Some problems have a well-defined set of boundaries because the causative agent exists and operates only within a specified terrain. The territory so bounded I loosely call a community. A change from dry to irrigated farming may extend the habitat of certain disease carriers if temperature and other requisites are present at the same time. In such cases, the boundaries of the problem community change, and the changes can usually be anticipated. Problems of day-to-day air pollution similarly have determinable boundaries. However, widely used contaminants that reach main water streams and high air currents typically spill over into separated and originally pollution-free areas and then become regional, national, continental or worldwide concerns. The boundaries of the places which produce the problem may often be precisely defined, but to set the boundaries of the community affected is quite another matter. If *origin* is used in the sense of place of origin of a specified tangible agent causing a problem, the definition of community is simple. But, if origin is used to include the forces that have led a community to use a pesticide or liberate radioactive material, any statement about the problem or ecological community boundaries will be complex. Similarly, using ecology in the full sense of including those affected by a problem, results in tremendous definitional problems, as the consequences spill from one subsystem onto the next or onto larger ones, often in quite different form.

Where systems-oriented analysis of a condition or disease reveals geographic, social, and other boundaries relevant to occurrence and thus to prevention or control, these boundaries become of significance for planning. In some cases, planning must embrace the whole nation—for example, when dealing with the automobile or with post-industrial era mobility. However, modifications even in such ubiquitous phenomena can sometimes be effected regionally if the appropriate boundaries and means are found.

The Community of Concern

The community of concern shares a social interest in a given issue and may not have political or geographic continuity, contiguity, or definition. Obviously, the community of concern can differ tremendously for each issue. It may be stimulated into being by the presence or absence of a community of need. If the problem is a block of street lights, the community of concern is usually the residents of the block, which is at the same time the community of need. The same community of concern may draw in nonresidents, outsiders who worry about crime, beauty, or other tangential considerations associated with the lack of adequate night-lighting in an area not ordinarily considered part of their territory or community.

The Community of Special Interest

A group of persons having no necessary geographic or even major social contiguity may still have a strong economic, social, or professional interest in common. The community of physicians, for example, scattered over a nation and socializing only in small, not-even-exclusively-physician groups, had such strong orientation in common from their work, training, background, and indoctrination that they were able successfully to hold back for decades almost every major threatened change in the distribution and economic pattern of their services.[63] Directed by a common purpose, they were able to weld a significant community of concern, including many other groups that feared social change for a variety of reasons. As a result, organized medicine remained a decisive inhibiting factor in national policy-making relating to this sphere of special interest, until their position finally became so far out of line with other social concerns and expectations that they could no longer gain and hold broad and mutually supportive allies.

The Community of Viability

For purposes of planning, the community of viability is the one that can effectively support the activity wanted. It is the one we most need to identify in terms of a needed activity. For example, a certain number of people in a relatively close geographic relationship (so many minutes or miles from the periphery to the hub) are necessary to support an acceptable all-around medical service that includes a reasonable array of specialties, facilities, and preventive, therapeutic, and rehabilitative services. Three times that number of people are probably required as a base to maintain a well-practiced preventive unit, blood bank, childhood growth and development evaluation unit, genetic service, special surgical skills, and so on. A community this large is also prerequisite to attracting a full array of qualified specialized personnel, providing enough clients to maintain and develop skills, and generating enough volume to allow reasonable overhead costs. Even at this size, a few skills and facilities will have to be utilized jointly with other communities, because they are only feasible when set up to serve clients on a million-person base. In other words, different minimal levels of community size provide a reasonable level of viability for different kinds of services.

The Community of Action Capability

The community of action capability concept may easily be confused semantically with the community of viability, but it has a totally different significance for planning. The community of action capability involves that grouping of people which can, or in fact does, mount action on any one issue at a given time. The grouping of people from which the desired movement can be anticipated or carried out does not necessarily coincide with any other type of community described here. From a volume, economic, or professional viewpoint, the group may not be a functionally viable base, but it may be the only group determined to get action. Because of attitudes, historically or socially inculcated, it may even be intent on doing so alone, in spite of an obvious resulting sacrifice of resources or quality. An example is the too-small, uneconomic, inadequate, all white, suburban hospital. The persons involved in the community of action capability for one specific need, such as the illconceived hospital mentioned, may not agree that the same community should serve as a base of action for other services. The need for many special districts often springs from these determined enclaves—for example, for insect control, hospitals, soil conservation, recreation centers, or fire protection.

The community of action capability, with all its potential vagaries, is the one that will bring into being voluntary or political entities which can raise money, proselyte, employ, and serve the cause. With clever planning, concerted pressures, and bargaining, it may thereby create a base many times larger than the original community of action capability. An encompassing city, county, or state which finds that heeding the appeal is politically necessary or expedient now becomes the new and greater community of action capability. On the other hand, a community may simply win for itself from the larger encompassing unit the right to set up independently. An example would be a municipal utility district that receives state permission to serve its public at their own expense and risk.

The Community of Political Jurisdiction

The community of political jurisdiction has finite geographical boundaries and basic powers of law making and enforcement, taxation, and provision of specified service. The interrelating transactions of the other types of community create a political jurisdiction whenever general agreement decides that a binding formal government unit is necessary to deal with salient needs. The community of action capability is often the most important in the creation of this political or implementation vehicle. The multiple choices among formal political jurisdictions include the tens of thousands of special districts created to extend, change, or subdivide the four customary types of governmental subdivisions, which do not always adequately cover the needs of different sized areas. These districts come into being when some or all of the various kinds of communities are brought to a focus to meet a given need—for example, a water supply, a police force, or a school system. The need is finally given specific geographic boundaries, and all of the residents there are forced, to a degree, by means of taxation to create what the community or communities of interest or concern wanted badly enough, and what the community or communities of functional viability, action capability, and resources could see as reasonably approximating their concern.

Political boundaries give to the community of political jurisdiction its purpose, responsibility, authority, and independence. The geographic boundaries give practical surface limits within which the political needs can be reasonably carried out and the burden proportionately distributed relative to those served by its purpose. What has finally come about is not, however, a satisfactory set of political mechanisms for introducing planned change. Roemer has documented the nightmarish set of political jurisdictions and formal administrative control agencies that are participants in determining the fate of California's physical environment, and that almost ensure the impossibility of effecting significant desired change unless done by the state legislature in a sweeping manner.[64] It is presently what might best be called a "Lindblom Delight."

The Community of Resources

Communities that come into being as a result of professional or political concern or need do not necessarily have a relationship with the kind of community that has the resources to enable satisfaction of needs. Communities of need, concern, special interest, action capability, and viability may coincide and create a community of political jurisdiction, but still be unable to muster the necessary resources. Although a majority of communities of more than a few hundred people could presumably support a classroom and one teacher for every 30 students, patently a good percentage of the nation's children still cannot get adequate schooling, largely because of lack of fundraising capacity. Presumably as a matter of concern with the general welfare, the state would assist its poorer and smaller communities in such matters. Because not all states can provide support and because many will not, the responsibility to provide the necessary resources to assist states has become national. The community of resources adequate to cope with a problem, therefore, may vary from a few families who need to drill a $100 well, to the three nations that would be required to create a $200 billion fresh water system for the West Coast of North America, if the water diverters have their way.

The Community of Solution

Many of us hold that democracy is strengthened when both the responsibility and authority for performing the social functions of government are placed as close to the people as the functional viability of the various issues will allow, so that the number of persons involved in policy-setting is expanded as much as possible. This is to say that the community capable of creating the major resources, usually the state or the nation, will not ordinarily be the template for the community of solution where the immediate planning or action is to be undertaken. I do not hold that the fiscal efficiency based on using the largest action base possible, "state or national agencies as the seat of action,"[65] is to be equated with the most effective, or even the most efficient, way of planning, governing, or delivering. But the localizing of responsibility can proceed only as far as allowed by the various types of coexisting communities that we have described.

The community of solution concept has been described by the National Commission on Community Health Services (NCCHS) as follows: "Planning, organization, and delivery of community health services by both official and voluntary agencies must be based on the concept of a *community of solution*—that is, environmental problem sheds and health-service marketing areas, rather than primarily on political jurisdiction."[66]

In terms of the ecological facts of life, the community of solution must maintain its focus on the boundaries of the natural sources, the patterns of living, and the human and vector bases shaping the problem that offer grounds for successful intervention to prevent occurrence of the problem or treat its undesirable consequences. This certainly embraces the community of identifiable need. The community of solution must, in addition, encompass the equivalent of the community of viability if the needed controls or services are to be operationally and economically feasible. The community of solution must also become the community of action capability in order to bring the needed activities into being, and it must be able to tap the community or communities of resources capable of keeping an activity going at the appropriate level. It must also be able to project from, or at least mesh with, the communities of concern and interest.

In some situations the objectives of the community of solution necessitate harnessing a great diversity of actors, guaranteeing conformity with standards that the consumer cannot easily understand or apply, or raising funds for a public good to which many might not contribute except through taxation. There is little doubt that the community of solution must, in such situations, have some if not most of the attributes of a political jurisdiction or be a creature very much under the guidance of a political jurisdiction (such as a public utility controlled by a political jurisdiction). Obviously, many neighborhoods will also be encompassed in the community of solution and innumerable communities of special interest will have been involved, whether they are based locally or nationally.

Taking these different community forces into account, I find the NCCHS statement difficult to interpret. Does it mean that each health need might best be planned and administered from a *different* sociogeographic base to be determined primarily by ecological or causative factors (problem shed) and by resources and transport routes (marketing area)? If either of these two elements or some mixture were to be the critical determinant of the area for the planning organization and the delivery of health services, some grievous situation would rise. How then are we to utilize the NCCHS recommendation which appears to carry the seed of a sensible solution to planning for the appropriate distribution of health promoting activities?

If the community of solution were considered as the base from which data collection and planning (but not necessarily servicing) must be done for each significant type of health problem, the primary focus would be on the ecological determinants. The area embraced by or contributing to the specific problem would be the minimum geographic area encompassed by an effectual community of solution, as its boundaries would describe the minimum planning base for coping with the problem. This area, however, may not offer sufficient resources to do the job; if it does not, the community of solution may need to draw on a larger area. How constant can a community of solution remain for even a single problem or a single purpose?

For example, providing a community water supply or sewage-removal facilities would necessitate changing the boundaries of the community of solution over time or in accordance with the time span chosen. In a short run approach, the problem may be kept manageable for five years by tapping a resource or disposal site in one direction to serve a single town. But growth projections for the next fifteen years may show that this investment will have to be abandoned and that another—lying in a different direction and requiring the cooperation of at least a dozen nearby towns—will have to be developed if any of the towns are to be served safely. What is the community of solution? For today it might be each household going it alone for a while longer, or for one town to set up a service which must be abandoned with a near total waste of its investment at the end of five years. Or is the community of solution the one necessary fifteen years hence—a unified regional endeavor that promises 100 years of good service for a dozen cities?

Other considerations raise similar issues. Assume that the problem is one of medical care services. Should the planning base be an area large enough to support a good 200-bed general hospital able to provide all but the scarcest and least-used special services and practitioners? Or should the planning base be large enough for a 400-bed hospital and include two adjacent towns because it is guided by other considerations, such as the base size needed for affiliation with a major regional center in order to provide continuing education of medical practitioners and student training? (The larger population base and the larger hospital also promise the local community a higher level and broader scope of care and ensure an adequate supply of well-trained professionals for the future, even though a trade-off of convenience and travel costs is involved.)

In these examples, we see the possible effects on the boundaries of the community of solution by changing the time base, on the one hand, and by changing the scope of concern on the other. Which community of solution is better? So far we have not even considered the issues of resources or of capability of action. Clearly the "market routes and environmental factors crucial to the problem" suggested by NCCHS are only the beginning in weighing boundary considerations for the community of solution.

At one time, each state was thought to be adequate in size and capability to mount resources for the health care of its people, and this was true as long as care cost little and was worth no more. Today, the provision of necessary effective skills and facilities overtaxes a high proportion of our counties and many of our states. Concern for financing and staffing the health needs of our citizens has, therefore, become national in scope. In terms of the actual ability to gather and distribute the dollars or to mount sufficient pressures for doing so, the federal political jurisdiction clearly becomes the vehicle of the national community of solution. But since we have already indicated that we are not likely to be well planned for or served if the nation is regarded as the sole community of solution, what then is the solution?

In determining how to define appropriate boundaries within which to plan in a way that will produce not only good design but implementation as well, one need not assume that planning boundaries must be identical with the area from which the service will be mounted. Each issue, having a different ecological base and its own points of intervention, helps define its own community of solution for planning purposes. If the same boundaries used for planning on each issue are to be used to establish the community of solution for providing services, we will see a multiplication of the single-purpose or sub-optimizing operating districts which we are desperately trying to avoid.

Part of the confusion can be overcome by realizing that there are three kinds of communities of solution: those for planning, those for action or political implementation, and those for creation or delivery of the desired product. Where we are fortunate, these three coincide; such is not always the case.

For Planning

The boundaries for planning communities of solution are determined on the basis of where issues can best be brought into focus by comprehensive planning bodies which have the intent of obtaining political implementation and product delivery. Neighborhood, city, county, metro, state, and multistate levels, as well as the national one, seem to be necessary, and have been extensively discussed in Chapter 10, where a case was made for interrelated sectoral planning centers at each of these levels.

For Action (Political Implementation)

Society cannot deal with the cross-effects of problems—such as rapid transit on freeways, of freeways on smog, of air pollution on incineration of wastes, or of alternatively requiring fill or polluting waterways—when each problem has a politically independent decision-making jurisdiction. As long as each issue has its own policy and control body, decisions will be made on an isolated all-or-none basis for each problem. And the public has no recourse except to vote for or against proposals or bonds, each specific for a one-purpose proposal, allowing no choice between alternative or balanced programs. A welter of single-purpose communities of solution for decision making presents a geofunctional balkanization and effectively precludes applying intelligent solutions. Without a multipurpose base of government the only recourse is to push decision making to higher and higher levels of government, at least to the level of the state. The states would then no doubt need to act through districts to create a suitable base for implementing the planned-for priorities (and ultimately might well be led into the provision of services). Under such circumstances, city and county jurisdictions would lose more autonomy, and local participation and the needed diversity of approaches would diminish further.

Political implementation of the outputs of comprehensive planning for health requires extending the scope of jurisdiction of existing multipurpose units of government and also minimizing the numbers and policy-making powers of singlepurpose units. In addition, multipurpose government is desperately needed at the metro level. When indicated by the ecological rationale, a pact among states may form a regional body, thus creating a community of solution for decision making as well as for planning or services. Federal support is available for these multistate operations.[67] In this case, authority is delegated to the multistate body from one or both of two routes: the state governments involved and the federal government. A national agency such as the Tennessee Valley Authority (TVA) is a longstanding example of a primarily federal creation that works closely with states in all three capacities: planning, decision making and product delivery. Similarly, planning, decision making, or service authority may be delegated to a metro from the local jurisdictions involved, may be created by state government decision, or may be created jointly from above and below.

For Production or Delivery of Services

The ecology of a problem—its origin, the distribution, control, service distribution, resources, public concern involved, and so on—is worked out among and between the various planning level bodies, and the political implementation for its control is obtained among the various levels of political communities. The actual service or delivery implementation may take place on similar or quite different bases. It is easy to visualize potentially innumerable other community-of-solution bases for distribution of services. For example, the matter of ensuring medical care (even though planned for and politically implemented as well as supervised from several other bases) might well best be delivered by private or quasipublic systems of a very local nature. Essentially this is the community of viability.

If the foregoing deductions about the three types of communities of solution are correct, then health planning bodies must move towards interrelating health planning levels, and they also must link health planning with other sectoral planning, so that planning bodies have flexibility to form and reform planning communities of solution (task forces). This method takes care of issues on realistic terms without recreating new planning bodies for each and every problem examined—for each problem has, as we have described, many and varying communities vitally involved.

Planning bodies must also create an output that assists the political implementation (action) communities of solution to work out ways of dealing with one another, so that planning outputs can be implemented politically. Their output must likewise take into account the possible delivery communities of solution where geographic or political boundaries may or may not parallel either the planning or political communities of solution. Because, not only implementation, but the very existence of planning body jurisdictions is a function of the political communities of solution, the latter remain the key.

The political community of solution is a common denominator for most of the separately visualized communities having any involvement in health. Contracts with an adjacent political community of solution can encompass problems in peripheral areas common to both. For single-purpose regional ventures of major importance, such as an airport, rapid transit, or sewage disposal, several political communities of solution of a general capacity can join in a contractual relationship to maintain the planning or servicing of the combined area, without necessarily giving up specific political concern or autonomy. They can, alternatively, give up or isolate the function into a still larger politically autonomous single-purpose community of solution which may, unfortunately, ultimately become a major obstruction to broader planning needs which are almost certain to keep arising.

It seems wisest, therefore, to place our hopes for centralizing effective planning and government, although not necessarily delivery, with the as yet almost nonexistent metropolitan unit of government. Such a unit is the key political and planning community of solution for the vast majority of planning concerns which will serve the vast majority of our people. Where the state can best serve as the metropolitan political and planning community of solution, it should be regarded as the metropolitan equivalent. Each geopolitical metro should include all the neighboring rural areas up to the periphery of those that fit more neatly into the next metro region. Rural areas with no real relationship to current metro regions can conceivably form their own metro type arrangement as the base from which to carry out those functions of government that local constituents cannot undertake independently. Friedmann and Miller provide guidance by relating cities and intermetropolitan peripheries to metropolitan cores within a single matrix.[68] The state or districts of the state also offer a good metro substitute solution for rural areas.

Whether metros should maintain a two- or three-tier form of government (new level plus preexisting cities and counties) is a moot point. Politically, the federal or multitier scheme seems like the only viable one in most states where resistance to metro government remains high for many and changing reasons.

All the discussion so far has indicated the apparent inevitability of a more centralized approach to planning and even to decision making, although emphasis has been on keeping the community of solution for operations as near to the people as possible. The requirement of comprehensive planning for the future as well as for the present, and the extension of our ability to control events, desirable or undesirable, make increasing centralization essential. At the same time, countervailing political devices are necessary if people and local needs are to be kept in mind. (This is the main reason for creating strong metro level of government as opposed to turning everything over to the state or nation.)

A major decentralizing device is the development of sublocal or neighborhood planning units, which can serve also as a clearing house for information about needs and ways of satisfying neighborhood requirements. If neighborhood service centers become common, they can also serve as a hub for health and well-being concerns by developing a network of community information and interaction and helping to bring individuals and local groups into decision-making. Neighborhood planning and development efforts offset the dangerous aspects of increased centralization by broadening the base of citizen participation and widening the horizon of choices. A metro, operating as the planning and service base of health, welfare, probation, guidance, counselling, employment, rehabilitation and the like, requires that neighborhood needs be understood, that delivery be performed at local points, and that it be made in such a way that people of each neighborhood can utilize services that they have helped to plan and govern.

In a document devoted to the problems of governance, Victor Jones had this to say:

> Concomitant with the thrust toward metropolitanization is another powerful thrust toward smaller areas where the influence, control and other objectives of political participation may be realized. . . . The creation or development of either a regional agency or a number of neighborhood agencies, or both, will increase the decision making points in a system of metropolitan governance. A regional agency should reduce the dysfunctional effects of very large governments now existing or soon to be created. . . . The Los Angeles City Charter Commission provides in its recommended charter for: "the formation of self-initiating neighborhood organizations (with populations between 5,000 and 30,000) with an elected board and an appointed neighborman, as a new institutional mechanism for communicating neighborhood needs and goals, involving citizens in city affairs, and reducing feelings of alienation." A neighborman would be the formal link among the elective Neighborhood Board, the residents of the neighborhood and city hall.[69]

PURSUING POLITICAL IMPLEMENTATION

In addition to pursuing a general strategy of doing well by its planning commitment, the planning body will have taken every opportunity to extend its audience, clients, and constituents and to amass the currency of power. In terms of political acceptance of each of its planning outputs (steps 4 and 5 in Figure 1.2) there are specific opportunities for aiding implementation that do not particularly involve dipping into the planning body's power bank. These usually depend on a clever analysis of the situation to determine what the history of the problem and its environment suggest about the possibilities of implementation.

Plan implementation which brings the proposed interventions into reality, formally proceeds on four broad successive levels. The first is adoption by community policy makers of one of the alternatives proposed by the planning body. The second is winning over (or coercing) the agencies and agents who must carry the planning into the realm of design for everyday operations. The third is converting policy into program, and includes the favorable involvement of those serving in the agencies. The fourth level is the change in those target groups whose attitudes, activities, habits, or behaviors must be affected. In actual practice, in order to get political implementation, the negotiations and planning will have already involved the ultimate consumers, workers in the delivery systems, and managers of the delivery systems.

The search for community adoption is continued in more specific terms. I have already discussed in general terms how to influence the policy-making machinery and the acquisition of clout by planning bodies. Now let us examine the requirements for pursuing political implementation of planning output as part of the planning process itself.

The roles most relevant to the strategy of achieving defined improvements were described in Chapter 9. The most important of these probably are Educator, Activator, and Power Modifier; to a lesser degree, Controller of Plan Implementation and each of the other roles— including those already utilized up through the stage of designing the output—have the potential of being used with forethought to advance political implementation. By outlining the kinds of concerns that would inhibit or favor implementation, a planning body intent on achieving selected improvements can carry out its activities in behalf of each of its roles in such a way that political implementation is kept in focus as much as the product design during the entire design phase. The watchword is the definition and analysis of goals and problems and the design of solutions in the light of political implementation as the major constraint, beyond the cause-and-effect knowledge needed to handle the situation.

Although the idea of health planning is currently attractive in the United States as a way out of our costly impasse over health care services and because of our not too remarkable accomplishments in health status, we must not overlook the deeply ingrained American resistance to having anyone remote, in whatever guise, telling us what to do. To quote Arnold and Welsh:

> There is a crucial question the answer to which is of fundamental importance to the health planner: "In a political system where nearly every adult may vote, but where knowledge, wealth, social position and access to officials and other resources are unequally distributed, who actually governs?"[70]
>
> Ideally, the answer to this question should aid the health planner in his broad and longer-range calculations concerning possible ways of using community resources and/or gaining access to resources outside the relevant community. The answer should help the planner better understand the issues on which the community might be persuaded to expend these resources and the perception that different groups within the community might have of the political costs and benefits from alternative uses of resources. More specifically, the answer to the question—who governs?—should help to identify and characterize the participants in political decision-making, determine who gains and loses from decision outcomes, and suggest how successful participation in the community's decision-making can be achieved.[71]

The sections which follow review some of these key political action determiners, which the planning body must not only understand but must work into its strategy for implementation. Mott stresses the gross inadequacies of the "rational decision model," the modest improvements made by the utilization of the "community action model," and the general inability of either to get the necessary parties to participate or to change, plus their inability to resolve basic conflict.[72] I can only agree with Mott's thesis that there can be no implementation of planning unless planning completely merges substantive issues with politics; in fact, that is our process definition of planning—the marriage broker for technology and politics.

Affecting Political Decision Making

In spite of the magnificent writings on how we are governed, it is very hard to put together anything like a satisfactory guide to the processes involved in political decision making. Yet this guide would be the foundation on which our planner is dependent for the political utilization of his outputs. We in the United States often marvel at the prestigious British commissions and study groups which are set up to provide a rounded study of a painful situation and bring in recommendations which are then often remarkably well-followed. (The Beveridge report is a well known example.)[73]

Of course, when we use the British study body as a political model, we are losing sight of the fact that such a study body is not ongoing with a life of its own, like our health planning body with its many chores. Rather, the British body represents the beginning of a solution—its appointment is an already determined political decision which has both acknowledged the existence of a painful and complex problem and the desire to do something about it. The committee is created to fill a clear major political need, and what it does is therefore awaited with some concern by the policy makers themselves.

In an excellently referenced article, Richard Bolan emphasizes utilizing the potential contributions of all relevant social science disciplines to community decision behavior.[74] He applies a set of variables which he calls decision field characteristics; these are reproduced here as Figure 11.5 because they are so central to our concerns with implementation. They summarize well many of the factors which have been observed as leading to or away from action and, thus, implementation. They seem to indicate that most of the steps indicated in participative and developmental planning advocated in this text have a history of leading to inaction. Fortunately, these were not observations made on conscious attempts to democratically carry out developmental planning. They are observations on social change which took place mostly under elitist or professional auspices. They do suggest, nonetheless, that developmental planning, like democratic government, is not necessarily a simple way of reaching wise decisions nor of obtaining their implementation.

Rogers, utilizing as his base the interrelationships between social structure and social relationships, provides another set of propositions:[75]

Social structure acts to impede or to facilitate the rate of diffusion and adoption of new ideas through system effects.

Diffusion can change the social structure of a social system.

Power elites act as gatekeepers to prevent restructuring innovations from entering a social system, while favoring functioning innovations that do not immediately threaten to change the system's structure.

A system's social structure helps determine the nature and distribution of the consequences of an innovation.

Top-down change in a system which is initiated by the power elites, is more likely to succeed than is bottom-up change.

Bottom-up change involves a greater degree of conflict than top-down change.

Bottom-up change is more likely to be successful at times of perceived crisis in a system.

Bottom-up change is more likely to be successful if a social movement is headed by a charismatic leader.

The role of the charismatic leader in a social movement decreases as the movement becomes institutionalized into a more highly structured organization.

The ingredients of public decision making by politicians are also critically important. Those commonly referred to include:

The intent to maximize the chances of returning to the elected

FIGURE 11.5
DECISION FIELD AND PLANNING STRATEGY IMPACTS ON DECISION OUTCOMES
(After Bolan)*

Decision Environment Characteristics	Tending Toward Action	Tending Toward Inaction
Formal-legal structure	Focused decision center	Dispersed decision centers
	Highly competent bureaucracy	Incompetent or lacking bureaucracy
	Articulated hierarchy	No hierarchy
Informal Structure	Strong party machine	Nonpartisan
	Elite or interest group dominance	Amorphous
Characteristics of polity	Homogeneous	Heterogeneous
	Crystallized	Noncrystallized
	Tradition-free	Tradition-laden
	Striving	Prosperous or settled

Decision Unit Characteristics	Tending Toward Action	Tending Toward Inaction
Source of power	Appointed body	Elected body
Accountability	Long term of office	Short term of office
	Large clientele	Small or specialized clientele
Group dynamics	Socially cohesive	Socially heterogeneous
	Significant reward-punishment schema	Insignificant reward-punishment schema
	High status	Low status
	High functional role differentiation	Little or no role differentiation
Group role	Focused	Comprehensive

Planning Strategies	Tending Toward Action	Tending Toward Inaction
Position variable	Attachment to power center	Independent and advisory
Position variable	Attachment to power center	Independent and advisory
Method variables	Ad hoc opportunism Problem-solving Incremental	Comprehensive Classical focus on interdependencies
Content variables	Immediate time horizon Means oriented Selected and focused information	Long-term time horizon Goal oriented Comprehensive information system
Action or intervention strategies	Efforts to maintain distribution of resources Efforts to change or modify individual behavior Efforts to bring about change with existing institutions and organizations	Efforts to reallocate distribution of resources Efforts to change or modify societal behavior Efforts to alter existing institutions and organizations

*Source: Richard S. Bolan "Hypothesis on the Impact of Planning Strategies on Decision outcomes." Reprinted, by permission, from the *Journal of the American Institute of Planners* 50 (September 25, 1969).

post, which includes the possibilities of favoring those who foot the bills, favoring those who vote favorably, avoiding overt favoritism so as not to antagonize too many and, thereby, offer an opposition candidate a ready-made platform.

Provision for the judgment and effort which will be best for the electing constituency generally.

Provision for the judgment and effort which will be best for the region and the country consistent with personal beliefs and under the constraints of the preceding points.

Putting out the best efforts for personal advancement and fame under the constraints of the preceding three points.[76]

All of these variables can be examined from many viewpoints. Economic theory assumes that constituents are as rational as their elected representative and that they weigh their vote for him against how well he has advanced their various values or positions. Sociopsychologic theory might give more credence to whether the constituent had derived a sense of participation, of worth, of not having been offended, perhaps of even having had the opportunity to do something for his representative or to give something to him or to his country as a result of the representative's actions. It would also take into account opportunities for social participation and gratification resulting from the constituent's support of his candidate.

Unfortunately these notions represent just the beginning of an analysis. Not only does the politician have his own internal tugs of war, but each constituent has his own. Things are even more complicated, because competing groups of citizens continually seek their representative's loyalties, and other political candidates compete with the current representatives for the citizen's loyalty. In addition, individuals deeply involved in the organization—either of political parties or of citizens' groups which carry on these competitions—also carry on the very personal games and problems of those whose fates are particularly tied up in such organizations, and thereby further complicate the relationships of citizens to their representatives.

Our concern in all of this is whether planning bodies can cleverly insert their output into this running set of games. Can they, on the one hand, influence the politicians' interests toward utilizing their deliberations and, on the other, so involve the citizen that his sense of his own best interests leads him to approve the planning output, and particularly to approve the legislator who supports its implementation?

At the local levels, such concurrence would seem more achievable. There the planning body, the public it can involve, the media, and the legislators all work close to one another and presumably can be brought to a modestly comparable view of what the planning body is doing and why its recommendations have come to be synonymous with what is wanted most.

At the metro, state, and particularly the national level, some overwhelming obstacles to this approach occur in the form of safe territories, some as large as states. Here a legislator can guarantee his long-term incumbency by working on only one issue that guarantees his meeting a dominant value of his constituency. They in return comfortably allow him to sell his vote or soul, even to carry on personal vendettas on any and all other issues without any danger of being brought to heel, even by a President who seeks to use the prestige of that office to unseat the legislator.

This brings us to another set of issues. Just what do various parts of the electorate actually envision as the kinds of persons they expect to take a hand in moving the government? If planning bodies are to take a hand, what are their limits? What are considered to be legitimate tools?[77] These questions are important to the planning body because there are no widely applicable answers. How their work at achieving implementation will be perceived is very much a situational affair, varying not only from place to place but from issue to issue.

From now on we will regard the planning body as a change agent, for that is what the successful strategic or implementative part of its work signifies. In this way we can more easily clarify the tasks and obstacles faced.

As a first step, the planning body will have to take into account the forces and powers at work; it must gently enlarge the scene, attract a positive constituency, generate its own seat of authority, and obtain power. Then, in part as the result of having power, it must generate further power by obtaining attention from various concerned interests, as well as from voters, and thus earn a hearing from legislators. If these are the same legislators whose work has simultaneously been aided by the fact-finding, goal-setting, and problem-solving activities of the planning change agent, they too will have independently awarded the planner their respect and an opportunity for a fair hearing.

Community Attributes That Determine Paths of Implementation

In pursuing the implementation of each of its planning activities, the planning body must turn to the specific communities of concern and see what they offer in the way of help or hindrance to implementation. This step, which is equally an analysis of resources of all kinds, must be taken to test the reality or feasibility of alternative proposals. There is absolutely no excuse for not addressing simultaneously the issue of the obstacles—beyond the traditional ones of time, money, manpower, and facilities—that may actually exist in men's minds. This means the categorical pursuit of information which tells of the probable political, social, and psychic possibilities for implementation. From analysis of the forces and dynamics that are likely to be at work on the issue, strategy takes form. Choosing the participants, labeling the issues, selecting the timing, reading the implications for various groups, grouping forces, and nullifying potential obstructions all become part of planning.

Historical Community Attributes

By means of a retrospective review, Wilson picks out key dimensions for success in community self-studies, which have much in common with planning undertakings.[78] He finds those that presage action are:

A basic fund of agreement on broad local aims.

A history of successful resolution of important community problems in the recent past.

A corps of interested persons involved in the consensus of aims and in recent successful actions.

An economic structure of sufficient vigor to enable leaders to go beyond sheer survival.

Some emergent awareness of the significance of well-being needs in community life.

Obviously, almost any and sometimes all of these strengths are missing in communities. Comprehensive planning will have to overcome serious gaps.

Current Community Attributes and Currents

After surveying the literature, Warren suggests four critical attributes which will describe a community's potential for change.[79] The strength of each of these four attributes tells a great deal about how the overall community is likely to react, and through which means.

The degree of local autonomy. In a study of the degree to which local communities finance municipal activities, it was found that the level of local fiscal autonomy permitted by state statute was the best indicator of actual municipal performance.[80]

Coincidence of service areas of local agencies. The likelihood of attacking issues effectively rises or falls with the unity or interrelatedness of service or "cause" agency boundaries. Where one kind of health agency serves two counties, another serves half of a county, and still another serves the isolated third of one of the two, or where welfare services are highly fractionated, or transport exists only along isolated ribbons, comprehensive planning may have to clear some monumental hurdles before it achieves implementation.

Psychological identification with the locality. When citizens identify strongly with the place in which they live, they have a concern for local resources and amenities and express this concern by willingness to tax themselves to support facilities and institutions. Problems are created if parts of a community, or the whole community, identifies with an overall geopolitical entity which cannot officially serve them— for example, if they relate to a city in another county or state. Failure to recognize one's parents, so to speak, may result in use of market, medical, cultural, financial, and recreational resources in a community where no support is contributed and in an unwillingness to create suitable institutions in the place of actual residence. The mobile middle and upper segments may get a free ride by doing this, and the poorer, less mobile persons may be left with no local community resources. In the area of education, this problem of alienation has become so exaggerated in many communities that citizens who are better off routinely send their children to private schools; the local school system, utilized only by those who traditionally get little from it, is left to starve. Sometimes nests of commuters who maintain double loyalties have peculiar effects on moves for local incorporation, community services, and so on. Usually executive commuter groups have more complex demands than labor pool areas.

Horizontal and vertical relationships. The horizontal pattern, or degree to which various local units (individuals and social systems) relate functionally and structurally, may be further complicated by the degree to which vertically directed interests become involved. Horizontal or essentially local relationships may continuously bump into vertically inspired directions that constrain some local groups. Demands of a national health agency that its chapters not affiliate with local "united giving" may affect not only the money-raising structure but may seriously impede the cooperation of various groups in other local causes. Long-standing attitudes, sometimes bolstered by edicts of professional societies that their members may not associate professionally with those of competitive organizations, may preclude necessary local programs. Attitudes of local chapters on race may defy national requirements and alienate locals or cause their inability to command national resources. Professionals almost automatically are forced to a heavy vertical commitment because their sources of education, professional status, journals, and annual meetings have a heavy national and on occasion international flavor, all based on the advancement of their science and their profession's welfare. Organized labor and political groups may have similar orientations.

The overlap of memberships in vertical and horizontal (locally oriented) organizations has the value of sparing most of us from a totally one-sided view. Hopefully, comprehensive planning will benefit from this duality of view. Local planning can clarify horizontal needs without overlooking vertically inspired concerns of members of the community; in return, vertically oriented groups can utilize their across-the-country connections and national positions to make various local needs understood.

Arnold and Welsh pick out another seven relationships,[81] a few of which are similar to Warren's:

The nature of the power structure. Is it concentrated or diffuse? Does it have an economic base or is the base dependent upon the type and scope of the issue? What prospects are there for change in the power structure?

The relationships between the governmental structure and the community's power relationships. What political ideologies are operative within the community?

How political leadership groups are formed in the community. Are they established with a strong organizational base? Are they integrated into the power structure? Are they based on interests or on political ideologies?

Shifts in the scope of government. Are local and national trends similar or different? Will they remain so?

The relationships between the socioeconomic system and the local political system. Are major economic decisions affecting the community made within the community or externally? What is the base from which the local political system is structured?

Relationships between the local political system and other political systems. Are county, state, regional, and national interests compatible with local interests? How much influence does each have on the other?

The manner in which issues are generally presented and their response from the community. Do issues dampen or arouse ideological competition?

Clark provides the most extensive set of propositions or guides for determining the elements likely to be involved in decision-making; these are derived from what he calls fundamental variables.[82]

Selection of Strategies

There are no end of strategies for a given situation, but a review of some of the more obvious requirements for strategy should be helpful.

General Propositions

Arnold and Welsh have condensed some of the major strategies into three groupings available to the partner in a transaction.[83] Choice among them depends on his needs and those of the other actors in the transaction.

Competition implies rivalry between two or more actors that is mediated by a third party; in other words, two or more parties can fulfill the needs of the third party and are competing to enter into a transactional relationship with him. Levine and White have suggested that health and welfare organizations may compete for clientele, for financial support, for functions to be performed, or even for a particular disease domain.[84]

Cooperative strategies may include bargaining, co-optation, or co-alition. In this case the transactions start from a point where both parties have needs to be fulfilled by each other. *Bargaining* implies a negotiation of an exchange between two or more individuals or groups. In order to make the transaction mutually attractive, each has to compromise and adjust to the other. *Co-optation* is the strategy of absorbing new elements into a leadership or policy-making structure of one group so that it may maintain its own position and stability. For example, the practice of placing a representative of organized medicine on a Board of Health is a co-optation strategy. Finally, *coalition* is the formation of a combined organization to serve a common purpose. "The enterprise that competes is not only influenced in its goal-setting by what the competitor and the third party may do but also exerts influence over both. Bargaining, likewise, is a form of mutual, two-way influence. Co-optation affects the co-opted as well as the co-opting party, and coalition clearly sets limits on both parties."[85]

Exclusion is a strategy where the transaction is avoided because it is to the advantage of the group not to enter into the transaction. There are two ways in which this can happen—either the actor is so highly rewarded through other social alternatives that the particular transaction has low salience, or the transaction would be so costly to the participant that he chooses to seek out other alternatives or do without the needs that could be served by the transaction.

Applications

From the assessment of who and what is involved in the various aspects of the planning purposes, the planning body or change agent (we use this appellation interchangeably because we want to stress this aspect of planning) will learn of the probable state of affairs.

Collaborative approaches. Where consensus is a practical goal, the planning body utilizes collaborative approaches, introducing, extending, smoothing over, explaining, in effect serving as enabler and catalyst until the plan is packaged and delivered as program activities.

A very popular model by Thompson and Tuden[86] later expanded by Thompson[87] and Arnold and Welsh,[88] provides further guidance in the area of cooperative strategies.

Where no agreement can be reached on either ends or means, the parties which intend to cooperatively reach a political decision or even a *modus vivendi* can only do so by avoiding the issues, keeping them from their agendas, or escalating them to a higher-systems-level set of concerns. Planning bodies as change agents must see this situation coming and work to prevent it or enlarge its scope through their planning negotiations—a necessity if they are to be of use to policy-makers. Naturally, destruction of cooperative arrangements and open conflict cannot always be avoided by these devices.

Where there is agreement about ends but not means, the model suggests that—even with a dominant factor or coalition—trial and error testing may be necessary, first on paper, as by forecasting. That may be followed by still further experimenting in practice, to develop one or more ways to proceed so that no group feels that an all-or-none loss is impending. The planning body can again help design for this possibility.

Where there is agreement about means, but not ends, compromise and bargaining are usually possible to determine what can be done, and the planning body can set the stage.

Most policy-making bodies have experience in overcoming these three disagreement situations in the cooperative strategies. However, because many required mechanisms for overcoming barriers are lethal to planning or to well planned proposals, the planning body had better participate in these mechanisms. Sometimes much of the planning can be salvaged by paving the way for introduction of proposals by one group rather than another, for initial hearing by one committee rather than another, or for prior involvement of key figures in the machinery. Warren and Hyman verify that, in fact, action systems in consensus situations do use collaborative strategies. (They also note that private sponsors tend to skirt seriously controversial issues but that government undertakes to carry them through to resolution.[89])

Unconcern. Where planners discern an absence of the impetus for change, they may determine that there is little interest in the issue, or a lack of understanding of its nature or significance, or that the issue does not have value relevance. By campaign type strategies, without direct pressure but with a clear focus on the pertinent groups, leaders, and those looking for a cause, an issue can be given visibility, and dissonance can be created for all by arousing awareness of value, goal, or expectation failures. Education, social affairs, mass media, study groups, and advertising may each be used appropriately. Potential opposition may even be silenced before it forms, either through co-optation of its potential leaders or by making the posture of potential opposition opprobrious. Opposition may of course light up, and the situation then becomes one of potential or real conflict.

Saliency sometimes results when an issue generalizes and is suddenly perceived as part of something that is highly value-charged. An ordinarily apathetic and disenfranchised group may go all out on an issue because it becomes a symbol for their smouldering revolt. An unconcerned business group may make housing development a top goal or a hated target when they discover the implications for property, profits, taxes and civil peace.

Conflict. The situation to be dealt with may rapidly reveal that it is one of potential or emerging conflict. Strategies open to the change agent vary according to whether opposition is isolated or comes from multiple sources. Splitting up the opposition, neutralizing it, bargaining with it, buying it off, threatening or pressuring it from respected or feared sources in the social, fraternal, employment, political, economic, or financial spheres—all these are relevant means to overcome opposition. On occasion, massive educational efforts and a show of force by friends of the issue can melt or turn away the opposition, which may come to dislike the measure less or fear opposing it more because its potential friends and sources of support have been removed. Saliency and the spread of other values have clearly sapped the organized opposition of the otherwise loyal and active supporters of the Roman Catholic church in the issue of family planning. The institution's followers may even come to resent interference by their customary leaders in the area given salience (for example, popular defiance of church denunciation of birth control in Puerto Rico and more recently throughout the world.)

Another approach to solving emerging conflict is to chip away at vulnerable areas where agreement is possible through accommodation or splitting the difference (compromise). One may concentrate on other areas among the priorities where the potential foes are not in disagreement. By continuing to make progress (and friends), proponents can gain status, momentum, and above all the trust and ability to reach the former opposition on a new footing. Preparation for handling the touchier areas at a later date needs to go on continuously. However, planners or change agents must beware of the enticing and traditional Community Council role of keeping everyone happy at the price of creating no significant change.

Haas provides a basic formulation for one type of conflict resolution that commonly escapes discussion: "the upgrading of the consumer interest," which amounts to a redefinition of the situation at a higher level of system or a broadened scope of concern.[90] For example, a large home builder may be opposed at zoning hearings because he makes no provision for land for schools or recreation. A solution which is suitable both for him and his neighbors may be worked out, so that an entire new zoning approach is taken, one in which he gives up land for public service entities that not only do not impose on his neighbors but assist them in obtaining services. His positive tradeoff for land loss is zoning for multiple and commercial land use which increases the value of his remaining land. McFarland gives other examples.[91] This level of resolution differs sharply from compromise (splitting the difference) or accommodation (agreeing on those items which are not in conflict).

Sometimes the best strategy may be to ignore the opposition. If not provoked or put on the spot, the opposition may well turn out to have less interest than tradition claimed. Sometimes the opposition may be predictably inactive because it is facing other battles that will require using up all of its accumulated resources and owed favors. (These battles can sometimes be prearranged.)

A similar issue is whether to acknowledge a power elite which is reluctant to accept a proposed plan. If the elitists have been wisely drawn in and utilized to the point where their egos or their welfare are satisfied, they are no longer a problem. If, on the other hand, involvement has not appeared wise, should their permission or their blessing ultimately be sought? It is probably just as wise to sidestep a reluctant elite unless they constitute a critical force. Their power is often imaginary, often for other issues, often ineffective. Acknowledging or paying homage to the power status of an elite group may have several harmful effects. A showing of respect, whether public or private, increases the status of the elite, makes them more formidable to deal with in future encounters, and may even make the proponents of a cause beholden to the elites, forever paying back a worthless, but nonetheless evidently acknowledged, favor.

Where conflict is underway or threatened, the change agent may choose to escalate the issues into an open confrontation and use appropriate strategies. Direct conflict may be the logical means of handling wavering opposition that cannot be neutralized. In health matters of public concern, change agent acceptance of conflict has usually been limited to confrontation through elections, recalls, referenda, or petitions, usually concerning public permission to do something, stop something, or expend new or increased monies. In fact, conflict has on occasion been the device for gaining issue salience among target groups, and thus building popular support for something not previously desired strongly nor demanded by the majority of the target group (for example, Medicare). Because such confrontations usually depend on a formal, public, or legislative decision, a loss may give saliency, but postponement or oblivion may also result. A win usually means creating a new service, institution, facility, or enforcement machinery, all of which are likely to perpetuate themselves and the servicing of the area at issue.

Conflict may be escalated to the level of legal and peaceful disruption, like picketing. It may extend to peaceful but illegal disruption, such as blocking streets and accepting the consequences of violating the law in order to call attention to the position or plight of a group.

When there is no redress from tyranny, conflict may be further escalated to include fighting and rioting, whether upheld by law or not.

Witness the American Revolution and secession from England. Planners are most unlikely to agree to the need for this way out, because planning should be able to resolve critical issues at an early stage and in a peaceful manner. However, planners need constant reminders that irrelevant planning may leave change agents other than planners with little choice but open conflict. (It is of interest that open conflict once resolved may leave a favorable milieu for dedication and growth.[92]) Gamson sees evidence that rancorous conflicts are associated with those places that are undergoing change, stimulation, and growth, and that communities free of such conflicts seem to be stagnating.[93]

Several interesting contributions to the theory and management of conflict are now available in the July-August 1972 special issue of the American Behavioral Scientist.[94]

Roles of the Change Agent

Planning, if it is sound, is the first step into action. Once it has analyzed the groups and issues facing it, the planning body will typically be operating in any or all but the two or three more aggressive conflict phases of the conflict-consensus spectrum. Even on the same issue at any one time, or seriatim, the change agent may be engineering resolution of conflicts with one group, searching for limited areas of agreement with others, attempting neutralization of conflict through pressures, seeking saliency for groups regarding themselves as uninvolved, and welding firm consensus among formerly unrelated but favorably inclined interests. Welding of support and a show of strength may be all that is needed in many issues. The firmed-up support also becomes the means of doing all-out battle with any remaining hard opposition that must be swept aside through legislative decisions or public goals.

In all of this, the characteristics of the change agent and of key actors will determine what means are used, as some people work better one way than another. Some change agents simply cannot pursue certain approaches.

It may come as something of a blow to follow Wilson's list of the circumstances under which he believes "centrally planned" change is "permitted" by communities:[95]

> When the major actors have an interest (their own?) in change.
> When the major actors have a common set of goals.
> When there is indifference by most parties to an issue.
> When the issue is made to appear so reasonable that anyone intending to oppose it is made to appear stupid or cheap.
> When crises make action seem less painful than inaction.
> When change is seen as inevitable.
> When influence resources have already been distributed at a

higher level and locals are unwilling to lose out on incentive bonuses and other such benefits.

When a group of actors have a mandated stranglehold on certain areas (and, as the California State Highway Commission did at one time, go where they will).

It may be relevant that Wilson really means *centrally* inspired change, in contrast to the wide-base involvement in planning advocated here. Because the latter has only infrequently been tried in the United States, it is unfair to assume, as Wilson does, that community change in the future will be limited to the situations typical of the past.

The realities of being involved in an intentional conflict presume an awareness of what is to be gained or lost. The chances of becoming involved unintentionally in conflict are also so great that it seems worth referring to Coleman's review of the development of controversy.[96]

One further consideration deserves mention here. In many situations where the change agent seeks to win power for a powerless or depressed constituency, no matter which issues he utilizes, the underlying purpose is community development or integration of the community, and how the specific issue is handled is subordinated to that primary consideration.[97] This is consistent with the traditional roles of the community worker as Enabler, Advocate, and Developer. In these roles he is teaching process rather than achieving specified community changes.[98]

PURSUING PROGRAMMATIC IMPLEMENTATION

Involving Producers and Purveyors

The next concern is for converting the politically implemented program or package into producer and agency policy and program, steps 5a and 6 in Figure 1.2. This second level of implementation can be described as the process of winning over the agencies and agents who must turn the plan into everyday operations. If the first level of community acceptance and political implementation was reasonably well designed, the two levels would have gone on simultaneously, because the producer and agency forces involved usually are the key vested interests who have more community, professional, and political holds on the resources (both tangible and normative) than almost any other group. Sometimes they will have been the opposition that was overcome. In either case, their inputs influence the selection of the designs to make the plans operationally suitable. Where they were included and supportive, all is well; where they were vanquished opponents, difficulties may be plentiful unless the reluctant producers and agency leaders have been swept away.

The third level of implementation—the conversion of accepted producer and agency policy and programs into client-affecting activities which really try to produce the outcomes originally planned—also includes the favorable involvement of those working for the producers and agencies. Hopefully, they will have been properly involved by their leaders and agency heads, so that subordinate workers will join their leaders in activating newly planned programs in which their interests have been reasonably considered and their participation significantly utilized. Because program leadership and worker involvement are at the heart of the concerns of administration, which has an ample literature of its own, these two subjects will not be discussed further.

Converting Accepted Planning Into Utilized Programs

This discussion pursues an eclectic approach to the conversion of planning efforts into agency programs which mesh with client behaviors. The development of any intervention must take into account, first, the analysis of the situation for those social, environmental, or personal elements likely to retard or advance personal acceptance of a proposed behavioral change and, second, the development of a strategy to overcome inertia or opposing influences and to mobilize supporting factors, so that a new plan will not founder for lack of participation by the persons for whom it was designed.

The issues involved in influencing or manipulating people come to mind as soon as one entertains the idea of planning in a democratic society. Yet, how can anyone plan seriously for health and health services, unless he simultaneously looks forward to facilitating, encouraging, or pressuring people to utilize unaccustomed procedures, change deleterious habits, and take up desirable ones? Because much of the major activity of our society is built on introducing interventions against illiteracy, crime, ill health, and so on, the democratic issue becomes one of offering choices for acceptance or rejection by the enfranchised members of our society. We undertake the phase of planning for individual behavior change on the assumption that the earlier phases of community acceptance and agency implementation have received public approval through the customary channels for the kind of program proposed—that is, the democratic processes for making a choice were duly followed.

The effectiveness of any design for comprehensive health services must depend, finally, on the human factors which will determine its acceptance. However broad the base, health programming needs to take into consideration the people—individuals, family units, and so-

cial groupings—for whom services are to be provided. Will they find
the services they need? Will they utilize the services offered? Will they
accept the patterns of health behavior prescribed for them, many of
which demand change in their accustomed living patterns?

Many different measures have been studied and advocated to influence behavior.[99] The change agent cannot accept the results of prior
studies uncritically: what is seen as a statistically significant variable in
a study is often of insignificant consequence as a practical matter.[100]

Beryl Roberts refers to the "decision making" of individuals as critical to their participation in health behavior or their utilization of
health programs.[101] She says:

> We realize that personal decisions are affected by much within the
> individual—the cognitive, affective, and conative elements—and
> by the situation in the sense of the total psychological field includ-
> ing, among other forces, significant persons, the message, the
> channel of communication, and the agent of education. Any de-
> cisional movement itself is embedded in a complex process and is
> difficult to isolate, for there are pre-decisional forces and events,
> the decision itself and post-decisional forces and events. For us in
> health work, the post-decisional forces are important for we have
> concern not only with the decision but also with the maintenance
> of action resulting from the decision.

Zaltman and Lin,[102] and Udry and Morris [103] provide lists of considerations affecting adoption of change that are in great part relevant
to individuals as well as to societies. The nominal group process used
by Delbecq and VandeVen in group situations is designed to bring
about the kind of involvement that presages action.[104]

Watson has summarized what he regards as the most important factors in the acceptance of change:[105]

Who brings the change? (1) Resistance will be less if persons
involved, teachers, board members, and community leaders feel that
the project is their own—not one devised and operated by outsiders;
(2) resistance will be less if the project clearly has wholehearted support from top officials of the system.

What kind of change? (1) Resistance will be less if participants
see the change as reducing rather than increasing their present burdens; (2) resistance will be less if the project accords with values and
ideals that have long been acknowledged by participants; (3) resistance will be less if the program offers the kind of new experience
which interests participants; (4) resistance will be less if participants
feel that their autonomy and their security are not threatened.

Procedures in instituting change: (1) Resistance will be less if
participants have joined in diagnostic efforts leading them to agree
on the basic problem and to feel its importance; (2) resistance will be
less if the project is adopted by consensual group decision; (3) re-

sistance will be reduced if proponents are able to empathize with opponents, to recognize valid objections, and to take steps to relieve unnecessary fears; (4) resistance will be reduced if it is appreciated that innovations are likely to be misunderstood and misinterpreted.

This summary is based on Watson's perceptions of the interaction of two sources of resistance. He categorizes these into resistances that were part of a given individual's makeup and those that could be said to be part of the fabric of the social system. The following material outlines other beliefs about what is needed to bring about changes in behavior on both an individual and a group basis. Suchman has a not dissimilar formulation.[106] (See Chapter 2 for a discussion of social change.)

Operating Premises to be Considered by Planners Acting as Change Agents

Behavior may seem consistent but is continuously changing as a result of experiences, physical and psychological maturation, degeneration, and so on.

Any one area of influence may be overwhelmingly effective.

Any one area of influence may be overwhelmingly inhibiting.

Some areas of influence are latent; of these, some are predictably hostile if we arouse them or if they are aroused by another source.

The more areas of influence acting in concert towards a particular event, the more likely the desired action will take place, although a sense of excessive pressure may alienate many.

It may be wise to reinforce some influences and dampen others, if we understand the situation clearly enough.

Action taken for whatever reason, or even if unintended, is likely to lead to rationalization about the desirability of the action, which might result in reinforcement for a desired or an undesired action.

Any one area of influence operating favorably in any of the three spheres, sociological, environmental or personal, may well create other favorable areas of influence in the same or in the other two spheres.

Each person is the product of heredity and of the previous experiences he has incorporated; these two influences make of him a total being who reacts to present environmental exposure, and the aggregate determines what reaction and therefore what action will take place. When the change agent wants to change health behavior, he tries, to some degree, to alter current environment and at the same time tries to make the target person a different person as a result of the encounter arranged for him. Of course, as the target person changes, he may also become unpredictable in some new ways. He is simultaneously getting other inputs, and these are the other sources of what may appear as irrational or unpredictable behavior.

Timing is a critical factor, because one area of influence may turn another one on or off, depending on where the readiness lies. Do not forget the old slogan: "Start where people are." One must listen to learn attitudes, fears, values, needs, desires, priorities, sources of information and influence. This also means going ahead with people on what they think they need first. And that may be something other than the goals which the change agent has in mind.

Target people obviously react to change in many different ways. Generally we can anticipate that:

—Compatibility with customary behavior or attitudes is a favorable omen.

—Giving up an existing action pattern may be harder than acquiring a new one.

—Ability to limit the activity or give it up later if desired is reassuring.

—Opportunity to try the activity on a partial or tentative basis is an inducive factor.

—Exchanging a new action pattern for an old one may be easier than stopping the old one.

—Ego involvement may become the major determining force.

—Any activity (action, motion) per se may be more desirable than a pattern of behavior minus some customary activity.

—Action patterns that carry threats to pleasure fulfillment may be hard to introduce.

—Actions tied in with elements of novelty, gimmickry, curiosity, pleasure, thrill, titillation, or even danger may be easier to initiate in some cultures and with some individuals.

—Actions dependent on gatekeeper approvals are more likely to encounter difficult obstacles.

—Actions encountering cultural distrust or fear of change are probably the most difficult to initiate.

—Known dreads in customary situations are more palatable for most persons than unknown dangers from new situations.

—Benefits will be weighed in absolute as well as in cost-comparative terms.

—Risk and uncertainty will be heavily weighed against acceptance.

—Clarity, lack of complexity, and ease of communicability of results will be favorable factors.

—The degree of privateness (versus publicness) of the desired actions may be of great consequence in enabling changes.

—The extent of dedication or commitment is certain to be a factor in acceptance.

Planning Steps Involved in Obtaining Individual or Group Action

Comprehensive health planning requires determination of the present attitudes and probable reaction of various target groups toward specific health objectives. What action is desired of each? What changes in attitude or behavior are required to effectuate the desired action? The answers to these questions will shape the strategy and will determine, for example, whether to mount a campaign of persuasion or to promote social and political action resulting in legal requirements.

Many analyses of community action (even analysis of analyses) exist.[107] The following outline is distilled from these as well as from more immediate sources and other parts of this chapter. We are concerned with all persons and groups whose behavior must be affected if planning is to result in change. Planning is not restricted to those who may be spared ill health; it is also concerned with needed changes in attitude and comprehension of all those impinging on the clients or targets of planning.

The following are steps taken in planning for this kind of group action:

Estimate and list groups by priority of significance for the action.

Provide the listing of priority factors to be achieved for each of the significant groups.

For each significant group outline: (1) key forces that make acceptances of the desired action easy for such persons; (2) key forces that make acceptance virtually impossible; (3) constellations of relevant and available forces that might be utilized for the desired and against the undesired.

Before planning the steps of the persuasion campaign survey and/or pretest to verify assumptions made in the assessment and analysis of the significant target groups. Some attributes may be found to be of greater or lesser importance than estimated; some groups unexpectedly may not be of consequence or may be all-important for the issue desired.

Involve all groups who must be active participants in any stage of the goal pursuit, if they are not already involved.

With the new participants, revise the list of target subgroups and priority factors. (The professionals who may be key persons in rendering the desired services are often the hardest to reach in terms of getting them to do their job in a new way that is acceptable to other groups who are to be involved or are to be recipients.)

Certain cautions must be observed:

There is always danger of substituting intellectual or intermediate action goals for final action goals (for example, if meetings, brochures or appeals become the center of concern). Proceedings may give a personal glow to the change agent and his allies, thereby becoming the tangible goal, but the basic goal may be forgotten.

Any suitably directed road may lead to action, but many less well marked can inadvertently lead away from it, because of half-knowledge, confused presentation, and so on.

Objectives or action for one desired end may of necessity be different for different persons or groups. What is involved for each target person or group must be clarified. In a campaign for family planning, for example, individual behavior cannot be the same for grandmother, mother, or father in the family. For each to assist with the overall objectives of a planned family, each has a different action to undertake, depending on tradition, role, available techniques, comprehension, and so on. Similarly, different community groups also carry a different role. Ministers, doctors, political parties, neighborhood organizations, and civic groups each do a different part of the job.

A high proportion of values and influences always remains hidden until after implementation is undertaken, and the multiplicity of such influences makes any prediction of reaction hazardous. Trial balloons and repeated polls may well have to be used in this area, just as they are before elections to test the reactions to tentative approaches.

Many target groups may have no one in their group who can or will participate as one with the planners; it may be necessary to create leadership, confidence, and skill among such groups before they can join the planners of the larger community. (Although community planning bodies usually visualize the disadvantaged as the target group whose ways are to be changed, often as great or greater change is required of the rest of the community in order to make it possible for target persons to participate.)

Bamberger has described approaches in Venezuela that probably are relevant anywhere.[108] These consist of organizing small, short-term, local projects to instill knowhow and confidence and develop community leadership through committee work, tapping all sectors so that the whole group can be mobilized. By setting up and continuing to foster working relationships with local government, private organizations, business, and so on, in establishing basic services, the small and large communities learn how to deal with one another, and a permanent selfsufficient institution is developed within the local group that is able to continue without aid from the larger community.

For objectives of a general nature, goals can and must ultimately be set by target groups in concert with change agents, professionals, and public and private agencies. For objectives of a technical nature, the experts (often synonymous with the change agent) may select or essentially dictate the terms or techniques of the service.

Figure 11.6, derived from Tannenbaum et al.,[109] indicates the relationships of a change agent and target person. Although the significance of this kind of community promotion may be more relevant to micro planning than to macro planning, the members of a planning body should be fully aware of the techniques of influence for change. At the far left, the change agent is depicted as having a strong role when he is carrying out something that is already authorized by force of law and thus prior public consent. In some issues and in some places, the force of custom or religion lends him similar authority.

Moving to the right on Figure 11.6, it can be foreseen that in other areas the change agent may have maximum freedom to tell, although not order, a receptive populace. For example, the doctor gives maternity advice to a group of pregnant women who listen. Moving further to the right, we come to situations, probably most typically those of personal health behavior problems, where the listener takes action only when he has been involved in the entire process of creating readiness for action. At the far right are the situations where relationships of change agent and target person are likely to be minimal indeed. In areas of religion, tribal customs, and so on, the customary health change agent may not even be allowed to enter into discussion except on the target person's terms.

Personal services which require personal initiative remain nearer the right. Change agents must truly join and hope to motivate the target person in his own behalf, so that he comes to believe in and carries out a particular health behavior desired by the change agent. Environmental services, which usually require a one-time popular or legislative approval, and thereafter only involve engineering and legal

FIGURE 11.6
THE CHANGE AGENT'S "AUTHORITY" VERSUS THE TARGET
PERSON'S "FREEDOM" IN COMMUNITY PROMOTION
(Adapted from Tannenbaum)

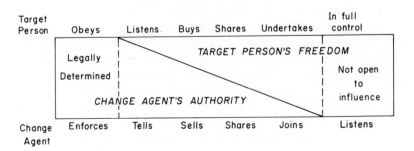

enforcement, depend less on personal initiative and more on legal guidance and institutional activities.

The change agent's practices are accordingly guided by whether there is need for a one-shot approval or for initiation of a long-term personal behavior pattern. This consideration will modify all prior strategic considerations. It can also be foreseen that a given health-promoting change agent may appear at many points along the spectrum of relationships with different target groups on different health issues at any one time or over the years. In the course of health change efforts with a single group, the change agent may also run the spectrum of roles: (1) He may only be *tolerated* as an observer initially, one whose advice is literally not tolerable until he is discovered to have some skill that the target group finds useful—often not in the area of his primary concern; (2) having earned acceptance, he may be allowed to *join* and help achieve mutually desired goals; (3) having proved his capacity and effective concern for what target people had on their agenda, he may be allowed to *introduce* the issues of greatest concern to him; (4) as a result of successful goal pursuit with the target group, he may establish himself as an expert in various areas and finally earn the right to *tell* and receive compliance from the target group which has finally granted him this position of authority in some areas.

The visible change agent—in the form of some person or group who introduces a subject, addresses a gathering, or informs a study group—must be carefully chosen. A group of practicing physicians can, for example, tolerate certain touchy subject matter best from an economist of repute, but other matters may have to be broached by a physician. Perhaps more scientific approaches can ultimately teach us more about what politically alert persons sense when they choose spokesmen for specific issues to be presented to selected groups.[110] An example of sizing up a community and becoming an effective health change agency has recently become available.[111]

Any given plan of attack will combine the general theoretic considerations involved and the specifics of the particular issue, group, time and place. Even the importation of professional promoters, community organizers and developers does not obviate the need for the analytic techniques outlined. Their advice must incorporate what local persons know about the matters described.

It is not untimely to point out that many people become paralyzed when they confront the veritable jungle, or at least thicket, of interests and interrelationships that will be revealed by community study. The reputed ties, conflicts of interest, and hidden but suspected motivations would never allow any major community to plan if each potentially significant factor were carefully catalogued and respected. Reasonable study commensurate with the importance and the presumed difficulties of the task is recommended. With this in mind, modest review of previous actions, public commitments, and major areas of interest would appear to be not too expensive as indicators for possible action. Using these as a base, and providing the appropriate interests with the opportunity to be involved and visible in significant community enterprises, has often set the stage for quite unexpected levels of support and participation.

REFERENCES

1. John Friedmann, "Notes on Societal Action," *Journal of the American Institute of Planners* 35 (September 1969), 311-18.

2. Cyril Roseman, "A Political Forecast for Health in the United States: 1990," School of Public Health, University of California, Berkeley, February 13, 1970, mimeographed.

3. Joseph L. Falkson and Demetrius J. Plessas, "Towards Rationalization and Integration of Urban Health Bureaucracies," *HSMHA Health Reports* 86 (June 1971), 495-500.

4. Aaron Wildavsky, "Does Planning Work?" *The Public Interest* 24 (Summer 1971), 95-104.

5. William H. Form, "Social Power and Social Welfare," *Centrally Planned Change: Prospects and Concepts,* ed. by Robert Morris (New York: National Association of Social Workers, 1964). Guy Benveniste, "Toward a Sociology of Planning," Department of Education, University of California, Berkeley, 1966, mimeographed. Warren F. Ilchman and Thomas Uphoff, *The Political Economy of Change* (Berkeley & Los Angeles: University of California Press, 1969), 81-89.

6. Rus Veljko, "Influence Structure in Yugoslav Enterprise," *Industrial Relations* 9 (February 1970), 148-60.

7. W. F. Ilchman, Ibid. no. 5, 81-89.

8. Terry N. Clark, "The Concept of Power," *Community Structure and Decision Making: Comparative Analyses,* ed. by Terry N. Clark (San Francisco: Chandler Publishing Company, 1968), Chapter 3.

9. John Walton, "Differential Patterns of Community Power Structure: An Explanation Based on Interdependence," *Community Structure and Decision Making: Comparative Analyses,* ed. by Terry N. Clark (San Francisco: Chandler Publishing Company, 1968), Chapter 21.

10. R. Veljko, Ibid. no. 6, 148-60. J. Walton, Ibid. no. 9, Chapter 21.

11. James D. Thompson, *Organizations in Action* (New York: McGraw-Hill, 1967), 25-38.

12. Andrew L. McFarland, *Power and Leadership in Pluralist Systems* (Stanford: Stanford University Press, 1969), 1-14.

13. Walter Buckley, *Sociology and Modern Systems Theory* (Englewood Cliffs, N. J.: Prentice-Hall, 1967), 176-205.

14. Edward W. Lehman, "Toward a Macrosociology of Power," *American Sociological Review* 34 (August 1969), 453-65.

15. Robert A. Dahl, *Modern Political Analysis* (Englewood Cliffs, New Jersey: Prentice-Hall, 1963), 32-74.

16. W. F. Ilchman, Ibid. no. 5, 81-89.

17. R. Veljko, Ibid. no. 6, 148-60.

18. Irving A. Spergel, *Community Problem Solving* (Chicago: University of Chicago Press, 1969), 106.
19. A. L. McFarland, Ibid. no. 12, 1-14.
20. R. A. Dahl, Ibid, no. 15, 32-74.
21. W. F. Ilchman, Ibid. no. 5, 81-89.
22. W. H. Form, Ibid. no. 5.
23. A. L. McFarland, Ibid. no. 12, Chapter 5.
24. E. A. Shils, "The Macrosociological Problem: Consensus and Dissensus in the Larger Society," *Trends in Social Science,* ed. by D. P. Ray (New York: Philosophical Library, 1961), 60-83.
25. G. Benveniste, Ibid. no. 5.
26. William A. Gamson, "Reputation and Resources in Community Politics," *Community Structure and Decision Making: Comparative Analyses,* ed. by Terry N. Clark (San Francisco: Chandler Publishing Company, 1968), Chapter 15.
27. Anthony Downs, *An Economic Theory of Democracy* (New York: Harper & Row, 1957), 85-107.
28. Mary F. Arnold and Isabel M. Welsh, "Community Politics and Health Planning," *Administering Health Systems: Issues and Perspectives,* ed. by Mary F. Arnold, L. Vaughn Blankenship, and John M. Hess (Chicago; New York: Aldine; Atherton, 1971), Chapter 10.
29. P. A. Miller, *Community Health Action* (East Lansing: Michigan State College Press, 1953).
30. Martin Rein, "Social Planning: The Search for Legitimacy," *Journal of the American Institute of Planners* 35 (July 1969), 233-44.
31. Richard S. Bolan, "Community Decision Behavior: The Culture of Planning," *Journal of the American Institute of Planners* 35 (September 1969), 301-09.
32. M. Rein, Ibid. no. 30, 233-44.
33. C. Wright Mills, *The Power Elite* (New York: Oxford University Press, 1956).
34. Floyd Hunter, *Community Power Structure* (Chapel Hill: University of North Carolina Press, 1953).
35. E. W. Lehman, Ibid. no. 14, 453-65.
36. Robert Lynd and Helen Merrell Lynd, *Middletown in Transition* (New York: Harcourt Brace & World, 1937). John Walton, "Substance and Artifact: The Current Status of Research on Community Power Structure," *American Journal of Sociology* 71 (January 1966), 430-38. Suzanne Keller, *Beyond the Ruling Class: Strategic Elites in Modern Society* (New York: Random House, 1963), 115.
37. James E. Curtis and John W. Petras, "Community Power, Power Studies and the Sociology of Knowledge," *Human Organization* 29 (Fall 1970), 204-18.
38. "Whom Does the Advocate Planner Serve," a Colloquium, *Social Policy* 1 (July-August, 1970), 33-41.
39. Donald B. Rosenthal and Robert L. Crain, "Structure and Values in Local Political Systems: The Case of Fluoridation Decisions," *Community Structure and Decision Making: Comparative Analyses,* ed. by Terry

N. Clark (San Francisco: Chandler Publishing Company, 1968), Chapter 10.

40. William A. Gamson, "Rancorous Conflict in Community Politics," *Community Structure and Decision Making: Comparative Analyses*, ed. by Terry N. Clark (San Francisco: Chandler Publishing Company, 1968), Chapter 9.

41. M. Rein, Ibid. no. 30, 233-44.

42. John P. Spiegel, "Campus Conflict and Professional Egos," *Trans-Action* 6 (October 1969), 41-50.

43. William J. Curran, "Health Planning Agencies: A Legal Crisis?" *American Journal of Public Health* 60 (February 1970), 359-60. Steven Sieverts, "Health Planning Agencies," *American Journal of Public Health* 60 (June 1970), 968-70. William J. Curran, "Are Planning Agencies Ready for Community Decision Making Role?" *Health Planning Perspectives* 6 (December 1970), 1. William J. Curran, "Health Planning with 'Clout': Certificate of Need Legislation," *American Journal of Public Health* 62 (November 1972), 1549.

44. San Francisco Comprehensive Health Planning Council; "Health Alliance," *The Scanner* 1 (November 1971), San Francisco, California.

45. Frank Stead, "Environmental Health and Natural Resources Planning," *Health Planning 1969*, by H. L. Blum and Associates (San Francisco: Western Regional Office, American Public Health Association, 1969), Chapter 20.

46. Vicente Navarro, "Methodology on Regional Planning of Personal Health Services," *Medical Care* 8 (September-October, 1970), 386-94. Vicente Navarro, "National Health Insurance and The Strategy for Change," *The Milbank Fund Quarterly* 51, (Spring 1973), 223-251.

47. W. C. Wheaton, "Integration at the Urban Level: Political Influence and the Decision Process," *The Integration of Political Communities*, ed. by P. Jacob and J. Toscano (Philadelphia: Lippincott, 1964), 130-32.

48. Robert E. Agger, et al., *Rulers and the Ruled* (New York: Wiley, 1964), 1-2.

49. Melvin M. Webber, "The Urban Place and the Non-Place Urban Realm," *Explorations into Urban Structure*, ed. by Melvin M. Webber (Philadelphia: University of Pennsylvania Press, 1964), 79-137.

50. G. A. Hillery, Jr., "Definition of Community: Areas of Agreement," *Rural Sociology* 20 (June 1955), 111-23.

51. Pranab Chatterjee and Raymond A. Kaleski, "The Concepts of Community and Community Organization: A Review," *Social Work* 15 (July 1970), 82-9.

52. Terry N. Clark, "Community or Communities?" *Community Structure and Decision Making: Comparative Analyses*, ed. by Terry N. Clark (San Francisco: Chandler Publishing Company, 1968), Chapter 4.

53. C. H. Cooley, *Social Organization: A Study of the Larger Mind* (New York: Scribner, 1969) J. Abu-Lughod, "The City Is Dead—Long Live the City: Some Thoughts on Urbanity," American Behavioral Scientist 10 (September 1966), 3-6.

54. Claude S. Fischer, "The Metropolitan Experience," Working Paper no.

195, Institute of Urban and Regional Development, University of California, Berkeley, November 1972.

55. Peter Marris, "A Report on Urban Renewal in the United States," *The Urban Condition*, ed. by L. J. Duhl (New York: Basic Books, 1963), 123-27.

56. John R. Seeley, et al., *Crestwood Heights* (New York: Basic Books, 1963). Herbert J. Gans, *The Levittowners* (New York: Random House, 1967).

57. Donald C. Klein, "The Meaning of Community in a Preventive Mental Health Program," *American Journal of Public Health* 59 (November 1969), 2005-1.

58. John R. Seeley, "The Slum: Its Nature, Use and Users," *Journal of the American Institute of Planners* 35 (February 1969), 7-14.

59. N. E. Cohen, "Summary Report on the Watts Riot: Two-year Study" (Institute of Government and Public Affairs, University of California at Los Angeles), *University Bulletin* 16 (August 14, 1967).

60. Phillip Felin and Eugene Litwak, "The Neighborhood in Urban American Society," *Social Work* 13 (July 1968), 72-80.

61. Paul R. Lazarsfeld and E. Katz, *Personal Influence* (Glencoe, Illinois: The Free Press, 1955).

62. U.S., Congress, Senate, Committee on Appropriations, "Children in Migrant Families," Robert submitted by the Department of Health, Education and Welfare, 1961.

63. R. Harris, "Annals of Legislation: Medicare," *The New Yorker* (July 2, 9, 16, 23, 1966).

64. Ruth Roemer, Jeanne E. Frink, and C. Kramer, "Environmental Health Services: Multiplicity of Jurisdictions and Comprehensive Environmental Management," *Milbank Memorial Fund Quarterly* 49 (October 1971), part 1, 419-508.

65. E. S. Redford, *Ideal and Practice in Public Administration* (Tuscaloosa: University of Alabama Press, 1958), 1-24.

66. National Commission on Community Health Services, *Health Is a Community Affair*, Report of the National Commission on Community Health Services (Cambridge: Harvard University Press, 1966), 2-4, 129.

67. J. M. Winters, *Interstate Metropolitan Areas*, Michigan Legal Publications (Ann Arbor: University of Michigan, 1962).

68. John Friedmann and John Miller, "The Urban Field," *Journal of the American Institute of Planners* 31 (November 1965), 312-19.

69. Victor Jones, "Representative Local Government: From Neighborhood to Region," *Public Affairs Report* (Bulletin of the Institute of Governmental Studies) 11 (April 1970).

70. Robert A. Dahl, *Who Governs?* (New Haven, Yale University Press, 1961), 1.

71. M. Arnold and I. Welsh, Ibid. no. 28, Chapter 10. ·

72. Basil J. F. Mott, "Political Needs of Planning: The Myth of Planning Without Politics," *American Journal of Public Health* 59 (May 1969), 797-803.

73. William Beveridge, *Social Insurance and Allied Service* (London: His Majesty's Printing Office, 1942).

74. R. S. Bolan, Ibid. no. 31, 301-09.

75. Everett N. Rogers, "Social Structure and Social Change," *American Behavioral Scientist* 14 (May/June 1971), 767-82.
76. John F. Kennedy, *Profiles in Courage* (New York: Harpers, 1956).
77. R. E. Agger, et al., Ibid. no. 55, 1-2.
78. R. N. Wilson, *Process Analysis: A Study of Community Structure and Health Action* (Washington, D.C.: Public Affairs Press, 1967).
79. Roland L. Warren, *The Community in America* (Chicago: Rand McNally, 1963), 12-14.
80. Y. H. Cho, "The Effect of Local Governmental Systems on Local Policy Outcomes in the United States," *Public Administration Review* 27 (March 1967), 31-38.
81. M. Arnold and I. Welsh, Ibid. no. 28, Chapter 10.
82. Terry N. Clark, "Community Structure and Decision Making," *Community Structure and Decision Making: Comparative Analyses*, ed. by Terry N. Clark (San Francisco: Chandler Publishing Co., 1968), Chapter 5.
83. M. Arnold and I. Welsh, Ibid. no. 28, Chapter 10.
84. Sol Levine and P. E. White, "Exchange as a Conceptual Framework for the Study of Interorganizational Relationships," *Administrative Science Quarterly* 5 (March 1961), 583-601.
85. James D. Thompson and William J. A. McEwen, "Organizational Goals and Environment," *Complex Organizations: A Sociological Reader*, ed. by Amitai Etzioni (New York: Holt, Rinehart & Winston, 1961),186; reprinted from *American Sociological Review* 23 (1958), 23-31.
86. James D. Thompson and Arthur Tuden, "Strategies, Structures and Processes of Organizational Decision," *Comparative Studies in Administration*, ed. by James Thompson, et al. (Pittsburgh: University of Pittsburgh Press, 1959), 195-216.
87. James D. Thompson, "Decision-Making, the Firm and the Market," *New Perspectives in Organizational Research*, ed. by W. W. Cooper, H. J. Leavitt, and M. W. Shelly (New York: Wiley, 1966), II, 334-48.
88. M. Arnold and I. Welsh, Ibid. no. 28, Chapter 10.
89. Roland L. Warren and Herbert H. Hyman, "Purposive Community Change in Concensus and Dissensus," *Community Structure and Decision Making: Comparative Analyses*, ed. by Terry N. Clark (San Francisco: Chandler Publishing Co., 1968), Chapter 19.
90. Ernst Haas, *Beyond the Nation State* (Stanford: Stanford University Press, 1964), 111.
91. A. L. McFarland, Ibid. no. 12, 1-14.
92. C. P. Loomis, "In Praise of Conflict and Its Resolution," *American Sociological Review* 32 (December 1967), 875-90.
93. W. A. Gamson, Ibid. no. 40, Chapter 9.
94. "Why Fight? Conflict Models for Strategists and Managers" *American Behavioral Scientist* 15 (July 1972), 809-927.
95. James Q. Wilson, "An Overview of Theories of Planned Change," *Centrally Planned Change: Prospects and Concepts*, ed. by Robert Morris (New York: National Association of Social Workers, 1964), 12-29.
96. James S. Coleman, *Community Conflict*, Publication of the Bureau of Applied Social Research, Columbia University (Glencoe, Illinois: The Free Press, 1957).

97. Murray Ross, *Community Organization: Theory and Principles*, 2nd ed. (New York: Harper & Row, 1967), 52.

98. I. A. Spergel, Ibid. no. 18, 106.

99. Edward A. Suchman, "Preventive Health Behavior: A Model for Research on Community Health Campaigns," *Journal of Health and Social Behavior* 8 (September 1967), 197-208. U.S., Department of Health, Education and Welfare, Public Health Service, Publication no. 572, "Public Participation in Medical Screening," by G. M. Hochbaum, 1958. Carol D'Onofrio, "Reaching Our Hard to Reach, The Unvaccinated," Seminar Proceedings, California State Department of Public Health, Berkeley, California, March 1965. Chester W. Douglass, "A Social-Psychological View of Health Behavior for Health Services Research," Health Services Research 6, Spring 1971, 6-14. R. M. Gray, J. P. Kesler, and P. M. Moody, "The Effects of Social Class and Friends' Expectations on Oral Polio Vaccination Participation," *American Journal of Public Health* 56 (December 1966), 2028-32.

100. R. M. Battistela, "Limitations in Use of the Concept of Psychologic Readiness to Initiate Health Care," *Medical Care* 6 (July/August 1968), 308-19.

101. Beryl J. Roberts, *Decision Making: An Illustration of Theory Building*, Health Education Monographs (Albany, N. Y., Society of Public Health Educators, Inc., November 9, 1960), 20-44.

102. Gerald Zaltman and Nan Lin, "On the Nature of Innovation," *American Behavioral Scientist* 14 (May/June 1971), 651-74.

103. J. Richard Udry and Naomi M. Morris, "A Spoonful of Sugar Helps the Medicine Go Down," *American Journal of Public Health* 61 (April 1971), 776-85.

104. Andre L. Delbecq and Andrew VandeVen, "A Group Process Model for Problem Identification and Program Planning," *Journal of Applied Behavioral Science* 7 (July/August 1971), 466-92.

105. Goodwin Watson, "Resistance to Change," *American Behavioral Scientist* 14 (May/June 1971), 745-66.

106. E. A. Suchman, Ibid. no. 99, 197-208.

107. R. L. Warren, Ibid, no. 79, 12-14. R. N. Wilson, Ibid. no. 78.

108. M. Bamberger, "A Defense of Urban Community Planning," *Community Development Journal* 2 (July 1967), 11-14. M. Bamberger, "Identifying Leaders in the Urban Community," *Community Development Journal* 2 (October 1967), 30-32.

109. Robert Tannenbaum, J. R. Weschler, and F. Masarik, *Leadership and Organization* (New York: McGraw-Hill, 1967), 69.

110. Robert Edward Mitchell, "Use of Content Analysis for Exploratory Studies," *Public Opinion Quarterly* 31 (Summer 1967), 230-41.

111. Thomas J. Rice and Stephen B. Bernstein, "The Process of Community Intervention in an Isolate Appalachian Mountain Hollow," *Medical Care* 9 (July/August 1971).

Part V

MEASURING THE IMPROVEMENTS
OBTAINED THROUGH PLANNING

12. Evaluation

THE NATURE OF EVALUATION

Planning of the kind described depends heavily on knowing the past and present state of affairs, and particularly the results of implemented activities from the last round of planning. I was taken with the succinctness of Mary Arnold's depiction of the Iterative Cycle of Planning—Implementing—Evaluating, which is presented here as Figure 12.1.[1] She introduces the figure as follows:

> In a sense, evaluation is the mirror-image of planning in that it is the process of looking back upon action, making a judgment about it in order to provide the necessary information for planning for the future. Thus, there is a cycle of evaluation-planning-implementation-evaluation that is a continual forward-moving process along a time continuum.

To quote Mary Arnold further:

> For practical purposes, evaluation is best considered as a feedback process whereby planned information is used to guide and direct organization (or individual) decisions. In the reality of organizational life there is an ongoing process of action, of adjustment, of change; a continual reformulation of directions and goals; and a never-ending flow of information. Much of this ongoing activity is

FIGURE 12.1
ITERATIVE CYCLE OF PLANNING—IMPLEMENTING—
EVALUATING

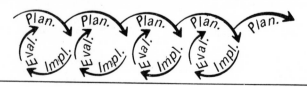

PA ST   FUTURE

542

considered to be standard operating procedure and little thought is given to the fact that every change, however minute, occurs as a product of evaluation. Evaluation is continuously going on; however, it is usually implicit and based on limited and non-generalizable experience.[2]

Evaluation is needed to tell us whether we are doing that which brings us what is wanted, whether we are doing it effectively and in an efficient way, whether our planning methods are any good, and what we should do the next time around. Evaluation can be applied not only to each or all of these issues, but also to small parts of them as well as to the whole—determining the place of a pamphlet in a clinic, the place of a clinic in the delivery system, or the utility of a delivery system in improving our health.

Andie Knutson makes one of the most terse characterizations of evaluation as "the questioning of programs before they are implemented."[3] However, this definition of evaluation is inclusive of nearly all the steps of planning shown in Figure 1.2. This definition would also be seen by forecasters as the sum and substance of their field, with evaluating as the process of getting feedback from the projected outcomes of a proposed plan.

However, Knutson reminds us of the most critical issue: What are we to evaluate for and against? Evaluation is not a specific set of arbitrary applications which tell us yes or no. Rather it is a rerun of the planning process after the results are in hand to learn whether we got what was intended, at the price, in the amounts, and in the way we specified, and whether we still want it. Expressed this way, evaluation can be no one test, nor any specified series of tests. Each plan undertaking was brought into being for its own set of reasons, and these reasons must be kept in mind during evaluation, not only in terms of achievement but for the validity of the assumptions made and for evidence of their continuing desirability.

This brings us to a current but needless controversy about whether evaluation should be done on a goal-attainment model or on a systems model.[4] As Etzioni uses a goal model,[5] he is referring to scrutinizing the attainment of objectives or outputs which an intervention or organizationally produced program was specifically designed to deliver. Therefore, he finds that the process of scrutiny of outputs one by one falls far short of revealing how well the system under study is making out. (He used the organization; we use the community or society as our reference system.) In other words, a system not only has to be able to produce the objective, but also to survive and even improve its conduct in the process. Thus, its performance cannot be evaluated solely on its products or output, nor can that output be evaluated as an entity unto itself, free of its effects on the system which is creating it.

We would go further in health planning and insist that if our community selected 25 goals and also used them as the criteria by which to select problems and by which to judge the virtue of proposed interventions, these same criteria of goodness generated by the community should be used to evaluate the outputs created by the interventions. Granted, new values may have arisen in the community, and some brand new goal or criterion may now have the greatest weight in evaluation even though it had not been thought of at the time the intervention was worked out. Is this fair? Totally, because the major utility of evaluation is not to guide us to what we once wanted, but to what we expect we will want tomorrow.

The Uses of Evaluation

The utilities of evaluation in planning need to be clarified. The term evaluation could, with justification, be assigned to the scrutiny of the worth or wisdom of almost every aspect of what has been covered as part of planning, but such intense study may or may not be a good use of resources. Evaluation could be applied to the processes called assessment and forecasting about the situation, to the selection and analysis of problems and interventions, and so on. I generally restrict the meaning of evaluation to the scrutiny of the outcomes that have resulted from application of the various activities of the planning process. However, it is often necessary to evaluate progress long before tangible outcomes have come to pass.

Spergel selects three concerns, impact of the program, program process, and program organization.[6] Sanazaro opens up the subject in terms of its application to medical care.[7] The first six uses shown on the following list represent the six levels of evaluation which I suggest embrace the logic needed to evaluate what we are doing to the system or to the community which we, as community health planners, are planning for. The seventh use is intended to advance the capacity and skills of planners. The eighth is to provide guidance for the next round of planning.

—Checking to See if Activity is Going On
—Checking to Determine if an Operation is Meeting Present Standards[8]
—Checking on the Efficiency of the Activity
—Checking to See if Activities Produced the Specific Objectives Set For Them (Effectivity)[9]
—Checking for Improvement Achieved (Outcome Validity)
—Checking for Improvement in the Functioning of the Encompassing System (Systemic Desirability)
—Testing Out and Extending Planning Wisdom and Technology

Planning considerations generally.   This is another area of validity testing; testing not the science which is at the heart of the situation— for example, immunology—but rather the process which the planner has utilized in handling the planned-for issue. How effective and suitable were the choices of the planning purposes operated under, the roles selected by the planners, and the choices of technologies, participants, and strategies? If effective, they are presumably illustrative of the knowledge and overall suitability of application of the planners' science. Perhaps this falls more into the area of planning research, but some planners do hold just such post mortems over their activities in order to learn more about the strengths and weakness of their science from the degree and nature of success attained. (One does need to be aware that satisfactory results may occur for the wrong reasons, from multiple factors at work, or just from the general pressure of the times.[10]

Analytic concerns.   Even with ideal social science data for the problem at hand, the planner's capacity to analyze a situation may be low, and a faulty analysis would not allow for useful applications of even the best of information. In evaluation it may not be easy to sort out which factor was more at fault, fact or analysis. But presumably the facts would be getting trials in the form of interventions applied elsewhere that would provide some clues, and a reanalysis or evaluation of the results in the situation being acted upon might provide others. One hopes to extend analytic capacity by seeing if analysis was adequate.

Design concerns.   This version of validity testing is directed to the quality of design rather than to the quality of scientific information and analysis. Again, this evaluation will be difficult because failure may be a result of poor assumptions, of poor systems analysis or poor intervention design, or of sloppy application. The comparison on paper of alternative analysis and design steps (one phase of forecasting) may indicate most weak points in advance of operating and should provide clues about which areas the evaluative efforts should be looking at. One hopes to extend design capacity by seeing if the design of interventions was adequate.

Goal selection concerns.   One hopes to extend capacity to select or design well-being goal measures by checking suitability of the well-being goal measures which have been chosen as the desired end-point of the planned for activity.

Testing Out and Extending Knowledge of the Real World as a Guide to the Next Round of Planning and Future Action

Substantive cause-and-effect considerations.   Although not unlike the other uses of evaluation which test validity, this has as its sole purpose proving the validity of the cause-effect hypotheses used, and extending the knowledge base by seeing if the knowledge applied to the situation was correct (validity or assumptions).[11] This search is infrequently used as the reason for evaluating and is rather more typical of research concerns. However, it will be in the back of the minds of health planners who are attempting to apply wisdom from many fields to interventions designed for specific situations.

The real world unveiled. Since the systems in which planners work are unbelievably complex, evaluation of interventions is one of the ways in which planners get a "feel" of what forces are at work, of what the real-life system is like. Clear cut cause and effect relationships are usually too much to ask for, but general sets or thrusts may be what the planner needs to know in order to proceed more wisely with his next attempt at intervening in the system. Better comprehension of the world he deals with is probably the major contribution of evaluation.

Along with Andie Knutson,[12] we repeat the question, "Evaluation for what?" and discover reasons other than the obvious and technical ones we have already advanced. These include:

> Justifying past or projected outlay of resources.
> Determining the cost of carrying out a plan.
> Obtaining evidence to demonstrate to others what planners claim was already known.
> Demonstrating that the planning product was worthwhile.
> Gaining support for more planning output.
> Gaining support for more planning.
> Satisfying demands for evidence that objectives are being reached.

These uses differ from the first eight listed, not so much in what they would reveal, as in the particular use to which the evaluatory information would be put. That is, the wording of these latter uses centers their impact on those watching the planners, rather than on concern with the impact of evaluation on the planners themselves. Self-education and satisfaction of the planners was the point of view of the last portion of our discussion of the utilities and needs for evaluation. However, planners must also be concerned with how the results of evaluation strike the onlookers who foot the bill. If questions are not worded so that the answers satisfy the public's general curiosity rather than the planners' more technical curiosity, evaluation may not contribute much to understanding planning or to its survival. Evaluative questions need not be rigged, however, just to satisfy the citizenry's questions and doubts. Evaluation can be done in such a way that it provides satisfaction to both the technicians and the public.

Can Evaluation be Considered As or Converted Into Research?

A word is in order about how evaluation differs from research, if it is knowledge-seeking for purposes other than immediate checking of outcomes. In many quarters evaluation is called either evaluatory research or just research. Is there a meaningful difference between research and evaluation? According to Schulberg,[13] when evaluation produces knowledge useful for application to operations, evaluation is suddenly transposed into research. Because one of the cardinal reasons for doing evaluation is further guidance for operations, there is no justification for taking the time to decide when evaluation is research of whether it is evaluatory research.

However, to clarify this commonly raised issue, we cite the situations in which evaluation is clearly also research.

>   Search for new substantive knowledge about the real world for application to further operations.
>   Search for new knowledge for application to concerns of planning capacity and skills.
>   Generalize planning theory from the specific situation.
>   Determine the real cause-and-effect relationships underlying the activities and results of the planning process machinery itself.
>   Put general planning theory to test by checking it against specific planning situations.

Whenever these purposes are tied in with evaluation, the operation may be considered as having a research component, and presumably it becomes significantly more valuable than it would be if used solely for guidance for operations. But it also becomes more demanding of competency, time, data, and money. It may become intolerable in terms of costs. More important, rarely can the research aspect of the effort be kept "clean" under the operational and political pressures for changes that will be met along the way, and which cannot be controlled against.[14] Notwithstanding, evaluation always holds a possibility for being partially converted into research. If its research limitations are honestly acknowledged, it is still, undoubtedly, one of the richest sources of new understanding. Witness the innumerable case studies on the urban scene which helped create a social science of urban areas.

HOW TO DO IT

The kind of evaluation that needs to be done in a given situation is not always as simple to determine as the nature of a project might indicate on a quick reading. What is wanted is likely to vary with the roles and beliefs of the persons interested in the evaluation. Ordinarily, the evaluator—whether part of the operations team, the planning team, the funding agency review staff, or an independent student—is not entirely free to evaluate just as he sees fit. Even the individual student with no agency pressures for any particular view has a first obligation to respect the intent of the project developers. How well what they meant to happen has actually taken place is open to evaluation.[15]

According To Whose Viewpoint?

For the Project Director

What the evaluator does for the program operator must surely be guided by the concerns of the operator. He may only want or only be able to use evaluation in one or a few areas, and light shed on other areas may be only of remote interest to him.[16] For example, evaluation may find that the project is of utility for specific purposes but is not societally appropriate. Because the donor of funds dictates the particular direction and the operator is willing to live within such a framework, he is little concerned whether his project is of significant societal consequence.

For Outside Evaluators with a Specific Stake in the Project

The donor of funds, prospective donors, the research office of a university, or a government unit considering a proposal may each justifiably ask for an evaluation. Irrespective of what the project director thinks, if such interests are to be allowed to evaluate, they may well have their own reasons for doing so. These may not coincide with the project's primary concerns, such as the effectivity of its activities for specific objectives. An outside interest may accept all other aspects but ask only for an efficiency evaluation which has been of no concern to the project operators up to this point. Other evaluators may wish to question the long-run appropriateness of the operation to society, even if it was set up for purposes of demonstrating efficiency and effectivity and is obviously achieving those purposes.

For Holders of Special Viewpoints

Physicians and other health professionals might want a delivery system evaluated for technological quality. Consumers might want it evaluated for access, acceptability, and connectivity; and the society, through its government, might want it evaluated for cost control and suitability of direction. (See Chapter 4 for a fuller discussion of different systemic outlooks.) The evaluator may, according to arrangements made by his client, take on any one or several evaluative tasks. If he is independent, he may do all or none of these evaluations, depending on his personal interests or source of funding.

It is legitimate to demand that the evaluator state the position he is taking. Is he evaluating accomplishments against his own values or goals or against some other specified set, and if so what are they? The evaluator sometimes identifies with ultimate clients, such as consumers, or with policy makers. If he does so, those utilizing his evaluation must know what the evaluator claims are the legitimate expectations that he is using as standards. If he is evaluating against the values and goals stated by the planners (those toward which the intervention is directed), it may be necessary to repeat them, clarify, state objectives and expected consequences, because persons carrying out the interventions may have misinterpreted, ignored, or substituted for what the planners intended.

When a plan—rather than its ultimate accomplishments—is being evaluated, it is fair for an evaluator to point out whether he would have proceeded as the planners did and whether he would have required and utilized the same resources, tools, and methodology. This issue is more fully discussed in the section of this chapter on evaluation of activities and outputs of comprehensive health planning bodies.

Six Levels of Evaluation

We have postulated that the major concern of evaluation is to check on what happened as a result of implemented planning. Almost all organized efforts have arisen as the result of someone's planning, and are, therefore, open to evaluation even if the planning processes are entirely hidden from general view or proceeded in a purely intuitive or wishful way. An activity or operation to be evaluated may be research, production, planning, education, or even a job of evaluation itself. Each such operation is open to the evaluatory scrutiny of how well it is doing what it promised to do.

Unfortunately, this is slightly more complex than it sounds at first.

Different evaluators want to look at different aspects of an operation's outcomes at different times or under different pressures. Because no one can, or even should, try doing every conceivable evaluatory task possible, I have broken down the possible major tasks of evaluation in accordance with the use intended. Any particular evaluatory study may have every reason to concentrate on any one of the levels of evaluation, given what is important to those desiring the evaluation; often the kind of evaluation that seems called for is substantially dictated by the stage of the operation. Each of the levels of evaluation discussed is relevant to any operation.

Deniston and his colleagues use a somewhat comparable set of levels of evaluation.[17] They use *appropriateness* as I do *validity*, and use *effectivity* and *efficiency* as I do. Understandably, they do not concern themselves with simple control nor with operational standard meeting—the two most commonly practiced but least informative of the levels. They insert a level of *adequacy* between effectivity and validity to take into account how much of a problem is being handled by an intervention. Because I am more system than goal oriented, I take for granted that the intervention was designed to do a specified aspect of system change, and feel that validity would cover direction while effectivity would cover quantity. They do not concern themselves at all with societal appropriateness at our sixth level. Yardy speaks of three levels in which he somewhat obscures but still considers all six levels utilized here.[18] Fleck describes the operational standard meeting level of evaluation as "ritualistic,"[19] and in general agrees with my feelings on the subject of standards expressed in this chapter and in Chapter 6.

Level One Evaluation—Activity
(Is the Operation Working?)

This level of evaluation may be exemplified by evaluation of a heating system which uses gas as input to a heater, the effector, to create heat, the output. Someone who makes decisions turns the heating system on or off according to how he feels about wanting heat. In terms of evaluation, this system allows simple spot checks to see if it is working. All that is being evaluated is whether the operation is in business—that is, whether the planned gas input is being used by the designed operation or organization (effector), and determination is made whether it is producing the heat output for which it was designed. A single criterion, that of operational activity, suffices.

Level Two Evaluation—Meeting Operational
Guidance Standards or Criteria

In the gas heater example, this level of evaluation is concerned with determining not only whether the system is working but whether it operates in a prespecified manner or according to specific criteria or standards. If the prescription calls for the heater to function from 8 a.m. to 6 p.m. so that 72 degrees is shown on a thermostat located at a particular position in a building, we would be able—by means of a spot check or continuous recording devices—to see that the heater-thermostat combination did act according to instructions. These criteria are typically unrelated to cost of unit of heat and are not even concerned with how comfortable people feel in the heated building.

For health care, operational criteria may be expressed in terms of access and acceptability to recipients, control of health care costs, units of particular activities (but not the outcomes caused by those activities), and the like. The question may be raised that such matters suggest standards, and if so, what about all the unpleasant things we have already said about standards? The distinction is that standards become meaningful when the community doing the evaluation converts aspects of the activity it desires into fixed, measurable qualities. For example, access to all shall be within 30 minutes, even by walking; acceptability shall show no less than 90% of the people indicating approval, as measured by a canvass asking specific questions in each neighborhood; or that increase in cost per capita shall not exceed 1% per year. These standards are not the same as the ritualistic standards whose weaknesses were amply discussed in Chapter 6. They are specific measures, designed for the situation at hand, which are accepted by the people of the area. These measures are the specifications of how adequate the operations of the project must be. Initially, they also provided guidance to the planners or designers of the delivery machinery. Now they guide the evaluators. What smack of ritualistic standards are the platitudinous specifications promulgated by the overriding larger region, state, or nation, which must be met if the local is to be allowed to operate. Even these standards become the kind we scoff at only when they set bottoms, not under services or quality for which they are guides, but under inputs—the number of dollars to be spent per capita, the number of beds to be available per capita, the number of doctors per capita, the number of nurses per doctor, the number of aides per nurse, or the number of gadgets per facility.

Input criteria which focus on amounts of money, resources, or manpower to be used, are obviously inferior to operational or throughput criteria. Yet inputs may be the best approximations or the best practically achievable surrogate criteria in some situations. Criteria come closer to being useful guides when they approach measuring the outputs, as by determining the throughputs or aspects of process like access, acceptability, scope of services, units of specified activities, or technological quality. Granted, in a societal sense, they may not be as useful as criteria directed to evaluating the achievement of the intended outputs themselves (level 4), which might focus on cures, fatalities, or untoward reactions.

When criteria are tailored to guide the design and are then to be used to measure desired outcomes for a given planned effort, they must be accompanied by a description of the circumstances under which they do and do not apply, as well as a description of the means of doing the measurements which are to show how well the criteria are being met.

Level Three Evaluation—Efficiency (Can the Cost Per Unit of Output be Improved? or Alternatively, Is the Operation Working at the Cost Agreed Upon?)

In terms of the heater analogy, a set of objectives concentrating on input-output relationships as they affect cost has been added at this level. The input is to be used in the least expensive way to gain a unit of heat output; or, alternatively, it is to produce the most heating within a prespecified cost ceiling, which in effect becomes a particular criterion. (If we say heating, we commence to include inseparable elements of effectivity—see the next level.) Again, by means of spot or continuous checks, the work—or in this case, heat output—is verified and the costs recorded. But much more has to be done, because less costly output units of heat (or of heating a given space) may be reached by means of adding a fan, changing the fuel, replacing the heater, or use of insulation, and these involve various calculations against available information or beliefs. Evaluation here can determine if a preset cost was reached, or it can be a planning-type scrutiny to see how cost can be reduced or how more heating can be produced for a preset cost. Evaluation is not directed to issues of how effectively the building is being heated nor how comfortable people feel who work in the building. In spite of its many limitations, the virtue of the efficiency criterion is supposedly apparent to all persons from money-oriented cultures.

Level Four Evaluation—Effectivity (How Well Is the Operation Producing the Net Outputs Specifically Desired?)

At this level we have added to the heater analogy another set of guiding criteria, the desired outputs. Perhaps we can say that the issue now is how well the building is being heated, or whether it is being heated, or whether it is being heated to meet preset criteria. Such guidance might have consisted of stipulations that there should be no more than two degree variation in temperature (no hot or cold spots), or that all persons shall be comfortable as a result of the heating. This is the effect that was presumably really wanted when the unit was installed. Again, by means of spot or continuous temperature checks and employee surveys, compliance to the objectives or the degree of failure is determinable. A research orientation might additionally explore how to achieve what was desired if there are failures. This level of evaluation determines the adequacy of the delivery of the specified product (in this case, uniform warmth) and is not unlike the old performance budgeting approach, so popular among administrators a few years ago—an approach which, in fact, continues to be one of the most useful management control devices. (It may have elements of level 2 evaluation.)

Level Five Evaluation—Outcome Validity (How Well Has the Intervention Achieved the Ultimate Consequences or Purposes for Which the Outputs Were Designed?)

Outcome validity evaluation is also very much a check on the validity of our understanding of the cause-effect relationships involved. In the heater analogy, let us say that the ultimate purpose of the desired effects is to keep workers warm and thus maximally free of respiratory illness, with the ultimate intent of reducing absenteeism caused by illness. Underlying reasons for setting up the heating system were presumptions that it would reduce respiratory illness and thus absenteeism. Obviously, recording not only has to be made as to whether the heater has been effective (really keeping the place warm as specified), recording must now include worker absenteeism due to respiratory illness, for this was the reason that set the whole matter in operation. All the preceding levels of evaluation by themselves would have shed light only on whether the heater worked, whether it worked as mechanically specified, whether its cost was at a certain level, whether it heated as required—but not whether it contributed to worker health and attendance.

We are now evaluating the supposed fact that health and subsequent absenteeism objectives are responsive to warmth which produces a decline in respiratory illness. Thus, observations about how suitable warmth did or did not significantly attain the objectives may lead to research type findings about the validity of warmth as a factor related to good health. This is the validification level of evaluation—do the outcomes that result from the outputs turn out as our knowledge led us to postulate?

Level Six Evaluation—Overall Desirability or System Appropriateness (Does the Desired Result Actually Serve the Overall Best Interest of the Encompassing System?)

The concept of overall goals or criteria relevant to systemic well-being was probably the major reason for and the central source of guidance to the planners when they set about designing the operation; now the same criteria must be used as a base against which to evaluate the accomplishments in the system. These objectives or criteria relate not just to what the operation can and will do, but to its final impact on the encompassing system of concern. In the heater analogy, system appropriateness raises the issue of whether overall systemically heating the building is good. Even if worker health has improved and there is less sickness-caused absenteeism, attaining these objectives does not necessarily indicate a more profitable future for the employers who operate the building and the business (the system desirability). The costs of operating the heater may exceed the gains to the company achieved by making employees healthier and reducing absenteeism. Gains in output from less illness may be more than offset by work losses due to dissatisfactions caused by some employees who now think they are too cold or too warm, those in other buildings who now insist that their building should be heated in the same way, and so on. In fact, the warmth associated with good health may have cut overall production by 10%, because no one feels like hustling in a comfortable environment.

In the six-level schema just presented, no issue was made as to whether each higher level of evaluation automatically included the lower level evaluation. It does not in fact follow that one must evaluate for efficiency as part of checking for validity. However, it would be hard to limit evaluation to validity without assuring oneself that the effectivity or specified impact had, in fact, been going on. It would, likewise, be hard to limit evaluation to system desirability without also checking on both effectivity and efficiency—the first to see if the effect was being delivered, and the second because cost is a critical item in terms of foregone opportunities, even if not in direct terms of affordability to the operating system concerned.

In our culture, issues of cost or efficiency have been of so much more day-to-day importance than issues of equity or ecology that over the years the criterion cost or efficiency has managed to procure for itself an honored place among the evaluatory tools (our level three). I believe that, by itself, it is no more and probably is a lot less important than any of the other levels of evaluation. (We could and do happily place it among the societal criteria—see Figure 6.1—as one of the minor indices by which to judge societal or systemic importance or desirability.) We simply are forced to give it a place by itself among evaluatory criteria because it is one fairly concise and meaningful aspect of evaluation, and not because of the emphasis that has been placed on it in the past. For example, among the excellent discussions of evaluation in Schulberg,[20] most authors take for granted that evaluation for efficiency is something particularly valuable, and George James used it as the basis for his entire schema of evaluation.[21] True, he takes validity for granted as a part of planning, but he does not suggest testing or evaluating for it.

What Applications Are Desirable?

Range of Applications of the Six Levels of Evaluation

Three examples of activities in the field of maternal and child health—varying from one with minute significance to one with great concern—help to clarify how each of the six levels of evaluation might be applied to each activity or operation when specific evaluatory objectives are to be met. George James used similar examples of evaluating programs primarily for efficiency (level 3) for each of several types of objectives varying in importance as shown here, but he did not concern himself with the other levels of evaluation.[22]

Application to a fairly broad and quite definitive type of objective. An antitoxemia, antiprematurity program of clinic services for women at risk (with the underlying objectives of reducing maternal morbidity and mortality, infant deaths and defective infants). *The major concern of evaluation at each of the six levels is:*
   Level One—evidence that the program is actually going on.
   Level Two—evidence that the program manifests the specified attributes and actually serves all the mothers for whom it is intended.
   Level Three—evidence that the program is delivered at the most reasonable cost per mother or per visit.
   Level Four—evidence that the incidence of toxemia of pregnancy and prematurity are lessened.
   Level Five—evidence that as a result of the lessened incidence of toxemia and prematurity there is reduction in the customary incidence of maternal morbidity and mortality and of infant deaths and defective infants among the serviced women at risk.
   Level Six—evidence that the reduction in maternal and infant damage is good for society.

Application to a limited, lower level, or intermediary subobjective. Provision of health education services in a prenatal clinic to improve nutrition during pregnancy. (The underlying rationale for this effort is that improved nutrition should reduce the incidence of toxemias and prematurity and thus their adverse maternal and infant consequences.) *The major concern of evaluation at each of the six levels is:*

   Level One—evidence that the program is actually going on.
   Level Two—evidence that all women at risk are coming to the clinic and receiving the specified health education.

Level Three—evidence that the women coming to the clinic get the service at the most reasonable cost.

Level Four—evidence that the women coming to the clinic get nutrition information that is meaningful and understood by them and that it changes their nutrition behavior favorably.

Level Five—evidence that among the serviced women at risk there is a reduction in the customary incidence of toxemia and prematurity.

Level Six—evidence that the health education services are overall a desirable feature of a maternal and child health clinic in terms of their health consequences and the nature of their side effects, and evidences that these services justified the opportunities foregone by using resources in this way.

Application to a very limited or low level subobjective. Creation of a pamphlet on "Nutrition During Pregnancy" to be used as a teaching device for all pregnant women receiving prenatal care. (The underlying objective being that exposure to this pamphlet will result in mothers following proper nutrition during pregnancy, with all the attendant benefits on maternal and infant health that should result.) *The major concern of evaluation at each of the six levels is:*

Level One—evidence that the pamphlet is available and being distributed.

Level Two—evidence that the pamphlet with specified qualities reaches all women at risk.

Level Three—evidence that the cost of this pamphlet and its distribution is at the most reasonable level.

Level Four—evidence that the pamphlet is readable, attracts attention, is accurate, is studied by all women receiving it, and that they learn from it what is correct.

Level Five—evidence that exposed women not only learn what is correct nutrition behavior during pregnancy but practice it.

Level Six—evidence that the nutrition pamphlet is overall a desirable feature of clinic nutrition education services because of its nutrition consequences and side effects on general clinic utilities, and that the pamphlet justifies the opportunities foregone because of this use of resources.

Choices as to Which Aspects of Activities are to be Subjected to Which Levels of Evaluation

For an operating entity, evaluation has the potential of focusing either on everything going on as part of that activity or on any one piece of the activity. Thus, decisions must be made about which aspects or objectives are to be evaluated, or whether it is all to be done.[23]

In addition, there is the possibility of evaluating each of the pieces of the activity at any of the six levels.

We must look at level six for the impact of the entire operation, that is, the appropriateness of the sum of the impacts of the pieces, if we want to see the major consequences of the operating entity to the larger or encompassing system—society.[24] In the example just used, appropriateness of the major objective of reducing maternal and infant morbidity and mortality would be determined by how the next higher level system looked at the issue. Is this successful reduction in maternal and infant morbidity and mortality good for our particular society at this time, given the program costs and the population, food, and production consequences? In the heater-heated building analogy, the level six appropriateness evaluation would be determined by whether the employing-producing system is better off by having the building heated, given the cost to the company and other consequences involved.

No one in his right mind would contemplate doing all the levels of evaluation on all of the pieces as well as checking for appropriateness of the total operating entity. Thus, much of the remainder of this chapter discusses which opportunities for evaluation should be seized, what kinds of evaluation should be done, at what expense, and under what circumstances.

From what has been said so far, how one goes about evaluation is clearly a personal or institutional choice. It may be the consequence of a subjective whim on the part of somebody who had a voice in the planning or decision-making path, which determined that a certain kind of evaluation was to be included. Typically, today, the designer of a project who seeks outside support has to incorporate evaluation. He needs guidance, because he will never be able to undertake all the possible evaluative thrusts that even a simple project might suggest. Just think of the evaluations a professor could do of his students' progress in a course. He might evaluate his assumptions about teaching and learning, about his facts, and about his techniques. Or as is more commonly done, evaluate the students' absorption of information, their comprehension, their ability to apply or utilize it, their ability to analyze it, their ability to synthesize from and with it, and their ability to do evaluations and apply the information.[25] Finally, our professor might wish to evaluate whether his course was a good thing for him, for the students, for their future employers, for the university, or for society. Are there any guides as to which types of evaluation are most useful in a given situation?

In all fairness to an activity, it should be measured in terms of whether it is achieving the effect for which it was mounted (level four), and then it should be evaluated to determine whether this objective is rational, valid, or causally sound, and whether it leads toward the underlying goals or objectives (level five) for which the activity was undertaken. However, in all cases it is perhaps wisest to do a quick evaluation at level one to determine if the activity has, in fact, ever taken place. If it has, evaluation at level two, if not very costly (and such data is usually collected by all operating units), may reveal whether most clients or only a rare one had the opportunity of receiving the activity as specified.

After doing levels one and two and finding reasonable activity, my preference would be to do a combined level four and five evaluation next. If level four seems bad, there is evidence that the methods of intervention are not suitable or that the cause-and-effect logic of the methodology is not really understood. If level four evaluation shows the activity is effective but level five shows that the anticipated outcomes did not occur, we can assume that the activity was carried out well but that the understanding of the cause-and-effect relationships of the products to the desired consequences from the products was inadequate. In the maternal and child health example, level four evaluation might show that toxemia and prematurity were reduced, but that this had no effect on reducing maternal and infant damage. Of course, one must also be aware of the possibility that some other or some new cause is contributing as much maternal and infant damage as our successful activity against toxemia and prematurity has actually prevented.

Level six would follow, if levels four and five indicated that effectivity and validity were either present or potential and that the intervention was justified. Level six evaluation is necessary because what was thought valuable, when the plan or intervention was designed just year or two before, may now strike us quite differently. For example, because of the spectacular reversals in ecological values over the past few years, what was applauded as a clever way of making building sites by filling in shallow bays now seems to be an abomination. Similarly, in many countries, monies previously allocated to feeding children now go to preventing their birth. (Confused understanding of the real world.)

The diversity of values or desirabilities is so extensive, so mixed up, and changing so rapidly, that the well-being of the system which encompasses the activity must be examined in terms of many criteria. What is superlatively good by one criterion may be bad by another— for example, our overwhelming concern for increased longevity is offset by our concern for overpopulation. Level six evaluation must always be carried out because, (like level five) conventional wisdom about what is good for society (or the system at hand) is probably not very trustworthy.[26] Where the capacity to evaluate is limited, level six would probably be the first and most important, after ascertaining that the activity is really in effect.

Naturally, cost per unit of output as well as per unit of effect (cost-effectiveness) is one aspect included in a thoroughgoing level six evaluation, as is total cost. In Figure 6.1 these, along with more than 20 other kinds of criteria, are listed as important in making societal-level evaluations. However, by itself, level three efficiency is, for many reasons, probably the last kind of evaluation to be done. If the activity has taken place or met operational standards (levels 1 and 2), it cannot sensibly be evaluated for efficiency until it further undergoes testing for effectivity or for validity and systemic suitability. However, if the activity is shown as acceptable at levels four, five, and six, then it should be subject to scrutiny for efficiency.

Evidence of failure at any level of evaluation does not automatically tell why or how the failure is occurring, unless the problem is obvious. Evaluation may or may not be extended to find out what is going wrong or what is involved in making the activity go right. The latter need only be done if there is still firm belief that the activity is both logical and reasonably feasible and that it merits further study.

For good and sufficient reason, any of the six levels may be what is wanted, and no particular order need be followed. However, it is unreasonable to check at level four (effectivity) without ascertaining by level two evaluation (operational criteria) that the machinery is indeed working in the specified way. No matter how it rubs us, it is similarly unnecessary to do a level four, five, or six evaluation if the policymakers refuse to consider funding any study or continuing any particular activity until its cost per unit (level three) evaluation is satisfactory to them.

There may be dozens or thousands of specific tasks or steps as part of what is done in one interventive instrument (for example, the hospital), and choice of what to evaluate is no simple matter. Comparative cost accounting and other devices give clues about where to look for inefficiencies, as do areas that are reputed to be the source of conflicts or unrest. However, more extensive operations research type studies may be required if extensive changes and new ways of running an institution or some major segment of it are to be explored.

Need for and Nature of Evaluation Vary Over Time and With Stage of Operation

The need for evaluation of an operation that is being brought into production may begin with a simple observation of how well its constituent pieces are being assembled or tested and whether it is keeping up with a prearranged schedule (such as PERT or CPM) which was used in the design.[27] Let us use the career of a planning body as an example of an operation to be evaluated. Its stage of development is critical to what can be examined and what can have progressed to any measurable point.[28] (Certainly, one would be a fool to wait 20 years to ascertain whether health status had improved due to the part played by a CHP body, because that source of improvements would probably be indistinguishable from a thousand other influences equally or more potently at work than a CHP.)

In the year after the birth of a CHP, one could observe first the goals and concerns selected, then the roles and functions assembled, and shortly thereafter, how well these were being practiced. At later dates, the actual immediate products of the enterprise—such as methods, criteria, standards, and plans—would successively emerge and could in turn be studied to derive a sense of the progress being made. At a still later time one could determine how well these planning outputs served to guide community operations. Some years later one could hope to see if these outputs were valid in terms of having aided society to move toward the desired well-being. The speed at which the agency assumed more advanced activities is another evaluatory criterion.

In another situation, the provision of care through Office of Economic Opportunity funded neighborhood health centers was examined by Sparer and Johnson. They made similar decisions about how they would assess progress in terms of the original objectives and basic policy mandates, and finally about what could be determined at the time they were evaluating the operations.[29] We will return to this study as one of the examples of applied evaluation.

Feedback and Data

Evaluation at any level has been described as requiring a five-step process which:

Redefines or clarifies the original goals and dependent or subsequent objectives of the activity to be evaluated.

Selects or designs measuring instruments or other procedures to collect data that will shed light on inputs, throughputs, and outputs.

Collects data.

Summarizes and analyzes data in a utilizable way.

Interprets data and concludes what they show about the degree, cost, adverse effects or unexpected bonuses of attainment of the original objectives.[30]

The machinery to produce evaluation is designed from this five step view of the process. The process of feedback is in many ways a restatement of what goes on in evaluation and may be defined even more broadly. Weiner describes it as "the property of being able to adjust to future conduct by past performance."[31] However, for our purposes feedback or the process of doing evaluation is accepted as carrying out these five steps. (These five steps involved in feedback must not be confused with the six levels of evaluation.)

PROBLEMS AND LIMITATIONS OF EVALUATION

The degree of investment in evaluation may well be determined by the kinds of limitations and difficulties that surround evaluation.

Are the Findings of Evaluation Likely to be Applied?
(Who Needs Them or Benefits from Them?)

One of the most interesting problems of evaluation is the potential unwillingness on the part of those whose work or organization is being evaluated to accept or utilize evaluatory findings (as any professor being rated by his students can attest). This difficulty reminds us to check who must be involved in carrying out evaluation so that they can or will be party to the changes suggested. We are also reminded that evaluation must promise something to those whose work is being evaluated beyond harder work, fewer frills, transfer, or loss of jobs. The evaluator who foresees becoming a hero by saving money or time or by improving output has different incentives for participating in evaluation than persons whose careers are likely to be altered, perhaps unfavorably. If the gains to the evaluator are pitted against the welfare of those being evaluated (unless the evaluator has total proprietary control) it is unlikely that his findings are going to be accepted—particularly when any and all studies are open to alternative interpretations by determined persons.

The acceptance of evaluative findings in several professional settings has been studied by Eaton in an interesting experiment in which workers were asked to comment on questions in the form of: "Supposing we found these situations, what would be your response?"[32] Interestingly enough, a high proportion of the professional social workers studied—persons who were very much in the business of regarding evaluation as part of their professional outlook and expectations—did not want to handle the simulated evaluatory findings, even to publicize or interpret them. Moreover, the studies were done in organizations whose attributes and records show good support of research, evaluations and free discussion. Eaton's experimental subjects rated high on interest in evaluatory research but rather poorly on readiness to interpret and on readiness to communicate about findings which, as they well knew, were only part of an attitudinal experiment. This observation—that persons who already believe in evaluation have their backs braced in principle against utilizing the results—suggests that even they would surely be formidable opponents in a real-life evaluation of their activities.

One wonders how more authoritarian types, such as physicians, would respond to other than intentionally experimental clinical evaluation (how well their experimentally intended efforts turn out). True, they do participate in extensive evaluation of day-to-day nonexperimental clinical results that heavily guide their choices of technology. But even there, many evaluatory non sequiturs occur, in that input standards are often developed for procedures. For example, "Mayo" indications for surgery of a specific kind may show a 1% mortality as compared to 10% for nonintervention. But someone not trained in the Mayo way or poorly trained generally, who follows these precepts and ostensibly applies the same techniques, may have a 20% mortality, which might then presumably go unquestioned. From such lessons we become concerned with quality review of outcomes, patient by patient, not quality of input criteria, procedure by procedure. The pains of such outcome evaluations are well described, and interesting reasons given for enduring them at the hands of one's peers in medical practice: (1) to improve quality of care, (2) to keep costs of care at reasonable levels, and (3) to prevent government or consumer groups from controlling medical practice.[33]

It is also important to determine whether procedures in nonemergency situations were properly timed for the patient's best functioning. Because this question introduces several new sets of parameters, such as evaluation for relevance to the patient and society (see Chapter 4), we are not at all sure that physicians would be interested in this kind of evaluative effort. Moreover, there is some doubt whether an exclusively physician group could carry out such an evaluation intelligently.

All of this is by way of saying that evaluation may be to the patient's advantage but not to that of some physicians. In other situations, the reverse might be true, and where probable outcomes can be guessed at, people may take vigorous positions for or against doing evaluation or doing it in particular ways. All of us have vivid memories of such impasses when an agency head or organization representative will go along with evaluation only if there is an unwritten but firm guarantee that some sacred piece of the activity is to be excluded from the evaluation, or measured in such a way that it can only appear adequate. This immunity, of course, is often achieved by checking exclusively on inputs rather than on outputs.

An interesting question arises: How well would operators go along with the results of evaluations if they were involved in setting up the studies? One of our assumptions about planning is that participation in the doing would ease the acceptance of new knowledge and altered values. The same kind of factors might be at work here. In many medical centers and "good" hospitals, outcome evaluations are well done in a participative way, although nonmedical participants are excluded. Ellis, however, provides a frank discussion of how local health department workers see themselves as providers of services and not as wasters of dollars on evaluation.[34] Given the cloudy definitions of their purposes, inadequate resources, day-to-day pressures, continuously changing technologies, incomplete acceptance of the need for evaluation, lack of knowing how to do it, and absence of a mandate to do it, this negative posture of public health workers toward evaluation is not illogical.

The literature is full of evaluatory studies in which little knowledgeable participation occurred but meaningful data was gathered. Estimates, however, of how well implementation of changes suggested by such evaluations took place varies so much with the source and nature of control of the efforts that were being evaluated, that the evidence pro and con on the effects of participation in implemention tends to be indeterminable. (Because of the nature of his study, Eaton did not have the opportunity to see whether participation in the design of the study would have influenced the willingness of workers to go further in utilizing evaluative results.[35])

At the higher levels of evaluation applied to community health, the primary concerns are the suitability of goals and the utility or societal desirability of programs. Here, implementation of evaluatory findings at the community level involves major agencies, pet programs of legislators, and legislated mandates. Both the friends of favorably evaluated programs and the enemies of poorly rated ones will be elated. We need not elaborate. Hopefully, under the stimulation of participative planning and evaluation, the bulk of the public and the legislators will be interested in the guidance available from the results of evaluation as much as from the planning effort of which it is a part. Goldman presents testimony to the fact that legislators currently need and welcome evaluatory findings.[36]

Evaluation which covers the outcomes of operational activities in order to apply them to the next round of planning is needed and will be wanted (1) by the community which bears the costs, (2) by the consumer who attempts or should attempt to utilize the services, and (3) by the purveyors, all of whom need to come abreast of the times as expressed in current needs, outcomes, and satisfactions. Evaluation at the validity and societal desirability levels should ultimately become even more attractive to the populace and policy makers. (The technical complexities and the historic vacuum of concern at these levels must be acknowledged.)

Above all, evaluation serves the immediate needs of the planners who have to be guided in the allocative, problem-solving, and future-building activities undertaken in behalf of the community. If the more extensive, research-type, evaluative tasks are undertaken, the planners will be the first to benefit, in the sense of gaining information which should enable them to offer a better product. But all of society would come out ahead. And so it is to be hoped that society will keep the pressure on planning bodies to do evaluation of this caliber, at least from time to time where capacity is present. However, in spite of proposed or evident desire for evaluatory results by policy makers, the allocation of money for evaluation is not a discernible trend below the national level at present.

Who Needs to be Involved In Evaluation?
Is There a Need for a Separate Evaluation Unit
In a Health Planning Body?

The question of who needs to be involved in evaluation sounds little different from the question of who needs to be involved in planning. The hope has just been expressed that evaluation would be better received when the key interests likely to be involved by the findings had a hand in shaping the direction of the evaluation. Weikel discusses this issue generally, pointing out that DHEW created evaluatory task forces using 50% membership from program level, 25% from agency level and 25% from the Office of the Secretary.[37] This effort, of course, is directed not at community but at agency concerns. There are other ways of approaching the subject of involvement in evaluation of community planning, which we shall now consider.

Those Who Can be Expected to Get Direct Benefit from Knowing About the Results of the Evaluation

The design of the evaluation should be adjusted to meet the needs of those who can be seen as needing to know about specific outcomes. This matter is often discovered after an evaluation is completed, and some of the information produced proves critical to one group, while other information is useful to another. Billings reports on this point in a health consumer feedback system in which the psychiatrists gained the most useful information from a delayed or postdischarge report while the administration got the most useful information from a pre-discharge report.[38] These need not be accidental discoveries. A perusal of what was wanted by various interests would direct one to where and under what circumstances a particular type of feedback vehicle would serve best. In other words, evaluation has to be specifically tailored for the concerns or needs of those who are to be influenced, and this is best done by involving such users in the evaluation.

The meaning of the term *benefit* in this context is not restricted to a special profit or gain out of the evaluatory knowledge; it may also include utility for the person, subsystem, or system needing the information to improve capacity or the means of doing whatever is wanted.

Diversity Needed to Enable Comprehension

For almost the identical technical reasons that were advanced in Chapter 7 for determining whom to involve in analysis of a problem, it is suggested that exactly those interests who represent the key actors on the operation stage—whether victims or providers—have to be present. In addition, representatives from other activities and sectors involved, as well as a goodly scattering of representation of general interest, are required if the levels of the planning and the criteria of effectivity and impact are to receive reasonably unbiased scrutiny.

Is There Need for a Separate Evaluating Unit in a Planning Body?

A good problem analysis and intervention design effort would have laid down much of what the evaluators have to do. That is, the problem analysis already has defined the nature of the general aims and the objectives (step one of feedback), and, therefore, the evaluatory body assigned to a given issue or problem may well be the same planning committee or task force whose analytic and design work was accepted for implementation originally. For the task force to continue into the evaluatory phase is logical, provided that they have technical assistance with evaluatory tools, from staff or by contract with outside experts, when the study is too complex for the task force to deal with by itself.

The question of whether the planning body needs a separate evaluatory unit is not answerable categorically. Evaluation of the ongoing interventive efforts in a given area, undertaken because the planning body is contemplating action or because it desires evaluation for its own recently implemented planning outputs in that area, suggests that the planning task force studying the area or problem might find that the effort of evaluation provides an important assist in its continued planning. Evaluation must also be built into the design of newly-planned interventions. For these two reasons it seems unwise to set up a single evaluation committee to handle all evaluatory tasks. Such a group cannot possibly understand all the issues involved in every planning effort without reliving much of the work of the particular planning task force and recreating a comparably diverse membership to participate in examining the results in the situation.

However, experience indicates that task forces may become wedded to the solutions they designed and protective of their planning outputs, and thus they may be poor evaluators. For this reason, a temporary group of evaluators theretofore not involved in the articular planning effort may be the best choice for looking over the results of significant interventions. The group can be augmented by a few members of the original planning task force, so that the new evaluatory group will be helped to understand what took place, and yet will not be engulfed by the history and viewpoints of the original planners.

Might there then be one key overall evaluation group (or is that not the planning body council itself?) which tries to relate what is learned through evaluation, not only to each specific intervention and thus to the problem attacked but also to the whole of health planning? There may well be room for a so-called policy study or directions committee of the planning body, and the bylaws might provide that such a policy committee be required to take cognizance of and report routinely on what is revealed by evaluative studies made by the health planning body or made available to it.

When and Under What Circumstances Should Evaluation Take Place?

The significant pieces or objectives of the interventive scheme should be built into each intervention as it is designed, so that evaluation is part of the operation. Similarly, the costs for recording, collecting, and analyzing the data must be planned for and made part of the budget of the operating agencies involved. At the same time, the planning body must plan and budget its own future so that its role will mesh with the evaluations built into the operating agencies. In this way a reasonable evaluation of the effects of the major programs it has designed can be assembled by the planning body.

Operating agencies will often be unable to do much about collecting data specifically relevant to level six. But because the planning body may and typically should through its general well-being assessment machinery, have antennae or probes constantly at work, these can be adjusted to try to tune in on any societal changes likely to occur as the result of major operational interventions designed by the planning body. And it is these observed changes which provide better understanding of the real world system which is being planned for.

Situations in Which Evaluation Seems Useless

It may in many ways be easier to spell out when evaluation ought not to be carried out, for these should be the exceptions:

When evaluation is essentially technically unattainable for a very popularly desired operation.

The most obvious situation in which evaluation may be ignored is where an activity is very much in demand and no one sees how to get useful feedback from it. Therefore, the activity is destined to be carried on without evaluation.

When an activity is proven "meaningless" but public desire keeps it in operation.

This situation occurs when an evaluation has been done, and the verdict of "useless effort" has been made clear to all policy makers and the public. If they then want the activity to continue on other grounds, such as esthetics, full employment of workers who would otherwise be out of a job, or a feeling of safety, clearly the operation does have some kind of value. It could then be evaluated for its utility against relevant criteria other than the ones which so-called rational evaluators have already used to measure some direct outputs which everyone knows the effort does not adequately create.

Where change obviously offers little gain by comparison to the expense or dangers that its introduction will be courting.

Evaluation may seem destined to show that change is called for on the usual evaluatory grounds, but in the given situation it is clear that no one will dare suggest carrying out the change which evaluation will surely indicate. This is a special case of the preceding situation where some higher or different value is not being considered by the evaluator. True, the evaluator may not regard an affront to the legislature, a guaranteed riot, or a strike as too high a price for some needed change. But those who employ him will have to consider such possibilities before authorizing evaluation. Decisions are also likely to be made against doing evaluation where little is likely to be saved or improved, but where something about the activity is highly symbolic and any derogatory evaluation or any proposed change will seriously jeopardize matters that the policy makers or citizenry find more important than the resources wasted in carrying out the evidently useless activity.

Where the cost of a suitable evaluation is a significant part of the costs of a total operation which "seems" to be working well.

All of the qualifying elements in the above statement are open not only to tremendous variation but to argument as well. If a proposal costs a million dollars a year and will presumably run on for decades if there is no evaluatory guidance, an evaluation investment of two or even ten million dollars may not be unduly expensive. This is particularly true if other communities seem likely to use a similar operation and, therefore, stand to gain from the knowledge (a tremendous justification for federal or even international support of key evaluatory studies). However, evaluation involving a recurring annual cost of half a million dollars for the same project, which means using up to half of the available money just for evaluation, seems out of line. If gross efficiency, outputs, or general impact of the operation are in serious doubt, the costly one-time route must be used to clarify the situation.

Situations in Which Evaluation is Called For

How much of ongoing operations should be routinely evaluated? An operation with a once documented most elegant payoff may run on its reputation long after its utility is gone. There are so many famous stories about such anachronisms that we can be sure that we are likely to overlook wasteful, but reassuring or pleasant, archaic practices for long periods of time. The answer here would seem to be to choose evaluation on the basis of several different kinds of considerations.

One rule of thumb would be to do a reasonable job of it whenever serious planning is to be applied to an area or package of operations.

A second rule would be to carry out evaluative efforts in any area which seems significantly out of line, by whatever criteria or information are brought to the planning body's attention, or as indicated by the amount of pressure put on the body to investigate an activity, even one that superficially seemed as useful as most other comparable activities. This would be a one-time evaluation unless reason were found to keep an eye on the particular operation.

A third rule would be for a substantial evaluation every two to five years for an activity which constitutes a sizable part of a community's budget.

An alternative rule would be to carry out evaluation on a continuing, but less in depth basis where significant resources are involved. The planners could select one or two key aspects thought crucial for each given major operation and run an annual check at the level of evaluation expected to be most revealing.

This is not a discussion of evaluation to be undertaken by each operating agency[39] (although there does not appear to be all that much difference in the logic). This discussion concerns what a planning body should be doing in the way of evaluation for those activities it is studying or has helped bring into being. If this advice were heeded, most operating agencies would be doing evaluation, and the planning body would need ask only for modifications, provide assistance, or cooperate with what is ongoing in the way of operating agency evaluation in order to get the evaluative information necessary for its community planning level overview.

How Rigorously Should Evaluation be Carried Out and What Is a Reasonable Cost?

There is another facet to what has already been touched on in discussion of when an investment should be made.

Rigor

Rigor is usually a major determinant of cost, and rigor is often the quality sacrificed when costs of evaluation are kept down. Rigor should be at least as much a function of what is being evaluated as of cost. For levels one and two, rigor in evaluation must not mean ridiculously trivial detail when only a few simple observations are needed. At level three, rigor will vary with the complexity of the operation, and truly skilled operations researchers may be needed to avoid serious mistakes that give a false set of indications as to what costs really are.

At levels four and five, rigor or skill may be very demanding, for the issue is no longer money but what was done and the effects. These concerns far supersede efficiency in terms of significance. Irrespective of efficiency, the outputs may be useless or even dangerous to the community. At level six, wisdom is more relevant than rigor. Wisdom differs with the viewpoint held, and so it is hard to prescribe for. The traditions and logic of democracy suggest a diversity of views, and that they will have to be correlated to obtain anything corresponding to wisdom.

Rigor is commensurate with a statistically and sociologically sound job. This may be simple for some issues and truly complicated for others. Once evaluation becomes more of a planning body concern, evaluation expertise will develop. The planning body will have to decide upon the degree of rigor needed to prevent the production of serious misinformation, the degree of good or harm at stake, and the cost of evaluation in relation to the cost of the operation as well as to the good or harm the operation seems capable of doing.

Bringing Evaluation to Bear on the Right Place

This is one aspect of rigor as well as of quality of evaluation and has partially been discussed under other considerations.

Conflicts.   One shortcut which can often take the evaluator to the heart of what most needs evaluation is to look for chronic conflicts in the activity under study and to make an analysis of the conflict his central task. Determining the precursors and consequences of the conflict provides an interesting type of evaluation, or at least serves to direct attention to the pieces of a system which need further evaluation. This sense of direction is important. Doing a whole system evaluation is expensive and generally impossible for the more complex systems, and simply guessing at which parts of an activity to check may not provide much of value.

Event Sequences.   When a series of linked events must occur in a particular order over time to create the machinery to turn out a product or to produce stages of the product, evaluation wisely looks at the earlier or formative events to see that they are really taking place at the time and in the way specified.[40] If not, the end product is not likely to occur, and waiting to do an elaborate evaluation at a later date is pointless, if an early check can give a valid prognosis.

Key products.   Where an activity is piggybacking on general processes that go on anyway, we can look at the "end of the line" to see whether what was wanted has shown up. If not, then we look among the steps of the intervention to see which ones were fouled up, which were erroneous, which were not done or were done wrongly, and whether piggybacking is really feasible after all.

Cost of Evaluation

The more that evaluation is built into future plans, the more the implementing agencies will carry the work and the costs of doing most of the feedback. But, as the planning body's output becomes implemented, it will be creating pressures on itself to insure evaluation of the specific operations that provide planned-for feedback and, at a mounting tempo, to see what the major societal impacts are. In addition, the more data the implementing agencies contribute, the more the planning body will find it timely to look at fifth and sixth level concerns, and these evaluations will be expensive until we have available some better methods of social accounting.[41]

Can the planning body do any useful evaluation if it utilizes 5%, 10%, or 50% of its budget, which now typically runs under 10-20 cents per capita for all health planning purposes.[42] If health planning bodies continue at the current levels of funding, as much as 25% of their resources must be devoted to evaluation if there is to be any evaluation, but this effort is still pathetic in terms of creating capacity for a new type of activity. (We note that health care costs are over $400 per capita per year.)

Evaluation will surely be a greater concern of the larger, and therefore better, totally funded planning bodies, particularly of the metros and the states. There will undoubtedly have to be huge federal inputs in the form of dollar resources and guidance for trials of evaluation to make this aspect of planning come to pass. Because health financing is moving toward a national base, and the benefits of much of the evaluation are widely applicable, shifting the costs of evaluation to the national level is logical. The one set of recommendations with which I am familiar indicates that an optimal level of annual funding for health planning (one dollar per capita for population groups under 150,000, to 20 cents per capita for those over 5 million persons) can only hope to make 5%-20% available for evaluation.[43] The U.S. Department of Transport in its experimental safety programs spends as much as 30% of the costs on evaluation, we are told. In many of its programs, DHEW assumes that 10% of program appropriations should be for evaluation.[44]

The newer, expensive health care delivery and ecological rectification programs will probably require such large chunks of money for rational evaluation that evaluation alone would dwarf the entire planning budget, although constituting only a modest percentage of the budgets for operating experiments. This means that, for political reasons, the planning body must get the bulk of funds for evaluation placed within the budgets of the large operating agencies whose activities it relates to, and not attempt to get all such moneys into its own budget. In order to put the role and cost of evaluating into proper perspective vis-a-vis the services for which it is meant to provide guidance, the planning body would do well to specify that costs of evaluation be written into the budget of each operating project it plans for or reviews.

EXAMPLES OF EVALUATIVE EFFORTS

A few examples are provided of how evaluation might be applied to subjects of concern to health planners.

Evaluation of the Outputs of Comprehensive Health Planning Bodies

It is reasonable to regard the outputs of a planning body as themselves requiring evaluation. This is a suitable activity for each state level planning agency which is "overseeing" the local agencies, because we believe the state agency must bear serious responsibility if there is to be any coherent planning in a state. It is also a suitable task for the federal health agency that has responsibility for the nationwide state and local efforts at health planning. This may be done on a 100% coverage or on a sampling basis from the national level, with a federal agency guiding each of the states so that each in turn evaluates some or all of its locals. Alternatively, an attempt may be made to do an annual nationwide canvass directly from the federal level. It is also a suitable activity for a research-oriented health planning institute or university center to undertake with federal support under federal requirements. (Justifiable questions have been raised about the use of highpowered think or design tank evaluatory teams who do mail order, itemized evaluations of dubiously comparable operations with which they remain unfamiliar. Some of these scrutinies are structured, but pointless, and seem at least equally intellectually offensive as the probably more relevant but poorly organized and uncorrelatable site visits and peer reviews of recent years.)

A planning body does not exist in a void and must contend with many factors in its environment by altering them or accepting them as constraints. The environment usually establishes for the planning body its basic structure and relationships, its degree of representativeness, and specific or legally defined capacities and duties as well as restrictions (to be sure, none are immutable). Within these boundaries, the planning body still has many choices of goals, purposes, roles, functions, activities, relationships, board membership, staff, and areas of health to be concentrated on. What it selects to do among these is subject to evaluation.

Local CHP bodies continue to come into existence, and if the nation is to be covered by them, the majority have yet to be founded. Because of the variations in age, it is important that they be evaluated in terms of where they are in their life cycle. Evaluation of CHP bodies might be done by stage of maturity, and this might correlate modestly with chronological age. In fact, some CHP bodies now in their seventh year of existence can hardly be said to be operative, while others less than a year old are obviously sophisticated and into the midst of extensive planning. Given the stage of maturity at which a planning body is functioning, another aspect of evaluation is to check on how well it is doing whatever is on its agenda. Slow maturation may give a different kind of prognosis than would a defective way of proceeding.

Prognostic (Evaluative) Criteria of Probable Success
Based on Forces Exerted by the External Environment

The following criteria are relevant at any of the stages of agency maturity but are critical for prognosticating the fate of the agency about to be activated. If we look for the presence or shape that the determinants of social change take in the situation under consideration (see Chapter 2), we can guess whether or not the planning agency is likely to be created for purposes of meaningful change. This evaluation is a prognosis or forecast of the future effectiveness of the agency and is essentially based on analysis of the environment spawning it. A review of what the environment holds and the effect it would have on the four determinants of social change would go about as follows:

Intensity and breadth of potential support (impetus determinants to social change). This is the general community climate towards planning.

Political structures, institutions, related agencies and organizations (structural control determinants to social change).

Source of energy, organizational support, cash (mobilization determinants to social change).

Sociocultural make up and traditions about using and participating in such things as planning (self-regulation determinants of social change).

Prognostic (Evaluative) Criteria of Probable Success
Based on the Initial Boundaries Prescribed
for the Planning Agency

For an agency about to come into being, the second set of key prognostic features involves those freedoms or capacities built in by charter or by legal mandate. Since there still is no real output to scrutinize at this stage, a prognostic evaluation based on this group of criteria is, of necessity, based on the scope of community-set goals placed on the organization, which include:

Role and functional freedom allotted the agency.

Prestige and visibility accorded the agency.

Representativeness demanded of the agency board.

Formal relationships to other planning agencies and units of government, both horizontally and vertically.

These criteria which speak to a good prognosis have been elaborated upon so extensively in the preceding chapters that it is not necessary to do more here.

Evaluative and Prognostic Criteria of Current and Probable Future Success Based on Operating Characteristics of the Planning Agency

The following criteria are applicable to the agency which has begun to involve itself in planning and has had time to organize itself in relationship to the tasks it feels are before it. Now a few specific attributes of its own making can be looked at. Perhaps the most tangible of these lie in the area of appointments made, and how the incumbents on the board and staff are behaving. Factors to be evaluated include:

Evidence of existence.

Evident sense of direction.

Clearcut definitions of responsibility between board and staff.

Feelings of satisfaction in board and staff.

Evidence of a representative board.

Evidence of suitable modes of choice of board members.

Evidence of participation in the activities of the board by the board members.

Evidence of board capacity.

Evidence of capacity of board members.

Evidence of board member commitment.

Evidence of overall board commitment.

Evidence of a suitable organizational structure (see Chapter 10).

Competency of the staff (see Figure 11.4: "Skills of Influence").

Evaluative and Prognostic Criteria of Current and Probable Future Success Based on Agency's Planning Procedures

The agency that has moved further along can be evaluated not only on the attributes of what are now historical or antecedent stages (which, of course, are still operant) but also on the immediate evidence at hand of what the planning body does about ostensible missions and its environment. (Moore describes this aspect of evaluation as normatively identifying how planning should be done and comparing agency performance against these normative standards.[45] Factors to be evaluated include:

Evidence that roles and functions undertaken are relevant to declared missions.

Identifiable and suitable processes used by which to decide what the problems are, order priorities, and decide which plans to implement.

Evidence that any concerned parties not already involved will be involved.

Evidence of reconciliation of long-range goals and problem-solving in adopted planning policies.

Evidence of awareness that proposals may be constrained by the values, goals, priorities, programs of the encompassing and encompassed systems (government at all levels, higher, lower, and parallel planning bodies, society, culture).

Evidence of a ready and visible means of communication with both the communities served and planning and policy-making structures.

Evidence of a mechanism to assess the relation between resources and programs.

Evidence that change strategies employed are relevant to the mission and the environment.

Evidence that relationships formed are relevant to roles and functions selected and change strategies adopted.

Evidence that activities undertaken to carry out selected functions and strategies will do the job and not create foolish or unwanted involvements.

Evaluative and Prognostic Criteria of Current and Probable Future Success Based on Evidence of Current Agency Planning Effectiveness

This level of evaluation is applicable to a well-established planning body which has had a planning output brought to the stage of implementation. Its most tangible record, of course, is its batting average on achieving implementation for its outputs. Because real consequences of most outputs may not be known for years, their social desirability and an intuitive feeling as to their success must supplement specific evidence that its implemented planning outputs are paying off. Factors to be evaluated include:

Perception by those in the agency's environment of its ability to get output implemented, and evidence that it has.

Evidence that it utilizes suitable organizational tactics.

Self-perceptions of the agency that jibe with those of the environment around it.

Planning accomplishments of the agency.

Planning of the planning body put into practice by its environment (implementation).

Additional important assignments are being given to the planning body.

Evidence that evaluation of its own activities and the consequences of its outputs are being suitably pursued.

Evaluative Criteria That Can be Applied a Few Years From Now

This kind of evaluation will become applicable to well established planning bodies whose maturity is such that their outputs have not only been implemented but have been made operant. The resulting products are then open to evaluation to see how well the planning body understood its tasks, the effectiveness of its designs and strategies in terms of the ensuing actual changes in the community served, and the desirability of these changes. Some of these criteria are:

Designs that have been implemented work reasonably well.

Results in terms of the objectives or the consequences are being achieved, such as, improved health care, more equitable distribution of care, or more efficiency.

Evidence of feedback from ongoing activities in operating agency programs which provides information by which to judge whether the desired objectives are occurring.

Evaluation is resulting in need for new studies, new problems are being identified, modification of existing plans or creation of new ones is proceeding.

Evidence that higher planning capacity is developing.

Evidence that the planning body has escalated its concerns from health care to health status.

Perhaps the quickest assessment of whether the operational planning body had been successful up to the date of evaluation, and therefore, whether it is likely to be successful in the future if it continues at the same level of competence, would be obtained by answering the following questions:

How good is the public image of the planning body?

Is the planning body staying ahead of what is being done (planning) or staying behind (reacting)?

Does the planning body's output seem to parallel the generally perceived priorities in the community or run counter to them?

Are community organization activities and services improving in response to the planning body output?

Is there evidence that health is apparently improving in response to planning body output? Some individual indices like infant death rate, tuberculosis or lead poisoning case rates which relate to this ultimate criterion can be applied early, but most may take a good many years to demonstrate perceptible change.

(A listing of evaluatory studies of CHP agencies is available.)[46]

Evaluation of Delivery System Proposals

Evaluation of delivery system proposals is an example of a typical and proper activity for a health planning body that has something in the way of a general aim or sense of direction about what health care involves, what the planning body constituency needs, and what that constituency has agreed that it desires (or, in the absence of expressed guidance from the community, what the representative planning body undertakes to accept in behalf of its community). A planning body, of course, cannot intelligently undertake evaluation of delivery system proposals until it has accepted for its territory what is, in effect, a set of guiding criteria for delivery systems built on long-range ideal goals.

Chapter 7 concluded with a set of normative goals and objectives which might be utilized as the beginning guides for policies by which health care systems must abide if they are to take us in the direction of desired health care goals.

Evaluation of Currently Operational
Health Care Delivery Systems

Evaluation of currently operational health care delivery systems also is a legitimate activity for any health planning body or research study unit. Two very useful studies have recently been reported which provide guidance. They each used different ways of proceeding, which is very helpful for our purposes of illustration.

The first study, that of Sparer and Johnson,[47] begins with the basic aims of the enabling legislation, which could be made tangible in eight major goals or objectives. The evaluators then proceeded to list a series of evaluative questions which correspond to each of the objectives. These are as follows:

Are the program concepts being implemented?

Who is being reached, and who is not being reached?

What services are being provided and to whom?

What is the quality of services?

What is the cost?

How does the community accept and relate to these services?

What changes have occurred in use of services?

How do various projects compare to each other on such factors as (1) utilization and client characteristics, (2) quality, (3) cost, and (4) community acceptance?

How does this concept of delivery compare to other options?

In order to answer these questions, tools and techniques were devised which would provide fairly specific answers and in turn tell how well Office of Economic Opportunity (OEO) centers did what they were "asked to do."

The tools and techniques devised were the following:

Site appraisal reviews.
Baseline health surveys.
Quality reviews.
Utilization reporting.
Cost reporting.
Special limited studies.

The tools and their applications are clearly described, as are the means of deriving the evaluative conclusions. Conclusions drawn for each of the eight basic goals are then boiled down to a few sentences about how well each area of intent is being met.

The second study, by Moorehead, Donaldson, and Seravalli,[48] was different in that it specifically set out to compare the services rendered by OEO neighborhood health centers with those of other health care providers. The methods used in the evaluation of quality are available in a separate paper by the senior author.[49] They are based on an audit of medical records that looks for some specifics which are felt to be correlatable with quality of care as described by the author.

For example, the scoreable components of adult medicine examinations used were grouped under four headings:

History.
Physical examination.
Laboratory and X-ray.
Time to assessment.

The audit items were applied to six types of health care providers:

Medical school affiliated.
OEO Neighborhood Health Centers.
Group practices.
Health department well baby clinics.
Children's Bureau maternal and infant care programs.
Children's Bureau children and youth programs.

The evaluators reviewed charts of patients attending three types of services:

Medicine.
Obstetrics.
Pediatrics.

The evaluators then provided audit scores which were arranged by each of the three types of service and then by each of the six types of institutional auspices. Conclusions permitted an evaluation of the OEO operations in terms of how well they performed medically compared to other providers of care. These conclusions were expressed in numerical form and were clearcut.

There is no particular point in criticizing either of these methodologies, for that is another issue in itself. But the two serve as different, practical, and generally acceptable approaches to determining how well a new set of agencies is doing. One study examines performance in a broad service or health care system sense that is relative to the aims of the law which set up the serving agencies. The other examines performance for three kinds of medical services based on more traditional criteria of quality, corresponding to the medical system view (see Chapter 4) of what good medical care embodies. Services given are then checked by a predesigned quality rating among the six kinds of competing service agencies to provide a comparative quality rating by which the OEO centers are evaluated.

Present day concern with evaluation of quality of care is exemplified by the efforts going into devices such as utilization reviews and Professional Standards Review Organizations. Donabedian spelled out the major considerations involved in quality evaluation several years ago in two classic articles.[50] What he had to say then about health care has been magnificently updated in a recent monograph.[51]

EVALUATION LEADS TO RECONSIDERATION OF ANY OR ALL PRIOR PLANNING STEPS

It is hardly any surprise that evaluation—which has as three of its declared purposes testing the quality of prior planning efforts, learning more about the real world, and setting planners off on the next round of planning—will lead to reconsideration of any or all of the preceding planning steps, shown in Figure 1.2, which are the contents of Chapters 5, 6, 7, 8, and 11, respectively. Evaluation may also lead to further evaluation. I do want to stress, however, that evaluation may be carried out for each phase of planning or its outputs, and need not return us to the immediately preceding step of planning, or to any other. The point to which it returns us is a function partly of the level of evaluation carried out and partly of the nature of the evaluator's findings.

Whatever evaluation or any one evaluator pronounces as a success at any one time may in due time or at the hands of another evaluator be considered a dismal failure. What any one person (or group) regards as good is very much a product of the times and the current pressing needs for survival, as accommodated by his general viewpoints or value scheme. Moreover, depending on the degree of farsightedness or upon the duration of time elapsed before evaluating, what is good may come to look quite differently. William Peterson presents these evaluative issues very well in an important discussion of the meaning of planning.[52]

REFERENCES

1. Mary F. Arnold, "Evaluation: A Parallel Process to Planning," *Administering Health Systems: Issues and Perspectives*, ed. by Mary F. Arnold, L. Vaughn Blankenship, and John M. Hess (Chicago; New York: Aldine; Atherton, 1971), Chapter 16.
2. Mary F. Arnold, "The Evaluative Process," College of Human Development, Pennsylvania State University, College Park, Pennsylvania, 1968, mimeographed.
3. Andie Knutson, "Pretesting: A Positive Approach to Evaluation," *Public Health Reports* 67 (July 1952), 199-203.
4. Herbert C. Schulberg, Alan Sheldon, and Frank Baker, eds., *Program Evaluation in the Health Fields* (New York: Behavioral Publications, 1969), Introduction and Chapter 35. Amitai Etzioni, "Two Approaches to Organizational Analysis: A Critique and a Suggestion," *Program Evaluation in the Health Fields*, ed. by Herbert C. Schulberg, Alan Sheldon, and Frank Baker (New York: Behavioral Publications, 1969), Chapter 8. Andrew C. Fleck, "Evaluation Research Programs in Public Health Practice," *Program Evaluation in the Health Fields*, ed. by Herbert C. Schulberg, Alan Sheldon, and Frank Baker (New York: Behavioral Publications, 1969), Chapter 7. Bernard Bergen, "Professional Communities and the Evaluation of Demonstration Projects in Community Mental Health," *Program Evaluation in the Health Fields*, ed. by Herbert C. Schulberg, Alan Sheldon, and Frank Baker (New York: Behavioral Publications, 1969), Chapter 9.
5. A. Etzioni, Ibid. no. 4, Chapter 8.
6. Irving A. Spergel, *Community Problem Solving: The Delinquency Example* (Chicago: The University of Chicago Press, 1969), 281-84.
7. Paul J. Sanazaro, "The Evaluation of Medical Care Under Public Law 89-239," *Medical Care* 5 (May/June 1967), 162-68.
8. Nathan Glazer, "Paradoxes of Health Care," *The Public Interest* (Winter 1971), 62-77. Daniel D. Roman, "The PERT System: An Appraisal of Program Evaluation Review Technique," *Program Evaluation in the Health Fields*, ed. by Herbert C. Schulberg, Alan Sheldon, and Frank Baker (New York: Behavioral Publications, 1969), Chapter 14.
9. Frances F. Piven and Richard A. Cloward, *Regulating the Poor: The Functions of Public Welfare* (New York: Pantheon Books, 1971).
10. Thomas S. Kuhn, *The Structure of Scientific Revolutions* (Chicago: The University of Chicago Press, 1962).
11. George James, "Education in Public Health Practice," *American Journal of Public Health* 52 (July 1962), 1145-54.
12. Andie L. Knutson, "Evaluation for What," *Program Evaluation in the Health Fields*, ed. by Herbert C. Schulberg, Alan Sheldon, and Frank Baker (New York: Behavioral Publications, 1969), 42-51.

13. H. C. Schulberg, Ibid. no. 4, Introduction and Chapter 35.
14. Martin Rein, "Social Planning: The Search for Legitimacy," *Journal of the American Institute of Planners* 35 (July 1969), 233-44.
15. Marvin C. Alkin, "Evaluation Theory Development," *Evaluation Comment* 2:1 (1972) 2-7, Center for the Study of Evaluation, University of California at Los Angeles.
16. E. Frank Ellis, "Evaluation of National Health Programs: A Disparity Between Desire and Practice in Local Health Departments," *American Journal of Public Health* 61 (September 1971), 1826-31.
17. O. L. Deniston, I. M. Rosenstock, and V. A. Getting, "Evaluation of Program Effectiveness," *Program Evaluation in the Health Fields*, ed. by Herbert C. Schulberg, Alan Sheldon, and Frank Baker (New York: Behavioral Publications, 1969), Chapter 13.
18. Karly D. Yardy, "Evaluation of National Health Programs on the Federal Level," *American Journal of Public Health* 61 (September 1971), 1803-08.
19. A. C. Fleck, Ibid. no. 4, Chapter 7.
20. H. C. Schulberg, Ibid. no. 4, Introduction and Chapter 35.
21. George James, "Evaluation in Public Health Practice," *Program Evaluation in the Health Fields*, ed. by Herbert C. Schulberg, Alan Sheldon, and Frank Baker (New York: Behavioral Publications, 1969), Chapter 2.
22. Ibid., Chapter 2.
23. John R. Moore, Jr., "Regional Health Services Planning: An Evaluation of the Planning Process," Final Report, Graduate School of Business, Stanford University, Stanford, California, February 1971, 30-31.
24. Herman E. Hilleboe and Morris Schaefer, "Evaluation in Community Health: Relating Results to Goals," *Bulletin of the New York Academy of Medicine* 2nd ser., 94 (February 1968), 140-158.
25. Benjamin S. Bloom, ed., *Taxonomy of Educational Objectives Handbook 1: Cognitive Domain Levels of Knowledge* (New York: David McKay Co., 1956).
26. John K. Galbraith, *The Affluent Society* (Boston: Houghton Mifflin, 1958), Chapter 2. Jay Forrester, *World Dynamics* (Cambridge, Mass.: Wright Allen Press, 1971).
27. D. D. Roman, Ibid. no. 8, Chapter 14.
28. J. R. Moore, Jr., Ibid. no. 23, 30-31.
29. Gerald Sparer and Joyce Johnson, "Evaluation of OEO Neighborhood Health Centers," *American Journal of Public Health* 61 (May 1971), 931-42.
30. Gary S. Dean, Sandra A. Robinson, Bruce E. Strein, and Jack E. Thompson, "Regional Medical Program Guidelines for Evaluation," Division of Design in Medical Education, University of Southern California School of Medicine, Los Angeles, March 1968, mimeographed.
31. Norbert Weiner, *The Human Use of Human Beings* (New York: Doubleday Anchor Books, 1964).
32. Joseph W. Eaton, "Symbolic and Substantive Evaluative Research," *Administrative Science Quarterly* 6 (March 1962), 421-42.
33. John G. Slevin, "What Is Peer Review?" *American Medical News* 14 (December 13, 1971), 4.
34. E. F. Ellis, Ibid. no. 16, 1826-31.

35. J. W. Eaton, Ibid. no. 32, 421-42.
36. LeRoy Goldman, "Evaluation of National Health Programs: A Political Perspective," *American Journal of Public Health* 61 (September 1971), 1809-11.
37. Keith Weikel, "Evaluation of National Health Programs: A Department View," *American Journal of Public Health* 61 (September 1971), 1801-03.
38. James E. Billings, "A Health Consumer Feedback System," *Researching a Growing Force for Social Change: Citizen Involvement in the 70's* (Minneapolis, Minn.: Health Services Research Center, American Rehabilitation Foundation, 1969), 7-22.
39. U.S., Department of Health, Education and Welfare, HSMHA, RMPS, Publication no. (HSM) 73-7021, *Quality Assurance of Medical Care,* Monograph, Feb., 1973.
40. B. D. Roman, Ibid. no. 8, Chapter 14.
41. Bertram M. Gross, special volume editor, "Social Goals and Indicators for American Society," *Annals of the American Academy of Political and Social Science* 371 (May 1967). Raymond A. Bauer, ed., *Social Indicators* (Cambridge: Massachusetts Institute of Technology, 1966).
42. Cyril Roseman, "A Resource Allocation Model for Region IX CHP 314[b] Applicant Agencies," prepared for Region IX, Office of Comprehensive Health Planning, Public Health Service, Department of Health, Education and Welfare, San Francisco, California, August 11, 1971.
43. Ibid.
44. K. Weikel, Ibid. no. 37, 1801-03.
45. J. R. Moore, Jr., Ibid. no. 23, 30-31.
46. *Health Planning Memorandum* 42 (Feb. 22, 1973), Community Health Inc., New York.
47. G. Sparer, Ibid. no. 29, 931-42.
48. Mildred A. Morehead, Rose S. Donaldson, and Mary A. Seravalli, "Comparisons between OEO Neighborhood Health Centers and Other Health Care Providers: Ratings of the Quality of Health Care," *American Journal of Public Health* 61 (July 1971), 1294-1306.
49. Mildred A. Morehead, "Evaluating Quality of Medical Care in the Neighborhood Health Center Program of the Office of Economic Opportunity," *Medical Care* 8 (March/April 1970), 118-31.
50. Avedis Donabedian, "Measurement of Quality in Health Care," *Quality in Health Care—Action Proposals and Discussions* (The 1968 National Forum, Los Angeles, March 15-17), II, 195-217. Avedis Donabedian, "Evaluating the Quality of Medical Care," *Program Evaluation in the Health Fields,* ed. by Herbert C. Schulberg, Alan Sheldon, and Frank Baker (New York: Behavioral Publications, 1969), Chapter 12.
51. U.S., Department of Health, Education and Welfare, Ibid. no. 39.
52. William Petersen, "On Some Meanings of Planning," *Journal of the American Institute of Planners* 32 (May 1966), 130-42.

Appendices

APPENDIX A
Health Future Mapping for a Two-County Community

This exercise is carried out with the understanding that all the non-health sectors have a much larger aggregate effect on health needs than the health sector—essentially, that they dictate the state of health.

To determine the probable extent of demands on the health sector, as well as the expected award of resources to it, a forecast must be made about the nature of general social objectives and thus the implied place of health and health care among the national priorities. The initial steps in determining what will be most needed and wanted in the way of health promotion and health care services involves anticipations about the major activities of the nation. From these are constructed parallel sets for a state, then for a metro and finally, for the local area. A set of fairly specific indices is used for the basic worksheets. A set of derived summary sheets which are useful for review and educational purposes can be prepared from the checked items on the basic worksheets. Many of these will be, in essence, composites of many related items.

Four general projections may be needed:

A_0—A *reference* projection, primarily what we anticipate will happen if things go on about as they have in the past.

A_1—An *advanced reference* projection, somewhat exploratory, of what we anticipate will happen if new, named, possible shifts in trends now on the horizon really take place.

A_2—The *wishful* projection, that is, the normative one we want to have come to pass.

A_3—The *planning* projection, the estimate of how far our planning can really take us toward A_2 and away from A_0 or A_1.

The size of the gaps between a desirable future A_2 and A_1 (or A_0), provides a quick review of what are likely to be the largest or most painful problems. Separate anticipations at each level may need to be developed for each major ethnic group which is thought to have significantly different attributes than the average for the population as a whole.

Suggested Technique

Estimates are first made for population composition and distribution.

Estimates are then made for the capacities and outputs of the major non-health sectors.

A forecast is also made about the nature of general social objectives.

From the general social aims the corresponding health goals are forecasted.

From the non-health sectoral estimates and general health goals, changes in levels of health status needs and consequent wants can be estimated.

From the estimates of needs, wants, and available resources, and the general health goals that will be desired, estimates can be made of the major unmet gaps.

All the sectoral estimates including the health ones must be re-examined by several rounds of anticipations with each estimate considered in the light of the probable influence of the others.

From a combination of the social objectives and the health gaps which are expected to cause concern, some specific objectives can be established for health and health care.

From the objectives for health care, alternative plausible organizational systems can be postulated to connect consumers to delivery by means of financing, technology, facilities, and manpower. Normative criteria of adequacy for each part of the system can also be postulated.

From these possibilities can be derived the types and numbers of manpower, the financing, technology, facilities, organization, and flexibility needed to meet the several futures that will have emerged from the forecasting at each level. For the local community being planned for, there will be the present forecasted sets of constraints, issues of distributive influences, resources and possible interventive methodologies.

Where numbers may not be available, or for any subject area where trends are of more interest, + may be used to indicate less than 2% change, + or - sign to indicate a change of 3% = 5% ++ or -- to indicate 6% = 10% change, +++ or --- to equal 11% = 20% change, and ++++ or ---- to mean 21% or more change.

Plus and minus signs refer to extent of change from the preceding ten years; they are not cumulative.

Suggested Indicators

The areas to be subject to forecasting are relatively simple in concept, very complex in actuality. Collections of other indicators are also available,[1] and a complex set of indicators of particular interest to comparisons among developing countries has also been produced.[2] Serious estimates of what the future holds have been made by Helmer,[3] and Kahn and Wiener,[4] among others.

Areas to be Examined

Distribution of people.

Distribution of non-health sector capacities and outputs in terms of:

(1) Educational status.

(2) Educational capacity.

(3) Natural resources, agriculture and physical environment.

(4) General technology and man-made physical environmental hazards.

(5) Transport and urban living.

(6) Economics.

(7) Politics and government.

Widely accepted *societal general aims* (scope and direction).

Widely accepted societal health aims (scope and direction including how health will be perceived).

Health needs, distribution of traditional physical and mental health afflictions.

Well-being needs, distribution of health capacity, social spiritual dissatisfactions.

Distribution of resources for both traditional health and well-being needs in terms of:

(1) Organization relevancy and consumer orientation.

(2) Manpower.

(3) Facilities and technology.

(4) Finances and financial practices.

(5) Environmental needs.

(6) Planning.

Distribution of the unmet health and well-being needs (not shown on the accompanying sheets).

Advanced Reference Projections

Anticipations Worksheets (Showing actual anticipated figures or anticipated changes from ++++ to ----)

The first worksheet, "Distribution of People," is shown in full. Only the stubs are shown for subsequent sheets. The column headings represent the parallel sets of anticipations which will be constructed: USA for the nation; Calif for the state; SFBA, San Francisco Bay Area, for the areawide figures; and EB, East Bay, for the two-county region in question. An asterisk means that the indicator is particularly useful for abstracting into the summary sheets.

FIGURE A.1   DISTRIBUTION OF PEOPLE

(separate sheet for each major race)

	1960				1970				1980				1990			
	USA	CALIF	SFBA	EB	USA	CALIF	SFBA	EB	USA	CALIF	SFBA	EB	USA	CALIF	SFBA	EB
Numbers																
*Total																
0-12 mos.																
1- 4 yrs.																
5-14 yrs.																
15-24																
25-34																
35-44																
45-54																
55-64																
65-74																
75+																
Distribution %																
*rural																
rural non-farm																
*urban																
suburban																
*under 20																
*over 65																
Competency																
% non-competent																
ages 15-34																
ages 35-54																
Average annual increase																

DISTRIBUTION OF NON-HEALTH SECTOR CAPACITIES AND OUTPUTS

EDUCATIONAL STATUS (separate sheet for each major race)	EDUCATIONAL CAPACITY	NATURAL RESOURCES, AGRICULTURE Physical Environment
Male age 50+ average years of education % below 8 years % below 12 years % BA or over 16 years % grad. degree or over 18 years	Output of college graduates relative to numbers at age 22 technical other overall	Abuses and pollution of *air *water *soil
Female age 50+ average years % below 8 years % below 12 years % BA or over 16 years % grad. degree or over 18 years	Output of high school graduates relative to numbers at age 18 technical other overall	Pollution health hazards in *food *water *air *Satisfactory waste disposal
Male age 30-50 average years % below 8 years % below 12 years % BA or over 16 years % grad. degree or over 18 years	Output of adult education courses relative to numbers at ages 25-65 technical other overall *Output of technicians for health relative to total population	Resources, adequacy duplication replacement renewal substitution *overall Shortages due to hazards to food production
Female age 30-50 average years % below 8 years % below 12 years % BA or over 16 years % grad. degree or over 18 years	Output of M.D. assist. relative to total population *Output of RN-type nurses relative to total population Output of RN assist. relative to total population	*Illness-producing agents carried by plants and animals Disease of plants and animals
*Male rural age 30+ average years		Average annual expansion in agricultural output

Housing

proportion of persons housed in dwellings with more than one person per room

proportion of persons housed in dwellings classified as dilapidated

proportion of persons housed in units without modern kitchen and bathroom plumbing

*Output of M.D.'s relative to total population

*Output of primary care M.D.'s relative to total population

Outputs of dentists, optometrists, podiatrists, midwives relative to total population

*Female rural age 30+ average years

*Male non-rural age 30+ average years

*Female non-rural age 30+ average years

ECONOMICS
(separate sheet for each major race for items below dotted line)

GNP average annual growth

GNP average annual growth per person

% GNP to taxes

Earnings

Capital investment

Savings

Inflation

Government capacity to borrow

Skill retraining mandatory before layoffs
....
Employment

TRANSPORT AND URBAN LIVING

Communications—ease

Transport—ease

Physical mobility
  elite
  middle
  poor

Congestion

Noise

Stress

*Disproportion of felt needs to resources

GENERAL TECHNOLOGY AND HAZARDS

Productivity advances in
electrification
communications
transport
agriculture
petrochemicals
ferrous metals
aerospace
other manufacturing
housing
worker skills
*service industry
*overall

Replacement of scarce resources

Demand on people
diversity of
stress of
career renewal

Hazards in
electrification
communications
transport
agriculture
petrochemicals
ferrous metals
aerospace
other manufacturing
housing
worker skills
service industry
*overall

agricultural

industrial

youth

*total

*Unemployment

Job Security

Prolonged Unemployment benefits

Age at Retirement

Social Security benefits

Income
*average
*% below $3,000
% below $5,000
*% over $15,000

POLITICS AND GOVERNMENT

*Citizen participation in government

Public information
*general level
*feedback about public to public
*social systems savvy

WIDELY ACCEPTED SOCIETAL GENERAL AIMS

*Democratic participation in decision-making

*Equability of opportunity

*Free education

WIDELY ACCEPTED SOCIETAL HEALTH AIMS

*Good health care for all

Good quality for all

All persons covered

All services covered

Respect for human dignity

Good health will be perceived primarily as

freedom from disability
freedom from disease
freedom from discomfort
internal satisfaction
external satisfaction
*capacity to participate
*increased life span

*Medical care as a right

*Reasonable personal liberties

*Justice

*Growth per se is good

Change per se is good

Technology per se is good

*Long-range plans are good

Short-range plans are good

*Prevention is better than cure

World considerations are of equal concern with national or international ones

Ecologic concerns are supreme

Work is imperative

social systems organized information exchange

Degree of citizen participation
*national level voting
*municipal level voting
*in planning
in political party work
*in demonstrations

*Voluntarism

Level at which planning done
*shift to national
shift to state
*shift to metro
shift to local
*shift to sublocal

*level at which decision making done
*shift to national
shift to state
*shift to metro
shift to local
*shift to sublocal

Level at which implementation done
shift to national
shift to state
*shift to metro
*shift to local
*shift to sublocal

589

Government acts as producer
Government acts as purchaser
Government acts as financer
Government acts as watchdog
Government acts as convener
Government acts as planner

HEALTH NEEDS—TRADITIONAL PHYSICAL & MENTAL AFFLICTIONS
(separate sheet for each major race)

*Need total

*Demand or felt need total

Effective demand total

Frequency of diseases, illness, disability
from:
old infections
new infections
old environmental hazards
new environmental hazards
old inappropriate behavior
new inappropriate behavior
metabolic—genetic factors
*aging—deterioration
*overall

WELL-BEING NEEDS
Health Capacity, Social, Spiritual Dissatisfactions

% Dependent socially at age
15-19
20-29
30-39
40-49
50-59
60-64
65+
*total

Delinquency
*male 14-20
*female 14-20
total 19-20

Crime, nonviolent
*male
*female

WELL-BEING NEEDS *(continued)*
(separate sheet for each major race)

Alcoholism
*male
*female
total

Soft drugs
male
female
total

Hard drugs
*male
*female
total

Sense of satisfaction
male over 40
male under 40

Malnutrition
*insufficient food
*imbalances

Mortality, ten major specified causes

1	6
2	7
3	8
4	9
5	10

*total

*Disabling morbidity, five major specified causes

1	4
2	5
3	*total

*Infant death rate
*Proportion noncompetent due to traditional causes

Expectation of life
*at birth
*at age 40

total

Child abuse
 male
 female
*total

Marital discord
*divorce
 other

female over 40
female under 40
*overall

Sense of belonging
 male over 40
 male under 40
 female over 40
 female under 40
*overall

Availability of recreation
 male over 40
 male under 40
 female over 40
 female under 40
*overall

Constructive use of recreation
 male
 female

Health knowledge

Health attitudes

Health behavior

FIGURE A.3
DISTRIBUTION OF RESOURCES FOR BOTH TRADITIONAL HEALTH AND WELL-BEING NEEDS

ORGANIZATION RELEVANCE AND CONSUMER ORIENTATION	MANPOWER**	FACILITIES & TECHNOLOGY
Accessibility	Primary care adequacy	Primary care facilities, adequacy
*rural	adequate number	number
urban middle class	adequate distribution	distribution
*urban ghetto	adequate preparation	connectedness
suburban	adequate production	*overall
overall	efficient use of	
	loss from practice	Acute hospital, adequacy
Connectedness	shift to use of assistants	number
rural	*overall	distribution
urban middle class		oversupply
urban ghetto	Specialists, adequacy medical and dental	unsuitable use
suburban	adequate number	*overall
*overall	adequate distribution	
	adequate preparation	Long-term care facilities, adequacy
Relevancy and acceptability	adequate production	number
*rural	efficient use of	distribution
urban middle class	loss from practice	connectedness
*urban ghetto	shift to use of assistants	unsuitable use
suburban	*overall	*overall
overall		

592

Equipment adequacy
  technology
  efficiency
  distribution
  *overall

Nurses, adequacy
  efficient use of
  loss from practice
  shift to use of assistants
  *overall

Others, adequacy
  efficient use of
  loss from practice
  shift to use of assistants
  *overall

Administrative capacity
  rural
  urban middle class
  urban ghetto
  suburban
  *overall

Acceptable alternative sources of care
  rural
  urban middle class
  *urban ghetto
  suburban
  overall

Consumer input at policy level
  rural
  urban middle class
  urban ghetto
  suburban
  overall

Consumer education re
  healthful living
  prevention
  overuse of care

593

FINANCES & FINANCIAL PRACTICES	ENVIRONMENTAL NEEDS	PLANNING

*Adequate amount
  coverage of all services
  coverage of all conditions
  coverage of all persons
  *overall
	Manpower adequacy
	  quantity
	  quality
	  *distribution
	  production
	  *overall
		Distribution and coverage
		  rural
		  urban
		  suburban
		  metro
		  local
		  sub-local
		  state
		  national
		  *overall

*Use of insurance	Facilities and equipment adequacy
	  quantity
	  quality
	  *distribution
	  production
	  *overall
		Agency capacity
		  financing
		  quantity of staff
		  quality of staff
		  technology
		  consumer input
		  professional input
		  vested interests input
		  political awareness
		  production of planners
		  jurisdiction
		  authority
		  *overall

Use of federal financing
  through insurance
  direct
  *overall
	*Appropriate decision-making structure	*Responsiveness of policy makers

*Shift from individual	Consumer-citizen input	

Cost control adequacy
  prepayment
  utility commission approach
  cost plus
  incentives
  insistence on connectedness
  increased competition
  removal of competition
  *overall
	*Consumer education	

*% of GNP	*Relevant human satisfaction standards	
*% of taxes	*Relevant human health standards	
*% of personal income	*Relevant technology	
	*Adequate funding	

**See "Educational Capacity."

APPENDIX B
Suggested Scoreboard Indicators

FIGURE B.1
TRADITIONAL HEALTH CONCERNS:
SUGGESTED SCOREBOARD INDICATORS

Prematurity Rate	
Infant death rate	0- 1 year
Lead poisoning rate	1- 4 years
Malnutrition rate	1- 4 years
	(a composite of ht, wt, hemoglobin)
Malnutrition rate	5-14 years
	(a composite of ht, wt, hemoglobin)
Apparent mental retardation rate	5- 9 years
	(school and institutional registration rate)
Dental DMF rate	5- 6 years
Dental DMF rate	14-15 years
Obesity rate	14-15 years
Auto accident death rate	
male	15-24 years
female	25-44 years
Occupational accidental death rate	
male	25-64 years
female	25-64 years
Other accidental death rate	
male	5-14 years
female	5-14 years
male	25-44 years
female	25-44 years
Maternal death rate	15-24 years
Cervical cancer death rate	25-44 years
Overall cancer death rate	
male	25-44 years
female	25-44 years
male	45-64 years
female	45-64 years
Coronary death rate	
male	45-64 years
female	45-64 years
Hypertension death rate	
male	45-64 years
female	45-64 years
Cancer of lung death rate	
male	45-64 years
female	45-64 years

Cirrhosis death rate	
male	45-64 years
female	45-64 years
Legal blindness rate	45-64 years
Emphysema death rate	
male	45-64 years
female	45-64 years

FIGURE B.2
SOCIAL, SPIRITUAL AND BEHAVIORAL CONCERNS:
SUGGESTED SCOREBOARD INDICATORS

Polio immunization level	5- 6 years
Pregnancy rate	12-14 years
Drug death rate	
male	10-14 years
female	10-14 years
male	15-24 years
female	15-24 years
Gonorrhea rates	10-14 years
	15-24 years
Hepatitis rates	
male	15-24 years
female	15-24 years
Abortions rate	
	15-24 years
	25-44 years
Completed suicides rate	
male	15-24 years
female	15-24 years
Homicide victims rate	
	15-24 years
	25-44 years
Alcoholism rate	
male	15-24 years
	(a new level-of-abuse index)
female	25-44 years
Mental illness rate	15-24 years
	(a new level-of-admissions- for-care index by severity)
	25-44 years
	45-64 years
Senility rate	65 + years
	(a new level-of-admissions- for-care index)
Internal satisfactions	15-24 years
	*(a new indicator: % of persons with lowest level

	of self-fulfillment or joy of living)
	25-44 years
External satisfactions, an overall indicator made up from the following 3 indicators	25-44 years *(a new indicator: % of persons with lowest level of satisfaction about living prospects)
Satisfaction with educational opportunities for children	25-44 years *(a new indicator: % of persons with lowest level of satisfaction)
Satisfaction with work opportunity	25-44 years *(a new indicator: % of persons with lowest levels of satisfaction)
Satisfaction with public safety and policing	25-44 years *(a new indicator: % of persons with lowest level of satisfaction)
Criminal convictions rate	
male	25-44 years
female	15-24 years
Unemployment rate	
male	20-24 years
female	20-24 years
male	25-44 years
female	25-44 years
AFDC rate	15-24 years 25-44 years
General education level	20-24 years 25-29 years
School dropout rate	15-19 years
Change of address rate	all ages (% move 1 or more times within 12 mos.)
Fertility rate	20-24 years

*Based on a 5 level scale.

FIGURE B.3
WELL-BEING SERVICES AND SOCIAL ENVIRONMENT: SUGGESTED SCOREBOARD INDICATORS

Preventive services availability rate	0- 1 years	
	1- 4 years	(% of population having
	5-14 years	all needed services at
	15-24 years	essentially no out-of-
	25-64 years	pocket expense)
	65 + years	

Corrective services availability rate	0- 1 years 1- 4 years 5-14 years 15-24 years 25-64 years 65 + years	(% of population having all needed services at essentially no out-of-pocket expense)
Geographic access rate	all ages	(% of population having essentially no physical access barriers)
Comprehensive (connectivity) access rate	all ages	(% of population having essentially no real barriers to all needed services)
Counseling access rate	all ages	(% of population having essentially no real barriers to living and health counseling)
Poverty rate	all ages	(% living below the poverty level)
Near-poverty rate	all ages	(% living above poverty level but below twice the poverty level)

FIGURE B.4
PHYSICAL ENVIRONMENT: SUGGESTED
SCOREBOARD INDICATORS

Dilapidated housing rate	*(% of persons living at bottom level)
Persons per room rate	*(% of persons living at bottom level)
Streets clean and maintained rate	*(% of persons living at bottom level)
Air cleanliness	*(% of persons living at bottom level)
Quietness	*(% of persons living at bottom level)
Park availability rate	(% urban dwellers with park available within 5 blocks)
Shopping availability rate	(% urban dwellers with shopping available within 5 blocks)
Public transport rate	(% urban dwellers with public transport within 3 blocks 18 hours per day)
Safe tasty water rate	(% persons with safe tasty water)

School access rate	(% persons 4-19 within 4 blocks of their school or free transport to their school)

FIGURE B.5
SUGGESTED FORMAT OF TABULATIONS FOR
EACH INDICATOR BY GEOPOLITICAL UNITS

As many as four or five indicators that are closely related could be shown on one tabulation. In the examples, Prematurity and Infant Death Rates are presented together in one table.

The codes used are as follows:

Race R1, R2, R3, and so on

Geopolitical Units

Nations U.S. = USA

Selected other countries = C1, C2, C3, and so on

States = S1, S2, S3, and so on

Planning regions or metros in a state = M1, M2, M3, and so on

Planning sub-units counties (or cities) in a metro= P1, P2, P3, and so on

Neighborhoods or aggregates of like census tracts in a county (or city) = N1, N2, N3, and so on

The same indicators calculated for ten years back and ten years forward would be very useful in contemplating trends. However, this is not meant to be a substitute for future mapping as shown in Appendix A.

EXAMPLE OF NATIONAL-LEVEL SCOREBOARD

Prematurity and Infant Death Rates, 1973, showing the United States, 10 selected nations, and the 50 states by major races.

	All races		*R1*		*R2*		*Etc.*
	Prem.	*Infant death*	*Prem.*	*Infant death*	*Prem.*	*Infant death*	
USA							
C1							
C2							
C3							
etc. to C10							
S1							
S2							
S3							
etc. to S50							

EXAMPLE OF STATE-LEVEL SCOREBOARD

Prematurity and Infant Death Rates, 1973, showing California and each metro or planning region level in the state as well as 5 selected states and the nation by major races.

USA							
Calif.							
State A							
State B							
State C							
State D							
State E							
M1							
M2							
M3							
etc. to M11							

EXAMPLE OF METRO-LEVEL SCOREBOARD

Prematurity and Infant Death Rates, 1973, showing the San Francisco Bay Area metro planning region, each of its subplanning units (counties), as well as five selected metros in the nation, the state and the nation by major races.

	All races		R1		R2		R3		Etc.
	Prem.	In-fant death	Prem.	In-fant death	Prem.	In-fant death	Prem.	In-fant death	
USA									
Calif.									
S.F. Bay Area									
Metro A									
Metro B									
Metro C									
Metro D									
Metro E									
P1									
P2									
P3									
etc. to P9									

EXAMPLE OF COUNTY-LEVEL SCOREBOARD

Prematurity and Infant Death Rates, 1973, showing the Alameda County planning level and each of its neighborhoods (or aggregate of like census tracts) as well as five selected counties in California, the San Francisco Bay Area Metro, the state, and the nation by major races.

USA

Calif.

S.F. Bay
Area

Ala. Co.

County A

County B

County C

County D

County E

N1

N2

N3

etc. to
N21

REFERENCES

1. John Oliver Wilson, *Quality of Life in the United States: An Excursion Into the New Frontier of Socio-Economic Indicators* (Kansas City, Mo.: Midwest Research Institute, MRI no. 1041, 1969). Center for Urban Studies, Wayne State University, *Social Reporting in Michigan: Problems and Issues*, Office of Planning Coordination, Bureau of Policies and Programs, Michigan Technical Report A-37, February, 1970.
2. United Nations, Economic and Social Council, *Second Development Decade: A System of Overall Review and Appraisal of the Objectives and Policies of the International Development Strategy* (May 1971).
3. Olaf Helmer, *On the Future State of the Union* (Menlo Park: Institute for the Future, Report R-27, May 1972).
4. Herman Kahn and Anthony J. Wiener, *The Year 2000: A Framework for Speculation on the Next Thirty-Three Years* (New York: Macmillan, 1970).

INDEX